I0042076

Machine and Human Together: Innovating Healthcare with Technology

Edited by

Shaweta Sharma

*Department of Pharmacy, School of Medical
and Allied Sciences, Galgotias University
Greater Noida, Uttar Pradesh-201310
India*

Akhil Sharma

*R. J. College of Pharmacy
Raipur, Uttar Pradesh-202165
India*

Shivkanya Fuloria

*Department of Pharmaceutical Chemistry
Faculty of Pharmacy, AIMST University
Bedong-08100, Kedah
Malaysia*

&

Anurag Singh

*School of Computing Science and Engineering
Galgotias University
Greater Noida, Uttar Pradesh-201310
India*

Machine and Human Together: Innovating Healthcare with Technology

Editors: Shaweta Sharma, Akhil Sharma, Shivkanya Fuloria & Anurag Singh

ISBN (Online): 979-8-89881-162-4

ISBN (Print): 979-8-89881-163-1

ISBN (Paperback): 979-8-89881-164-8

© 2025, Bentham Books imprint.

Published by Bentham Science Publishers Pte. Ltd. Singapore, in collaboration with Eureka Conferences, USA. All Rights Reserved.

First published in 2025.

BENTHAM SCIENCE PUBLISHERS LTD.

End User License Agreement (for non-institutional, personal use)

This is an agreement between you and Bentham Science Publishers Ltd. Please read this License Agreement carefully before using the ebook/echapter/ejournal (**"Work"**). Your use of the Work constitutes your agreement to the terms and conditions set forth in this License Agreement. If you do not agree to these terms and conditions then you should not use the Work.

Bentham Science Publishers agrees to grant you a non-exclusive, non-transferable limited license to use the Work subject to and in accordance with the following terms and conditions. This License Agreement is for non-library, personal use only. For a library / institutional / multi user license in respect of the Work, please contact: permission@benthamscience.org.

Usage Rules:

1. All rights reserved: The Work is the subject of copyright and Bentham Science Publishers either owns the Work (and the copyright in it) or is licensed to distribute the Work. You shall not copy, reproduce, modify, remove, delete, augment, add to, publish, transmit, sell, resell, create derivative works from, or in any way exploit the Work or make the Work available for others to do any of the same, in any form or by any means, in whole or in part, in each case without the prior written permission of Bentham Science Publishers, unless stated otherwise in this License Agreement.
2. You may download a copy of the Work on one occasion to one personal computer (including tablet, laptop, desktop, or other such devices). You may make one back-up copy of the Work to avoid losing it.
3. The unauthorised use or distribution of copyrighted or other proprietary content is illegal and could subject you to liability for substantial money damages. You will be liable for any damage resulting from your misuse of the Work or any violation of this License Agreement, including any infringement by you of copyrights or proprietary rights.

Disclaimer:

Bentham Science Publishers does not guarantee that the information in the Work is error-free, or warrant that it will meet your requirements or that access to the Work will be uninterrupted or error-free. The Work is provided "as is" without warranty of any kind, either express or implied or statutory, including, without limitation, implied warranties of merchantability and fitness for a particular purpose. The entire risk as to the results and performance of the Work is assumed by you. No responsibility is assumed by Bentham Science Publishers, its staff, editors and/or authors for any injury and/or damage to persons or property as a matter of products liability, negligence or otherwise, or from any use or operation of any methods, products instruction, advertisements or ideas contained in the Work.

Limitation of Liability:

In no event will Bentham Science Publishers, its staff, editors and/or authors, be liable for any damages, including, without limitation, special, incidental and/or consequential damages and/or damages for lost data and/or profits arising out of (whether directly or indirectly) the use or inability to use the Work. The entire liability of Bentham Science Publishers shall be limited to the amount actually paid by you for the Work.

General:

1. Any dispute or claim arising out of or in connection with this License Agreement or the Work (including non-contractual disputes or claims) will be governed by and construed in accordance with the laws of Singapore. Each party agrees that the courts of the state of Singapore shall have exclusive jurisdiction to settle any dispute or claim arising out of or in connection with this License Agreement or the Work (including non-contractual disputes or claims).
2. Your rights under this License Agreement will automatically terminate without notice and without the

need for a court order if at any point you breach any terms of this License Agreement. In no event will any delay or failure by Bentham Science Publishers in enforcing your compliance with this License Agreement constitute a waiver of any of its rights.

3. You acknowledge that you have read this License Agreement, and agree to be bound by its terms and conditions. To the extent that any other terms and conditions presented on any website of Bentham Science Publishers conflict with, or are inconsistent with, the terms and conditions set out in this License Agreement, you acknowledge that the terms and conditions set out in this License Agreement shall prevail.

Bentham Science Publishers Pte. Ltd.
No. 9 Raffles Place
Office No. 26-01
Singapore 048619
Singapore
Email: subscriptions@benthamscience.net

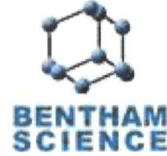

BENTHAM SCIENCE

CONTENTS

Akanksha Sharma, Shaweta Sharma, Ashish Verma, Sunita, Shilpa Thukral and
Akhil Sharma

Ashish Verma, Akhil Sharma, Shaikh Yahya, Shivkanya Fuloria and *Shaweta
Sharma*

FOREWORD

Welcome to the future of healthcare, a future where human ingenuity intertwines seamlessly with technological innovation to redefine the very essence of patient care. "Machine and Human Together: Redefining Healthcare with Innovations" embarks on a journey through this dynamic landscape, where the convergence of human expertise and cutting-edge technologies reshapes the boundaries of what is possible in healthcare delivery. In the pages that follow, you will discover a world where artificial intelligence, machine learning, robotics, and data analytics converge to revolutionize every aspect of healthcare. Through captivating examples and insightful analyses, this book showcases how these advancements empower healthcare professionals, enhance diagnostic accuracy, and personalize treatment regimens like never before.

However, innovation does not come without its challenges. As we navigate this brave new world, we must confront ethical dilemmas, privacy concerns, and the ever-present need to ensure that technology remains a tool for good. As you embark on this journey, envision a future where human compassion and technological prowess harmonize to provide healthcare that is not only efficient and effective but also deeply empathetic and patient-centered. Together, let us embrace the possibilities of tomorrow and redefine healthcare for the betterment of humanity.

Neeraj Kumar Fuloria
Department of Pharmaceutical Chemistry
Faculty of Pharmacy, AIMST University
Semeling Campus, Jalan Bedong–Semeling 08100 Bedong
Kedah Darul Aman
Malaysia

PREFACE

In "Machine and Human Together: Redefining Healthcare with Innovations" we embark on a journey into the future of healthcare, where human ingenuity and technological advancement converge to reshape the landscape of patient care. This book is composed from a profound acknowledgment of the transformative potential inherent in the collaboration between human expertise and cutting-edge technologies. Within these chapters, readers will encounter a myriad of examples illustrating how artificial intelligence, machine learning, robotics, and data analytics are revolutionizing healthcare delivery. From streamlining diagnostic processes to personalizing treatment plans, the possibilities are both awe-inspiring and boundless.

Nevertheless, amidst the excitement of innovation, we must remain mindful of the ethical considerations and disparities that may arise. This preface invites readers to engage in critical reflection on these challenges and to explore pathways toward responsible and equitable integration of technology in healthcare. As we delve into the world of "Human + Machine," let us embrace the vision of a future where technology amplifies human compassion and enhances patient-centered care. Together, let us navigate the complexities of healthcare innovation with a shared commitment to improving health outcomes for all.

Shaweta Sharma
Department of Pharmacy, School of Medical
and Allied Sciences, Galgotias University
Greater Noida, Uttar Pradesh-201310
India

Akhil Sharma
R. J. College of Pharmacy
Raipur, Uttar Pradesh-202165
India

Shivkanya Fuloria
Department of Pharmaceutical Chemistry
Faculty of Pharmacy, AIMST University
Bedong-08100, Kedah
Malaysia

&

Anurag Singh
School of Computing Science and Engineering
Galgotias University
Greater Noida, Uttar Pradesh-201310
India

List of Contributors

Akhil Sharma	R. J. College of Pharmacy, Raipur, Uttar Pradesh-202165, India
Afroz Khan	Department of Pharmacy, School of Medical and Allied Sciences, Galgotias University, Greater Noida, Uttar Pradesh-201310, India
Akanksha Sharma	R. J. College of Pharmacy, Raipur, Uttar Pradesh 202165, India
Amit Raj Singh	Department of Pharmacy, School of Medical and Allied Sciences, Galgotias University, Greater Noida, Uttar Pradesh-201310, India
Aryan Kumar	Department of Pharmacy, School of Medical and Allied Sciences, Galgotias University, Greater Noida, Uttar Pradesh-201310, India
Ashish Verma	Department of Pharmacy, Mangalmay Pharmacy College, Greater Noida, Uttar Pradesh-201306, India
Anurag Singh	School of Computing Science and Engineering, Galgotias University, Greater Noida, Uttar Pradesh-201310, India
Arfa Shams	Department of Pharmacy, School of Medical and Allied Sciences, Galgotias University, Greater Noida, Uttar Pradesh-201310, India
Chanchla Devi Haldkar	Shri Rawatpura Sarkar Institute of Pharmacy, Jabalpur, Madhya Pradesh-482001, India
Ganna Rajan	Department of Pharmacy, SGRR University, Dehradun, Uttarkhand-248001, India
Gunjan	Department of Pharmacy, School of Medical and Allied Sciences, Galgotias University, Greater Noida, Uttar Pradesh-201310, India
Jyoti Pandey	Department of Pharmacy, School of Medical and Allied Sciences, Galgotias University, Greater Noida, Uttar Pradesh-201310, India
MD Kaif	Department of Pharmacy, School of Medical and Allied Sciences, Galgotias University, Greater Noida, Uttar Pradesh-201310, India
Naga Rani Kagithala	Department of Pharmacy, School of Medical and Allied Sciences, Galgotias University, Greater Noida, Uttar Pradesh-201310, India
Niranjan Kaushik	Department of Pharmacy, School of Medical and Allied Sciences, Galgotias University, Greater Noida, Uttar Pradesh-201310, India
Priyanka Dubey	Department of Pharmacy, Banasthali Vidyapith, Vanasthali, Rajasthan-304022, India
Pushpak Singh	Department of Pharmacy, School of Medical and Allied Sciences, Galgotias University, Greater Noida, Uttar Pradesh-201310, India
SK Abdul Rahaman	Department of Pharmacy, School of Medical and Allied Sciences, Galgotias University, Greater Noida, Uttar Pradesh-201310, India
Sagar Pamu	Pharmacy Practice Department, Institute of Pharmacy, Nirma University, Ahmedabad, Gujarat-380001, India
Sarvesh Paliwal	Department of Pharmacy, Banasthali Vidyapith, Vanasthali, Rajasthan-304022, India
Shivangi Bhardwaj	Department of Pharmacy, Banasthali Vidyapith, Vanasthali, Rajasthan-304022, India

Shivkanya Fuloria Department of Pharmaceutical Chemistry, Faculty of Pharmacy, AIMST University, Jalan Bedong—Semeling 08100 Bedong, Kedah, Malaysia

Shilpa Thukral Dnyan Ganga College of Pharmacy, Thane, Maharashtra-400615, India

Shekhar Singh Faculty of Pharmacy, Babu Banarasi Das Northern India Institute of Technology, Lucknow, Uttar Pradesh-226028, India

Shekhar Singh Faculty of Pharmacy, Babu Banarasi Das Northern India Institute of Technology, Lucknow, Uttar Pradesh-226028, India

Shaweta Sharma Department of Pharmacy, School of Medical and Allied Sciences, Galgotias University, Greater Noida, Uttar Pradesh-201310, India

Sunita R. J. College of Pharmacy, Raipur, Uttar Pradesh 202165, India

Swapnil Sharma Department of Pharmacy, Banasthali Vidyapith, Vanasthali, Rajasthan-304022, India

Swati Verma Department of Pharmacy, Banasthali Vidyapith, Vanasthali, Rajasthan-304022, India

Shaikh Yahya Department of Pharmaceutical Chemistry, School of Pharmaceutical Education and Research, Jamia Hamdard, New Delhi-110062, India

Yatindra Kumar Department of Pharmacy, GSVM Medical College, Kanpur, Uttar Pradesh-208002, India

CHAPTER 1

Synergy of Humans and Machines in Healthcare

Amit Raj Singh[1] and **Shaweta Sharma**[1,*]

[1] *Department of Pharmacy, School of Medical and Allied Sciences, Galgotias University, Greater Noida, Uttar Pradesh-201310, India*

Abstract: This chapter explores the synergy of humans and machines in health care, focusing on how they work together to enhance outcomes in medical practice. By combining human creativity and judgment with the precision and data-processing capabilities of machines, this partnership addresses key shortcomings in contemporary medical practices. It discusses various applications of AI and ML in health care: drug discovery, diagnosis, predictive analysis, telemedicine, and remote patient monitoring. Innovations in technology are revolutionizing the spheres where quicker drug development, enhanced diagnostic accuracy, and cost-cutting are evident. The integration of AI in treatment facilitates personalized medicine through the assessment of vast volumes of data, predicting outcomes, and developing the most optimal treatment plans for each patient. Technologies enhance telemedicine access to healthcare by providing real-time monitoring of chronic disease management and wearable devices equipped with IoT sensors. It will conclude the chapter by stating how this human-machine synergy will revolutionize healthcare delivery and enhance patient care, while also providing innovative solutions in medical research.

Keywords: Artificial intelligence, Drug discovery, Machine learning, Predictive analysis, Remote patient monitoring, Telemedicine.

INTRODUCTION

The term "synergy" is derived from the Attic Greek word synergia, which is derived from synergos, meaning "working together." The effect of this synergy of humans and machines is that both produce something that can easily turn out to be more than the potential of the single result if one of them works alone; it occurs largely in that people add, creativity and judgment with appropriate context, while computers can better process information and execute actions with high accuracy for innovative and improved productivity in health care and many aspects of manufacturing, scientific investigation, *etc.*

---
* **Corresponding author Shaweta Sharma:** Department of Pharmacy, School of Medical and Allied Sciences, Galgotias University, Greater Noida, Uttar Pradesh-201310, India; E-mail: shawetasharma@galgotiasuniversity.edu.in

Shaweta Sharma, Akhil Sharma, Shivkanya Fuloria & Anurag Singh (Eds.)
All rights reserved-© 2025 Bentham Science Publishers

Technological breakthroughs are revolutionizing nearly every sector, with the health care business poised to gain significantly from these innovations. Significant developments in technology and financing have led to the widespread adoption of machines in healthcare facilities for various activities, including next-generation sequencing, electronic data collection and storage, as well as diagnosis and treatment recommendations. The gathering and analysis of big data have reached extraordinary levels, surpassing human analytical and interpretative capacities, thanks to sensors and innovative algorithms that enable the continuous measurement and storage of patients' health metrics. The conversion of AI technologies and big data into actionable biological and clinical information has expanded, facilitating precision medicine. These algorithms now possess the potential to learn and thus enhance over time. The benefits of employing AI algorithms or neural networks in healthcare are increasingly evident in numerous healthcare systems, resulting in reduced diagnostic errors, resource conservation, and enabling doctors to address the needs of additional patients [1, 2].

The collaboration between humans and AI is becoming a potent tool to rectify the existing deficiencies in medicine.

These deficiencies encompass inadequate prediction accuracy, vulnerability to critical diagnostic and therapeutic mistakes, unexpected repercussions of empirical decision-making, and inefficient hospital procedures, frequently culminating in inferior patient care. AI is poised to transform how urologists provide care for their patients. AI encompasses the scientific, engineering, and developmental processes of systems that replicate human intellect and behaviour. Effective AI encompasses unique insights in perception, pattern recognition for text, audio, and images, as well as decision-making and problem-solving capabilities. Significant progress has been achieved in creating synergistic human-machine systems that leverage the advantages of both human and AI-generated reasoning [3].

The key areas in healthcare include human and machine drug discovery & drug development, diagnosis & predictive analysis, telemedicine and remote patient monitoring, robot-assisted surgery, and hospital management. This book chapter will discuss these topics in detail and how human and machine synergy have impacted them, as well as their future perspectives.

DRUG DISCOVERY & DEVELOPMENT

Finding and developing drugs is a lengthy process that involves searching, designing, and testing new drugs to fulfill fundamental health needs. Once a candidate molecule is identified, it is also tested in preclinical and clinical studies, where its safety, efficacy, and potential side effects are determined. Such procedures may take years and have to be done with cooperative efforts from scientists, doctors, regulatory agencies, and drug manufacturers. Despite all these problems, successful drug discovery will lead to novel therapies, thereby enhancing the condition of patients and improving medical science [4, 5].

In recent years, technological advancements have significantly transformed the majority of factors involved in the drug discovery process, facilitating and accelerating individual phases. High-throughput screening techniques enable scientists to rapidly evaluate thousands of chemicals for potential therapeutic benefits, thereby significantly accelerating the primary discovery phase [6].

Furthermore, computational strategies, including AI, are increasingly finding applications in predicting the properties and behaviors of drug candidates, thereby reducing the reliance on the traditional trial-and-error approach [7, 8]. ML is a significant area within AI, allowing machines to learn from data without being programmed [9]. ML algorithms have been very effectively applied in various niches of drug discovery, such as genomics, proteomics, and transcriptomics, having revealed important molecular pathways and molecular biomarkers related to the pathologies of many diseases. This has enabled the validation and prioritization of tractable drug targets. ML may one day eradicate, if not minimize, testing on live animals [10]. Fig. (**1**) shows the various applications of AI in drug discovery and development.

A study by Margulis [11] and his group is one such example of the use of ML in drug discovery. The aim was to explore how ML can be useful in identifying highly bitter compounds in the early stages of drug development. The aim was to understand if a specific ML algorithm can be used as an alternative to *in vivo* testing to predict the bitterness of different drug molecules. Eighty percent of the bitter compounds present were matched to those associated with a brief access taste aversion (BATA) test, indicating that the above research was successful. This experiment, following the BATA test, revealed that toxicity should not be directly linked to being bitter, as scientists had hypothesized over time. This denotes how ML can produce required outputs with new knowledge simultaneously. Fig. (**2**) represents machine learning in drug design.

The study by Raschka *et al.* [12, 13] shows the functionality and applicability of ML technology in GPCR ligand recognition, which is an important concern regarding drug design. The task is to determine if older-fashioned technology used for blocking Sea Lamprey Receptor 1 (SLOR1) receptor signal inhibiting tests can be replaced with newly attained results from the ML algorithm, as validated by the described use of these tests. The results generated by the algorithm were close to the benchmark set; therefore, the novel algorithm could replace the older one for identifying other drugs' features.

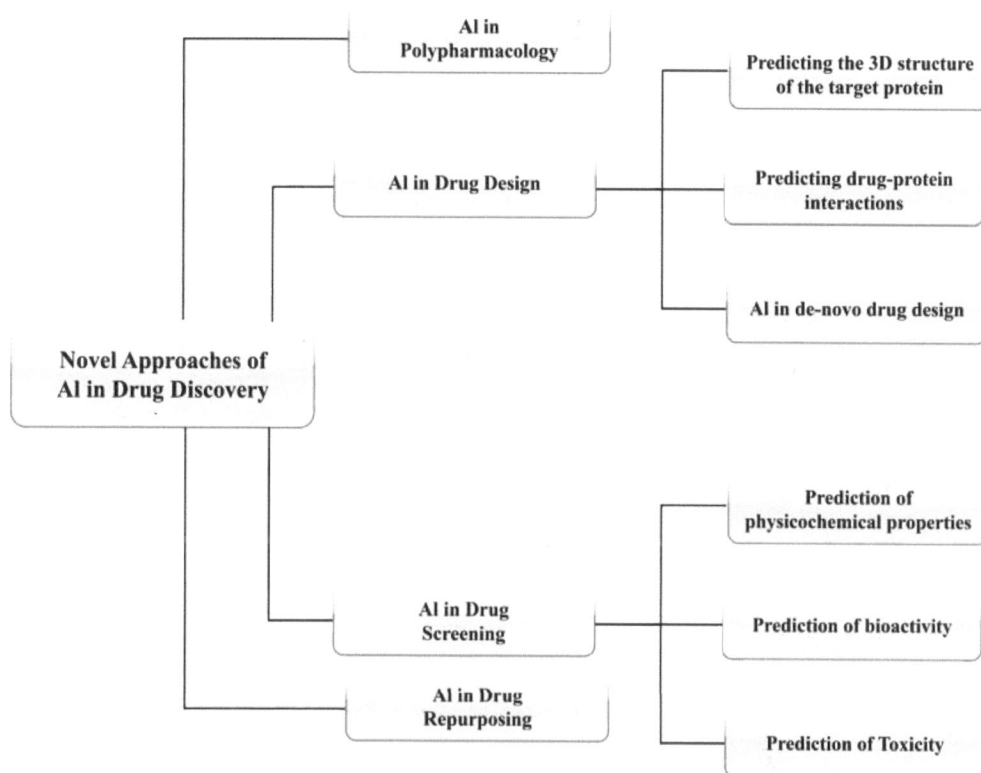

Fig. (1). Applications of AI in drug discovery & development..

Two experiments, conducted by Rantanen and Khinast [14] and Turki and Taguchi [15], respectively, fall into other groups of ML and are therefore best compared. The paper published by Turki and Taguchi was a reinforcement learning exercise that utilized three necessary frameworks to sustain ML, along with its two sister approaches, supervised and unsupervised learning, aimed at accelerating the search for potentially useful drugs. Conversely, Zhavoronkov and Mamoshina applied transfer learning to predict the response of myeloma patients to an existing drug. Transfer learning is an ML problem that involves the application of knowledge learned in one environment to a similar situation. Turki and Taguchi revealed that the drug design procedure required about 46 days, much less compared to traditional approaches. The research conducted by Zhavoronkov and Mamoshina yields superior prediction accuracy compared to their baseline measurements. Turki and Taguchi determined that enhancements in algorithm coding are necessary to guarantee that synthesized compounds possess distinct formulas compared to existing market products; conversely, Zhavoronkov and Mamoshina asserted that the algorithm's scope should be broadened through the integration of hybrid and deep learning models, as the data gathered for individuals is not representative of a wider population. Table **1** shows some more studies that used ML for drug design.

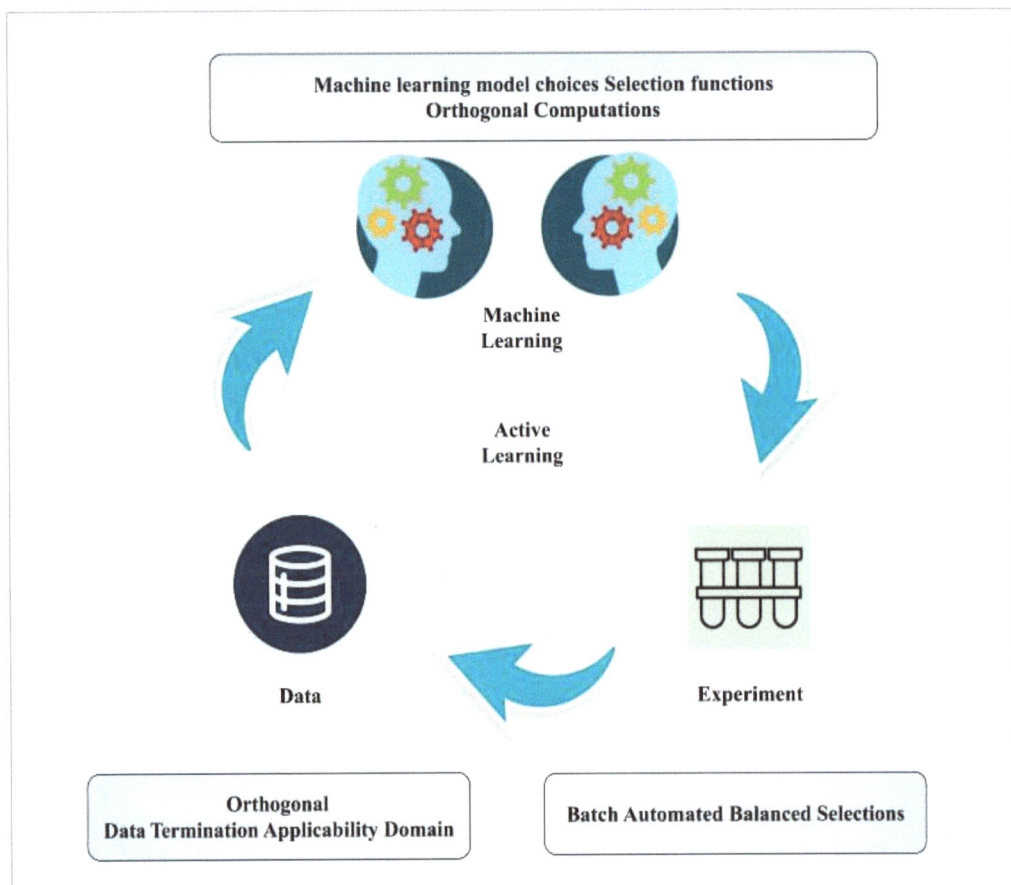

Fig. (2). ML in drug design..

Table 1. An overview of studies that used ML for drug design.

Technique	Application	Methods	Accuracy
Traditional reinforcement learning	New drug development	Employing various ML methodologies to synthesize novel compounds	Highly accurate (95% of compounds were determined to be viable)

(Table 1) cont.....

Technique	Application	Methods	Accuracy
Transfer learning	Emulating biological processes	Employing regression-based transfer learning to model responses to anticancer therapeutics	Extremely precise
Multitask learning	Drug development and testing	Employing regression-based transfer learning to model responses to anticancer therapeutics Employing genetic and pharmacological data to track the signals among the pathways traversed by the medication molecules.	Precise
Multitask analysis	Drug-target interaction	Employing various ML algorithms and subcategories to study and monitor the interactions between the medicine and its target.	Precise
Multitask learning	Post-manufacture drug reviews	Employing multitask learning and analytical algorithms to conduct large-scale data analysis	Highly precise (4,200 evaluations during a brief period)

Fig. (**3**) illustrates the various areas of supervised ML-based drug design. This synergy between human expertise and machine intelligence revolutionizes the drug discovery process by integrating data-driven accuracy with scientific ingenuity. ML expedites discovery, reduces expenses, and reveals innovative insights, whereas human supervision ensures ethical considerations, contextual comprehension, and strategic implementation. Collectively, they facilitate more efficient, precise, and significant therapeutic progress.

DIAGNOSIS & PREDICTIVE ANALYSIS

The complexity of chronic diseases necessitates a shift from a disease-centric perspective to a more patient-centered approach. Considering the extensive patient data available, the established data storage framework, and the progress in data analytics, AI has emerged as the primary tool that provides a conducive framework for addressing the challenges of patient-focused treatment plans [16]. ML constitutes a fundamental element of AI in medical care. The adaptability and efficacy of ML algorithms, coupled with readily available computer capabilities, are crucial. They can identify patterns, distinctions, and connections within information to estimate the probability of unexpected results in intricate care environments. ML models have been employed as an auxiliary tool to recognize specific diseases and conditions [17], as well as tumor classifications derived from the examination of clinical data [18]. ML-based methodologies have proven effective in creating polygenic risk scores that assist in identifying people with elevated genetic susceptibility to a disease [19]. ML has demonstrated efficacy in elucidating the effects of drugs and chemicals on cellular characteristics [20]. ML algorithms can yield dependable learning models if the quality of the utilized data is adequate. Nonetheless, these models are challenging to comprehend, as they require an understanding of how input data is converted into results. The 'black box' issue can be detrimental, resulting in diminished confidence and fostering apprehension and dispute regarding the reliability of ML. The deficiencies in understanding the model and the learning process [21] necessitate the explicit incorporation of algorithmic outcomes into the medical decision-making process. Moreover, greater emphasis should be placed on elucidating the results derived from the ML models.

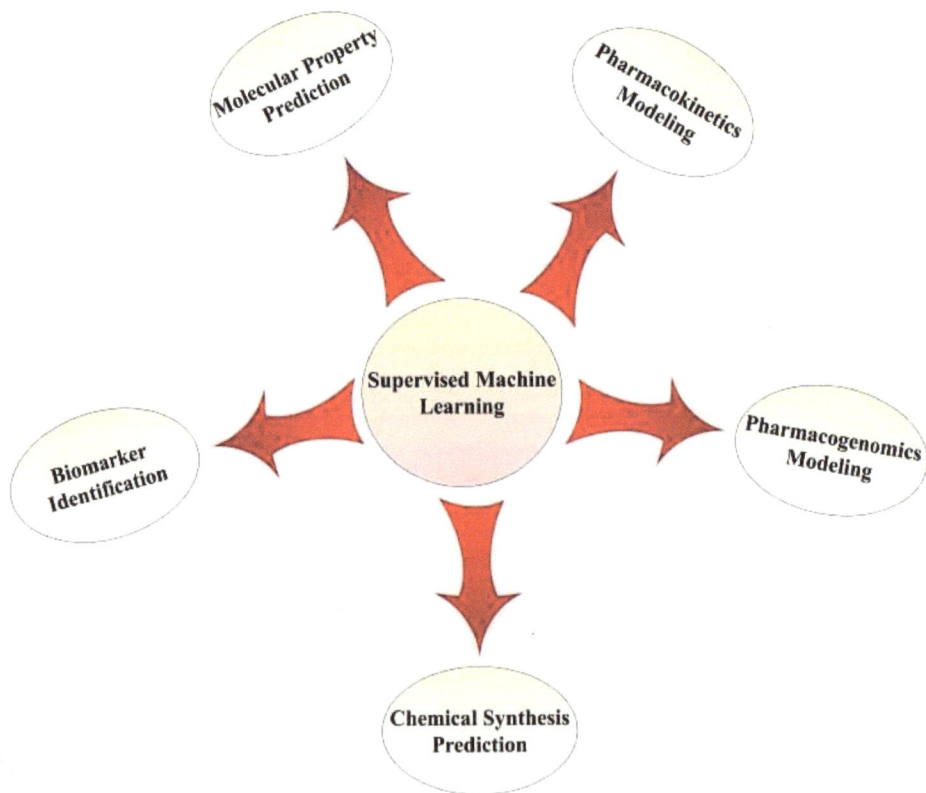

Fig. (3). Supervised ML-based areas in drug design..

This collaboration between human expertise and machine intelligence cultivates a balanced methodology wherein data-driven insights augment clinical judgment to enhance decision-making. By integrating ML outputs with contextual understanding, doctors can ensure more precise, transparent, and ethically robust outcomes. This collaboration fosters trust in AI systems and improves the accuracy of medical care.

TELEMEDICINE & REMOTE PATIENT MONITORING (RPM)

Telemedicine is defined by the United States Department of Health and Human Services as the application of electronic information and telecommunication technologies to support and improve remote clinical healthcare, health-related education for patients and professionals, as well as public health and administration. Numerous telemedicine technologies have emerged in healthcare, enabling the conservation of resources for both patients and clinicians while enhancing the quality of care [22]. Telemedicine facilitates access to healthcare professionals in environments where such access might be impractical or even unattainable. Remote Patient Monitoring (RPM) is a modality of telemedicine that facilitates direct visual interaction between a medical practitioner and a patient within a hospital setting [23, 24].

It is an approach that enables direct visual interaction between an expert and a patient in a hospital environment [25]. It encompasses diverse technologies, including wearable devices, mobile health applications, and Internet of Things (IoT)-enabled sensors, which monitor vital signs, physical activity, and medication compliance [26]. Through the utilization of these instruments, RPM provides a more adaptable method of healthcare delivery, especially for patients necessitating long-term monitoring without the necessity for regular trips to healthcare institutions [27]. The scope of RPM has considerably broadened with the incorporation of big data technology, establishing it as a crucial element in patient-centered care models, especially for the control of chronic diseases such as diabetes, hypertension, and cardiovascular disorders (CVDs) [28].

Monitoring the metabolic and hemodynamic parameters of patients is essential to assess their health condition during therapy, including body temperature, heart rate, blood pressure, and oxygen levels, particularly for those with moderate indications who are quarantined at home [29]. Moreover, chronic conditions such as CV ailments and diabetes result in a significant number of fatalities annually, including arteriosclerosis, diabetes, coronary heart disease, and hypertension, which can be effectively mitigated with preliminary diagnosis and prolonged continuous observation. Nonetheless, consistently monitoring the aforementioned physiological signs at home using conventional clinical methods/devices is challenging due to their limited feasibility and substantial costs [30 - 33].

Healthcare Wearable Devices (HWDs) are defined as gadgets that are worn on the body or on garments [34]. These devices comprise a target receptor and a transducer. The receptor identifies the target analyte and reacts appropriately [35]. The transducer converts the response from the receptor into a functional signal. Numerous studies have demonstrated the applicability of HWDs across various domains; thus, these devices have yielded encouraging outcomes in healthcare owing to their deformability and compliance. These HWDs enhance comprehension of physiological changes within the human body and assist in the prevention and treatment of disorders. Biosensors were originally employed as intrusive instruments in regulated laboratory environments prior to their incorporation into wearable sensors. In 1956, Leland C. Clark, recognized as the "father of biosensors," was the first individual to use electrodes for measuring blood oxygen (O_2) levels. This gadget was designed for the constant and real-time monitoring of O_2 levels in operating room environments during CV surgery [36]. Originally developed on Leland C. Clark's electrochemical biosensor, the first glucose analyzer was commercialized in 1975 thanks to the arrival of electrodes in healthcare [37].

The shrinking of electronics, resulting in micro- and nanoelectronics, along with breakthroughs in materials science, has led to the emergence of integrated healthcare wearable devices (HWDs). These HWDs comprise electronic devices for collecting, processing, and disseminating data. Traditional, stiff, and heavy electronic items, such as Printed Circuit Boards (PCBs), are unsuitable for HWDs; consequently, significant progress has been made in recent years regarding the materials, fabrication techniques, processing circuits, and transceivers of electronic devices to improve their compatibility with HWDs [38 - 40].

Due to the swift advancement of flexible electronics, wearable skin-like devices exhibiting exceptional plasticity and skin-suitable characteristics have been described and considered vital for healthcare applications [41 - 50]. Currently, numerous innovative medical devices have been investigated for the detection of body temperature, blood pressure, heart rate, and glucose utilizing thermoelectric effects, piezoelectric/piezoresistive mechanisms, capacitive effects, or electrocatalytic/electrochemical principles [51 - 55]. Notably, these observational gadgets can be incorporated into garments or timepieces for continuous healthcare, thereby facilitating home-based telehealth monitoring [56 - 58].

Numerous elements must be evaluated before developing a health monitoring device. Biocompatibility necessitates that the components do not interact with or harm organs and tissues, which is a critical factor in material selection. Secondly, breathability is intrinsically linked to comfort, particularly in the context of continuous health monitoring. Health monitoring gadgets featuring porous architecture and hydrophilicity are highly sought after to facilitate the release of perspiration expelled from the body, thereby preventing dermatological irritation.

Thirdly, flexibility and elasticity characteristics dictate the potential for the device to be integrated into garments or patches; thus, flexible organic polymers with superior mechanical properties are suitable choices for substrate films. Fourthly, sensitivity and accuracy, response time, detection limit, and the disparity between responding signals and actual physiological counterparts significantly influence the practical medical applications. Fifthly, stability and durability are critical considerations for commercialization and industrialization. Moreover, the self-sustaining and repairing functionalities of HWDs are essential for their practical applications [59].

This synergy between human expertise and advanced technologies fosters a seamless healthcare ecosystem where clinicians leverage machine-driven insights to provide timely and personalized interventions. The integration of wearable devices and telemedicine not only enhances remote monitoring but also empowers patients to manage their health actively. Together, human oversight and machine precision drive a transformative approach to healthcare, bridging access gaps and improving outcomes.

ROBOTICS IN HEALTHCARE

Since the onset of the COVID-19 pandemic, the healthcare sector has been inundated with innovative technologies to facilitate care in extraordinary conditions [60, 61]. Staff vacancy rates rose [62, 63], social restrictions limited conventional care delivery methods [64], and the introduction of rigorous infection control protocols created new barriers to human-provided care [65]. Despite the alleviation of numerous pandemic-induced issues in healthcare, staff burnout [66], an aging demographic, and backlog pressures resulting from the outbreak have led to ongoing personnel shortages in healthcare systems globally [67, 68]. Robotic systems have consistently been recognized for their potential to mitigate workforce demands, particularly in healthcare [69].

These systems may include remotely operated robots for virtual consultations or transportation robots for the automated transportation of items within healthcare facilities. Besides aiding hospitals, robotic devices can enhance clinical practice across several disciplines. Examples encompass exoskeletons that help stroke patients with mobility and surgical robots that enable surgeons to perform surgeries remotely. Understanding the panorama of robotic jobs in healthcare is crucial for guiding future research and development [70]. Table **2** provides an overview of different robot groups, the most frequently used robots, and the tasks at hand.

Table 2. Most common robots used in healthcare.

Robot Group	Description	Total Number of Robots Used	Most Frequently Used Robot(s)
Rehabilitation and mobility	Robots that can physically evaluate and help patients accomplish a task	102	Lokomat® (Hocoma, Switzerland)
Surgical	Robots that aid surgeons during operations	19	Da Vinci Surgical System (Intuitive Surgical, USA)
Telepresence	Robots that enable people to be physically present through the use of the robot	10	Remote Presence (RP) (InTouch Technologies, USA)
Pharmacy	Robots that facilitate the administration and distribution of pharmaceutical services	10	APOTECA Chemo (Loccioni Humancare, Italy); ROWA Vmax (BD Rowa, Germany)
Socially assistive	Robots manifest in various configurations, including humanoid and animal forms, to assist in domains traditionally occupied by humans, such as companionship and the delivery of services	9	Paro (AIST Japan)
Interventional	Robots are employed to aid in interventional procedures	9	Niobe (Stereotaxis, USA)
Imaging assistance	Robots are employed for their capacity to facilitate imaging across various domains of medicine	8	Soloassist® (AKTORmed, Germany); Freehand® (Freehand, UK)
Disinfection	Robots are employed to sanitize clinical environments, including hospital wards and outpatient facilities	2	Lightstrike™ (Xenex, USA); Ultra Violet Disinfection Robot® (UVD-Robot) (Clean Room Solutions)
Radiotherapy	Robots are employed to facilitate the administration of radiotherapy	1	Cyberknife (Accuracy, USA)
Delivery and transport	Robots are employed for the relocation of objects across different zones	1	TUG (Aethon, USA)

Surgical robots can aid in executing surgical procedures. Their specialized functions in surgery are diverse, encompassing instrument manipulation to automated surgical table adjustments.

The da Vinci Surgical System is the most widely used robot and, as such, possesses the most extensive body of literature supporting it. The device offers instruments that a surgeon can use *via* a control panel to execute minimally invasive surgeries. This technique finds application in surgical procedures including cholecystectomy, pancreatectomy, and prostatectomy. Jensen *et al.* [71]

conducted a retrospective cohort study involving 103 subjects, comparing robot-assisted anti-reflux operations utilizing the da Vinci Surgical system with traditional laparoscopy, and assessed perioperative results. Additional robots examined constitute the ROBO DOC® Surgical System (Curexo Technology, USA), utilized in bone surgery for the planning and execution of total knee replacement [72], and the Robotized Stereotactic Assistant (ROSA®) (Zimmer Biomet, France), that aids in neurological surgeries such as intracranial electrode implantation [73]. Certain robots can also aid in biopsy procedures.

The iSR'obot™ Mona Lisa (Biobot Surgical, Singapore) enhances the process of visualization and robotic needle navigation in the context of prostate biopsy procedures [74].

Robots for rehabilitation and mobility are designed to provide physical assistance or evaluate patients to facilitate the attainment of objectives. The Lokomat, a widely recognized robotic gait orthosis, serves as a valuable tool in the rehabilitation of various disorders, including stroke. The primary objective is to improve strength and flexibility in the lower limbs [70].

Unlike their surgical counterparts, robots in this category are used to assist in interventional operations. These techniques include ablation for atrial fibrillation, percutaneous coronary intervention (PCI), and neuroendovascular intervention. Their role may encompass catheter guiding and stent positioning. Nine robots exist, predominantly the Niobe System (Stereotaxis, USA) and the Hansen Sensei Robotic Catheter System (Hansen Medical, USA), succeeded by the Corpath systems (GRX and 200) (Corindus, USA). The Niobe system utilizes robotically controlled magnets to enhance the precision of catheter navigation [75].

A cohort of robots is designated to facilitate the administration and distribution of pharmaceutical services. This includes the inventory, dispensing, and manufacturing of pharmaceuticals. A robot might aid in the production of toxic medications to decrease errors and mitigate operator risk. The BD Rowa Vmax is an automated system designed for the storage and delivery of medication at the user's request. Berdot *et al.* [76] employed this system in a teaching hospital pharmacy and assessed the return on investment, including the incidence of dispensing errors. The APOTECA Chemo system facilitates the automation of chemotherapeutic treatment. Buning *et al.* [77] investigated the environmental pollution associated with APOTECA Chemo in comparison to traditional medication compounding.

The synergy of human expertise and robotic precision enables healthcare workers to provide care with improved efficiency, accuracy, and safety. Robotic technologies enable doctors to concentrate on patient-centered care by automating repetitive chores and facilitating intricate procedures. This collaborative dynamic not only tackles workforce concerns but also facilitates innovative, accessible, and tailored healthcare solutions. One issue that must be considered is the ethical implications of these advancements from the viewpoints of the patient, caregiver, family member, care provider, physician, and hospital [78]. Frequently, robots are built and developed by engineers who neglect ethical considerations. Involving ethicists in the design of assistive robots is crucial for evaluating ethical considerations from the perspectives of diverse stakeholders [79].

HOSPITAL MANAGEMENT

Hospital management faces significantchallenges, including the handling of extensive patient data, the optimization of resource allocation, and the assurance of operational efficiency. The reliance on manual processes and outdated systems characteristic of conventional management approaches frequently leads to inefficiencies, elevated operational costs, and diminished patient care [80]. These inefficiencies are exacerbated by the complexity and volume of data generated in hospitals, creating a significant challenge for administrators seeking to make informed decisions and manage resources effectively. Additionally, the growing pressures on healthcare systems necessitate creative solutions to uphold high levels of patient care while enhancing performance. Optimizing operations, AI has surfaced as a groundbreaking technology in numerous sectors [81]. The current global pandemic has highlighted the critical need for effective resource allocation, as healthcare systems around the world face increasing patient numbers and limited resources [82].

AI-powered predictive analytics at a leading healthcare organization in the United States. Through the examination of patient information, the system can forecast patient admissions and optimize bed distribution, resulting in a 20% decrease in waiting periods and an increase in patient satisfaction [83]. A medical facility in Asia demonstrates the effectiveness of AI-driven chatbots in enhancing patient engagement and streamlining administrative processes. The chatbots were accessible for support 24/7, answering patient inquiries, arranging appointments, and dispatching reminders. This resulted in a 30% rise in patient satisfaction and a significant decrease in administrative expenses [84].

Several shared elements play a crucial role in the effective execution of AI in medical facilities. These factors include strong leadership backing, extensive staff training initiatives, robust data governance structures, and ongoing assessment and oversight of AI systems. Hospitals that invest resources in these areas are more likely to utilize AI technologies to enhance management and patient care [85].

The implementation of AI-powered inventory management systems at the Mayo Clinic has enabled the prediction of healthcare product needs and streamlined supply restocking, resulting in a 20% decrease in inventory expenses and a notable reduction in stock shortages, thereby ensuring the continuous availability of essential supplies [86].

The application of AI for appointment scheduling has proven effective in lowering no-show rates and enhancing schedule efficiency. For instance, the adoption of an AI-based scheduling system at a large healthcare institution resulted in a 30% decrease in no-show rates and a 25% increase in the utilization of appointment slots.

This synergy between human expertise and AI-driven technology transforms hospital management, enabling administrators to make data-informed decisions while alleviating manual burdens. AI improves operational efficiency through predictive analytics and automation, while humans address the ethical implications, adaptability, and strategic alignment. Together, they form a balanced framework that optimizes resource utilization, enhances patient outcomes, and sustains high-quality care delivery in an ever-changing healthcare landscape.

CONCLUSION

This synergy of human expertise and machine intelligence, then, holds transformative potential for healthcare. It enhances not only the efficiency and accuracy of clinical practices but also addresses major problems in the healthcare industry, such as diagnostic errors and resource allocation. This chapter illustrates how the integration of AI and ML into numerous aspects of healthcare, such as drug discovery, diagnosis, telemedicine, and RPM, could bring better outcomes and even more personalized care to the patient. With the further evolution of AI systems, it promises to make things easier, cheaper, and more innovative when handling complex medical problems. This would have to be weighed by human judgment against machine-driven insights in order to hold in place the ethical considerations and contextual understanding of clinical decision-making. Thus, the future of medicine will be determined both by humans and machines, and hence, set forth more enhanced patient care and delivery systems in healthcare. This synergy will be embraced as the key to overcoming deficiencies that exist in healthcare, paving the way for a more integrated and responsive medical landscape.

REFERENCES

[1]   Chen CT, Ackerly DC, Gottlieb G. Transforming healthcare delivery: Why and how accountable care organizations must evolve. J Hosp Med 2016; 11(9): 658-61.
[http://dx.doi.org/10.1002/jhm.2589] [PMID: 27596543]

[2]   Hackbarth AD, Hackbarth AD. Eliminating waste in US health care. JAMA 2012; 307(14): 1513-6.
        [http://dx.doi.org/10.1001/jama.2012.362] [PMID: 22419800]

[3]   Bhandari M, Reddiboina M. Augmented intelligence: A synergy between man and the machine. Indian
        J Urol 2019; 35(2): 89-91.
        [http://dx.doi.org/10.4103/iju.IJU_74_19] [PMID: 31000911]

[4]   Sarkar C, Das B, Rawat VS, *et al.* Artificial intelligence and machine learning technology driven
        modern drug discovery and development. Int J Mol Sci 2023; 24(3): 2026.
        [http://dx.doi.org/10.3390/ijms24032026] [PMID: 36768346]

[5]   Aly M, Alotaibi AS. Molecular property prediction of modified gedunin using machine learning.
        Molecules 2023; 28(3): 1125.
        [http://dx.doi.org/10.3390/molecules28031125] [PMID: 36770791]

[6]   Mak KK, Wong YH, Pichika MR. Artificial intelligence in drug discovery and development. Drug
        Discov Eval Saf Pharmacol Assays 2024; pp. 1461-98.
        [http://dx.doi.org/10.1007/978-3-031-35529-5_92]

[7]   Fu R, Yu Z, Zhou C, *et al.* Artificial intelligence-based model for dose prediction of sertraline in
        adolescents: a real-world study. Expert Rev Clin Pharmacol 2024; 17(2): 177-87.
        [http://dx.doi.org/10.1080/17512433.2024.2304009] [PMID: 38197873]

[8]   Marchetti F, Moroni E, Pandini A, Colombo G. Machine learning prediction of allosteric drug activity
        from molecular dynamics. J Phys Chem Lett 2021; 12(15): 3724-32.
        [http://dx.doi.org/10.1021/acs.jpclett.1c00045] [PMID: 33843228]

[9]   Rustam F, Reshi AA, Mehmood A, *et al.* COVID-19 future forecasting using supervised machine
        learning models. IEEE Access 2020; 8: 101489-99.
        [http://dx.doi.org/10.1109/ACCESS.2020.2997311]

[10]   Elbadawi M, Gaisford S, Basit AW. Advanced machine-learning techniques in drug discovery. Drug
        Discov Today 2021; 26(3): 769-77.
        [http://dx.doi.org/10.1016/j.drudis.2020.12.003] [PMID: 33290820]

[11]   Margulis E, Dagan-Wiener A, Ives RS, Jaffari S, Siems K, Niv MY. Intense bitterness of molecules:
        Machine learning for expediting drug discovery. Comput Struct Biotechnol J 2021; 19: 568-76.
        [http://dx.doi.org/10.1016/j.csbj.2020.12.030] [PMID: 33510862]

[12]   Raschka S, Kaufman B. Machine learning and AI-based approaches for bioactive ligand discovery and
        GPCR-ligand recognition. Methods 2020; 180: 89-110.
        [http://dx.doi.org/10.1016/j.ymeth.2020.06.016] [PMID: 32645448]

[13]   Raschka S. Automated discovery of GPCR bioactive ligands. Curr Opin Struct Biol 2019; 55: 17-24.
        [http://dx.doi.org/10.1016/j.sbi.2019.02.011] [PMID: 30909105]

[14]   Rantanen J, Khinast J. The Future of Pharmaceutical Manufacturing Sciences. J Pharm Sci 2015;
        104(11): 3612-38.
        [http://dx.doi.org/10.1002/jps.24594] [PMID: 26280993]

[15]   Turki T, Taguchi Y. Machine learning algorithms for predicting drugs–tissues relationships. Expert
        Syst Appl 2019; 127: 167-86.
        [http://dx.doi.org/10.1016/j.eswa.2019.02.013]

[16]   Cacciaguerra L, Storelli L, Rocca MA, Filippi M. Current and future applications of artificial
        intelligence in multiple sclerosis. In: Augmenting neurological disorder prediction and rehabilitation
        using artificial intelligence. Academic Press 2022; pp. 107-144.
        [http://dx.doi.org/10.1016/B978-0-323-90037-9.00012-6]

[17]   Tiwari S, Jain A, Sapra V, *et al.* A smart decision support system to diagnose arrhythymia using
        ensembled ConvNet and ConvNet-LSTM model. Expert Syst Appl 2023; 213: 118933.
        [http://dx.doi.org/10.1016/j.eswa.2022.118933]

[18] Triberti S, Durosini I, Pravettoni G. A "Third wheel" effect in health decision making involving artificial entities: a psychological perspective. Front Public Health 2020; 8: 117.
[http://dx.doi.org/10.3389/fpubh.2020.00117] [PMID: 32411641]

[19] Khera AV, Chaffin M, Aragam KG, *et al.* Genome-wide polygenic scores for common diseases identify individuals with risk equivalent to monogenic mutations. Nat Genet 2018; 50(9): 1219-24.
[http://dx.doi.org/10.1038/s41588-018-0183-z] [PMID: 30104762]

[20] Schork NJ. Artificial intelligence and personalized medicine. In: Von Hoff D, Han H, Eds. Precision medicine in cancer therapy. Cancer treatment and research, vol. 178. Cham: Springer; 2019. p. 265-83.
[http://dx.doi.org/10.1007/978-3-030-16391-4_11]

[21] Sandhu S, Lin AL, Brajer N, *et al.* Integrating a machine learning system into clinical workflows: qualitative study. J Med Internet Res 2020; 22(11): e22421.
[http://dx.doi.org/10.2196/22421] [PMID: 33211015]

[22] Sasangohar F, Davis E, Kash BA, Shah SR. Remote patient monitoring and telemedicine in neonatal and pediatric settings: Scoping literature review. J Med Internet Res 2018; 20(12): e295.
[http://dx.doi.org/10.2196/jmir.9403] [PMID: 30573451]

[23] Rincon F, Vibbert M, Childs V, *et al.* Implementation of a model of robotic tele-presence (RTP) in the neuro-ICU: effect on critical care nursing team satisfaction. Neurocrit Care 2012; 17(1): 97-101.
[http://dx.doi.org/10.1007/s12028-012-9712-2] [PMID: 22547040]

[24] Garingo A, Friedlich P, Tesoriero L, Patil S, Jackson P, Seri I. The use of mobile robotic telemedicine technology in the neonatal intensive care unit. J Perinatol 2012; 32(1): 55-63.
[http://dx.doi.org/10.1038/jp.2011.72] [PMID: 21617643]

[25] Bitsaki M, Koutras C, Koutras G, *et al.* ChronicOnline: Implementing a mHealth solution for monitoring and early alerting in chronic obstructive pulmonary disease. Health Informatics J 2017; 23(3): 197-207.
[http://dx.doi.org/10.1177/1460458216641480] [PMID: 27102885]

[26] Pereira T, Oliveira T, Cabeleira M, *et al.* Comparison of low-cost and noninvasive optical sensors for cardiovascular monitoring. IEEE Sens J 2013; 13(5): 1434-41.
[http://dx.doi.org/10.1109/JSEN.2012.2236549]

[27] Plachkinova M, Vo A, Bhaskar R, Hilton B. A conceptual framework for quality healthcare accessibility: a scalable approach for big data technologies. Inf Syst Front 2018; 20(2): 289-302.
[http://dx.doi.org/10.1007/s10796-016-9726-y]

[28] Rodbard D. Continuous glucose monitoring: A review of successes, challenges, and opportunities. Diabetes Technol Ther 2016; 18(Suppl 2) (Suppl. 2): S3-13.
[http://dx.doi.org/10.1089/dia.2015.0417] [PMID: 26784127]

[29] Xu Q, Fang Y, Jing Q, *et al.* A portable triboelectric spirometer for wireless pulmonary function monitoring. Biosens Bioelectron 2021; 187: 113329.
[http://dx.doi.org/10.1016/j.bios.2021.113329] [PMID: 34020223]

[30] Libanori A, Chen G, Zhao X, Zhou Y, Chen J. Smart textiles for personalized healthcare. Nat Electron 2022; 5(3): 142-56.
[http://dx.doi.org/10.1038/s41928-022-00723-z]

[31] Chen G, Xiao X, Zhao X, Tat T, Bick M, Chen J. Electronic textiles for wearable point-of-care systems. Chem Rev 2022; 122(3): 3259-91.
[http://dx.doi.org/10.1021/acs.chemrev.1c00502] [PMID: 34939791]

[32] Zhou Y, Zhao X, Xu J, *et al.* Giant magnetoelastic effect in soft systems for bioelectronics. Nat Mater 2021; 20(12): 1670-6.
[http://dx.doi.org/10.1038/s41563-021-01093-1] [PMID: 34594013]

[33] Zhao X, Zhou Y, Xu J, *et al.* Soft fibers with magnetoelasticity for wearable electronics. Nat Commun

2021; 12(1): 6755.
[http://dx.doi.org/10.1038/s41467-021-27066-1] [PMID: 34799591]

[34]   Xie J, Chen Q, Shen H, Li G. Review—Wearable Graphene Devices for Sensing. J Electrochem Soc 2020; 167(3): 037541.
[http://dx.doi.org/10.1149/1945-7111/ab67a4]

[35]   Kozitsina A, Svalova T, Malysheva N, Okhokhonin A, Vidrevich M, Brainina K. Sensors based on bio and biomimetic receptors in medical diagnostic, environment, and food analysis. Biosensors (Basel) 2018; 8(2): 35.
[http://dx.doi.org/10.3390/bios8020035] [PMID: 29614784]

[36]   Bhalla N, Jolly P, Formisano N, Estrela P. Biosensor Technologies for Detection of Biomolecules. Biosci Rep 2016; 60(1): 1-10.

[37]   Kim J, Campbell AS, de Ávila BEF, Wang J. Wearable biosensors for healthcare monitoring. Nat Biotechnol 2019; 37(4): 389-406.
[http://dx.doi.org/10.1038/s41587-019-0045-y] [PMID: 30804534]

[38]   Someya T, Bao Z, Malliaras GG. The rise of plastic bioelectronics. Nature 2016; 540(7633): 379-85.
[http://dx.doi.org/10.1038/nature21004] [PMID: 27974769]

[39]   Salim A, Lim S. Recent advances in noninvasive flexible and wearable wireless biosensors. Biosens Bioelectron 2019; 141: 111422.
[http://dx.doi.org/10.1016/j.bios.2019.111422] [PMID: 31229794]

[40]   Stylios GK. Novel smart textiles. Materials (Basel) 2020; 13(4): 950.
[http://dx.doi.org/10.3390/ma13040950] [PMID: 32093274]

[41]   Phillips JW, Prominski A, Tian B. Recent advances in materials and applications for bioelectronic and biorobotic systems. VIEW 2022; 3(3): 20200157.
[http://dx.doi.org/10.1002/VIW.20200157]

[42]   Li A, Ho HH, Barman SR, Lee S, Gao F, Lin ZH. Self-powered antibacterial systems in environmental purification, wound healing, and tactile sensing applications. Nano Energy 2022; 93: 106826.
[http://dx.doi.org/10.1016/j.nanoen.2021.106826]

[43]   Singh SU, Chatterjee S, Lone SA, *et al.* Advanced wearable biosensors for the detection of body fluids and exhaled breath by graphene. Mikrochim Acta 2022; 189(6): 236.
[http://dx.doi.org/10.1007/s00604-022-05317-2] [PMID: 35633385]

[44]   Nguyen N, Lin ZH, Barman SR, *et al.* Engineering an integrated electroactive dressing to accelerate wound healing and monitor noninvasively progress of healing. Nano Energy 2022; 99: 107393.
[http://dx.doi.org/10.1016/j.nanoen.2022.107393]

[45]   Wang B, Wang C, Yu X, *et al.* General synthesis of high-entropy alloy and ceramic nanoparticles in nanoseconds. Nature Synthesis 2022; 1(2): 138-46.
[http://dx.doi.org/10.1038/s44160-021-00004-1]

[46]   Safaei J, Wang G. Progress and prospects of two-dimensional materials for membrane-based osmotic power generation. Nano Research Energy 2022; 1(1): e9120008.
[http://dx.doi.org/10.26599/NRE.2022.9120008]

[47]   Lin Z, Zhi C, Qu L. *Nano Research Energy* : An interdisciplinary journal centered on nanomaterials and nanotechnology for energy. Nano Research Energy 2022; 1(1): e9120005.
[http://dx.doi.org/10.26599/NRE.2022.9120005]

[48]   Gu J, Peng Y, Zhou T, Ma J, Pang H, Yamauchi Y. Porphyrin-based framework materials for energy conversion. Nano Res Energy 2022; 1(1): 1-8.

[49]   Zhou Z, Chen K, Li X, *et al.* Sign-to-speech translation using machine-learning-assisted stretchable sensor arrays. Nat Electron 2020; 3(9): 571-8.
[http://dx.doi.org/10.1038/s41928-020-0428-6]

[50]   Lin Z, Zhang G, Xiao X, *et al.* A personalized acoustic interface for wearable human–machine interaction. Adv Funct Mater 2022; 32(9): 2109430.
[http://dx.doi.org/10.1002/adfm.202109430]

[51]   Zhou Y, Mazur F, Fan Q, Chandrawati R. Synthetic nanoprobes for biological hydrogen sulfide detection and imaging. VIEW 2022; 3(4): 20210008.
[http://dx.doi.org/10.1002/VIW.20210008]

[52]   Lin H, He M, Jing Q, *et al.* Angle-shaped triboelectric nanogenerator for harvesting environmental wind energy. Nano Energy 2019; 56: 269-76.
[http://dx.doi.org/10.1016/j.nanoen.2018.11.037]

[53]   Zheng Q, Peng M, Liu Z, *et al.* Dynamic real-time imaging of living cell traction force by piezo-phototronic light nano-antenna array. Sci Adv 2021; 7(22): eabe7738.
[http://dx.doi.org/10.1126/sciadv.abe7738] [PMID: 34039600]

[54]   Lin Z, Sun C, Liu W, *et al.* A self-powered and high-frequency vibration sensor with layer-powde--layer structure for structural health monitoring. Nano Energy 2021; 90: 106366.
[http://dx.doi.org/10.1016/j.nanoen.2021.106366]

[55]   Peng M, Li Z, Liu C, *et al.* High-resolution dynamic pressure sensor array based on piezo-phototronic effect tuned photoluminescence imaging. ACS Nano 2015; 9(3): 3143-50.
[http://dx.doi.org/10.1021/acsnano.5b00072] [PMID: 25712580]

[56]   Lin H, Liu Y, Chen S, *et al.* Seesaw structured triboelectric nanogenerator with enhanced output performance and its applications in self-powered motion sensing. Nano Energy 2019; 65: 103944.
[http://dx.doi.org/10.1016/j.nanoen.2019.103944]

[57]   Shi S, Jiang Y, Xu Q, *et al.* A self-powered triboelectric multi-information motion monitoring sensor and its application in wireless real-time control. Nano Energy 2022; 97: 107150.
[http://dx.doi.org/10.1016/j.nanoen.2022.107150]

[58]   He M, Lin YJ, Chiu CM, *et al.* A flexible photo-thermoelectric nanogenerator based on MoS2/PU photothermal layer for infrared light harvesting. Nano Energy 2018; 49: 588-95.
[http://dx.doi.org/10.1016/j.nanoen.2018.04.072]

[59]   Dai B, Gao C, Xie Y. Flexible wearable devices for intelligent health monitoring. VIEW 2022; 3(5): 20220027.
[http://dx.doi.org/10.1002/VIW.20220027]

[60]   Budd J, Miller BS, Manning EM, *et al.* Digital technologies in the public-health response to COVID-19. Nat Med 2020; 26(8): 1183-92.
[http://dx.doi.org/10.1038/s41591-020-1011-4] [PMID: 32770165]

[61]   Dunlap DR, Santos RS, Lilly CM, *et al.* COVID-19: A gray swan's impact on the adoption of novel medical technologies. Humanit Soc Sci Commun 2022; 9(1): 232.
[http://dx.doi.org/10.1057/s41599-022-01247-9]

[62]   Schmitt N, Mattern E, Cignacco E, *et al.* Effects of the Covid-19 pandemic on maternity staff in 2020 – a scoping review. BMC Health Serv Res 2021; 21(1): 1364.
[http://dx.doi.org/10.1186/s12913-021-07377-1] [PMID: 34961510]

[63]   White EM, Wetle TF, Reddy A, Baier RR. Front-line nursing home staff experiences during the COVID-19 pandemic. J Am Med Dir Assoc 2021; 22(1): 199-203.
[http://dx.doi.org/10.1016/j.jamda.2020.11.022] [PMID: 33321076]

[64]   Chiesa V, Antony G, Wismar M, Rechel B. COVID-19 pandemic: health impact of staying at home, social distancing and 'lockdown' measures—a systematic review of systematic reviews. J Public Health (Oxf) 2021; 43(3): e462-81.
[http://dx.doi.org/10.1093/pubmed/fdab102] [PMID: 33855434]

[65]   Luciani LG, Mattevi D, Cai T, Giusti G, Proietti S, Malossini G. Teleurology in the time of COVID-

19 pandemic: Here to stay? Urology 2020; 140: 4-6.
[http://dx.doi.org/10.1016/j.urology.2020.04.004] [PMID: 32298686]

[66]   Lluch C, Galiana L, Doménech P, Sansó N. The impact of the COVID-19 pandemic on burnout, compassion fatigue, and compassion satisfaction in healthcare personnel: A systematic review of the literature published during the first year of the pandemic. Healthcare (Basel) 2022; 10(2): 364.
[http://dx.doi.org/10.3390/healthcare10020364] [PMID: 35206978]

[67]   Duffy SW, Seedat F, Kearins O, *et al.* The projected impact of the COVID-19 lockdown on breast cancer deaths in England due to the cessation of population screening: a national estimation. Br J Cancer 2022; 126(9): 1355-61.
[http://dx.doi.org/10.1038/s41416-022-01714-9] [PMID: 35110696]

[68]   Jin YP, Canizares M, El-Defrawy S, Buys YM. Backlog in ophthalmic surgeries associated with the COVID-19 pandemic in Ontario 2020. Can J Ophthalmol 2023; 58(6): 513-22.
[http://dx.doi.org/10.1016/j.jcjo.2022.06.020] [PMID: 35905943]

[69]   Abdi J, Al-Hindawi A, Ng T, Vizcaychipi MP. Scoping review on the use of socially assistive robot technology in elderly care. BMJ Open 2018; 8(2): e018815.
[http://dx.doi.org/10.1136/bmjopen-2017-018815] [PMID: 29440212]

[70]   Morgan AA, Abdi J, Syed MAQ, Kohen GE, Barlow P, Vizcaychipi MP. Robots in healthcare: A scoping review. Current Robotics Reports 2022; 3(4): 271-80.
[http://dx.doi.org/10.1007/s43154-022-00095-4] [PMID: 36311256]

[71]   Jensen JS, Antonsen HK, Durup J. Two years of experience with robot-assisted anti-reflux surgery: A retrospective cohort study. Int J Surg 2017; 39: 260-6.
[http://dx.doi.org/10.1016/j.ijsu.2017.02.014] [PMID: 28216290]

[72]   Stulberg BN, Zadzilka JD. Active robotic technologies for total knee arthroplasty. Arch Orthop Trauma Surg 2021; 141(12): 2069-75.
[http://dx.doi.org/10.1007/s00402-021-04044-2] [PMID: 34259928]

[73]   De Benedictis A, Trezza A, Carai A, *et al.* Robot-assisted procedures in pediatric neurosurgery. Neurosurg Focus 2017; 42(5): E7.
[http://dx.doi.org/10.3171/2017.2.FOCUS16579] [PMID: 28463617]

[74]   Miah S, Servian P, Patel A, *et al.* A prospective analysis of robotic targeted MRI-US fusion prostate biopsy using the centroid targeting approach. J Robot Surg 2020; 14(1): 69-74.
[http://dx.doi.org/10.1007/s11701-019-00929-y] [PMID: 30783886]

[75]   Arya A, Zaker-Shahrak R, Sommer P, *et al.* Catheter ablation of atrial fibrillation using remote magnetic catheter navigation: a case-control study. Europace 2011; 13(1): 45-50.
[http://dx.doi.org/10.1093/europace/euq344] [PMID: 21149511]

[76]   Berdot S, Korb-Savoldelli V, Jaccoulet E, *et al.* A centralized automated-dispensing system in a French teaching hospital: return on investment and quality improvement. Int J Qual Health Care 2019; 31(3): 219-24.
[http://dx.doi.org/10.1093/intqhc/mzy152] [PMID: 30007301]

[77]   Werumeus Buning A, Geersing TH, Crul M. The assessment of environmental and external cross-contamination in preparing ready-to-administer cytotoxic drugs: a comparison between a robotic system and conventional manual production. Int J Pharm Pract 2020; 28(1): 66-74.
[http://dx.doi.org/10.1111/ijpp.12575] [PMID: 31489970]

[78]   Bouazzaoui S, Castelle K, Witherow MA. Ethics and robotics. In: Long S, Ng EH, Downing C, Nepal B, Eds. Proceedings of the American Society for Engineering Management; 2016 Oct 26-29; Charlotte, NC, USA. Huntsville (AL): American Society for Engineering Management; 2016.

[79]   Khan A, Anwar Y. Robots in Healthcare: A Survey. In Arai K, Kapoor S, editors, Advances in Computer Vision - Proceedings of the 2019 Computer Vision Conference CVC. Springer Verlag. 2020. p. 280-292. (Advances in Intelligent Systems and Computing).

[http://dx.doi.org/10.1007/978-3-030-17798-0_24]

[80]   Mi D, Li Y, Zhang K, Huang C, Shan W, Zhang J. Exploring intelligent hospital management mode based on artificial intelligence. Front Public Health 2023; 11: 1182329.
[http://dx.doi.org/10.3389/fpubh.2023.1182329] [PMID: 37645708]

[81]   Božić V. Integrated risk management and artificial intelligence in hospital. J AI 2023; 7: p. (1)63-80.
[http://dx.doi.org/10.61969/jai.1329224]

[82]   Arab Momeni M, Mostofi A, Jain V, Soni G. COVID19 epidemic outbreak: operating rooms scheduling, specialty teams timetabling and emergency patients' assignment using the robust optimization approach. Ann Oper Res 2022; 1-31.
[http://dx.doi.org/10.1007/s10479-022-04667-7] [PMID: 35571378]

[83]   Nizam V, Aslekar A. Challenges of applying AI in healthcare in India. J Pharm Res Int 2021; 33(36B): 203-9.
[http://dx.doi.org/10.9734/jpri/2021/v33i36B31969]

[84]   Rathore Y, Chaturvedi VM, Karwande VS, Rokade AH, Nagargoje Y. Patient engagement and satisfaction in AI-enhanced healthcare management. In: 2023 International Conference on Artificial Intelligence for Innovations in Healthcare Industries (ICAIIHI); 2023; Raipur, India. Piscataway (NJ): IEEE; 2023. p. 1-7.
[http://dx.doi.org/10.1109/ICAIIHI57871.2023.10489712]

[85]   Guo H, Wu Y, Zhao R, *et al.* Leveraging AI for strategic management in healthcare: Enhancing operational and financial performance. Journal of Intelligence and Knowledge Engineering 2024; 2(3): 1-20.
[http://dx.doi.org/10.62517/jike.202404301]

[86]   Alhaider AA, Lau N, Davenport PB, Morris MK. Quantitative evidence supporting distributed situation awareness model of patient flow management. Proceedings of the International Symposium on Human Factors and Ergonomics in Health Care 2020; 238-41.
[http://dx.doi.org/10.1177/2327857920091000]

Artificial Intelligence in Clinical Decision Support

Gunjan[1] and **Shaweta Sharma**[1,*]

[1] Department of Pharmacy, School of Medical and Allied Sciences, Galgotias University, Greater Noida, Uttar Pradesh-201310, India

Abstract: Artificial Intelligence (AI) is revolutionizing the healthcare industry by improving medical research, diagnosis, therapy, and patient care. AI systems use machine learning, natural language processing, and computer vision to analyze vast volumes of medical data, assist physicians in making informed decisions, and develop individualized treatment regimens. AI is also crucial for early illness detection, health outcome prediction, and process improvement in the medical field. However, to fully leverage AI in healthcare, several problems must be resolved, including patient data protection, ethical considerations, and legal constraints. AI has the potential to revolutionize healthcare by assisting physicians in making more informed decisions, enhancing patient safety, and mitigating the impact of staffing shortages. Regulators and politicians are concerned about the reliability of Clinical Decision Support Systems (CDSSs) and Artificial Intelligence (AI), as well as whether users trust them. This study examines these disparities with a particular focus on physicians' perceptions of AI and trust in CDSS. Clinical Decision Support Systems (CDSS) are currently successfully using AI, which can be classified into two categories: data-driven and knowledge-based. AI is particularly helpful for tasks like determining the reasons for cardiac enlargement, evaluating ECG data, and detecting electrolyte imbalances. However, AI has drawbacks, such as a lack of accountability for incorrect medical judgments or treatment outcomes. An ageing population is predicted to make the skilled labor shortage in the healthcare industry worse, and AI-based Clinical Decision Support Systems (AICDSS) have shown benefits in reducing workload and enhancing healthcare. AICDSS has gained recognition for its ability to use both organized and unorganized clinical data to help patients and healthcare professionals in various circumstances. However, AI-based AICDSS must be more effectively incorporated into existing healthcare practices to use vast amounts of data while adhering to stringent privacy regulations and ensuring user satisfaction. To promote the application of AI-CDSS in clinical settings and achieve wider acceptance, a comprehensive understanding of the variables influencing physicians' inclination to use AI-CDSS and their relationships with each other is needed.

Keywords: Artificial intelligence, Clinical decision support systems, Diagnosis, Machine learning, Medical data analysis, Patient care.

* **Corresponding author Shaweta Sharma:** Department of Pharmacy, School of Medical and Allied Sciences, Galgotias University, Greater Noida, Uttar Pradesh-201310, India; E-mail: shawetasharma@galgotiasuniversity.edu.in

Shaweta Sharma, Akhil Sharma, Shivkanya Fuloria & Anurag Singh (Eds.)
All rights reserved-© 2025 Bentham Science Publishers

INTRODUCTION

First launched in the 1980s [1], AI-CDSS are technologies that use clinical expertise, patient data, and wellness data to improve medical decision-making [2]. These systems provide vital information and intelligent tools to identify, treat, and enhance health concerns, which benefits patients, carers, and medical professionals [3]. Advanced AI technology is used by modern AI-CDSS to evaluate patient information from digital medical records, provide rational evaluations or suggestions, and assist medical professionals in making informed decisions [4], as well as assessing data that humans cannot comprehend or understand [5]. In the healthcare industry, AI-CDSS is frequently utilized for activities including patient management, diagnosis, treatment, prevention, and decision-making. They are thought to be crucial for raising the standard of healthcare since several systems have been demonstrated to improve physician performance [6]. Researchers have investigated the application of AI-CDSS in several healthcare domains. According to Hansen *et al* [7], AI-CDSS enhanced the precision and comprehensiveness of nursing interventions. According to Alsharqi *et al.* [8], these systems use machine learning to analyze and interpret echocardiogram images efficiently. By examining their data, Islam *et al.* [9] showed how AI-CDSS assists diabetic patients in tracking and controlling their insulin levels. In anaesthesiology, AI-CDSS are commonly used to help minimize inhaled anesthetics, increase preoperative use of beta-blockers and antibiotics, and aid with anesthesia billing and recordkeeping [10 - 12]. Doctors are the primary clients of AI-CDSS, and their adoption of these systems depends on their desire to utilize them. Concerns about undeveloped technology, data privacy, a lack of human interaction, and mistrust of new systems are among the reasons why some physicians have a favorable opinion of AI-CDSS, while others are apprehensive. According to Wagner *et al.* [13], only 54.9% of family physicians were amenable to diagnosing patients with AI. According to a study by O'Leary *et al.* [14], 82% of healthcare experts polled found AI useful for detecting uncommon disorders. According to a 2020 survey of 156 American radiology students conducted by Park *et al.* [15], more than 75% of the respondents believed AI would have a big influence on medicine in the future, with 66% anticipating it would have a significant impact on diagnostic radiography. AI reduced the students' interest in radiology, according to nearly half of them (44.2%). 71% of 632 academics and students from the areas of ophthalmology, radiology, and dermatology in a study by Scheetz *et al.* [16] thought AI would advance medicine, and 85.7% thought it would affect the demand for healthcare workers in the next ten years. According to a South Korean poll by Oh *et al.* [17], only 5.9% of doctors were quite knowledgeable about AI, despite the fact that the majority of them believed it to be useful. Similarly, UK medical students feel unprepared to deal with AI, according to 2020 research by Sit *et al.* [18]. Concerns about technology replacing human labor are the key reason why many experts have conflicting opinions regarding AI in healthcare. According to Poon and Sung's [19] research, doctors' scepticism regarding AI in clinical settings hindered advancement due to a lack of confidence. Since there are still high expectations for AI-CDSS, it is essential to research physicians' inclination to use these systems and understand the factors that affect their utilization in order to successfully integrate them into clinical practice. Prior studies have demonstrated that the application of AI in diagnosis and treatment is constrained by factors such as worries about professional autonomy. Doctors in underdeveloped nations were less inclined to adopt AI-CDSS because they believed their independence would be threatened. Still, their desire to do so rose when they were involved in the system's planning and design, according to Sambasivan *et al.* [20]. Compared to physicians in large hospitals, Laka *et al.* [21] found that primary care physicians identified patient preferences, autonomy issues, and time restrictions as the main obstacles to using AI-CDSS. The majority of current research focuses on the individual elements that influence physicians' usage of AI-based clinical decision support systems (AI-CDSS). Still, it doesn't examine how these aspects combine or function as a whole. Studies that examine every element influencing physicians' choices to use AI-CDSS and how they relate to one another are also lacking. Our study employs fsQCA to investigate the combined impacts of many factors on Chinese doctors' desire to adopt AI-CDSS in order to assist in promoting its usage in healthcare.

FRAMEWORK FOR AI-CDSS ADOPTION INTENTION

The Unified Theory of Acceptance and Use of Technology (UTAUT) was proposed by Venkatesh *et al.* [22] in 2003 to explain the variables that influence an individual's desire to embrace new technology. The four primary components of the UTAUT—performance expectation, effort expectancy, social influence, and enabling conditions—all have an intentional impact on behaviour [23]. The UTAUT also considers the impact of age, experience, gender, and voluntary usage on the adoption of technology. The hypothesis was first created to examine the practical advantages of implementing new technology in businesses. With the rise of AI technologies, an increasing number of academics are using the UTAUT to study how people use AI. According to Tornatzky *et al.*'s [24] Technology-Organization-Environment (TOE) model, organisations' adoption and implementation of new technologies are also influenced by organisational, technological, and external environmental variables. Fig. (**1**) shows the framework for AI-CDSS adoption intention.

Technical Factors Influencing the Adoption of AI-CDSS by Doctors

One important component of the UTAUT model, which explains and forecasts how people will embrace technology, is performance expectation [25] It shows how many medical professionals in hospitals believe that utilizing new technologies would enhance their ability to perform their jobs [26]. Performance expectation, which is similar to the concept of perceived utility in the technology adoption paradigm, has been the subject of previous studies. It is significant for physicians implementing AI-CDSS [27]. Compared to other technology use cases, doctors are more likely to focus on how technology affects their ability to perform their jobs. AI technology can improve work performance, eliminate pointless chores, and assist in decision-making [28, 29]. Nevertheless, some problems impact labour productivity, such as hurdles to communication between doctors and AI technology. The efficacy of AI in the workplace has not yet been thoroughly established [30]. Thus, doctors' inclination to use AI technology is still significantly influenced by performance expectations.

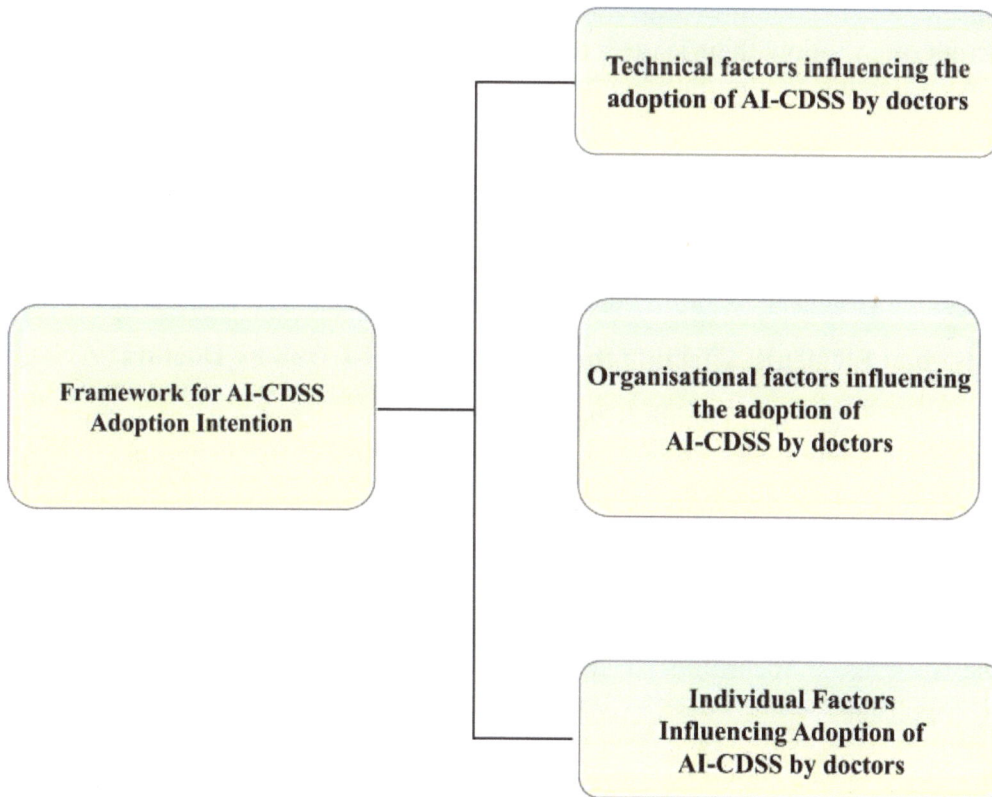

Fig. (1). Framework for AI-CDSS adoption intention.

Physicians' sense of unease when utilizing technology to complete tasks and exchange data is known as perceived risk [31]. A lot of data, frequently from several different sources like people and businesses, is necessary for AI technology to function. Physicians' readiness to embrace AI technology may be significantly impacted by moral, ethical, and legal considerations if there is a risk of data leakage.

Organisational Factors Influencing the Adoption of AI-CDSS by Doctors

Social influence refers to how doctors are affected by their social environment when deciding whether to adopt a certain behaviour. It is an important factor in the UTAUT model that impacts people's inclination to use new technology [27]. In a work setting, doctors are often influenced by their colleagues and leaders, and they feel more connected by following the group. When faced with new technologies like AI, there might not be enough information to make a fully informed choice, so doctors are more likely to be influenced by their peers. Leaders also play a role in doctors' decisions to adopt AI technology [32]. They have the power to approve promotions, rewards, and punishments. As a result, doctors often follow their leaders to gain recognition. Another component of the UTAUT model, facilitating conditions, refers to how much physicians believe their organisation has the resources and support they require to use new technologies [27]. This impacts their readiness to embrace AI technology. Organisations must provide resources like technology, funds, and expertise for new technologies to succeed. The likelihood that doctors will adopt AI technology increases with the ease and convenience of the support. According to research, favourable circumstances influence physicians' inclination to use AI [33, 34].

Individual Elements Affecting the Adoption of AI-CDSS by Doctors

The dread or concern people have when utilizing new technology is known as technology anxiety. People feel anxious when they think the technology will test their talents or confidence, which reduces their likelihood of embracing it [25]. People are becoming more nervous about AI technology than they are about other technologies because of its increasing potential to replace human talent. Consequently, our framework includes technological anxiety as a component of our study. The desire to explore new things is referred to as personal innovativeness. According to the innovation diffusion hypothesis, people's intentions and actions differ according to how innovative they are. According to some research, being creative in consumer situations encourages individuals to use self-service technology [35]. Given that AI is a disruptive technology, doctors' inventiveness plays a significant role in encouraging them to embrace it. Therefore, we think that doctors' propensity to employ AI technology is significantly influenced by their own level of innovation.

BACKGROUND AND FUNDAMENTAL CONCEPTS

Three phases make up the medical AI life cycle [36], which adheres to best practices: (a) the design and assessment of models; (b) the generation and gathering of data; and (c) the security of AI. We examined recent developments in interpretability and explainable AI in medicine, as well as existing techniques and data. To aid in understanding the subjects covered later, this section gives an overview of the primary ideas in these fields. The techniques discussed here are derived from those applied in the papers chosen as part of the systematic review procedure.

Common AI Methods Applied to Clinical Data for Patient Monitoring

The three primary categories of Machine Learning (ML) approaches are reinforcement learning, unsupervised learning, and supervised learning. Labeled data is used to train the model in supervised learning (*e.g.*, identifying known categories). The model operates in unsupervised learning (*e.g.*, clustering) without any prior knowledge of the target variable. Another type of machine learning often used in clinical decision support is reinforcement learning, which interacts with its surroundings to learn to accomplish predetermined objectives.

Through observation of the present state of its surroundings, action, and feedback from those actions, an agent in Reinforcement Learning (RL) gradually learns to maximize rewards [37]. Reinforcement Learning (RL) is based on a Markov Decision Process (MDP) [38] Where the agent learns an optimal policy (π\pi^*π) to maximize cumulative rewards, it does this by exploring the environment, defined by the probabilities of states and actions ($p(s, a, s')p(s, a, s')p(s, a, s')$) and rewards ($rrr$), and using inherent awareness of the surroundings, symbolized by value functions ($V\pi V$_\piV$\pi$ or $Q\pi Q$_\piQ$\pi$) and a discount factor ($\gamma\gamma\gamma$). A Markov Decision Process (MDP) has frequently been used to represent clinical decision-making. More recent techniques concentrate on Q-learning variants like Fitted-Q-Iteration (FQI) [39] and Deep Q-Networks (DQN) [40]. Earlier approaches employed dynamic programming. In cardiovascular monitoring, Reinforcement Learning (RL) has been applied to tasks such as choosing measures and figuring out when and how much to treat patients. Numerous Prognostic and diagnostic duties in the medical field industry depend on supervised machine learning models, including Logistic Regression (LR), Support Vector Machines (SVM), and ensemble techniques like additional trees and Random Forests (RAF) [41 - 44]. AI algorithms are frequently used to process time-independent tabular patient data. Techniques including Natural Language Processing (NLP), deep learning, Convolutional Neural Networks (CNNs), and Recurrent Neural Networks (RNNs) are frequently employed for more complicated data types, like text, time series, and medical images [45 - 47]. In this discipline, simple datasets are frequently used to test more complex classifiers, such as Logistic Regression (LR) and decision tree techniques [48, 49].

- ***Logistic Regression***: One supervised machine learning technique for resolving binary classification issues is logistic regression [50]. It uses a mathematical function known as the sigmoid or logistic function to make probability-based predictions about the future. Based on a predetermined decision boundary, this function assists in estimating the probability that a data item falls into one of two categories.
- ***Support Vector Machines***: Depending on the complexity of the data, Support Vector Machines (SVMs) [51]. Those are methods for supervised machine learning. They seek to determine the optimal dividing line (or hyperplane) to divide data points into one, two, or more dimensions. With an emphasis on the support vectors—the points that are closest to the hyperplane—the objective is to maximize the margin, or distance, between various classes of data points. As a result, fresh, unseen data may be classified more accurately.
- ***Ensemble Algorithms and Decision Trees***: For classification tasks, decision trees employ a framework akin to a flowchart to generate judgments based on input data [52]. Using a single feature, a choice is made at each stage on whether to forecast or proceed to the next feature. The tree's leaves contain the results or forecasts. To increase prediction accuracy, ensemble techniques, such as random forest, integrate many decision trees, each constructed using random data samples [53].
- ***Gradient Boosting and Categorical Boosting***: Gradient boosting combines the predictions of many weak models, usually random forests or decision trees, and is applied to both classification and regression applications [54]. The CatBoost algorithm outperforms existing gradient boosting techniques and is more efficient for categorical data [55].
- ***Recurrent Neural Networks***: Recurrent Neural Networks (RNNs) are designed to operate on sequential input and capture intricate connections across time, in contrast to typical feedforward neural networks, which handle time-independent data. RNNs store information from earlier stages in hidden states. The data from the preceding stage is processed at each time point in addition to the current input. For applications like patient monitoring, RNN models, such as the Gated Recurrent Unit (GRU) and Long Short-Term Memory (LSTM), are frequently utilized [56]. Hochreiter and Schmidhuber first proposed LSTM in 1997 [57]. Its purpose is to detect patterns in sequential data, including clinical time series, that are both in the short-term and long-term. LSTMs allow the model to retain

important data across multiple time periods by controlling the information flow through cells that have input, output, and forget gates.

- *Natural Language Processing*: Textual patient information, including Electronic Health Records (EHRs), may be automatically analyzed using Natural Language Processing (NLP). NLP is made up of AI-based methods that can recognize textual patterns in order to comprehend human language. NLP is used to process Electronic Health Records (EHRs) and other patient data that is kept in databases like the Medical Information Mart for Intensive Care (MIMIC) [58, 59]. In clinical and medical settings [60].

Conventional Scoring Methods That Have Been Established for Critical Care

Several scoring systems, including APACHE, SOFA, and MPM, are often used to evaluate and manage patients' status in Intensive Care Units (ICUs), in addition to the ongoing patient monitoring conducted by intensivists and other medical personnel. Because they provide trustworthy standards for comparison, these scoring systems are helpful for studies on novel AI techniques in clinical decision-making.

APACHE [61] and Mortality Prediction Models (MPMs) [62] are mathematical models that use patient information, including demographics, medical diagnoses, and physiological indicators, to calculate the likelihood that individuals in the critical-care unit who are severely ill will die. Each model predicts mortality using a distinct set of factors and methods. Although these models have limits and should be used with clinical judgment, they aid in identifying risk factors, guiding clinical decisions, and evaluating ICU performance. Before being used in clinical settings, MPMs must be verified and modified as their accuracy might differ based on the model and patient population.

A scoring system is used to monitor organ dysfunction in patients in the critical care unit, called the Sequential Organ Failure Assessment (SOFA) [63]. With values ranging from 0 to 4, it assesses the respiratory, cardiovascular, hepatic, renal, coagulation, and neurological systems; higher scores indicate more dysfunction. Each patient's total SOFA score, which varies from 0 to 24, is calculated daily. SOFA is a beneficial predictor of death in critically sick patients and is often utilized in clinical research and ICU quality improvement.

Modalities of Medical Data for Critical Patient Care

There are two parts of medical information: unstructured data, such as Electronic Health Records (EHRs) and medical imaging, and structured data, with or without timestamps. For AI and ML techniques, numerical data, such as patient demographics (weight, age), may be utilized to generate feature vectors. Clinical time series data should be created by including the timestamp in the analysis of time-dependent data, such as vital signs and lab findings. This section provides an overview of the various data types used in this review. Clinical time series are among the most often handled data types by medical professionals and computerized systems for monitoring patients in critical care units and Electrocardiograms (ECGs). Open-access databases also aid in assessing the effectiveness of AI techniques applied in this domain.

Clinical time series data: Many measures are taken at various timestamps as a result of ongoing patient monitoring. Regardless of the ailment, patient monitoring may be done using a variety of time-based datasets, such as test results, vital signs, Electronic Health Records (EHR), diagnoses, and treatment records [64].

Electrocardiograms (ECGs): William Einthoven created Electrocardiograms (ECGs) in 1902 [65]. These are non-invasive recordings of a patient's body that display the electrical activity of the heart. Particularly in cardiac intensive care units, ECGs are frequently utilized to diagnose cardiac issues.

Open Access Datasets

Replicating techniques are essential in data science and typically call for data sharing. However, sharing patient data raises ethical questions because it is extremely sensitive and private in the clinical and medical domains. The requirement for research reproducibility must be weighed against these worries. This highlights the importance of publicly available datasets for medical research. A few popular public datasets for critical patient care are introduced in this section.

A popular platform for biomedical research and teaching, PhysioNet offers open-source software, instructional courses, and free access to large quantities of physiological and clinical data [66]. Notable datasets available through this platform include the eICU [67] dataset, the Medical Information Mart for Intensive Care (MIMIC-II, MIMIC-III, and MIMIC-IV) [68 - 70], and the High Time-Resolution ICU Dataset (HiRID) [71]. Some of the most popular clinical data sets on PhysioNet for ICU studies are listed below. De-identified electronic health information from more than 60,000 adult intensive care unit patients at Beth Israel Deaconess Medical Centre is available to the public in the MIMIC database. It contains demographic, diagnostic, laboratory, pharmaceutical, and clinical note data collected from sources such as hospital systems and bedside monitors. MIMIC is frequently used in machine learning and clinical research to create predictive models, find risk variables, and enhance patient outcomes. Access is freely available through PhysioNet, an MIT data repository, but requires an application and Institutional Review Board permission.

The requirement for regular, thorough patient monitoring makes Intensive Care Units (ICUs) a major source of time series data. Time-stamped, nurse-verified physiological parameters, such as hourly records of heart rate, blood pressure, and breathing rate, are frequently included in publicly accessible intensive care unit datasets. Additional instances include fluid balances, records of continuous intravenous medicine, and progress comments from healthcare professionals [68].

Healthcare AI Interpretability and Explainability

AI systems usually support decision-making in critical patient care by offering risk assessments and forecasts, which physicians must then evaluate, comprehend, and confirm. AI developers and physicians employ a variety of higher-level evidence for assessment in order to guarantee the dependability of these systems [72]. According to earlier research and a few chosen experiments [73], an AI system has to be validated both technically and clinically before being deployed in a clinical context [74 - 77]. Validation uses a consistent procedure to guarantee the correctness and reliability of a system. To ensure openness, it is also critical to offer post hoc explanations that highlight the AI system's main areas of concentration. In medical AI, this is particularly crucial for patient monitoring [78]. Making the workings of "black box" algorithms intelligible and interpretable for people is known as transparency [79]. Ensuring traceability entails giving sufficient information to enable precise replication of procedures and outcomes in data analysis. AI audibility is becoming a crucial instrument for safe and open innovation.

Medical AI frequently uses techniques like Recursive Feature Elimination (RFE) and Shapley Additive Explanations (SHAP) to mitigate the "black box" nature of AI models with complicated structures and understand their conclusions. Until the required number of features is obtained, RFE begins with all input features and ranks them according to relevance at each stage, eliminating the least important ones [80]. SHAP links credit allocation with local explanations by assigning each input characteristic a priority value for a particular prediction [81]. It is based on game theory and is used to explain the outputs of machine learning models. The majority of traditional techniques, such as RFE and SHAP, offer explainability at the model level, which aids in understanding how a model arrives at a conclusion but lacks the semantic context required for explanations that are comprehensible to humans. Medical expertise, such as explaining things at the symptom level, often drives the demand for explainability in medical applications, as the terminology used by doctors is a key factor [82].

An Alternative Reality: AI Supporting and Preserving Clinical Judgement

The patient may have looked up potential diagnoses and located care using an AI-based symptom checker like Symptomate before visiting the emergency room. After entering the patient's symptoms, the program suggested contacting an ambulance because of the risk of pneumothorax or pulmonary embolism. After the clinical history has been entered into an electronic health record, possibly with the help of an AI scribe, AI technologies can aid doctors by using natural language processing as well as additional information, including physiological measures and biomarkers. These methods can identify patients who are more likely to worsen, ensuring that crucial factors are taken into account, and assist in generating a differential diagnosis [83, 84]. In order to facilitate patient flow and service planning, the hospital can use normal clinical data gathered from a patient's presentation at the emergency room to forecast the need for admission [85]. AI technologies that are tailored to a particular study or multimodal tools that combine several data inputs help clinicians improve test interpretation. While physicians usually depend on established reference ranges for interpretation, AI can provide more individualized interpretations of blood results and find distinct patterns for each individual [86]. Artificial Intelligence (AI) techniques are becoming increasingly accessible to help doctors identify conditions, often equal to or even exceeding the accuracy of skilled clinicians. For instance, PM cardio may test for 38 cardiovascular illnesses by digitizing a paper ECG for AI analysis. Artificial Intelligence (AI) models have also been created to diagnose pathology on chest X-rays. These models include models unique to a given condition, such as those for early SARS-CoV-2 diagnosis, to more all-encompassing options, such as Annalise Enterprise CXR, which can recognise 124 different radiographic abnormalities represented in Fig. (2)

It is hard to believe that this patient's pneumothorax could have gone unnoticed at first if such instruments had been accessible. Although there was no patient injury in this instance, anticoagulation has dangers, and it is possible that proper care was delayed.

AI: A Flawed Companion to a Flawed Medical Professional

Although AI can assist physicians in avoiding cognitive biases, it is crucial to be mindful of the possible drawbacks of its application:

- *Overreliance on AI*: Automation bias is the tendency to over-rely on AI systems and assume they are faultless, which can result in errors. In order to identify errors or inaccurate predictions, clinicians need to remain critical and closely inspect the AI tool [88].

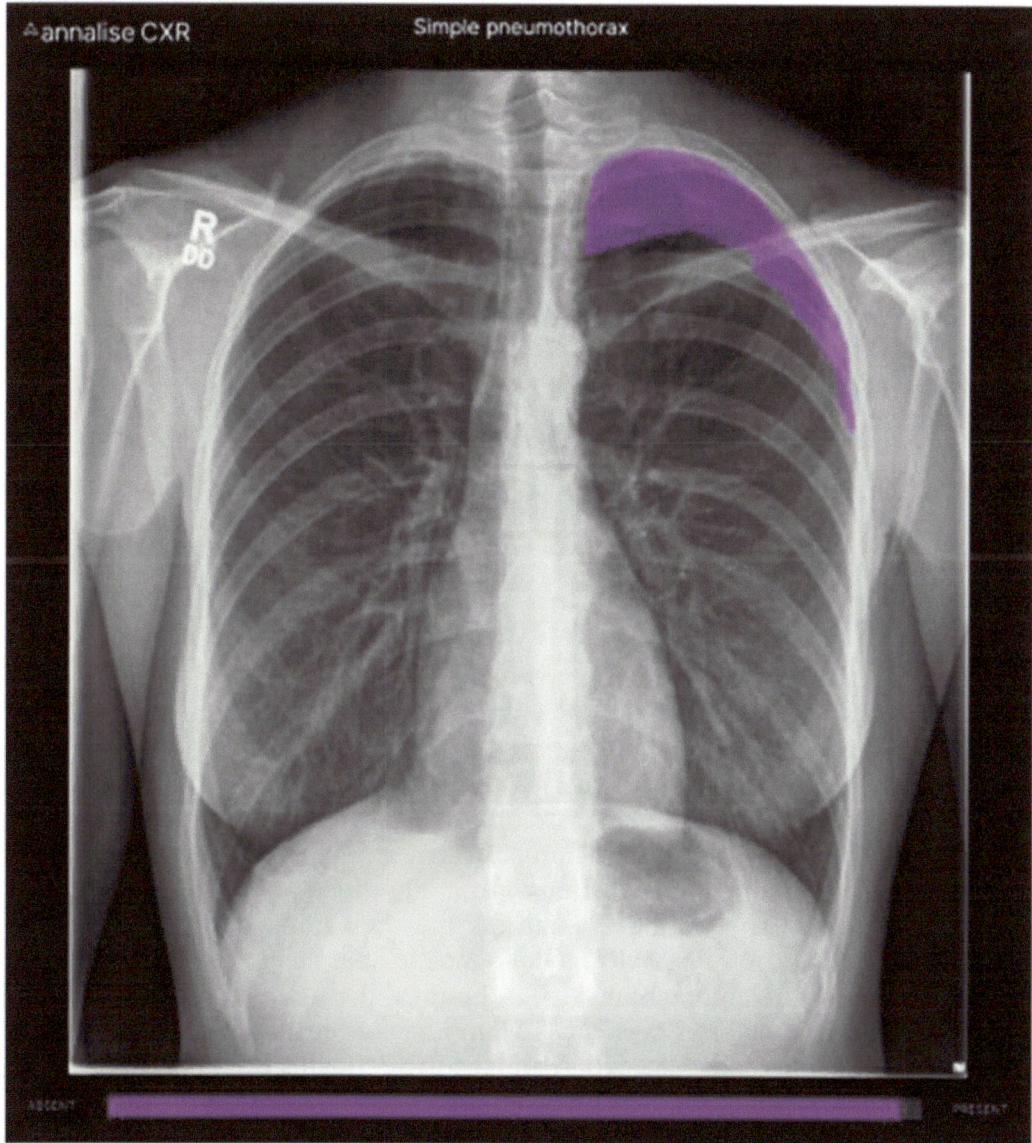

Fig. (2). The chest radiograph of this patient is shown in Annalise Enterprise CXR (Annalise; Sydney, Australia), with the AI-identified pneumothorax finding superimposed [87].

- ***Biased AI***: Biases in the methods or data that are used to train AI systems might cause bias. Clinicians need to be conscious of these biases and take steps to stop the AI from perpetuating or reinforcing them [89].

- *Data Quality*: An AI system's effectiveness can be significantly impacted by the quality of the data used to train it. The AI system is more likely to produce accurate predictions or suggestions if the data is comprehensive, accurate, objective, and applicable in a variety of healthcare contexts.
- *Interpretation of Results*: Clinicians must comprehend the algorithms and statistical techniques employed, as well as the constraints of the data and system, in order to appropriately interpret the outcomes from AI systems [90, 91].
- *Legal and Ethical Considerations*: There are ethical and legal issues with using AI in therapeutic settings, particularly with regard to informed consent and privacy. One major concern is automated decision-making, especially when AI systems are used to make choices that have an impact on a patient's health. The GDPR enforces strict guidelines on automated judgments, including the right of persons to question and understand the reasoning behind them [92]. Clinicians need to make sure that patients are given clear explanations of AI-driven judgments and that the use of AI in decision-making is transparent.
- *Liability*: The doctor is ultimately in charge of a patient's treatment; thus, while utilizing AI, they must exercise caution to make sure the best available data and knowledge support their choices. Simultaneously, people creating and deploying AI systems need to make sure they are impartial, accurate, dependable, and used ethically.

RELATED WORK

Only a small number of the several XAI techniques that have been developed recently are suited to certain application domains. For instance, LIME [93] and SHAP [94] are two of the most widely used XAI techniques. LIME and SHAP offer local explanations that demonstrate how each feature affects the model's output, aligning with the XAI approach covered in this study [95]. Both approaches can produce explanations from any black-box AI model [96], independent of the application domain, as they are both model-agnostic and application-agnostic. While XAI's model-agnostic approach offers flexibility, its application-agnostic approach means it ignores the unique requirements of customers in other sectors [97]. Our XAI approach is in line with new research that creates XAI methods especially suited for the medical domain [98 - 100]. These approaches emphasize the special qualities and applications of healthcare data or include medical expertise in the explanation process [101 - 103]. The majority of approaches do not provide explanations with the end-user in mind, unless doctors are involved in the AI development process [104], even though this study starts to meet the demands of healthcare professionals. Few have also examined the efficacy of their explanations with medical experts. Ideally, doctors should be able to modify their confidence to reflect the AI system's true dependability [105] by being informed about clinical Decision Support System

(DSS) recommendations [106]. From total mistrust to an excessive dependence on AI, there are a number of levels of trust. Concerning AI-based clinical DSSs, extremes of both types have been seen. On the one hand, several studies have demonstrated that doctors frequently depend too much on automated recommendations, showing little initiative [107] or accepting inaccurate diagnoses that AI suggests [108]. Automation bias is the term for this phenomenon, which may be especially harmful in crucial fields like health [109, 110]. However, doctors may be susceptible to algorithmic aversion [111], reflecting the human propensity to reject algorithmic guidance [112], and are hesitant to trust algorithms since they do not understand them [113, 114]. Due to ambiguous liability regimes, clinicians are also concerned about potential legal ramifications if something goes wrong, which contributes to their mistrust of the applications of artificial intelligence in medicine [115, 116]. This study examines how consumers' trust in algorithmic suggestions in the healthcare setting is affected by AI explanations. Our experimental setup makes it possible to determine whether an explanation boosts confidence in AI when its proposal is accurate. An experimental environment like this provides some preliminary understanding of how artificial intelligence explanation might affect the process of trust calibration. By using a co-design strategy to enhance the usability of the explanation interface, we also leverage participant input to inform its design and boost the AI system's usefulness and trust. The AI system's openness is communicated through the user interface [117], and with the introduction of XAI, the system uses the interface to explain its suggestions [118]. An HCI lens must be used to examine the design of this kind of interface since its quality is crucial [119]. Although an AI model's interface has no bearing on its capabilities, early research has demonstrated the connection between interface design and user trust. Indeed, users' perceptions of the AI interface's capabilities and level of confidence in its judgment can be influenced by its design [120]. Additionally, it has been demonstrated that some interface elements, such as usability and simplicity, may enhance users' confidence in automation [121]. In addition, design decisions for explanation interfaces, including the gradual exposure of information, can aid users in making decisions [122].

SHARED DECISION MAKING AND ARTIFICIAL INTELLIGENCE

In a doctor-patient relationship, patients and doctors work together to manage the patient's health. Together, they strive to deliver the best treatment possible while honouring the patient's autonomy, outlining alternatives in detail, and obtaining consent before acting [123]. Respect for the patient's free will and effective communication are the two most important facets of the doctor-patient interaction [124]. Whether or not AI is used, these are the fundamental prerequisites for Shared Decision-Making (SDM). However, preserving these essential components can become more difficult with the advent of AI. It is necessary to consider how doctors and AI interact, as well as how this is conveyed to patients.

AI-Doctor Autonomy and Communication

To arrive at a diagnosis during the clinical assessment procedure, physicians examine a variety of intricate medical data. When AI is used, its suggestions are included in this procedure. Because AI's recommendations impact, shape, and occasionally contradict doctors' judgments, they can have a greater impact on their decisions than they may be aware of. This raises the question of who is actually in charge of making decisions [125]. The widespread impact of AI may restrict the autonomy of physicians [126]. As a result, some medical professionals fear AI poses a "threat to professional autonomy" and might "decrease their control over making choices " [127]. Professional autonomy is a prerequisite for physicians to exercise their clinical judgment freely when providing patient care. Physicians must be able to make decisions about their patients' treatment [128]. This liberty also means that doctors must give their patients the best treatment possible [129]. Since doctors are granted autonomy for the good of society, which guarantees that they can deliver quality treatment, their autonomy and responsibility are closely related [130]. Professional autonomy is crucial for doctors because it gives them the freedom to make judgments and exercise their judgment while also holding them responsible for those decisions. Because it benefits society, this autonomy must be preserved. Doctors' autonomy to choose how AI is utilized in their practice and to use their clinical judgment to act in patients' best interests rather than their own is under jeopardy [131]. The collaborative nature of Shared Decision-Making (SDM) necessitates that patients and physicians maintain their capacity for autonomous and well-informed decision-making. Since doctors actively participate in SDM, they must be able to make independent clinical judgments and decisions. Respecting the autonomy of both patients and physicians is necessary for this. Two things determine a doctor's autonomy: their proficiency with clinical skills and AI, as well as their ability to base judgments on situational and clinical facts. Skilled medical professionals work alongside AI, evaluating its suggestions and looking for mistakes [132]. Determining the degree of knowledge required by physicians to successfully integrate AI's recommendations into their everyday practice while maintaining critical thinking skills is essential. Physicians will be better able to evaluate AI's recommendations and determine whether to accept them in their decision-making if they understand the ramifications and underlying presumptions. Physicians should therefore try to understand the logic underlying AI's suggestions in order to assess their correctness and communicate to patients their part in the clinical evaluation [133]. The black box problem, or the opacity of certain AI systems, is one obstacle to doctors' comprehension. Because black box AI doesn't explain how it operates or how it makes judgments, it makes communication more challenging [134]. The interaction between AI and doctors can be improved by addressing the black box problem. However, AI explainability can only be mandated if the explanations are not only mathematical but also take into consideration the unique context, background knowledge, and interests of doctors [135]. Several elements, including premises, implications, and the AI's output in connection with the real-life situation, should be incorporated into the explanation process [136]. But it's crucial to understand that this isn't a straightforward solution. Doctors may not fully appreciate the ramifications of utilizing AI or its assumptions if they provide causal explanations for AI behavior and comprehend the linkages between input and output. In a similar vein, evaluating AI's suggestions may not necessarily require a grasp of its causal reasoning. The most crucial aspect is that medical professionals understand the potential and constraints of AI in their particular setting. Therefore, doctors would benefit from knowing the underlying assumptions, but they don't need to be fully informed about how AI makes recommendations. For instance, does AI modify risk evaluations by examining comparable data or taking family history into account?

Although explainability has its uses, concentrating too much on the black box problem may obscure other aspects that may be equally or even more important in restricting physicians' use of AI. Training physicians to comprehend and evaluate AI's output effectively enough to preserve their autonomy and make decisions about when, how, and if to incorporate AI into their clinical judgment is still a challenge, even with a completely transparent and effective AI system. Making AI understandable alone does not guarantee that physicians and patients, or AI and doctors, can communicate effectively. Time restraints and motivation could also be important issues that require attention. Another essential element of effective AI-doctor collaboration and maintaining physicians' professional autonomy is the supporting role of these tools—they are intended to inform, assist, and educate clinicians, not substitute them [137]. In the near future, AI is not expected to take the position of humans as the primary decision-makers in the healthcare industry [138]. Despite this, there is a widespread perception that AI poses a danger to physicians and challenges their competence. For example, a venture investor from Silicon Valley once predicted that "radiologists will be obsolete in five years" and that "machines will replace 80% of doctors" [139]. Even if these claims were made a while ago, they haven't materialized; AI can now only be used as a tool, not a substitute, by physicians [140]. It is not a good idea to introduce AI as a new partner in clinical practice by characterizing it as an independent and competitive agent. In the end, the historical and emotional intelligence needed to make judgements in high-risk, emotionally charged, and uncertain scenarios is lacking in present AI tools: "Some judgements go beyond basic survival-based logic" [141]. Waiting for Artificial Intelligence to become "intelligent" enough to make decisions on its own is not the answer. On the one hand, this could be something we never want to happen, but on the other side, underutilizing AI might put people at risk for injury and add needless complexity [142]. Although physicians shouldn't avoid employing AI, it is also not a good idea to keep them out of clinical decision-making. Clinical practice will likely embrace human-in-the-loop models, in which physicians collaborate with AI systems, supervise their application, and determine what, when, how, and why to utilize AI's outputs to inform clinical judgment [143]. A cooperative relationship between AI and physicians—in which AI systems collaborate with people rather than compete with them—should be encouraged [144]. Through this partnership, physicians would be able to preserve their independence while addressing issues like empathy, risk communication, and comprehending patients' beliefs, hopes, anxieties, and expectations—aspects that even an ideal algorithm cannot handle [145] while simultaneously guaranteeing improved performance [146]. Together, doctors and AI could deliver better treatment than anyone could on their own [147]. This is crucial as Shared Decision-Making (SDM) with AI depends on the professional autonomy of physicians. Doctors can only support patients' autonomy by maintaining their own, which will allow them to speak candidly with patients and clarify complicated material [148]. As a result, even with AI, patients are in a better position to engage in the SDM process. In fact, some experts worry that physicians may start acting more as communicators of AI's outputs than as decision-makers [149]. An integral component of the SDM process is a physician's capacity for independent decision-making. Thus, effective AI-doctor communication is crucial for both SDM and the autonomy of doctors.

AI-powered Autonomy and Communication Between Doctors and Patients

Physicians may be obliged to notify their patients when AI is used in clinical evaluations, as AI might significantly influence their decisions [150]. Giving patients this sort of information can improve their comprehension of the prognosis, available options, and the rationale for a diagnosis. As a result, patients would be able to participate more actively in the decision-making process. As previously said, explainability is not sufficient to safeguard patients' autonomy, even though it can help physicians understand and assess AI's suggestions. In addition to evaluating AI's recommendations, doctors also need to be competent and eager to interact with patients. AI cannot provide effective doctor-patient collaboration unless both parties are willing to interact. As long as doctors are prepared to talk about and expose AI, patients' autonomy is not in danger. Clear communication between physicians and AI is the cornerstone of this. As a result, AI-doctor communication not only supports the independence of physicians but also enables them to include patients in the decision-making process, thereby fostering patient autonomy. AI might lead to the emergence of a new kind of paternalism in which the "computer knows best" [151]. This is conceivable as AI's suggestions might not consider patients' values; for example, its only goal might be to maximize lifetime. Not all patients prioritize prolonging their lives, even if this might be considered a shared priority. For example, at the same stage of a terminal disease, one patient may select palliative care. At the same time, another may prefer more therapy [152]. There cannot be a one-size-fits-all decision threshold in clinical settings [153]. Clinical data is only one aspect of the decision-making process in medicine; other elements that must be taken into account include risk tolerance, values, and personal preferences [154]. By considering the patient's preferences and unique situations, AI can help them more effectively. Although physicians are essential in inquiring about patients' preferences and making sure they are taken into account, patients would feel more secure knowing that their values are being upheld if the AI's assessment already took their preferences into account.

Currently, the values that inform AI judgments are hidden within the algorithm and are shaped by organisations and businesses rather than by patients [155]. Finding and exposing the values ingrained in AI is the first essential step. As a result, physicians (and possibly patients) must be aware of these fundamental principles and make sure that, in the end, patients' values are upheld and given precedence over other viewpoints. In order to support Shared Decision-Making (SDM) between patients, physicians, and AI, clinicians need to ensure that the unique preferences of their patients are taken into account. One option is to incorporate the algorithm's recommendations for treatments with patient preferences and risk tolerance. "Respecting the autonomy of patients means that their beliefs should guide the decision-making process" [154]. Achieving the optimal AI-doctor-patient relationship would be the second stage, in addition to efficient AI-doctor-patient communication. In order to avoid paternalism and enable patients to actively engage in Shared Decision-Making (SDM), AI must respect patients' autonomy.

TECHNOLOGIES FOR MACHINE LEARNING AND ARTIFICIAL INTELLIGENCE IN HCI

Interactions with AI systems have long piqued the attention of Human-Computer Interaction (HCI). As machine learning technologies have evolved and been used outside of academic research, this curiosity has only increased. One important use for AI/ML-based systems is still healthcare. We focus on studies conducted within the last ten years, which corresponds to the emergence of deep-learning neural networks. This time frame has seen, for example, a large number of workshops on HCI in AI-driven healthcare applications, including "Realising AI in Healthcare: Challenges Appearing in the Wild" [156]. A couple of examples are Patient-clinician communication: the path for HCI [157] and Recognizing obstacles and possibilities in Human-AI Collaboration in Healthcare [158], both of which included several articles examining pertinent topics. Similarly, the work presented at the 2017 and 2018 AAAI Spring Colloquium on designing machine learning tools' experience [159] served as the basis for the Special Topic on Designing AI [160] in the November–December 2018 edition of Interactions. The creation of transparent, explainable, responsible, and understandable systems was a key focus [161], partly fuelled by DARPA's Explainable AI (XAI) initiative [162]. Additionally, we referenced earlier research on AI-enabled CDS systems that were put into use in the wild, including the work by Cai *et al*. [163]. Vereschak *et al*. [164] defined AI-assisted decision-making as a field of study in which "humans make decisions using their expertise alongside recommendations from an AI-based algorithm." This idea—how people and AI work together to make decisions—is the focus of our publication. The significance of providing doctors with the necessary training to let them comprehend and work with AI CDS has been the subject of recent studies [163, 165] Cai *et al*. [163] stress how crucial it is to convey an AI assistance system's subjective viewpoint, overarching design goal—what it is optimized for—and its acknowledged advantages and disadvantages. By first pointing out the challenge of having a single design emphasis and then detailing the several goals physicians take into account when suggesting T2DM medication, we expand on the idea of design objectives in this work. Future technologies that facilitate human-AI collaboration are advocated by Wang *et al*'s [166] investigation of an AI-supported Clinical Decision System (CDS) for diagnosis and prescription recommendations in rural China. According to their recommendations, AI systems must be "cooperative," assisting physicians, blending in with the local environment, integrating with current IT infrastructure, and improving workflow efficiency. In order to provide more individualized advice, they also urge AI systems to adhere to common decision-making criteria and take patients' social, cultural, and personal circumstances into account. These are significant but challenging objectives that require an in-depth, situation-specific study. In this work, we investigate how the US healthcare system influences the usage of AI-supported CDS, particularly in the treatment of diabetes. We pay special attention to personalization misalignments, highlighting how difficult this work is in the "art of medicine."

WORKFLOWS FOR HEALTHCARE PROVIDERS AND THE WORK OF ELECTRONIC HEALTH RECORDS (EHR)

The Electronic Medical Records (EHR) [167], sometimes referred to as digital patient or medical records, are a key piece of technology in the healthcare industry. EHRs offer a number of other functions in addition to storing digital patient records, such as dashboards for care gap checklists, secure email, e-prescribing, and care management data. Veinot *et al.* [168] describe many usage categories in their research of doctors' use of an EHR system for diabetes treatment, including "stimulating, organising, evaluating, educating, and carrying on." These categories show how EHRs are used to guide the sequence of questions, documentation, resource sharing, and next actions during the actual consultation as well as for pre-tasking (such as reminding doctors about a patient's recent medical history or creating questions for the appointment). In order to complement Veinot *et al.*'s "informing" category of clinical consultation, the prototype that we looked at in this study was designed to integrate with an EHR system. Researchers in HCI have also looked at technologies that facilitate communication between patients and clinicians. Several studies [169 - 172] have demonstrated that power and knowledge disparities are among the main reasons why patient-clinician communication might be challenging during a therapeutic interaction. Mamykina *et al.* [173] created MAHI, a health monitoring application, as a first step to encourage collaborative reflection and learning. Its purpose is to assist newly diagnosed diabetes patients in developing reflective thinking abilities through connections with diabetes educators. Individuals were able to address self-management issues and gain more self-efficacy in controlling their diabetes by promoting introspection and continuing discussions with educators, which helped them move towards a more powerful internal locus of control. The extreme time constraints on clinical decision-making will be one of the major obstacles facing clinical technologies. A primary care physician would need to work more than twenty-four hours a day [174]. Only to provide treatment that is indicated by guidelines, while the average practitioner spends extremely little time with patients, sometimes less than ten minutes [175]. The suggested method of shared decision-making (*e.g.*, [176, 177]), in which patients and physicians jointly consider treatment choices, is put to the test by this time constraint. Our study examines the need for implementing an AI-assisted clinical decision support tool in this highly time-constrained setting, where providers have little time to use information-intensive EHR tools, receive more than 900 technological alerts daily, and have little time to delve into and thoroughly review the details in the documents [178]. By examining how an AI-assisted CDS presents additional difficulties for physicians in the areas of explainability and trust, we contribute to the corpus of knowledge in HCI. Additionally, we describe how, in these time-limited circumstances, these issues intersect with the objectives of the physician.

SYSTEMS FOR CLINICAL DECISION SUPPORT (CDS) IN HEALTHCARE ENVIRONMENTS

The subject of clinical decision support systems has long been of great interest to researchers in the field of technology. According to the method that "provides clinicians, employees, patients or other individuals with knowledge and Person-specific data, intelligently filtered or presented at appropriate times for improving health and health care" [179]. By providing insights specific to a patient's characteristics in a given clinical context, CDS systems aid in clinical decision-making. These systems can help with several healthcare-related tasks, including warnings for certain medical issues, help with diagnosis or treatment, and reminders for preventive care. A CDS tool, for instance, assists by providing physicians, staff, patients, or others with pertinent knowledge and tailored information that is intelligently filtered and provided at the appropriate times to enhance health and care outcomes [179]. In order to produce suggestions for the user, CDS systems evaluate patient-specific data pertaining to the clinical scenario using algorithms like rules-based decision trees or machine learning models. These systems may help with a number of healthcare tasks, such as condition monitoring, diagnosis, treatment, and prevention; they can also fix coding errors [180] and notify doctors of possible medication interactions [181]. The extensive usage of CDS tools in clinical settings raises the crucial question of how much confidence doctors and other consumers place in them. These tools can operate independently or be linked to EHRs. It has been challenging to create CDS systems that work. The "five rights" of CDS—delivering the right information to the right person, in the right format, over the right channel, and at the right place in the workflow—are the culmination of years of expertise [182]. Alarm fatigue, on the other hand, can lead to overrides, workarounds, and clinical burnout if a CDS is poorly constructed [183]. The fact that very few CDS trials have demonstrated better patient outcomes is even more concerning [183, 184]. For many CDS technologies, achieving the "five rights" is still a goal [182]. Clinical decision assistance based on artificial intelligence has existed for many years [185, 186]. Large volumes of health data might now be used to train Artificial Intelligence models for CDS over a manageable period because of advancements in computing power. The ethics and intelligibility of AI-based CDS are more complex than those of rules-based CDS (such as an alarm that is generated when an individual has an allergy to a given drug). For example, data confounding might perpetuate hidden biases, and physicians may find it challenging to comprehend the generalizability of the CDS due to the lack of ability in certain AI models [185]. In fact, AI models frequently behave as "black boxes," with little clarity surrounding the "rules" that guide their decision-making [187]. Clinicians must decide whether to follow the CDS based on the model for their patient, but the lack of transparency in how an AI model generates an output undermines their faith [187].

CONCLUSION

The chapter talks about how Artificial Intelligence (AI) is revolutionizing the use of Clinical Decision Support Systems (CDSS) in the medical field. By using natural language processing, machine learning, and computer vision to evaluate vast amounts of medical data, it demonstrates how AI improves healthcare research, examination, and patient care. In addition to helping with early disease identification and health outcome prediction, this results in better decision-making and individualized treatment regimens. The protection of patient data, ethical ramifications, and legal problems are only a few of the major obstacles to the widespread adoption of AI in healthcare. Healthcare workers must have faith in AI systems because many of them express doubts about their dependability. The paper highlights how crucial it is to comprehend doctors' attitudes and the factors affecting their readiness to use AI-CDSS. It implies that in order to promote wider acceptability, these issues must be addressed holistically, with an emphasis on fostering trust and guaranteeing successful integration into current procedures. Overall, even though AI can improve patient safety and reduce staffing shortages, its effective application depends on removing obstacles pertaining to professional autonomy, privacy, and trust. In order to encourage the use of AI in therapeutic settings, the paper recommends more investigation into how these aspects interact.

REFERENCES

[1] Sutton RT, Pincock D, Baumgart DC, Sadowski DC, Fedorak RN, Kroeker KI. An overview of clinical decision support systems: benefits, risks, and strategies for success. NPJ Digit Med 2020; 3(1): 17.
[http://dx.doi.org/10.1038/s41746-020-0221-y] [PMID: 32047862]

[2] Osheroff JA, Teich J, Levick D, *et al.* Improving outcomes with clinical decision support: An implementer's guide. 2nd ed. Chicago (IL): HIMSS Publishing; 2012.
[http://dx.doi.org/10.4324/9781498757461]

[3] Shankar P, Anderson N. Advances in sharing multi-sourced health data on decision support science 2016-2017. Yearb Med Inform 2018; 27(1): 16-024.
[http://dx.doi.org/10.1055/s-0038-1641215] [PMID: 30157504]

[4] Lu Y, Melnick ER, Krumholz HM. Clinical decision support in cardiovascular medicine. BMJ 2022; 377: e059818.
[http://dx.doi.org/10.1136/bmj-2020-059818] [PMID: 35613721]

[5] Ackerhans S, Huynh T, Kaiser C, Schultz C. Exploring the role of professional identity in the implementation of clinical decision support systems—a narrative review. Implementation Science. 2024 Feb 12;19(1):11.

[6] Ash JS, Sittig DF, Guappone KP, *et al.* Recommended practices for computerized clinical decision support and knowledge management in community settings: a qualitative study. BMC Med Inform Decis Mak 2012; 12(1): 6.
[http://dx.doi.org/10.1186/1472-6947-12-6] [PMID: 22333210]

[7] Hanson LC, Zimmerman S, Song MK, *et al.* Effect of the goals of care intervention for advanced dementia: a randomized clinical trial. JAMA Intern Med 2017; 177(1): 24-31.

[http://dx.doi.org/10.1001/jamainternmed.2016.7031] [PMID: 27893884]

[8] Alsharqi M, Upton R, Mumith A, Leeson P. Artificial intelligence: a new clinical support tool for stress echocardiography. Expert Rev Med Devices 2018; 15(8): 513-5.
[http://dx.doi.org/10.1080/17434440.2018.1497482] [PMID: 29992841]

[9] Islam R, Sultana A, Tuhin MN, Saikat MSH, Islam MR. Clinical decision support system for diabetic patients by predicting type 2 diabetes using machine learning algorithms. J Healthc Eng 2023; 2023(1): 6992441.
[http://dx.doi.org/10.1155/2023/6992441] [PMID: 37287539]

[10] Nair BG, Peterson GN, Newman SF, Wu WY, Kolios-Morris V, Schwid HA. Improving documentation of a beta-blocker quality measure through an anesthesia information management system and real-time notification of documentation errors. Jt Comm J Qual Patient Saf 2012; 38(6): 283-AP3.
[http://dx.doi.org/10.1016/S1553-7250(12)38036-7] [PMID: 22737780]

[11] Nair BG, Peterson GN, Neradilek MB, Newman SF, Huang EY, Schwid HA. Reducing wastage of inhalation anesthetics using real-time decision support to notify of excessive fresh gas flow. Anesthesiology 2013; 118(4): 874-84.
[http://dx.doi.org/10.1097/ALN.0b013e3182829de0] [PMID: 23442753]

[12] Freundlich RE, Barnet CS, Mathis MR, Shanks AM, Tremper KK, Kheterpal S. A randomized trial of automated electronic alerts demonstrating improved reimbursable anesthesia time documentation. J Clin Anesth 2013; 25(2): 110-4.
[http://dx.doi.org/10.1016/j.jclinane.2012.06.020] [PMID: 23333782]

[13] Wagner G, Raymond L, Paré G. Understanding prospective physicians' intention to use artificial intelligence in their future medical practice: configurational analysis. JMIR Med Educ 2023; 9: e45631.
[http://dx.doi.org/10.2196/45631] [PMID: 36947121]

[14] O'Leary P, Carroll N, Richardson I. The practitioner's perspective on clinical pathway support systems. In: 2014 IEEE International Conference on Healthcare Informatics (ICHI); 2014 Sep 15-17; Verona, Italy. Piscataway (NJ) 2014. p. 194-201.
[http://dx.doi.org/10.1109/ICHI.2014.33]

[15] Park CJ, Yi PH, Siegel EL. Medical student perspectives on the impact of artificial intelligence on the practice of medicine. Curr Probl Diagn Radiol 2021; 50(5): 614-9.
[http://dx.doi.org/10.1067/j.cpradiol.2020.06.011] [PMID: 32680632]

[16] Scheetz J, Rothschild P, McGuinness M, et al. A survey of clinicians on the use of artificial intelligence in ophthalmology, dermatology, radiology and radiation oncology. Sci Rep 2021; 11(1): 5193.
[http://dx.doi.org/10.1038/s41598-021-84698-5] [PMID: 33664367]

[17] Oh S, Kim JH, Choi SW, Lee HJ, Hong J, Kwon SH. Physician confidence in artificial intelligence: an online mobile survey. J Med Internet Res 2019; 21(3): e12422.
[http://dx.doi.org/10.2196/12422] [PMID: 30907742]

[18] Sit C, Srinivasan R, Amlani A, et al. Attitudes and perceptions of UK medical students towards artificial intelligence and radiology: a multicentre survey. Insights Imaging 2020; 11(1): 14.
[http://dx.doi.org/10.1186/s13244-019-0830-7] [PMID: 32025951]

[19] Poon AIF, Sung JJY. Opening the black box of AI-Medicine. J Gastroenterol Hepatol 2021; 36(3): 581-4.
[http://dx.doi.org/10.1111/jgh.15384] [PMID: 33709609]

[20] Sambasivan M, Esmaeilzadeh P, Kumar N, Nezakati H. Intention to adopt clinical decision support systems in a developing country: effect of Physician's perceived professional autonomy, involvement and belief: a cross-sectional study. BMC Med Inform Decis Mak 2012; 12(1): 142.
[http://dx.doi.org/10.1186/1472-6947-12-142] [PMID: 23216866]

[21] Laka M, Milazzo A, Merlin T. Factors that impact the adoption of clinical decision support systems (CDSS) for antibiotic management. Int J Environ Res Public Health 2021; 18(4): 1901.
[http://dx.doi.org/10.3390/ijerph18041901] [PMID: 33669353]

[22] Venkatesh V, Morris MG, Davis GB, Davis FD. User acceptance of information technology: Toward a unified view. Manage Inf Syst Q 2003; 27(3): 425-78.
[http://dx.doi.org/10.2307/30036540]

[23] Bendary N, Al-Sahouly I. Exploring the extension of unified theory of acceptance and use of technology, UTAUT2, factors effect on perceived usefulness and ease of use on mobile commerce in Egypt. J Bus Retail Manag Res 2018; 12(2)
[http://dx.doi.org/10.24052/JBRMR/V12IS02/ETEOUTOAAUOTUFEOPUAEOUOMCIE]

[24] Tornatzky LG, Klein KJ. Innovation characteristics and innovation adoption-implementation: A meta-analysis of findings. IEEE Trans Eng Manage 1982; EM-29(1): 28-45.
[http://dx.doi.org/10.1109/TEM.1982.6447463]

[25] Menon D, Shilpa K. "Chatting with ChatGPT": Analyzing the factors influencing users' intention to Use the Open AI's ChatGPT using the UTAUT model. Heliyon 2023; 9(11): e20962.
[http://dx.doi.org/10.1016/j.heliyon.2023.e20962] [PMID: 37928033]

[26] Venkatesh V, Thong JYL, Xu X. Consumer acceptance and use of information technology: extending the unified theory of acceptance and use of technology. Manage Inf Syst Q 2012; 36(1): 157-78.
[http://dx.doi.org/10.2307/41410412]

[27] Lambert SI, Madi M, Sopka S, *et al.* An integrative review on the acceptance of artificial intelligence among healthcare professionals in hospitals. NPJ Digit Med 2023; 6(1): 111.
[http://dx.doi.org/10.1038/s41746-023-00852-5] [PMID: 37301946]

[28] Kaplan A, Haenlein M. Siri, Siri, in my hand: Who's the fairest in the land? On the interpretations, illustrations, and implications of artificial intelligence. Bus Horiz 2019; 62(1): 15-25.
[http://dx.doi.org/10.1016/j.bushor.2018.08.004]

[29] Xu P, Xu X. Change logic and analysis framework of enterprise management in the era of artificial intelligence. Manag World 2020; 1: 122-9.

[30] Qiu Y, He Q. Research on the progress the impact of Artificial Intelligence on Employment and the theoretical analysis framework in Chinese context. Hum Resour Dev China 2020; 37: 90-103.

[31] Pillai R, Sivathanu B. Adoption of artificial intelligence (AI) for talent acquisition in IT/ITeS organizations. Benchmarking (Bradf) 2020; 27(9): 2599-629.
[http://dx.doi.org/10.1108/BIJ-04-2020-0186]

[32] Chatterjee S, Bhattacharjee KK. Adoption of artificial intelligence in higher education: a quantitative analysis using structural equation modelling. Educ Inf Technol 2020; 25(5): 3443-63.
[http://dx.doi.org/10.1007/s10639-020-10159-7]

[33] Sohn K, Kwon O. Technology acceptance theories and factors influencing artificial Intelligence-based intelligent products. Telemat Inform 2020; 47: 101324.
[http://dx.doi.org/10.1016/j.tele.2019.101324]

[34] Chen LSL, Wu KIF. Antecedents of intention to use CUSS system: moderating effects of self-efficacy. Serv Bus 2014; 8(4): 615-34.
[http://dx.doi.org/10.1007/s11628-013-0210-1]

[35] Chen J, Li R, Gan M, Fu Z, Yuan F. Public acceptance of driverless buses in China: an empirical analysis based on an extended UTAUT model. Discrete Dyn Nat Soc 2020; 2020(1): 1-13.
[http://dx.doi.org/10.1155/2020/4318182]

[36] Ng MY, Kapur S, Blizinsky KD, Hernandez-Boussard T. The AI life cycle: a holistic approach to creating ethical AI for health decisions. Nat Med 2022; 28(11): 2247-9.
[http://dx.doi.org/10.1038/s41591-022-01993-y] [PMID: 36163298]

[37]   Sutton RS. Introduction: The challenge of reinforcement learning. In: Sutton RS, Ed. Reinforcement learning. The Springer international series in engineering and computer science, vol. 173. Boston (MA): Springer; 1992. pp 1-3.
[http://dx.doi.org/10.1007/978-1-4615-3618-5_1]

[38]   Moazemi S, Vahdati S, Li J, *et al.* Artificial intelligence for clinical decision support for monitoring patients in cardiovascular ICUs: A systematic review. Front Med (Lausanne) 2023; 10: 1109411.
[http://dx.doi.org/10.3389/fmed.2023.1109411] [PMID: 37064042]

[39]   Riedmiller M. Neural fitted Q iteration–first experiences with a data-efficient neural reinforcement learning method. 2005; 16th European Conference on Machine Learning 2005 Oct 3-7; Porto, Portugal: Springer 2005; pp. 317-28.
[http://dx.doi.org/10.1007/11564096_32]

[40]   Mnih V, Kavukcuoglu K, Silver D, *et al.* Playing Atari with deep reinforcement learning. arXiv preprint arXiv:13125602 2013.

[41]   Parsi A, Glavin M, Jones E, Byrne D. Prediction of paroxysmal atrial fibrillation using new heart rate variability features. Comput Biol Med 2021; 133: 104367.
[http://dx.doi.org/10.1016/j.compbiomed.2021.104367] [PMID: 33866252]

[42]   Yu Y, Peng C, Zhang Z, *et al.* Machine learning methods for predicting long-term mortality in patients after cardiac surgery. Front Cardiovasc Med 2022; 9: 831390.
[http://dx.doi.org/10.3389/fcvm.2022.831390] [PMID: 35592400]

[43]   Chen WT, Huang HL, Ko PS, Su W, Kao CC, Su SL. A simple algorithm using ventilator parameters to predict successfully rapid weaning program in cardiac intensive care unit patients. J Pers Med 2022; 12(3): 501.
[http://dx.doi.org/10.3390/jpm12030501] [PMID: 35330500]

[44]   Bodenes L, N'Guyen QT, Le Mao R, *et al.* Early heart rate variability evaluation enables to predict ICU patients' outcome. Sci Rep 2022; 12(1): 2498.
[http://dx.doi.org/10.1038/s41598-022-06301-9] [PMID: 35169170]

[45]   Madinei HS, Keyvanpour MR, Shojaedini SV. An Attention-Based Model for Clinical Time Series Prediction: Enhancing ICU Readmission Prediction. In 14th International Conference on Computer and Knowledge Engineering (ICCKE) 2024 Nov 19 (pp. 119-124).

[46]   Qin F, Madan V, Ratan U, *et al.* Improving early sepsis prediction with multi-modal learning. arXiv preprint arXiv:210711094 2021.

[47]   Baral S, Alsadoon A, Prasad PWC, Al Aloussi S, Alsadoon OH. A novel solution of using deep learning for early prediction cardiac arrest in Sepsis patient: enhanced bidirectional long short-term memory (LSTM). Multimedia Tools Appl 2021; 80: 32639-64.
[http://dx.doi.org/10.1007/s11042-021-11176-5]

[48]   Lin YW, Zhou Y, Faghri F, Shaw MJ, Campbell RH. Analysis and prediction of unplanned intensive care unit readmission using recurrent neural networks with long short-term memory. PLoS One 2019; 14(7): e0218942.
[http://dx.doi.org/10.1371/journal.pone.0218942] [PMID: 31283759]

[49]   Lin WT, Chen WL, Chao CM, Lai CC. The outcomes and prognostic factors of the patients with unplanned intensive care unit readmissions. Medicine (Baltimore) 2018; 97(26): e11124.
[http://dx.doi.org/10.1097/MD.0000000000011124] [PMID: 29952954]

[50]   Cox DR. The regression analysis of binary sequences. J R Stat Soc Series B Stat Methodol 1958; 20(2): 215-32.
[http://dx.doi.org/10.1111/j.2517-6161.1958.tb00292.x]

[51]   Cortes C, Vapnik V. Support-Vector Networks. Mach Learn 1995; 20(3): 273-97.
[http://dx.doi.org/10.1023/A:1022627411411]

[52] Quinlan JR. Induction of decision trees. Mach Learn 1986; 1(1): 81-106.
[http://dx.doi.org/10.1023/A:1022643204877]

[53] Breiman L. Random Forests. Mach Learn 2001; 45(1): 5-32.
[http://dx.doi.org/10.1023/A:1010933404324]

[54] Friedman JH. Greedy function approximation: A gradient boosting machine. Ann Stat 2001; 29(5): 1189-232.
[http://dx.doi.org/10.1214/aos/1013203451]

[55] Dorogush AV, Ershov V, Gulin A. CatBoost: Gradient boosting with categorical features support. arXiv preprint arXiv:181011363 2018.

[56] Sherstinsky A. Fundamentals of recurrent neural network (RNN) and long short-term memory (LSTM) network. Physica D 2020; 404: 132306.
[http://dx.doi.org/10.1016/j.physd.2019.132306]

[57] Hochreiter S, Schmidhuber J. Long short-term memory. Neural Comput 1997; 9(8): 1735-80.
[http://dx.doi.org/10.1162/neco.1997.9.8.1735] [PMID: 9377276]

[58] Johnson AEW, Pollard TJ, Shen L, *et al.* MIMIC-III, a freely accessible critical care database. Sci Data 2016; 3(1): 160035.
[http://dx.doi.org/10.1038/sdata.2016.35] [PMID: 27219127]

[59] Johnson AEW, Bulgarelli L, Shen L, *et al.* MIMIC-IV, a freely accessible electronic health record dataset. Sci Data 2023; 10(1): 1.
[http://dx.doi.org/10.1038/s41597-022-01899-x] [PMID: 36596836]

[60] Huang K, Altosaar J, Ranganath R. ClinicalBERT: Modeling clinical notes and predicting hospital readmission. arXiv preprint arXiv:190405342 2019.

[61] Ho KM, Dobb GJ, Knuiman M, Finn J, Lee KY, Webb SAR. A comparison of admission and worst 24-hour Acute Physiology and Chronic Health Evaluation II scores in predicting hospital mortality: a retrospective cohort study. Crit Care 2006; 10(1): R4.
[http://dx.doi.org/10.1186/cc3913] [PMID: 16356207]

[62] Higgins TL, Teres D, Copes WS, Nathanson BH, Stark M, Kramer AA. Assessing contemporary intensive care unit outcome: An updated Mortality Probability Admission Model (MPM0-III). Crit Care Med 2007; 35(3): 827-35.
[http://dx.doi.org/10.1097/01.CCM.0000257337.63529.9F] [PMID: 17255863]

[63] Vincent JL, de Mendonça A, Cantraine F, *et al.* Use of the SOFA score to assess the incidence of organ dysfunction/failure in intensive care units. Crit Care Med 1998; 26(11): 1793-800.
[http://dx.doi.org/10.1097/00003246-199811000-00016] [PMID: 9824069]

[64] Jabali AK, Waris A, Khan DI, Ahmed S, Hourani RJ. Electronic health records: Three decades of bibliometric research productivity analysis and some insights. Inform Med Unlocked 2022; 29: 100872.
[http://dx.doi.org/10.1016/j.imu.2022.100872]

[65] Ali IM, Abd O, Ahmed EA, Ebraheim MN. Nurses' performance regarding electrocardiography application and its interpretation: suggested nursing guideline. Egypt J Health Care 2021; 13(4): 281-295.

[66] Goldberger AL, Amaral LAN, Glass L, *et al.* PhysioBank, PhysioToolkit, and PhysioNet: components of a new research resource for complex physiologic signals. Circulation 2000; 101(23): E215-20.
[http://dx.doi.org/10.1161/01.CIR.101.23.e215] [PMID: 10851218]

[67] Pollard TJ, Johnson AEW, Raffa JD, Celi LA, Mark RG, Badawi O. The eICU Collaborative Research Database, a freely available multi-center database for critical care research. Sci Data 2018; 5(1): 180178.
[http://dx.doi.org/10.1038/sdata.2018.178] [PMID: 30204154]

[68] Yan Z, Quan G, Jia-Hui X. Criticality of Nursing Care for Patients With Alzheimer's Disease in the ICU: Insights From MIMIC III Dataset. Clinical Nursing Research. 2024 Nov;33(8):630-7.

[69] Jung J, Kim D, Hwang I. Exploring Predictive Factors for Heart Failure Progression in Hypertensive Patients Based on Medical Diagnosis Data from the MIMIC-IV Database. Bioengineering. 2024 May 23;11(6):531.

[70] Saeed M, Villarroel M, Reisner AT, *et al.* Multiparameter Intelligent Monitoring in Intensive Care II: A public-access intensive care unit database. Crit Care Med 2011; 39(5): 952-60.
[http://dx.doi.org/10.1097/CCM.0b013e31820a92c6] [PMID: 21283005]

[71] Yèche H, Kuznetsova R, Zimmermann M, Hüser M, Lyu X, Faltys M, *et al.* HiRID-IC--Benchmark—A comprehensive machine learning benchmark on high-resolution ICU data. arXiv preprint arXiv:211108536 2021.

[72] Shaban-Nejad A, Michalowski M, Buckeridge DL. Explainability and interpretability: keys to deep medicine. In: Shaban-Nejad A, Michalowski M, Buckeridge DL, Eds. Explainable AI in healthcare and medicine. Studies in computational intelligence, vol. 914. Cham: Springer; 2021. p. 1-9.
[http://dx.doi.org/10.1007/978-3-030-53352-6_1]

[73] Antoniadi AM, Du Y, Guendouz Y, *et al.* Current challenges and future opportunities for XAI in machine learning-based clinical decision support systems: a systematic review. Appl Sci (Basel) 2021; 11(11): 5088.
[http://dx.doi.org/10.3390/app11115088]

[74] Moazemi S, Kalkhoff S, Kessler S, *et al.* Evaluating a recurrent neural network model for predicting readmission to cardiovascular ICUs based on clinical time series data. Eng Proc 2022; 18(1): 1.
[http://dx.doi.org/10.3390/engproc2022018001]

[75] Zhao QY, Wang H, Luo JC, *et al.* Development and validation of a machine-learning model for prediction of extubation failure in intensive care units. Front Med (Lausanne) 2021; 8: 676343.
[http://dx.doi.org/10.3389/fmed.2021.676343] [PMID: 34079812]

[76] Jentzer JC, Kashou AH, Lopez-Jimenez F, *et al.* Mortality risk stratification using artificial intelligence-augmented electrocardiogram in cardiac intensive care unit patients. Eur Heart J Acute Cardiovasc Care 2021; 10(5): 532-41.
[http://dx.doi.org/10.1093/ehjacc/zuaa021] [PMID: 33620440]

[77] Andersson P, Johnsson J, Björnsson O, *et al.* Predicting neurological outcome after out-of-hospital cardiac arrest with cumulative information; development and internal validation of an artificial neural network algorithm. Crit Care 2021; 25(1): 83.
[http://dx.doi.org/10.1186/s13054-021-03505-9] [PMID: 33632280]

[78] Kiseleva A, Kotzinos D, De Hert P. Transparency of AI in healthcare as a multilayered system of accountabilities: between legal requirements and technical limitations. Front Artif Intell 2022; 5: 879603.
[http://dx.doi.org/10.3389/frai.2022.879603] [PMID: 35707765]

[79] Srinivasu PN, Sandhya N, Jhaveri RH, Raut R. From blackbox to explainable AI in healthcare: existing tools and case studies. Mob Inf Syst 2022; (1): 1-20.
[http://dx.doi.org/10.1155/2022/8167821]

[80] Guyon I, Weston J, Barnhill S, Vapnik V. Gene selection for cancer classification using support vector machines. Mach Learn 2002; 46(1-3): 389-422.
[http://dx.doi.org/10.1023/A:1012487302797]

[81] Lundberg S, Lee SI. A unified approach to interpreting model predictions. arXiv preprint arXiv:170507874 2017.

[82] Pesquita C. Towards semantic integration for explainable artificial intelligence in the biomedical domain. In: Proceedings of the 14th International Joint Conference on Biomedical Engineering Systems and Technologies (BIOSTEC 2021); 2021; Vienna, Austria. SciTePress; 2021. p. 747-53.

[http://dx.doi.org/10.5220/0010389707470753]

[83] Giordano C, Brennan M, Mohamed B, Rashidi P, Modave F, Tighe P. Accessing artificial intelligence for clinical decision-making. Front Digit Health 2021; 3: 645232.
[http://dx.doi.org/10.3389/fdgth.2021.645232] [PMID: 34713115]

[84] Noor K, Roguski L, Bai X, *et al.* Deployment of a free-text analytics platform at a UK national health service research hospital: Cogstack at University College London Hospitals. JMIR Med Inform 2022; 10(8): e38122.
[http://dx.doi.org/10.2196/38122] [PMID: 36001371]

[85] King Z, Farrington J, Utley M, *et al.* Machine learning for real-time aggregated prediction of hospital admission for emergency patients. NPJ Digit Med 2022; 5(1): 104.
[http://dx.doi.org/10.1038/s41746-022-00649-y] [PMID: 35882903]

[86] Kline A, Wang H, Li Y, *et al.* Multimodal machine learning in precision health: A scoping review. NPJ Digit Med 2022; 5(1): 171.
[http://dx.doi.org/10.1038/s41746-022-00712-8] [PMID: 36344814]

[87] Brown C, Nazeer R, Gibbs A, Le Page P, Mitchell ARJ. Breaking bias: the role of artificial intelligence in improving clinical decision-making. Cureus 2023; 15(3): e36415.
[http://dx.doi.org/10.7759/cureus.36415] [PMID: 37090406]

[88] Coppola F, Faggioni L, Gabelloni M, *et al.* Human, all too human? An all-around appraisal of the "artificial intelligence revolution" in medical imaging. Front Psychol 2021; 12: 710982.
[http://dx.doi.org/10.3389/fpsyg.2021.710982] [PMID: 34650476]

[89] Challen R, Denny J, Pitt M, Gompels L, Edwards T, Tsaneva-Atanasova K. Artificial intelligence, bias and clinical safety. BMJ Qual Saf 2019; 28(3): 231-7.
[http://dx.doi.org/10.1136/bmjqs-2018-008370] [PMID: 30636200]

[90] Miller DD. The medical AI insurgency: what physicians must know about data to practice with intelligent machines. NPJ Digit Med 2019; 2(1): 62.
[http://dx.doi.org/10.1038/s41746-019-0138-5] [PMID: 31388566]

[91] Sendak MP, Gao M, Brajer N, Balu S. Presenting machine learning model information to clinical end users with model facts labels. NPJ Digit Med 2020; 3(1): 41.
[http://dx.doi.org/10.1038/s41746-020-0253-3] [PMID: 32219182]

[92] Pesapane F, Volonté C, Codari M, Sardanelli F. Artificial intelligence as a medical device in radiology: ethical and regulatory issues in Europe and the United States. Insights Imaging 2018; 9(5): 745-53.
[http://dx.doi.org/10.1007/s13244-018-0645-y] [PMID: 30112675]

[93] Ribeiro MT, Singh S, Guestrin C. Why should I trust you?. Proceedings of the 22nd ACM SIGKDD International Conference on Knowledge Discovery and Data Mining 2016; 1135-44.

[94] Bakır R, Orak C, Yüksel A. Optimizing hydrogen evolution prediction: A unified approach using random forests, lightGBM, and Bagging Regressor ensemble model. Int J Hyd Ener. 2024 May 20; 67: 101-10.

[95] Covert I, Lundberg S, Lee SI. Explaining by removing: A unified framework for model explanation. J Mach Learn Res 2021; 22(209): 1-90.

[96] Molnar C, Casalicchio G, Bischl B. Interpretable machine learning–a brief history, state-of-the-art and challenges. In: Koprinska I, Kamp M, Appice A, *et al.*, Eds. ECML PKDD 2020 workshops. Communications in computer and information science, vol. 1323. Cham: Springer; 2020. p. 417-19.
[http://dx.doi.org/10.1007/978-3-030-65965-3_28]

[97] Arya V, Bellamy RKE, Chen PY, *et al.* One explanation does not fit all: A toolkit and taxonomy of AI explainability techniques. arXiv preprint arXiv:190903012 2019.

[98] Metta C, Guidotti R, Yin Y, Gallinari P, Rinzivillo S. Exemplars and counterexemplars explanations

for image classifiers, targeting skin lesion labeling. 2021 IEEE Symposium on Computers and Communications (ISCC) 2021; 1-7.
[http://dx.doi.org/10.1109/ISCC53001.2021.9631485]

[99]   Panigutti C, Guidotti R, Monreale A, Pedreschi D. Explaining multi-label black-box classifiers for health applications. Precision Health and Medicine: A Digital Revolution in Healthcare 2020; 97-110.
[http://dx.doi.org/10.1007/978-3-030-24409-5_9]

[100]   Panigutti C, Perotti A, Panisson A, Bajardi P, Pedreschi D. FairLens: Auditing black-box clinical decision support systems. Inf Process Manage 2021; 58(5): 102657.
[http://dx.doi.org/10.1016/j.ipm.2021.102657]

[101]   Barnett AJ, Schwartz FR, Tao C, *et al.* A case-based interpretable deep learning model for classification of mass lesions in digital mammography. Nat Mach Intell 2021; 3(12): 1061-70.
[http://dx.doi.org/10.1038/s42256-021-00423-x]

[102]   Choi E, Bahadori MT, Song L, Stewart WF, Sun J. GRAM: Graph-based attention model for healthcare representation learning. Proceedings of the 23rd ACM SIGKDD International Conference on Knowledge Discovery and Data Mining 2017; 787-95.
[http://dx.doi.org/10.1145/3097983.3098126]

[103]   Zhang M, King CR, Avidan M, Chen Y. Hierarchical attention propagation for healthcare representation learning. Proceedings of the 26th ACM SIGKDD International Conference on Knowledge Discovery & Data Mining 2020; 249-56.
[http://dx.doi.org/10.1145/3394486.3403067]

[104]   Signoroni A, Savardi M, Benini S, *et al.* BS-Net: Learning COVID-19 pneumonia severity on a large chest X-ray dataset. Med Image Anal 2021; 71: 102046.
[http://dx.doi.org/10.1016/j.media.2021.102046] [PMID: 33862337]

[105]   Marusich LR, Files BT, Bancilhon M, Rawal JC, Raglin A. Trust Calibration for Joint Human/AI Decision-Making in Dynamic and Uncertain Contexts. In: International Conference on Human-Computer Interaction. Cham: Springer Nature Switzerland 2025: pp. 106-120.
[http://dx.doi.org/10.1007/978-3-031-93412-4_6]

[106]   Wu Y, Dong Y, Mou Y, Kim KJ. How the Algorithmic Transparency of Search Engines Influences Health Anxiety: The Mediating Effects of Trust in Online Health Information Search. InProceedings of the 2025 CHI Conference on Human Factors in Computing Systems 2025 Apr 26 (pp. 1-10).

[107]   Levy A, Agrawal M, Satyanarayan A, Sontag D. Assessing the impact of automated suggestions on decision-making: Domain experts mediate model errors but take less initiative. Proceedings of the 2021 CHI Conference on Human Factors in Computing Systems 2021; 1-13.
[http://dx.doi.org/10.1145/3411764.3445522]

[108]   Harada Y, Katsukura S, Kawamura R, Shimizu T. Effects of a differential diagnosis list of artificial intelligence on differential diagnoses by physicians: An exploratory analysis of data from a randomized controlled study. Int J Environ Res Public Health 2021; 18(11): 5562.
[http://dx.doi.org/10.3390/ijerph18115562] [PMID: 34070958]

[109]   Lee JD, See KA. Trust in automation: designing for appropriate reliance. Hum Factors 2004; 46(1): 50-80.
[http://dx.doi.org/10.1518/hfes.46.1.50.30392] [PMID: 15151155]

[110]   Skitka LJ, Mosier KL, Burdick M. Does automation bias decision-making?. Int J Hum Comput Stud 1999; 51(5): 991-1006.
[http://dx.doi.org/10.1006/ijhc.1999.0252]

[111]   Dietvorst BJ, Bharti S. People reject algorithms in uncertain decision domains because they have diminishing sensitivity to forecasting error. Psychol Sci 2020; 31(10): 1302-14.
[http://dx.doi.org/10.1177/0956797620948841] [PMID: 32916083]

[112]   Logg JM, Minson JA, Moore DA. Algorithm appreciation: People prefer algorithmic to human

judgment. Organ Behav Hum Decis Process 2019; 151: 90-103.
[http://dx.doi.org/10.1016/j.obhdp.2018.12.005]

[113] Tsai CC, Kim JY, Chen Q, Rowell B, Yang XJ, Kontar R, Whitaker M, Lester C. Effect of artificial intelligence helpfulness and uncertainty on cognitive interactions with pharmacists: Randomized controlled trial. Journal of Medical Internet Research. 2025 Jan 31;27:e59946.

[114] Shinners L, Aggar C, Grace S, Smith S. Exploring healthcare professionals' understanding and experiences of artificial intelligence technology use in the delivery of healthcare: An integrative review. Health Informatics J 2020; 26(2): 1225-36.
[http://dx.doi.org/10.1177/1460458219874641] [PMID: 31566454]

[115] Neri E, Coppola F, Miele V, Bibbolino C, Grassi R. Artificial intelligence: Who is responsible for the diagnosis?. Radiol Med (Torino) 2020; 125(6): 517-21.
[http://dx.doi.org/10.1007/s11547-020-01135-9] [PMID: 32006241]

[116] Strohm L, Hehakaya C, Ranschaert ER, Boon WPC, Moors EHM. Implementation of artificial intelligence (AI) applications in radiology: hindering and facilitating factors. Eur Radiol 2020; 30(10): 5525-32.
[http://dx.doi.org/10.1007/s00330-020-06946-y] [PMID: 32458173]

[117] Kizilcec RF. How much information? Effects of transparency on trust in an algorithmic interface. Proceedings of the 2016 CHI Conference on Human Factors in Computing Systems 2016; 2390-5.
[http://dx.doi.org/10.1145/2858036.2858402]

[118] Bansal G, Wu T, Zhou J, *et al.* Does the whole exceed its parts? The effect of AI explanations on complementary team performance. Proceedings of the 2021 CHI Conference on Human Factors in Computing Systems 2021; 1-16.
[http://dx.doi.org/10.1145/3411764.3445717]

[119] Ehsan U, Riedl MO. Proceedings of HCI International 2020: 22nd International Conference On Human-Computer Interaction 2020; 449-66.

[120] Küper A, Krämer N. Psychological traits and appropriate reliance: Factors shaping trust in AI. International Journal of Human–Computer Interaction. 2025 Apr 3;41(7):4115-31.

[121] Hoff KA, Bashir M. Trust in Automation. Hum Factors 2015; 57(3): 407-34.
[http://dx.doi.org/10.1177/0018720814547570] [PMID: 25875432]

[122] Buçinca Z, Malaya MB, Gajos KZ. To trust or to think: cognitive forcing functions can reduce overreliance on AI in AI-assisted decision-making. Proc ACM Hum Comput Interact 2021; 5(CSCW1): 1-21.

[123] Ha JF, Longnecker N. Doctor-patient communication: a review. Ochsner J 2010; 10(1): 38-43.
[PMID: 21603354]

[124] Ward P. Trust and communication in a doctor-patient relationship: a literature review. Arch Med (Oviedo) 2018; 3(3): 36.

[125] Taddeo M, Floridi L. How AI can be a force for good. Science 2018; 361(6404): 751-2.
[http://dx.doi.org/10.1126/science.aat5991] [PMID: 30139858]

[126] Shortliffe EH, Sepúlveda MJ. Clinical decision support in the era of artificial intelligence. JAMA 2018; 320(21): 2199-200.
[http://dx.doi.org/10.1001/jama.2018.17163] [PMID: 30398550]

[127] Wong DA, Kumar A, Jatana S, Ghiselli G, Wong K. Neurologic impairment from ectopic bone in the lumbar canal: a potential complication of off-label PLIF/TLIF use of bone morphogenetic protein-2 (BMP-2). Spine J 2008; 8(6): 1011-8.
[http://dx.doi.org/10.1016/j.spinee.2007.06.014] [PMID: 18037352]

[128] Wilson-Nash C. Locked-in: the dangers of health service captivity and cessation for older adults and their carers during COVID-19. J Mark Manage 2022; 38(17-18): 1958-82.

[http://dx.doi.org/10.1080/0267257X.2022.2078861]

[129] Stylianou N, Buchan I, Dunn KW. A review of the international Burn Injury Database (iBID) for England and Wales: descriptive analysis of burn injuries 2003–2011. BMJ Open 2015; 5(2): e006184.
[http://dx.doi.org/10.1136/bmjopen-2014-006184] [PMID: 25724981]

[130] McAndrew S. Internal morality of medicine and physician autonomy. J Med Ethics 2019; 45(3): 198-203.
[http://dx.doi.org/10.1136/medethics-2018-105069] [PMID: 30665950]

[131] Emanuel EJ, Pearson SD. Physician autonomy and health care reform. JAMA 2012; 307(4): 367-8.
[http://dx.doi.org/10.1001/jama.2012.19] [PMID: 22274681]

[132] Grote T, Berens P. On the ethics of algorithmic decision-making in healthcare. J Med Ethics 2020; 46(3): 205-11.
[http://dx.doi.org/10.1136/medethics-2019-105586] [PMID: 31748206]

[133] Diprose WK, Buist N, Hua N, Thurier Q, Shand G, Robinson R. Physician understanding, explainability, and trust in a hypothetical machine learning risk calculator. J Am Med Inform Assoc 2020; 27(4): 592-600.
[http://dx.doi.org/10.1093/jamia/ocz229] [PMID: 32106285]

[134] Johann to Berens P, Molinier J, Molinier J. Formation and recognition of UV-induced DNA damage within genome complexity. Int J Mol Sci 2020; 21(18): 6689.
[http://dx.doi.org/10.3390/ijms21186689] [PMID: 32932704]

[135] Páez A. The pragmatic turn in explainable artificial intelligence (XAI). Minds Mach 2019; 29(3): 441-59.
[http://dx.doi.org/10.1007/s11023-019-09502-w]

[136] Arbelaez Ossa L, Starke G, Lorenzini G, Vogt JE, Shaw DM, Elger BS. Re-focusing explainability in medicine. Digit Health 2022; 8.
[http://dx.doi.org/10.1177/20552076221074488] [PMID: 35173981]

[137] Salwei ME, Carayon P. A sociotechnical systems framework for the application of artificial intelligence in health care delivery. J Cogn Eng Decis Mak 2022; 16(4): 194-206.
[http://dx.doi.org/10.1177/15553434221097357] [PMID: 36704421]

[138] Birch J, Creel KA, Jha AK, Plutynski A. Clinical decisions using AI must consider patient values. Nat Med 2022; 28(2): 229-32.
[http://dx.doi.org/10.1038/s41591-021-01624-y] [PMID: 35102337]

[139] Pappas H, Frisch P. The Rise of the Intelligent Health System. Boca Raton, FL: CRC Press 2024.
[http://dx.doi.org/10.4324/9781032690315]

[140] Krittanawong C. The rise of artificial intelligence and the uncertain future for physicians. Eur J Intern Med 2018; 48: e13-4.
[http://dx.doi.org/10.1016/j.ejim.2017.06.017] [PMID: 28651747]

[141] Liu X, Keane PA, Denniston AK. Time to regenerate: the doctor in the age of artificial intelligence. J R Soc Med 2018; 111(4): 113-6.
[http://dx.doi.org/10.1177/0141076818762648] [PMID: 29648509]

[142] Floridi L, Cowls J, Beltrametti M, *et al.* AI4People—an ethical framework for a good AI society: opportunities, risks, principles, and recommendations. Minds Mach 2018; 28(4): 689-707.
[http://dx.doi.org/10.1007/s11023-018-9482-5] [PMID: 30930541]

[143] Rajpurkar P, Park A, Irvin J, *et al.* AppendiXNet: deep learning for diagnosis of appendicitis from a small dataset of CT exams using video pretraining. Sci Rep 2020; 10(1): 3958.
[http://dx.doi.org/10.1038/s41598-020-61055-6] [PMID: 32127625]

[144] Bebbington E, Miles J, Young A. Exploring the similarities and differences of burn registers globally: Results from a data dictionary comparison study. Burns. 2024 May;50(4):850-65.

[145] Liu M. Progress in documenting the complexities of citation practice: a review of citation studies. J Doc 1993; 49(4): 370-408.
[http://dx.doi.org/10.1108/eb026920]

[146] Li J, Ye J, Luo Y, Xu T, Jia Z. Progress in the application of machine learning in CT diagnosis of acute appendicitis. Abdom Radiol (NY). 2025 Sep;50(9): 4040-4049.

[147] Patel BN, Rosenberg L, Willcox G, *et al.* Human–machine partnership with artificial intelligence for chest radiograph diagnosis. NPJ Digit Med 2019; 2(1): 111.
[http://dx.doi.org/10.1038/s41746-019-0189-7] [PMID: 31754637]

[148] Farzaneh N, Ansari S, Lee E, Ward KR, Sjoding MW. 21 Optimizing AI-physician collaboration for enhanced diagnostic accuracy: A case study on acute respiratory distress syndrome detection using chest X-ray imaging. J Clin Trans Sci 2025; 9(s1): 7-8.
[http://dx.doi.org/10.1017/cts.2024.712]

[149] Nilashi M, Baabdullah AM, Abumalloh RA, Ooi KB, Tan GW, Giannakis M, Dwivedi YK. How can big data and predictive analytics impact the performance and competitive advantage of the food waste and recycling industry?. Anna Oper Res 2025; 348(3): 1649-90.
[http://dx.doi.org/10.1007/s10479-023-05272-y]

[150] Lorenzini G, Shaw DM, Arbelaez Ossa L, Elger BS. Machine learning applications in healthcare and the role of informed consent: Ethical and practical considerations. Clin Ethics 2023; 18(4): 451-6.
[http://dx.doi.org/10.1177/14777509221094476]

[151] McDougall J. The calculation of the terms of the optical spectrum of an atom with one series electron. Proc R Soc Lond A Math Phys Sci 1932; 138(836): 550-79.

[152] Onifade M, Adebisi JA, Zvarivadza T. Recent advances in blockchain technology: Prospects, applications and constraints in the minerals industry. Int J of Min, Reclam Envir. 2024 Aug 8;38(7):497-533.

[153] Sharma A, Malviya R, Awasthi R, Sharma PK. Artificial intelligence, blockchain, and internet of medical things: New technologies in detecting, preventing, and controlling of emergent diseases. In: Advances in Multidisciplinary Medical Technologies— Engineering, Modeling and Findings: Proceedings of the ICHSMT 2019. Cham: Springer International Publishing 2020; pp. 127-154.
[http://dx.doi.org/10.1007/978-3-030-57552-6_10]

[154] Ghosh A, Ahmed F, Ferdous MJ, *et al.* Strain-induced changes in the electronic, optical and mechanical properties of the inorganic cubic halide perovskite Sr3PBr3 with FP-DFT. J Phy Chem Solids 2024; 191: 112053.
[http://dx.doi.org/10.1016/j.jpcs.2024.112053]

[155] Liu M. Progress in documentation the complexities of citation practice: a review of citation studies. J Doc 1993; 49(4): 370-408.
[http://dx.doi.org/10.1108/eb026920]

[156] Osman Andersen T, Nunes F, Wilcox L, Kaziunas E, Matthiesen S, Magrabi F. Realizing AI in healthcare: challenges appearing in the wild. Extended Abstracts of the 2021 CHI Conference on Human Factors in Computing Systems 2021; 1-5.
[http://dx.doi.org/10.1145/3411763.3441347]

[157] Vorobeva D, El Fassi Y, Costa Pinto D, Hildebrand D, Herter MM, Mattila AS. Thinking skills don't protect service workers from replacement by artificial intelligence. J Serv Res 2022; 25(4): 601-13.
[http://dx.doi.org/10.1177/10946705221104312]

[158] Park SY, Kuo PY, Barbarin A, Kaziunas E, Chow A, Singh K, *et al.* Identifying challenges and opportunities in human-AI collaboration in healthcare. Companion Publication of the 2019 Conference on Computer Supported Cooperative Work and Social Computing 2019; 506-10.
[http://dx.doi.org/10.1145/3311957.3359433]

[159] Kuniavsky M, Churchill E, Steenson MW. Designing the user experience of machine learning

systems. AAAI spring symposium Proceedings (technical report SS-17-04) 2017; 27-9.

[160] Burgess ER, Jankovic I, Austin M, Cai N, Kapuścińska A, Currie S, *et al.* Healthcare AI treatment decision support: design principles to enhance clinician adoption and trust. Proc 2023 CHI Conf Hum Factors Comput Syst 2023; 1-19.
[http://dx.doi.org/10.1145/3544548.3581251]

[161] Abdul A, Vermeulen J, Wang D, Lim BY, Kankanhalli M. Trends and trajectories for explainable, accountable and intelligible systems: an HCI research agenda. Proc 2018 CHI Conf Hum Factors Comput Syst 2018; 1-18.
[http://dx.doi.org/10.1145/3173574.3174156]

[162] Tun HM, Rahman HA, Naing L, Malik OA. Trust in Artificial Intelligence–Based Clinical Decision Support Systems Among Health Care Workers: Systematic Review. Journal of Medical Internet Research. 2025 Jul 29;27:e69678.

[163] Cai CJ, Winter S, Steiner D, Wilcox L, Terry M. "Hello AI": uncovering the onboarding needs of medical practitioners for human-AI collaborative decision-making. Proc ACM Hum Comput Interact 2019; 3(CSCW): 1-24. [CSCW].
[http://dx.doi.org/10.1145/3359206]

[164] Vereschak O, Bailly G, Caramiaux B. How to evaluate trust in AI-assisted decision making? A survey of empirical methodologies. Proc ACM Hum-Comput Interact 2021; 5(CSCW2)

[165] Cai CJ, Winter S, Steiner D, Wilcox L, Terry M. Onboarding materials as cross-functional boundary objects for developing AI assistants. Extended Abstracts of the 2021 CHI Conference on Human Factors in Computing Systems 2021.
[http://dx.doi.org/10.1145/3411763.3443435]

[166] Wang D, Wang L, Zhang Z, Wang D, Zhu H, Gao Y, *et al.* Brilliant AI Doctor. Proc 2021 CHI Conf Hum Factors Comput Syst 2021.

[167] Evans RS. Electronic health records: then, now, and in the future. Yearb Med Inform 2016; 25(S 01) (Suppl. 1): S48-61.
[http://dx.doi.org/10.15265/IYS-2016-s006] [PMID: 27199197]

[168] Veinot TC, Zheng K, Lowery JC, Souden M, Keith R. Using electronic health record systems in diabetes care: emerging practices. Proc 1st ACM Int Health Inform Symp 2010; 240-9.
[http://dx.doi.org/10.1145/1882992.1883026]

[169] Berry ABL, Lim C, Hartzler AL, *et al.* Creating conditions for patients' values to emerge in clinical conversations: perspectives of healthcare team members. Proc 2017 Conf Designing Interact Syst 2017; 1165-74.
[http://dx.doi.org/10.1145/3064663.3064669]

[170] Berry ABL, Lim C, Hirsch T, *et al.* Getting traction when overwhelmed: implications for supporting patient-provider communication. Companion of the 2017 ACM Conf Comput Support Coop Work Soc Comput 2017; 143-6.
[http://dx.doi.org/10.1145/3022198.3026328]

[171] Burgess ER, Kaziunas E, Jacobs M. Care frictions: a critical reframing of patient noncompliance in health technology design. Proc ACM Hum-Comput Interact 2022; 6(CSCW2): 1-31.
[http://dx.doi.org/10.1145/3555172]

[172] Lim C, Berry ABL, Hirsch T, Hartzler AL, Wagner EH, Ludman E, *et al.* It just seems outside my health. Proceedings of the 2016 ACM Conference on Designing Interactive Systems 2016; 1172-84.
[http://dx.doi.org/10.1145/2901790.2901866]

[173] Mamykina L, Mynatt E, Davidson P, Greenblatt D. MAHI: investigation of social scaffolding for reflective thinking in diabetes management. Proceedings of the SIGCHI Conference on Human Factors in Computing Systems 2008; 477-86.
[http://dx.doi.org/10.1145/1357054.1357131]

[174] Porter J, Boyd C, Skandari MR, Laiteerapong N. Revisiting the Time Needed to Provide Adult Primary Care. J Gen Intern Med 2023; 38(1): 147-55.
[http://dx.doi.org/10.1007/s11606-022-07707-x] [PMID: 35776372]

[175] Ouajdouni A, Chafik K, Allioui S, Jbene M. Patient satisfaction with the mawiidi hospital appointment scheduling application: insights from the information systems success model and technology acceptance model in a moroccan healthcare setting. big data and cognitive computing. 2024 Dec 3; 8(12): 180.

[176] Eslami S, Mazaheri Habibi MR, Abadi FM, Tabesh H, Vakili-Arki H, Abu-Hanna A. Evaluation of patient satisfaction of the status of appointment scheduling systems in outpatient clinics: Identifying patients' needs. J Adv Pharm Technol Res 2018; 9(2): 51-5.
[http://dx.doi.org/10.4103/japtr.JAPTR_134_18] [PMID: 30131937]

[177] Montori VM, Gafni A, Charles C. A shared treatment decision-making approach between patients with chronic conditions and their clinicians: the case of diabetes. Health Expect 2006; 9(1): 25-36.
[http://dx.doi.org/10.1111/j.1369-7625.2006.00359.x] [PMID: 16436159]

[178] Kizzier-Carnahan V, Artis KA, Mohan V, Gold JA. Frequency of Passive EHR Alerts in the ICU: Another Form of Alert Fatigue?. J Patient Saf 2019; 15(3): 246-50.
[http://dx.doi.org/10.1097/PTS.0000000000000270] [PMID: 27331600]

[179] Osheroff JA, Teich JM, Middleton B, Steen EB, Wright A, Detmer DE. A roadmap for national action on clinical decision support. J Am Med Inform Assoc 2007; 14(2): 141-5.
[http://dx.doi.org/10.1197/jamia.M2334] [PMID: 17213487]

[180] Bell CM, Jalali A, Mensah E. A decision support tool for using an ICD-10 anatomographer to address admission coding inaccuracies: A commentary. Online J Public Health Inform 2013; 5(2): 222.
[http://dx.doi.org/10.5210/ojphi.v5i2.4813] [PMID: 23923104]

[181] Nanji KC, Seger DL, Slight SP, et al. Medication-related clinical decision support alert overrides in inpatients. J Am Med Inform Assoc 2018; 25(5): 476-81.
[http://dx.doi.org/10.1093/jamia/ocx115] [PMID: 29092059]

[182] Osheroff JA, Teich J, Levick D, et al. Improving outcomes with clinical decision support: An implementer's guide. 2nd ed. Chicago (IL): HIMSS Publishing 2012.
[http://dx.doi.org/10.4324/9780367806125]

[183] Jankovic I, Chen JH. Clinical Decision Support and Implications for the Clinician Burnout Crisis. Yearb Med Inform 2020; 29(1): 145-54.
[http://dx.doi.org/10.1055/s-0040-1701986] [PMID: 32823308]

[184] Garg AX, Adhikari NKJ, McDonald H, et al. Effects of computerized clinical decision support systems on practitioner performance and patient outcomes: a systematic review. JAMA 2005; 293(10): 1223-38.
[http://dx.doi.org/10.1001/jama.293.10.1223] [PMID: 15755945]

[185] Magrabi F, Ammenwerth E, McNair JB, et al. Artificial Intelligence in Clinical Decision Support: Challenges for Evaluating AI and Practical Implications. Yearb Med Inform 2019; 28(1): 128-34.
[http://dx.doi.org/10.1055/s-0039-1677903] [PMID: 31022752]

[186] Shortliffe EH, Davis R, Axline SG, Buchanan BG, Green CC, Cohen SN. Computer-based consultations in clinical therapeutics: Explanation and rule acquisition capabilities of the MYCIN system. Comput Biomed Res 1975; 8(4): 303-20.
[http://dx.doi.org/10.1016/0010-4809(75)90009-9] [PMID: 1157471]

[187] Durán JM, Jongsma KR. Who is afraid of black box algorithms? On the epistemological and ethical basis of trust in medical AI. J Med Ethics 2021; 47(5): medethics-2020-106820.
[http://dx.doi.org/10.1136/medethics-2020-106820] [PMID: 33737318]

CHAPTER 3

Robotics in Surgical and Medical Procedures

Swati Verma[1,*]**, Sarvesh Paliwal**[1]**, Swapnil Sharma**[1]**, Shivangi Bhardwaj**[1] **and Priyanka Dubey**[1]

[1] *Department of Pharmacy, Banasthali Vidyapith, Vanasthali, Rajasthan-304022, India*

Abstract: Recent advancements in artificial intelligence and robotics have transformed mechanized surgical techniques. Robotic technology improves surgical precision, consistency, and agility. Robots use computed tomography and magnetic resonance imaging in image-guided procedures to guide instruments to the treatment area. This necessitates the development of novel algorithms, user interfaces, and sensors to register the patient's anatomy with preoperative image data and to develop the procedure. The use of remotely controlled robotics in minimally invasive surgery enables surgeons to access internal organs and tissues without the need for extensive incisions. Sensing technology and specialized mechanical designs are necessary to optimize dexterity in the face of these constraints. Currently, a variety of surgical procedures employ robots. In the field of neurosurgery, image-guided machines are capable of performing biopsies on brain lesions with minimal collateral damage. Orthopaedic surgeons frequently employ robotics to shape the femur, ensuring it is in ideal alignment with a prosthesis during a hip joint replacement procedure. Although the initial clinical outcomes are promising, numerous unresolved questions remain, including physician acceptability, excessive capital expenditures, performance validation, and safety concerns. This chapter discusses how robotics can be utilized to enhance the accuracy and speed of surgery by enabling AI systems to make informed decisions and implement real-time adjustments across multiple procedures. Medical research has undergone significant enhancements as a result of robotics, and this chapter examines the evaluation of the relevance of robotics.

Keywords: AI, Healthcare, Robotics, Surgeons, Surgical assistants, Tele-surgery, Transition in surgery.

INTRODUCTION

Surgical procedures and other medical therapies have evolved in conjunction with the expansion of global scientific knowledge. In recent years, technological advancements and the introduction of new surgical techniques have dramatically altered numerous aspects of surgical procedures [1]. The intricate integration of

---

* **Corresponding author Swati Verma:** Department of Pharmacy, Banasthali Vidyapith, Vanasthali, Rajasthan-304022, India; E-mail: verma22swati@gmail.com

Shaweta Sharma, Akhil Sharma, Shivkanya Fuloria & Anurag Singh (Eds.)
All rights reserved-© 2025 Bentham Science Publishers

data with physical activity provided by robotic systems has resulted in a significant cultural shift. Some of the numerous applications include industrial production, quality control and inspection, laboratory automation, exploration, field service, rescue operations, surveillance, healthcare, and medicine. In recent decades, people have utilized robots to automate or enhance specific tasks, such as installing test devices or electrical circuits. Nevertheless, their most substantial economic impact often results from their role as essential intermediaries for integrating computers into comprehensive manufacturing or service operations [2].

Soon, robot hardware and computer-integrated surgical systems might make it possible to create medical treatments that are less invasive, more precise, and more focused. Robotic technology can perform surgical procedures with a reduced risk of complications, less blood loss, and quicker recovery periods for patients [3]. By connecting data sources, such as medical images, to operations performed in the operating room, robotic technology has the potential to improve the efficiency of clinical processes. Thanks to advancements in imaging and other sensor data that transcend human motion control, robots may soon be capable of performing surgical procedures that are physically impossible for humans to complete. Medical robots could significantly enhance the field of interventional medicine by simplifying the use of various components within larger computer-based systems. These systems can aid in diagnosis, pre-surgical planning, precautionary measures during and after surgery, hospital logistics and scheduling, as well as long-term monitoring and quality control. Modern surgical procedures have undergone significant transformations as a result of the integration of robotics. The surgical process has become more straightforward as technology has advanced and new instruments have been developed, leading to numerous enhancements in surgical techniques. Neurosurgery and other medical disciplines have made significant strides in recent years, largely due to the advancement of image-guided surgery [4].

The utilization of surgical robotics in hospitals and universities has experienced substantial expansion. Surgical robotics has evolved into a multibillion-dollar industry over the past two decades. Today, thousands of surgical operations worldwide utilize robots deployed in over 1,000 locations. The initial recorded robotic surgical treatment was the catalyst for the development, expansion, and widespread adoption of surgical robotics [5].

Some individuals may perceive robotic systems and surgical robots as "smart" surgical instruments that assist human surgeons in providing more effective, safer, and minimally invasive treatments to individual patients. Additionally, the information infrastructure and consistency of medical robots and computer-integrated surgery in health care are as critical as CIMS is to industrial production (Fig. **1**) [6]. The orthopedic surgery subspecialty has advanced significantly due to the introduction of new technologies and research. The orthopedic industry has experienced significant benefits as a result of the development of CRIGOS, or miniature robotics for image-guided orthopedic surgery. This technology has inspired a significant number of individuals to undergo foot surgery. Robotics was initially implemented in the field of orthopedics; however, they have since infiltrated other medical disciplines. Robots have revolutionized neurosurgery, in addition to benefiting ocular surgery. Scientific advancements have enabled the attainment of new levels of precision and proficiency in medical research, thereby significantly enhancing patient satisfaction [7].

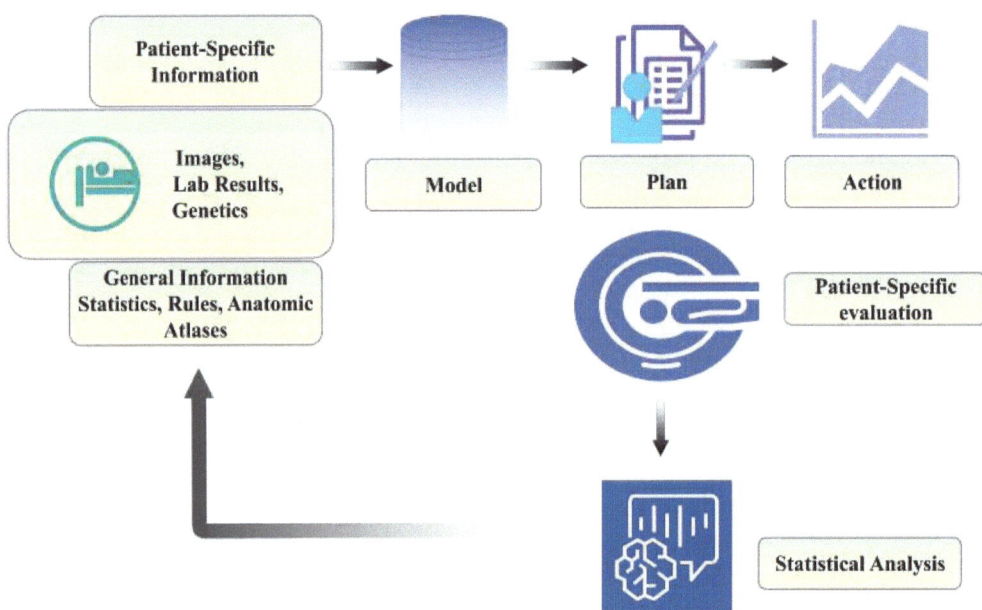

Fig. (1). Work-flow of computer-integrated surgery.

Before robots can realize their full potential in interventional medicine and surgery, significant advancements in hardware design, software, and clinical integration are required. The hardware side is perpetually engaged in the process of reducing the size, enhancing safety, and ensuring that robotic devices comply with imaging standards. The development of control and planning algorithms that consider tissue deformations, uncertainty in sensing and motion, and other factors is a focus of extensive software research in Artificial Intelligence (AI) for robotic surgical instruments. The translation of these innovations into clinical practice is contingent upon the development of user-friendly visual and tactile interfaces for physicians. Microscale interventions and noninvasive tissue access through natural orifices are two examples of novel therapies that robotics researchers are currently developing [8].

The primary objective of this chapter is to comprehend the connections between more general concepts such as computers, interface technology, and systems, as well as rehabilitative, assistive, and surgical robotics. Current and future research may allow surgical robots to achieve semi-autonomy while still granting physicians complete control over the procedures. The majority of surgical robotics currently in use aims to enhance a physician's capabilities [9].

CLASSIFICATION OF ROBOTICS

Following the worldwide standard ISO 8373:2012, the International Federation of Robotics (IFR) classifies robotics as industrial or service. Factories often view industrial robots as multi-purpose manipulators, capable of automatic programming and control, which can move along a predetermined path or autonomously. Service robots resemble driving mechanisms, capable of performing useful tasks, yet they are not suitable for factory automation. To meet the specific requirements of different industries, the IDR has classified service robots into many subcategories [10].

Surgical Robotics

Surgeons are required to make more decisions, have a broader field of vision, and be more flexible in doing minimally invasive surgery and proper intervention. This led to the development of surgical robots. In addition to providing high-definition images of the surgery site with an advanced 3D imaging system and augmented reality technology, it can also display vital anatomical features, such as the locations of blood vessels and nerves, in real-time. As a result, surgeons can utilize robots to aid them in performing precise treatments. By carefully planning their operations, advanced autonomous medical robots can utilize navigation and image-guiding technology to perform precise surgical procedures. Table **1** shows the differences between robot-assisted and traditional surgery [11].

Additionally, compared to a free hand, the robotic arm provides greater stability and precision. It can now do small, delicate treatments with fewer human errors due to fatigue, tremors, and a lack of competence. The surgical robot also features AI technology, enabling it to perform autonomous diagnostic analysis, adapt surgical techniques, and utilize deep learning to create personalized surgical plans [12, 13]. To enhance their sensing and image-directing capabilities, surgical robots may utilize technologies such as vision, speech recognition, telecommunications, 3D imaging, and artificial intelligence. This increases the reliability and accuracy of surgical operations by overcoming the constraints of manual techniques. Researchers hypothesize that robotic-assisted surgery could potentially decrease pain, recuperation time, and trauma in comparison to conventional surgery [14].

Table 1. Surgical robot-assisted surgery v/s conventional surgery.

	Robot-assisted surgery	**Conventional Surgery**
Advantages	Motion on a scale A high degree of geometric precision Infection and radiation resistance are both present Maintaining a steady and unflagging pace Capable of being sterilized The ability to control using a variety of sensors	Simple haptic skills Sound reasoning Adaptable and versatile Able to include a wide range of data Capable of using qualitative data More skilled Excellent precision of hand and eye Simple to train and evaluate
Limitations	Incapable of using qualitative data Refrain from passing judgment Expensive Additional research is required Rapidly evolving technology Lack of feeling	Easily infected and vulnerable to radiation Strictly limited geometric precision Strictly limited geometric precision Poor sterility

Additionally, it operates continuously without fatigue, reduces the workload of medical personnel, minimizes the occupational exposure of surgeons, and enables remote surgery [15]. The commercialization stage of medical robots has been progressively passed, and they are already being deployed in clinical settings (Table **2**). Thanks to its exceptional hand-eye coordination, magnification, and precision, the da Vinci system has become the most famous surgical robot. Surgeons can do minimally invasive procedures on a wide range of complicated problems [16, 17].

Table 2. Representative examples of commercially available surgical robotics.

Company	**Name of Robotics**	**Application field**	**References**
Computer Motion Inc.	Aesop	Laparoscopy	[18]
Intuitive Surgical Inc.	Da Vinci	Laparoscopy	[19]
Renishaw	NeuroMate	Neurosurgery	[20]
Computer Motion Inc.	Zeus	Laparoscopy	[21, 22]
Curexo Technology	ROBODOC	Orthopedics	[23]
Stryker	Acrobat	Orthopedics	[24]
Hansen Medical	Sensei	Vascular surgery	[25]

(Table 2) cont.....

Company	Name of Robotics	Application field	References
Endocontrol Medical	Viky	Laparoscopy	[26]
Mazor Robotics	Spine Assist	Spine surgery	[27]
Medrobotics	Flex	Endoluminal; surgery	[28]
Smith & Nephew	BlueBelt Navio	Orthopedics	[29]
Stryker	Mako	Orthopedics	[30]

As a distinct anatomical structure, the mouth has its own set of challenges during dental treatment, including limited visibility, a small operating space, and the potential disturbance of saliva and the tongue. Consequently, dental procedures are intricate and rely significantly on the surgeon's ability and knowledge, which may be difficult for inexperienced surgeons to acquire. Doctors are beginning to explore the viability of using the da Vinci robotic system for craniofacial surgery, following its successful application in laparoscopic surgery. Fixing cleft palates, treating Obstructive Sleep Apnea-Hypopnea Syndrome (OSAHS), and removing tumors from the mouth and throat are some of the procedures that the Da Vinci robot can perform [31, 32]. The oropharyngeal anatomy is complex, and the da Vinci system's many robotic arms limit the surgeon's field of view, making the procedure less effective. Oropharyngeal surgery may now utilize FDA-licensed flexible robots, such as The Flex, following the lifting of a prior ban. Orthognathic and dental implant surgeries, as well as those involving the skull and facial bones, are not possible with the da Vinci system. There has been a consistent increase in the number of studies examining the use of robotics in dental implant surgery since its inception in 2001. It is possible to use dental implant robots to place zygomatic implants alongside more conventional implant surgeries [33, 34].

Medical Robotics

Los Angeles Hospital in the US used the Puma 200 robot to inject needles during a Computed Tomography (CT)-guided brain biopsy in 1985, marking the beginning of the era of medical robot applications. Surgical, nursing, and rehabilitation are just a few of the many fields that have made substantial use of medical robots, which have been steadily improving for over 40 years and offering a wide range of remarkable advantages [35, 36].

Yang [6 - 8, 37] classified medical robot autonomy into six levels: zero autonomy (level 0), no autonomy, robot assistance, task autonomy, conditional autonomy, high autonomy, and total autonomy. Level 0 robots, such as the da Vinci system (Intuitive Inc., California, USA), operate entirely under human supervision. These humans are responsible for all aspects of the robot's operation, including observation, decision-making, and generating performance alternatives. While the robot provides direction based on positional constraints at level 1, humans are required to lead it at level 2 [38]. Orthopedic surgery makes use of Mako Smart Robotics, for instance. At the second level, the robot can follow operator instructions and preprogrammed procedures to perform certain tasks autonomously, but humans still need to guide it occasionally. At this tier, we have robots like the ROBODOC, which can replace both the hip and the knee. Level 3 autonomy allows robots to follow predetermined protocols throughout operations and to dynamically adjust their schedules in response to changes in the intraoperative position of the target item. One example of such robotics is the CyberKnife radiation therapy robot, which can monitor breathing. The robot becomes more than simply a medical device with higher degrees of autonomy, especially at levels 5 and possibly even 4, when it can practice medicine, something that is currently off-limits due to ethical, legal, and regulatory concerns [39].

Robots that provide surgical procedures, rehabilitation, nursing, medical transportation, patient consultations, and other services by integrating traditional medical diagnostic methods with cutting-edge technology like AI and big data are known as medical robotics, according to the International Federation of Robotics (IFR). Based on their intended use, medical robots may be classified into five distinct types: surgical, rehabilitative, diagnostic, laboratory analysis automation, and other [40].

Diagnostic Robotics

To improve diagnostic precision, convenience, non-invasiveness, and safety, diagnostic robots aid physicians in doing tests and making diagnoses. For instance, Given Imaging (now Medtronic) developed wireless capsule endoscopy, which enables less intrusive examinations of the gastrointestinal tract. A medically feasible alternative to classic interventional endoscopy is the usage of pill cams, which allow patients to capture photos deep within the intestines, revolutionizing gastrointestinal endoscopy. In addition, wearable robots are quickly becoming an integral part of medical diagnostics by monitoring a wide range of health indicators non-invasively.

Rehabilitation Robotics

Surgical robots are the most well-known area of medical robotics research and development, but rehabilitation robotics is rapidly gaining ground. Therapeutic robots and assistive robotics are the two main types of rehabilitation robots. Patients may get physical or mental treatment from therapeutic robots to help them improve certain skills. Physical therapy, functional rehabilitation of disabled patients, and behavioral induction to improve social skills in autistic youngsters are common uses for them [40]. By restoring or augmenting movement and function, assistive robots aim to improve the lives of people with musculoskeletal or neuromuscular impairments [20, 41, 42]. For instance, Handy1, developed by Mike Topping, assists the severely disabled with several everyday activities [43]. A similar device, ReWalk, developed in Israel, assists individuals with spinal cord injuries in walking, turning, climbing, and descending stairs by utilizing motorized hip and knee movement [44]. HAL is a powered prosthesis developed in Japan. It lets users control their joint movements by combining bioelectrical impulses measured on the skin surface with pressure sensors in the feet [45].

FACTORS AFFECTING THE ACCEPTANCE OF MEDICAL ROBOTS

Research in the field of medical robotics is, at heart, focused on practical applications. Despite the high level of innovation that goes into medical robotic systems and the potential for groundbreaking technical advancements, the public must see tangible benefits from these devices before they will embrace and use them. These advantages may vary in importance to different groups, be difficult to measure at times, and require a considerable amount of time to assess, which only exacerbates the situation [46, 47].

The advantages of medical robots are substantial. For instance, by combining human and robotic expertise, medical robots have the potential to significantly enhance surgeons' technical capabilities in implementing therapies. One can program a medical robot to surpass a human in accuracy and geometric precision. Due to their exceptional dexterity, they can perform minimally invasive therapies within the patient's body, even in potentially hazardous radioactive environments. These traits not only make previously impossible surgeries feasible but also enhance the ability of a routine surgeon to perform procedures typically reserved for the most highly trained surgeons [48].

Another comparable capability is that medical robots can enhance surgical safety (Table 3). The surgeon achieves this through both their enhanced technical performance and active assists, such as virtual fixtures or no-fly zones, which prevent surgical instruments from accidentally damaging delicate structures. Integrating medical robots into the CIS system's information architecture may also provide surgeons with online decision support and enhanced monitoring, both of which could increase safety [49].

Table 3. A comparison of safety and limitations supplied by robots versus humans.

	Strengths	Limitations
Robots	Ionizing radiation will not affect them capable of integrating data from a variety of sources, including numerical and sensor data Excellent precision in geometrical terms Consistent and unflappable Has the capability of being built to function at a wide variety of motion and payload scales	The haptic sense is limited Inadequate judgment Having trouble with hand-eye coordination A restricted capacity to integrate and analyze information that is quite complicated Decreased manual skill A challenge to adjust to new circumstances
Humans	Able to integrate and act on multiple information sources Excellent judgment Easily trained Excellent hand-eye coordination Versatile and able to improvise	Because of the tremor, the fine motion control is limited It is impossible to see through tissue A restricted degree of geometric correctness Extremely prone to exhaustion and interaction Radiation and infection may affect Bulky end-effectors Hand dexterity and limited manipulation capabilities beyond the normal scale

By gathering detailed information online, CIS systems and medical robots design surgeries to be more consistent. Accuracy is crucial when it comes to quality, whether it's in the positioning of components in joint reconstructions or the spacing and tensioning of sutures. The information recorded and regularly reviewed by a medical robot's light data recorder can be used for statistical studies of multiple cases to improve surgical planning, assess the morbidity and mortality caused by major surgical mishaps, and for other similar purposes. In addition to serving as a database for developing systems to evaluate and certify surgeons' skills, such data may also be valuable input for surgical simulators [50 - 52].

THE DESIGN AND INSTALLATION OF ROBOTIC MEDICAL SYSTEMS

Interface technology bridges the virtual reality of computer models with the actual reality of the patient, operating room, and surgical staff. In contrast, computer-based modeling and analysis of images, patient anatomy, and surgical plans facilitate the coupling of these components in a modular and robust manner, ensuring safe and predictable performance. These three areas constitute the research that supports these systems [53].

Modeling and Analysis

Computational modeling and analysis will play an increasingly important role in the advancement of medical robots. A large and diverse group of researchers is actively involved, covering a wide range of topics and methods. Finding computationally efficient methods to construct models of individuals and groups of patients from various data sources and then use these models to aid in real-world tasks is the main challenge [54]. Simulating not only the tasks themselves but also the performance environment of these tasks, such as a house, a clinic, a critical care unit, or an operating room, presents an associated challenge [55]. Medical image segmentation and fusion are used to build and maintain anatomical models unique to each patient, which is a common theme. The field encompasses the characterization of treatment plans and individual task steps, such as suturing and needle insertion, the registration of images and computational models to patient reality, optimization methods for treatment planning and system control, and biomechanical modeling for surgical planning, control, and rehabilitation [56].

There is no way to separate or undermine the usefulness of these concepts. A notable example is the close relationship between registration methods and modern medical image segmentation algorithms. Medical robots have always relied heavily on statistical methods, and this reliance is only increasing. A few examples are: Initially, we employed these methods to "deformably" align atlases with specific patient images, thereby creating "most likely" patient models based on the available data [57]. These models include historical data on potential treatment methods, biomechanical models, and anticipated outcomes, all without requiring any effort on your part. After that, statistical "atlases" will be made to examine the variation in anatomy across large populations. Because they are naturally organized, these atlases are ideal for collecting a wide range of information, including medical conditions, the outcomes of biochemical models, surgical procedures, and their effects [58]. Furthermore, by integrating data from treatment plans and procedure execution, important aspects that affect outcome and safety can be identified. Following that, Statistical atlases can be used to create more accurate biopsy plans for each patient, convert 2D x-ray images into 3D models of bones, and examine the variations in different hip replacement procedures. Another example is the statistical modeling of the prostate cancer location using histology specimens [36].

While patient-specific models for rehabilitation planning have been underutilized so far, there is considerable promise in using similar atlas-based techniques that incorporate biomechanical simulations.

Interface Technology

For robotic systems to function effectively, there must be seamless connections between the digital and physical realms. To that end, robotics has traditionally drawn from a broad variety of academic fields and fields of study. The primary goal in the challenging and limited field of medical robotics is to enhance robots' capabilities in sensing, mobility, and adapting to human environments.

Specialized Mechanism Design

Commonly adjusted for safety and cleanliness, early medical robots (*e.g.*, [36, 59 - 62]) used ordinary industrial manipulators. Despite its many advantages, this method remains a frequent choice in labs and for rapid prototyping; however, it requires specific considerations regarding workspace, dexterity, compactness, and working conditions for surgical and rehabilitative applications. This has led to a rise in the popularity of personalized layouts. Procedures like percutaneous needle insertion and laparoscopic surgery often involve passing or handling tools around a shared entry point into the patient's body. As a result, two primary layouts have seen widespread use. One uses a passive wrist to allow the tool to rotate around its insertion point; the Aesop and Zeus robots utilize this [62, 63]. Several organizations have adopted the second method, which requires the surgical tool to rotate around a distant center of motion (RCM) (distal to the robot's structure).

Another concern is the increasing miniaturization and scarcity of the areas within the patient's body that need high levels of dexterity. Conventional wisdom suggests that cable-actuated wrists are the most effective solution. Nevertheless, several teams have explored bending structural components, shape-memory alloys, micro-hydraulics, and other methods to overcome the challenges of scaling these designs to extremely small dimensions. For epicardial or endoluminal applications, many organizations have developed semi-autonomous moving robots (*e.g.*, [64 - 67]) in response to the difficulty of accessing surgical sites within the body. To address the demand for assistive or rehabilitative robots that respect human biomechanics and physical limitations, researchers have developed specialized designs [68, 69].

Teleoperation and hands-on control

Teleoperated surgical robots are commonly incorporated into medical practices. Two key drawbacks of these robots, which necessitate significant changes to the surgical process, are the removal of the surgeon from the operating table and the requirement for supplementary equipment, such as a master control station. In their early experiences with ROBODOC and other surgical robots [70, 71]. Surgeons discovered a form of hands-on (admittance control) that allowed the robot to move in reaction to forces applied directly to the surgical end-effector. Since then, other institutions have adopted this concept for precise surgical tasks; two notable examples are the Imperial College Acrobot orthopaedic system [72] and the Johns Hopkins University Steady Hand microsurgical robot [73]. By eliminating physiological tremors and enhancing the surgeon's inherent kinesthetic sense and eye-hand coordination, these devices provide extremely high rigidity and accuracy. Other teams have developed entirely manual instruments that can identify and actively counteract physiological tremors. Some groups have developed semiactive or passive techniques to aid surgeons with the use of tools or human body parts [74 - 76].

Human–Machine Cooperative Systems

The ability to move an instrument freely and deftly is a common goal of both teleoperation and hands-on control; however, the fact that a computer controls the robot's mobility opens up numerous new possibilities. The most basic kind is a no-fly zone or safety barrier that blocks the robot's tool from reaching certain parts of the work area. More recent versions have included virtual springs, dampers, or complex kinematic constraints to assist surgeons in tasks such as tool alignment and force maintenance. The Acrobat system is an effective clinical application of this concept, commonly referred to as virtual fixtures [77 - 80]. In active cooperative control, the surgeon and robot switch roles at various points during a surgical procedure, as research from several groups has shown [81 - 83]. These modes will play an increasingly important role in surgical assistant applications as computers' ability to model and monitor surgical processes continues to improve.

Assistance systems for individuals with disabilities and those undergoing rehabilitation also utilize teleoperation and hands-on control. When it comes to rehabilitation and helping people with mobility issues, limited hands-on devices are lifesavers. We anticipate that teleoperation, cognitive task following, and control will drive future advancements in assistive technology for individuals with significant physical disabilities.

Augmented Reality Interfaces

When a surgical procedure starts, the surgeon focuses on the patient's anatomy. Surgeons used to rely on their innate hand-eye coordination when operating, either by looking directly at the patient or, more recently, by watching endoscopic videos. In the past, a light box in the operating room displayed additional information, such as medical imaging data. The computer's ability to record and display photos, models, and other task-specific data might greatly enhance the surgeon's ability to integrate and utilize all this information. Consequently, much of the research and development efforts have gone into creating AR data displays and adding interactive capabilities to surgical assistant devices, such as laser pointers. Similar interfaces, also used in rehabilitation systems, may guide a patient's movements during exercise.

Systems Science

Computing, sensors, mechanics, and human-machine interfaces are just a few of the interrelated subsystems that comprise medical robots. Therefore, they share the same essential needs for top-notch engineering and system design, such as modularity and clearly defined interfaces. However, certain requirements arise due to their use in therapeutic settings or direct human interaction. Of these, maintaining the safety standards proves to be of utmost importance. Even if several valid approaches to robot safety exist across various contexts, some universal ideas prevail; among these, redundancy is paramount, given that no medical robot should ever lose control or put a patient at risk due to a single point of failure [84, 85]. The second, and often more important, idea is that the virtual workspace must be a replica of the physical one. This is of the utmost importance for robotic systems that operate on images taken before surgery. It is possible to significantly reduce the likelihood of the robot escaping or performing unwanted actions with careful planning and implementation. However, until the patient's physical, virtual, and robotic coordinate systems are all in sync, it won't be of much benefit. Ensuring a well-designed and executed process is equally important. Not all surgical robots are human. Surgeons must use these surgical tools correctly. Therefore, the surgeon must have a thorough understanding of the robot's strengths and weaknesses. Keep in mind that surgical robots have the potential to increase patient safety in many cases. One potential benefit of using a robot is the increased control it offers over process variables (such as accuracy and force) that govern the final product. Furthermore, unlike human operators, robots seldom exhibit brief lapses in attention. Thirdly, virtual limits may be programmed into a robotic system such that the surgical tool cannot access a restricted region unless the surgeon deliberately bypasses the restriction. Thorough testing and validation, in addition to meticulous design, are necessary to achieve these advantages [85].

Concerns voiced by regulatory bodies regarding the safety of medical robotics include the need for extensive documentation and rigorous procedures throughout the development, testing, and maintenance of these devices. Surgical robots present unique challenges in terms of sterility and biocompatibility, which may restrict material choices and other design aspects. Different parts of the system are important for real-world applications, especially for developers and researchers. Integration test beds play a pivotal role, which is the most important one. Without access to all the necessary components to run comprehensive trials, it is very difficult to design medical systems, especially those that need image guidance.

ROBOTIC TECHNIQUES FOR SURGERY

The use of robots is on the rise due to several current developments in surgery. The widespread availability of 3D imaging data and the increasing emphasis on minimally invasive surgical methods are key factors to consider. Other robotic properties, such as stability and the ability to operate on microscopic scales, motivate the development of new robotic applications.

Image-Based Procedures

Robotic surgery has become increasingly popular due to advancements in non-invasive imaging techniques, such as Computed Tomography (CT) and magnetic resonance imaging, as well as 2D approaches like ultrasonography, fluoroscopy, and standard X-ray radiography. These pictures may help pinpoint exactly where diseases are located, which will enable the creation of computer and mechanical methods that can target treatments specifically at the disease while leaving healthy tissue unaffected. Biopsy and excision of brain tumors are frequent examples [86]. It is possible to locate the tumor within the skull with high precision using preoperative magnetic resonance imaging. Once the surgeon, whether human or robotic, opens the skull, they can use the imaging data to guide instruments directly to the tumor. Preoperative imaging carefully plans the instrument path, reducing the risk of collateral damage to brain tissue and avoiding important brain structures. Planning, registration, and navigation are the three primary concerns that must be addressed to execute this type of operation [87].

Planning

Before being sent to the surgeon in the right format, preoperative images must undergo processing to reveal the important structures. Some systems analyze imaging data using path-planning algorithms and then provide the surgeon with the results for validation [88, 89]. Segmenting image data into physiologically relevant parts is a common first step in the planning process. There is considerable interest in automated segmentation. However, current systems enable the physician to perform this procedure cognitively. One of the methods being studied currently is statistical categorization. Other physiological techniques include modeling developmental trends to predict organ shape and matching anatomical atlases with imaging data [90 - 92]. Finding the exact position and borders of a brain tumor and then segmenting it from the rest of the brain is no easy task. To avoid removing good tissue while leaving behind cancer, precise segmentation is essential.

After the imaging data has been analyzed, the surgeon receives it to evaluate the patient's anatomy and arrange the procedure. The user interface for brain tumor surgery must allow users to select the incision site and instrument path, as well as interactively display 3D imaging data on a 2D computer screen. Computer algorithms create a perfect treatment plan and send it to the doctor for approval for certain procedures, including hip replacement surgery [93 - 95]. Due to the necessity of planning strategies that account for the specific characteristics of the organs involved and the treatment procedure, various approaches to the computational and user interface components have emerged.

Registration

The imaging data has to be registered with the patient's anatomy to implement this preoperative plan during the operation [46]. Registration establishes a relationship between points on the operating table and points in the patient's preoperative imaging data. Two primary methods have been established for this purpose: systems based on fiducials and systems based on shapes. The appropriate anatomical structure is marked with fiducials or markers before imaging. By analyzing the image data, the robot's control computer can ascertain the location of the disease in the fiducials. While the surgeon operates, a sensor gadget transmits the precise location of the marks to a laptop. A variety of sensing technologies may be used to determine the fiducial location. One straightforward method involves a probe attached to the robot manipulator. Upon making contact with a fiducial, the probe immediately detects the location of the object in the robot's coordinate space. By creating comprehensive spatial transitions with multiple fiducials, it is possible to transition seamlessly from the preoperative image to the patient. Surgical procedures make use of several sensing techniques [96]. Among these, optical trackers are among the most common. Equipped with light-emitting diodes or reflecting targets, a probe is monitored from specified locations by a succession of cameras or optical sensors. After that, the location of each target in the robot's coordinate frame can be determined *via* triangulation, allowing for submillimeter resolutions to be readily achievable.

Electromagnetic transceivers, articulated probe arms, laser and ultrasonic rangefinders, and other similar devices are also used for sensing. Commercial image-guided treatment systems use a lot of these tracking approaches. The attachment of the markers before imaging could be a major surgical procedure, which is a potential drawback of fiducial-based registration. As an example, the ROBODOC system utilizes fiducials, which are pins inserted into the proximal and distal ends of the femur, during hip replacement surgery. This not only makes the robotic therapy more expensive and time-consuming, but it also causes the patient excruciating pain. As an alternative, form-based registration may match the shape of anatomical characteristics acquired from intraoperative measurements to preoperative imaging data, thereby removing these problems. It is possible to collect patient measurements using a variety of sensing techniques, such as evaluating video footage, scanning the surface with a laser range finder, or drawing curves on the required anatomical structure using an optical tracker probe. The final product is a patient-specific description of the structure's shape [96].

Following this, a computational approach identifies the spatial transformation that minimizes the disparity between the preoperatively perceived shape and the shape extracted from the imaging data collected during the operation. The registration problem may be expressed in several ways. Using readily accessible 2D ultrasound or X-ray photographs as a sensing tool during surgery is one approach that may be beneficial. Following this, the 3D preoperative imaging data is used to match the produced anatomical "slices" or projections. Making adjustments for patient movement or tissue deformation during surgery is a major challenge in registration. This is of the utmost importance in neurosurgery since it prevents post-cranial hematoma swelling. Some have proposed biomechanical models that include the edema process or deformable template matching as a way to overcome this obstacle. To keep track of patients' whereabouts in real-time, some monitoring methods utilize video images [96]. It has also become clear that research into checking the accuracy of registration methods is crucial. Registration has recently garnered significant academic attention because it is crucial for establishing fundamental accuracy limits. It is therefore necessary in all areas of image-guided therapy.

Navigation

After registration, either a human or a robot surgeon may use the preoperative plan and imaging data for navigation or guidance. To control the instrument's motion in a fixed coordinate frame, a robotic manipulator uses its kinematic model in conjunction with sensors in its joints. Thanks to the patient and imaging data recorded with this frame, the control computer can link the motions of the instruments to the patient's anatomy and preoperative plan. As they use handheld instruments, human surgeons get instructions. The surgeon can precisely reach the affected area because of sensors that track the instruments' movements and computer-generated motion commands [97]. Whether to use robotic or manual navigation depends on several factors, including cost, implementation challenges, clinical acceptance, and safety concerns. Both systems utilize sensors and computers to modify quantitative image data in ways that people can't. In the future, more manual operations will be able to be performed robotically thanks to further improvements in robotic technology that are expected to decrease development and system costs while enhancing accuracy.

Minimally Invasive Procedures

Minimally invasive surgery, often referred to as minimally invasive surgery, has revolutionized several branches of surgery over the last decade [98]. Laparoscopic cholecystectomy, also known as gallbladder excision, is a common surgery that almost always employs minimally invasive surgical methods. The surgeon makes three or five incisions, each about 1 cm long. The surgeon uses a video laparoscope to view the internal working region and long-handled instruments to grab and cut tissue within the body. Because this procedure does not involve cutting a huge hole in the abdominal wall, patients can recuperate more quickly than with conventional open surgery [99]. Reduced convalescence and hospitalization costs, improved cosmesis, less time lost from work, and much less discomfort are all advantages. Arthroscopic knee repair and thoracoscopic lung resection are only two of many additional minimally invasive procedures that have shown comparable results. Handheld instruments can only perform a limited number of surgeries, and working *via* a few fixed incisions greatly restricts the dexterity of manipulation. The incision acts as a fulcrum, preventing the instrument shaft from moving laterally. The surgeon's hand movements at the instrument tip invert as a result, and the mechanical advantage shifts as the instruments enter and exit the body. Because the endoscope and the monitor are in different orientations, it is difficult to mentally switch between visual and motor coordinate frames, which is especially problematic when the video display is on the opposite side of the patient [100].

The use of robotic manipulators might provide solutions to some of these problems. Creating gadgets that require a tremendous amount of manual dexterity and intuitive control, and can be implanted through very small holes, is the challenge. Developing versatile systems that can perform a range of general procedures, such as thoracic and gynecological surgeries, is one objective [101 - 103]. Different approaches are now being developed to address specific access methods, such as transurethral prostate removal and percutaneous needle puncture. Other systems operate at microscopic scales and utilize robots to perform stable and repetitive tasks, such as endoscope pointing and organ retraction.

Interaction Modes

There are many methods by which surgeons may interact with robots. A crucial criterion is the robot's level of autonomy. In a few procedures, the robot follows a preoperative plan without direct human intervention. It would be very difficult for a human surgeon to accurately follow the complex or repetitive optimal pathways suggested in procedures such as radiosurgery and hip joint replacement due to their inherent complexity [36, 66]. The surgeon meticulously plans and executes the procedure, closely monitoring the team to ensure adherence to safety protocols.

An interactive or assisted procedure occurs when a surgeon and a robot collaborate, such as a robotic instrument cutting bone during knee replacement procedures [32, 79]. During the surgical procedure, a low-impedance robot manipulator attaches a cutting tool to reshape the bone, allowing it to fit the prosthetic joint. While the surgeon is working, the robot monitors their movements, allowing them to freely move within the designated cutting zone while applying pressure to areas where bone removal is not necessary. This allows the surgeon to oversee and control the robot with the same level of intuition and experience as a person while simultaneously implementing "active limitations" to enhance the accuracy and safety of the cutting process. Since the surgeon remains in charge throughout the procedure, this approach has the potential to enhance the acceptance of robotic systems among both surgeons and patients. In the face of changing workloads, most robots are designed with high stiffness to ensure geometric accuracy at the tip; however, innovative manipulator designs may be necessary for assistive control applications. Due to this, developing a sensor and control method that enables the robot to mimic the surgeon's hand movements without introducing undue strain or significant delays is a formidable challenge. On the other hand, surgeons often exercise open control over the minimally invasive surgical robot systems mentioned earlier, which represent the other extreme of the autonomy continuum. The surgeon creates all motion commands using sensory data gathered from the surgical site, often in the form of video footage or still photographs. Even though the surgeon is typically present in the operating room with the surgical robot, the term teleoperation is used to describe this control mode because the master manipulator is physically separate from the robot [67]. Scientists are hopeful that this innovation may allow surgeons to treat patients remotely [31, 62].

REVIEW OF SURGICAL ROBOTIC SYSTEMS

Neurosurgery

By inserting a needle or probe into a precisely bored hole in the skull, one can detect brain tumors and other abnormalities. This method is minimally invasive for treating brain lesions, involving the removal of only a small section of brain tissue under imaging supervision. The exact manipulation of the needle to reach the tumor region is of the utmost importance during these biopsy operations, which require the expert use of small instruments. Moving brain tissue during surgery is another significant challenge, which is why microsurgery or image-guided robot-assisted technologies are crucial. This serves as the blueprint for the fundamental structure of stereotactic brain biopsy. The needle can be positioned and moved along three spatial axes: x and y for precise placement on the biopsy arena and z for achieving the correct depth. Medical robotics began with the use of the Unimate Puma 560, an industrial robot, for stereotactic brain surgery. The surgeon guides the robot to the damaged area. To get straight-line access to the tumor, the surgeon burrs a hole in the skull after the correction and inserts a biopsy probe [104]. Other industrial robots, such as Minerva (University of Lausanne, Lausanne, Switzerland) and NeuroMate (Integrated Surgical Systems, Sacramento, CA), also played a role in the early days of neurosurgery. The FDA approved the sale of NeuroMate, the first neurosurgery robot. It used an arm and an image guidance system to perform surgeries.

The University of Lausanne's Minerva used a real-time 3D CT scanner to pinpoint the surgical area, even in cases where the brain or skull had undergone changes in shape. Prosurgics in the UK (formerly Armstrong Healthcare) developed the 6-DoF PathFinder, a brand-new neurorobotic device currently available in Europe. It is configured to detect fiducial markers autonomously and can align its instrument holder to the desired trajectory with an accuracy of 1 mm or better [105]. CT and MRI imaging technology has improved over the years, making it possible to make computer-based stereotactic frameworks that are more accurate and easier to use [106]. Chan *et al.* presented a neurosurgical robotic system prototype, named NISSTM, in 2009 [107. 108]. The NISSTM outperforms two FDA-authorized commercial robotics systems, PathfinderTM and NeuroMateTM, in terms of both speed and operational appropriateness. The latest commercially available neurorobotic technology, Cyberknife (Accuray, Inc., Sunnyvale, CA), offers a less invasive alternative to traditional open surgery for lesions that would otherwise be unreachable. Its components include a computer-controlled robotic manipulator with six degrees of freedom and an X-ray image-guiding system [109]. CyberKnife serves not only in neurosurgery but also in pediatric, prostate, pancreatic, renal, and lung surgeries.

Gynaecologic Surgery

The four main subspecialties of gynecologic surgery are reproductive surgery, reconstructive pelvic surgery, general gynecology, and gynecologic oncology. The therapies all make use of various non-surgical methods. Three main types of robotic systems are used: laparoscopic holders, robotic integrated surgical systems, and immersive telerobotic surgical systems. Gynecology was the first to use a laparoscopic surgical holder and its ancillary equipment. Computer Motion

Inc. of Goleta, CA, developed the AESOP laparoscopic holder, an active voice-controlled device, as the first robotic technology in gynecology. During surgery, this device enables surgeons to adjust the laparoscope and camera attachment for enhanced visibility. Computer Motion Inc. of Goleta, USA, developed the first AESOP laparoscopic camera holder. With FDA approval, it finds widespread use in surgical systems [110]. Remote robot-assisted surgery is the main application of the Zeus and da Vinci robotic systems. The FDA has approved both systems for use in various minimally invasive surgeries [111].

In 1998, six female pigs underwent microsurgical uterine horn anastomoses, marking the first application of the Zeus approach in gynecologic oncology [22]. With its precise motor movements, 3D vision, and motion scaling, the robotic system aided microsurgery. After that, eleven people who had undergone tubal ligation had laparoscopic tubal suturing [112]. Tubal reanastomosis was done with the Zeus surgical system. Other fields that extensively utilize the da Vinci surgical system include gynecology and telesurgery [113]. The first gynaecology feasibility study examined eight patients [114]. This study demonstrated that a remote 3D vision robotic system can perform laparoscopic microsurgical tubal reanastomosis. The automation of operating processes may speed up operations compared to open microsurgical techniques.

Orthopaedic Surgery

Some of the surgical treatments that may benefit from the use of robots include osteotomy, tendon or ligament restoration, spine surgery, and total joint or knee replacement. Integrated Surgery Systems, Inc. of Canada developed the first commercially available orthopedic surgery robot, RoboDoc [115]. RoboDoc frequently functions in conjunction with OrthoDoc, a supplementary robotic device that serves as a preoperative planning station equipped with a CT scanner. This tool provides precise and efficient data to the surgical robot before an orthopedic procedure [116]. The patient's leg must be securely attached to the surgical framework to avoid any movement during the hip replacement treatment, both before and during the operation. After that, the surgeon uses a handheld interface to guide the robot to the correct spot and then controls it while it scrapes the femoral head. To make room for the femoral implant, the robotic end-effector spins a cutter. Early tests of RoboDoc revealed that operations took a long time and resulted in significant blood loss [117, 118]. Newer research suggests that these problems may have been resolved, along with improved implant placement and more precise production of femoral components. Another integrated robotic system developed by OrtoMaquet of Germany for knee surgery is CASPAR, which stands for Computer Assisted Surgical Planning and Robotics. A preoperative CT scan is necessary for the extraction and transfer of image data to the planning operations, much as with the robotic systems mentioned before. With the use of 3D CT-scan data that can be exported for use with the CASPAR system, Petermann *et al.* provided exact preoperative planning to ensure a flawless graft insertion location and placement [119].

Urologic Surgery

In urologic surgery, the organs are far more pliable than in orthopedic surgery, where the physician encounters more rigid structures. Robotics applications have garnered more attention from neurosurgeons and orthopedic surgeons compared to urologic specialists. It wasn't until early 1987 that Imperial College in London constructed the first urologic robot, or URobotics. The goal of the writers was to remove the prostate *via* the urethra. Johns Hopkins University's urology department utilized the LARS robot—a urologic robot—to facilitate renal access and biopsies, leveraging its integrated Remote Center of Motion (RCM). The development of mechatronics and robotic surgery has enabled the surgical completion of several urologic procedures, including nephrectomy, cystectomy, sacrocolpopexy, vasovasostomy, and laparoscopic prostatectomy [120, 122].

Ophthalmologic Surgery

The eye is a delicate and small organ. Thus, any surgical treatment requires precise positioning and the use of instruments. Robotically Assisted Microsurgery (RAMS) systems assist microsurgeons with delicate procedures, eliminate hand tremors, accurately position microsurgical instruments, and provide haptic feedback on the surgical field [123]. For use in eye surgeries, Hunter *et al.* developed a pioneering robotic system in ocular microsurgery [124]. The authors also created a digital environment that mimicked the anatomy, optics, and surgical procedures of the eye by using a continuum model and its related mechanics. Before performing the complex operation on a real patient, the operator might learn and practice it in this virtual environment [124]. Johns Hopkins University researchers Taylor *et al.* [72] developed "steady hand," an ophthalmologic surgical robot capable of micromanipulation. It was designed to help achieve these goals by functioning as both a robot-assisted system for eye surgery and a tool to assist microsurgical operators in performing force scaling and positioning procedures with reduced tremor.

Cardiac Surgery

Heart surgery has changed a lot when it comes to coronary artery disease, congenital disabilities, valvular disease (including surgeries on the mitral valve and arterial septal defect), transplants, assistive devices, cardiopulmonary surgeries, arrhythmia, and figuring out how to treat these conditions [125]. Once upon a time, Off-Pump Coronary Artery Bypass (OPCAB) *via* a sternotomy was the gold standard for valve surgery and coronary artery bypass grafting. Because the patient's chest is open during the procedure, this method is classified as open-chest surgery; hence, the recovery period is somewhat prolonged. Fewer stresses during surgery and smaller cuts mean less harm and faster recovery. For this reason, experts have suggested minimally invasive procedures such as angioplasty, endoscopic surgery, and laparoscopic surgery as alternatives [126 - 131]. Systems like AESOP, Zeus, and da Vinci are intelligent systems designed for telemanipulation. At the same time, surgeon-assistant tools like AESOP photograph the operating theatre and hold and position surgical instruments during surgery. Surgical robots often use the AESOP voice-controlled imaging arm in conjunction with Zeus-based systems. In fact, among various cardiac operations, the Zeus, AESOP, and da Vinci surgical systems were the most frequently used. In 1998, a team at Germany's Munich-Grosshadern University Hospitals used AESOP and the Zeus robotic microsurgical system to perform coronary bypass surgery by voice-controlling an endoscope [63]. A mitral valve surgery and coronary artery bypass grafting were being conducted, using the da Vinci system to facilitate minimally invasive cardiac surgery [132, 133]. Later, the Zeus and da Vinci surgical systems were used, among others, for more cardiac procedures [6, 134 - 136].

Gastrointestinal Surgery

A team using the 'Mona' (Intuitive Surgical) master-slave system performed the first telesurgical laparoscopic cholecystectomy at St. Blasius Hospital in March 1997 [97]. An obese patient had the first gastric banding procedure using this approach in September 1998 [137]. By 2001, three years later, 146 cases of robotic laparoscopic surgery had been documented, with 39 involving antireflux procedures, 48 involving cholecystectomies, and 10 involving obesity-related gastroplasties [138]. More dexterity, better ergonomics, more tooltip mobility, a reasonable operating time and hospital stay, and no system-related morbidity were among the benefits they found while using this laparoscopic robotic procedure. To implement computer-assisted Nissen fundoplication for gastroesophageal reflux, Cadiere *et al.* performed a series of robot-assisted laparoscopy procedures using the 'Mona' system in conjunction with conventional laparoscopy on a total of 21 patients [139]. According to the study, telesurgery was made possible by using a computer connection to connect the surgeon and patient. The telesurgical group had a lengthier procedure, but both groups had the same amount of morbidity and no deaths. While there will be an increase in operating time, Melvin *et al.* demonstrated that computer-assisted laparoscopic antireflux is safe after operating on 20 patients [140]. Some gastrointestinal operations that have been reported to benefit from robot-assisted procedures include gastric bypass, oesophagectomy, oesophageal leiomyoma, colorectal surgery, intragastric resection, distal gastrectomy, splenectomy, Heller myotomy, and oesophagectomy [141 - 145].

EVALUATION OF ROBOTIC SYSTEMS IN SURGERY

The medical business has grown in tandem with the advancements in research. Surgical methods have become more sustainable and efficient because of the development of robots, which has led to several advancements in medical research. Orthopedic treatment is now more reliable due to advancements in robotics and image-guided surgery. Patients have benefited from the therapeutic use of small robots for image-guided orthopedic surgery (CRIGOS) as their accuracy has increased. The CRIGOS modulation system, which includes a tiny parallel robot and a software system for operation planning, monitors the delicate parts. To ensure accuracy with the help of robots and technology, they must provide them with efficient instructions and guide them correctly [37, 146].

Surgical robots have enhanced not only the quality of surgical procedures but also the system design concept, which includes the definitions, functions, and interfaces of the many components. Medical research has reached new heights thanks to developments in human-computer interface design and methods for collecting calibrated X-rays [147]. Several areas of medical study have utilized robotics technology to assist surgeons with their precise technical skills, thereby improving understanding and efficiency. The robotics facility provides doctors with more specific data about the patient's needs, serving as a tool to help carry out planned and accurate surgical operations. Robotic technology helps with post-operative verification and situational status monitoring for patients [148].

There are several ways in which medical procedures have become more flexible as research has advanced. With the advent of Computer-Integrated Surgery (CIS), physicians can now achieve more accurate results during surgical procedures. Because it provides the surgeon with efficient assistance, computer-guided medical surgery increases the chances of success [149, 150]. Computer-integrated facilities enable the tailoring of surgical procedures to meet the unique demands of each patient, resulting in significant improvements, as they have a major impact on correctly planning the operation. The patient in the preoperative state benefits from modifications to the computer-integrated surgical services system. Because the CIS system, under the surgeon's supervision, assumes that role during the intraoperative stage, patients need extra care and attention at this time. Additionally, depending on the patient's needs, the CIS assists the surgeon and the patient during the post-operative period [151].

By adapting to each patient's needs, medical research has become more reliable because of these technological advancements [152]. Thanks to advancements in image-guided surgery, doctors are now better able to implement life-saving operations. Technology aids both patients and physicians during this type of surgery, thereby increasing the success rate of the process and necessitating effective support [153, 154]. Calibrated X-ray services, which have been recently used in the medical field, have improved results by providing accurate test results. The introduction of new technologies into the field of medical sciences has increased both the success rate of surgeries and the money generated by such procedures [155, 156].

The use of modern technology has also increased the effectiveness and efficiency of eye surgery. Technological advancements have enabled the conduct of precise eye examinations. Essential tests that require more nuanced attention are now easier to perform than in the past due to technological advancements that enhance the quality of patient examinations. Surgeons have benefited from modern technology, such as computerized equipment, in the vitally important fields of neurosurgery and ophthalmology. Working with the human skeleton requires precise and accurate orthopedic treatments. Patients have been more content as a result of the technological tools that have helped surgeons. The medical field has benefited from these technological advances; however, they are still fragile and require specific guidelines to function as intended [157 - 159].

LIMITATIONS AND CHALLENGES OF ROBOTIC SURGERY

Several factors limit the use of surgical robots. Particularly for minimally invasive procedures performed in confined spaces, the present mechanical architecture of manipulators limits dexterity. More efficient and compact actuator and transmission technologies, along with numerous opportunities for advancements in kinematic configurations, are on the horizon. When it comes to detecting and controlling, robots face many of the same challenges as humans, particularly in autonomous operation due to their computer-controlled nature. Robots can only follow instructions verbatim; they lack the cognitive capacity for abstract reasoning, cannot integrate data from many sources, and cannot make sound decisions. Despite the ability to preprocess complex 3D image data for precise tasks, robots are still unable to control their behavior by utilizing data from all sensors throughout a procedure. While faster processors can improve robot control, they also make these systems more complex and challenging to develop and debug.

The high cost of robotic surgery might prevent many hospitals from implementing such a program. The price tag includes everything from the robot itself to annual repairs, disposable surgical tools, operating room time, medication, hospitalization, and the cost of medical staff. The dVSS is too expensive for many medical schools, costing $1.2 million upfront and $100,000 per year in maintenance fees. Furthermore, Steinberg *et al.* estimate that teaching just one person to proficiency would require an additional $217,000.

The steep learning curve of the dVSS is even more problematic. The original running duration for RALRP was 360 minutes, as reported by Menon *et al.* We also know that on average, it takes 74 occasions to become competent. Residents have limited opportunities to train with the system due to increased patient expectations, medico-legal issues, and performance optimization constraints imposed by hospital administration. The lack of a clearly defined competency-based training program stands out even more, as it has been brought up repeatedly.

CONCLUSION

A major step forward in modern medicine is the automation of surgical procedures *via* the use of robots and artificial intelligence. These technologies have demonstrated precision, safety, and success in a wide range of surgeries, from simple to complex procedures. Surgeons may potentially enhance their skills by utilizing robotic tools and algorithms for machine learning. This improves patient outcomes while decreasing the number of mistakes and difficulties they experience.

Robotic surgery is quickly integrating a broad range of common medical procedures. Shortly after robotic surgery became standard practice in hospitals, a trend toward more reliance on the robotic platform emerged, which was associated with less reliance on preexisting minimally invasive techniques like laparoscopic surgery, this pattern persisted across many different types of surgeries, including those where robotic surgery offers no therapeutic benefit to the patient and conventional laparoscopic surgery is the current gold standard. The researchers' findings underscore the importance of continuously monitoring the expansion of robotic surgery to ensure that enthusiasm for new technology doesn't overshadow the evidence required for its use in the most favorable clinical scenarios.

Future developments in robotics and artificial intelligence will greatly influence the level of integration of these technologies into surgical procedures. To encourage more widespread usage, researchers may aim to enhance autonomous methods, make them more accessible, and remove legal constraints in the future. To properly harness the revolutionary power of new technology, we will need the combined efforts of multiple fields, including academia, medicine, engineering, and related disciplines.

REFERENCES

[1] Alterovitz R. Surgical Robotics [TC spotlight]. IEEE Robot Autom Mag 2009; 16(2): 16-7.
[http://dx.doi.org/10.1109/MRA.2009.932616]

[2] Lanfranco AR, Castellanos AE, Desai JP, Meyers WC. Robotic Surgery. Ann Surg 2004; 239(1): 14-21.
[http://dx.doi.org/10.1097/01.sla.0000103020.19595.7d] [PMID: 14685095]

[3] Rashid HH, Leung YYM, Rashid MJ, Oleyourryk G, Valvo JR, Eichel L. Robotic surgical education: A systematic approach to training urology residents to perform robotic-assisted laparoscopic radical prostatectomy. Urology 2006; 68(1): 75-9.
[http://dx.doi.org/10.1016/j.urology.2006.01.057] [PMID: 16844450]

[4] Murphy DG, Hall R, Tong R, Goel R, Costello AJ. Robotic technology in surgery: current status in 2008. ANZ J Surg 2008; 78(12): 1076-81.
[http://dx.doi.org/10.1111/j.1445-2197.2008.04754.x] [PMID: 19087046]

[5] Abboudi H, Khan MS, Aboumarzouk O, *et al.* Current status of validation for robotic surgery simulators – a systematic review. BJU Int 2013; 111(2): 194-205.
[http://dx.doi.org/10.1111/j.1464-410X.2012.11270.x] [PMID: 22672340]

[6] Mohr FW, Falk V, Diegeler A, *et al.* Computer-enhanced "robotic" cardiac surgery: Experience in 148 patients. J Thorac Cardiovasc Surg 2001; 121(5): 842-53.
[http://dx.doi.org/10.1067/mtc.2001.112625] [PMID: 11326227]

[7] Duchene DA, Moinzadeh A, Gill IS, Clayman RV, Winfield HN. Survey of residency training in laparoscopic and robotic surgery. J Urol 2006; 176(5): 2158-67.
[http://dx.doi.org/10.1016/j.juro.2006.07.035] [PMID: 17070283]

[8] Smith AL, Schneider KM, Berens PD. Survey of obstetrics and gynecology residents' training and opinions on robotic surgery. J Robot Surg 2010; 4(1): 23-7.
[http://dx.doi.org/10.1007/s11701-010-0176-0] [PMID: 27638568]

[9] Schreuder HWR, Wolswijk R, Zweemer RP, Schijven MP, Verheijen RHM. Training and learning robotic surgery, time for a more structured approach: a systematic review. BJOG 2012; 119(2): 137-49.
[http://dx.doi.org/10.1111/j.1471-0528.2011.03139.x] [PMID: 21981104]

[10] International Organization for Standardization. ISO 8373:2021, Robotics—Vocabulary [Internet]. Geneva: ISO. 2021. https://cdn.standards.iteh.ai/samples/75539/1bc8409322eb4922bf680e15901852d2/ISO-8373-2021.pdf

[11] Wang Y, Butner SE, Darzi A. The developing market for medical robotics. Proc IEEE 2006; 94(9): 1763-71.
[http://dx.doi.org/10.1109/JPROC.2006.880711]

[12] Liu Y, Xie R, Wang L, *et al.* Fully automatic AI segmentation of oral surgery-related tissues based on cone beam computed tomography images. Int J Oral Sci 2024; 16(1): 34.
[http://dx.doi.org/10.1038/s41368-024-00294-z] [PMID: 38719817]

[13] Alemzadeh K, Raabe D. Prototyping artificial jaws for the robotic dental testing simulator. Proc Inst Mech Eng H 2008; 222(8): 1209-20.
[http://dx.doi.org/10.1243/09544119JEIM402] [PMID: 19143415]

[14] Kazanzides P, Fichtinger G, Hager GD, Okamura AM, Whitcomb LL, Taylor RH. Surgical and interventional robotics - core concepts, technology, and design. IEEE Robot Autom Mag 2008; 15(2): 122-30.
[http://dx.doi.org/10.1109/MRA.2008.926390] [PMID: 20428333]

[15] Khan K, Dobbs T, Swan MC, Weinstein GS, Goodacre TEE. Trans-oral robotic cleft surgery (TORCS) for palate and posterior pharyngeal wall reconstruction: A feasibility study. J Plast Reconstr

Aesthet Surg 2016; 69(1): 97-100.
[http://dx.doi.org/10.1016/j.bjps.2015.08.020] [PMID: 26409954]

[16]   Nadjmi N. Transoral robotic cleft palate surgery. Cleft Palate Craniofac J 2016; 53(3): 326-31.
[http://dx.doi.org/10.1597/14-077] [PMID: 26120882]

[17]   Vicini C, Dallan I, Canzi P, Frassineti S, La Pietra MG, Montevecchi F. Transoral robotic tongue base
resection in obstructive sleep apnoea-hypopnoea syndrome: a preliminary report. ORL J
Otorhinolaryngol Relat Spec 2010; 72(1): 22-7.
[http://dx.doi.org/10.1159/000284352] [PMID: 20173358]

[18]   Ewing DR, Pigazzi A, Wang Y, Ballantyne GH. Robots in the operating room--the history. Semin
Laparosc Surg 2004; 11(2): 63-71.
[PMID: 15254644]

[19]   Maeso S, Reza M, Mayol JA, *et al.* Efficacy of the Da Vinci surgical system in abdominal surgery
compared with that of laparoscopy: a systematic review and meta-analysis. Ann Surg 2010; 252(2):
254-62.
[http://dx.doi.org/10.1097/SLA.0b013e3181e6239e] [PMID: 20622659]

[20]   Liu C, Liu Y, Xie R, Li Z, Bai S, Zhao Y. The evolution of robotics: research and application progress
of dental implant robotic systems. Int J Oral Sci 2024; 16(1): 28.
[http://dx.doi.org/10.1038/s41368-024-00296-x] [PMID: 38584185]

[21]   Leal Ghezzi T, Campos Corleta O. 30 years of robotic surgery. World J Surg 2016; 40(10): 2550-7.
[http://dx.doi.org/10.1007/s00268-016-3543-9] [PMID: 27177648]

[22]   Falcone T, Goldberg J, Garcia-Ruiz A, Margossian H, Stevens L. Full robotic assistance for
laparoscopic tubal anastomosis: a case report. J Laparoendosc Adv Surg Tech A 1999; 9(1): 107-13.
[http://dx.doi.org/10.1089/lap.1999.9.107] [PMID: 10194702]

[23]   Abdul-Muhsin H, Patel V. History of robotic surgery. In: Kim K, Ed. Robotics in General Surgery.
New York, NY: Springer 2014; pp. 3-8.
[http://dx.doi.org/10.1007/978-1-4614-8739-5_1]

[24]   Jakopec M, Rodriguez Baena F, Harris SJ, Gomes P, Cobb J, Davies BL. The hands-on orthopaedic
robot "acrobot": early clinical trials of total knee replacement surgery. IEEE Trans Robot Autom
2003; 19(5): 902-11.
[http://dx.doi.org/10.1109/TRA.2003.817510]

[25]   Reddy VY, Neuzil P, Malchano ZJ, *et al.* View-synchronized robotic image-guided therapy for atrial
fibrillation ablation: experimental validation and clinical feasibility. Circulation 2007; 115(21): 2705-
14.
[http://dx.doi.org/10.1161/CIRCULATIONAHA.106.677369] [PMID: 17502570]

[26]   Voros S, Haber GP, Menudet JF, Long JA, Cinquin P. ViKY robotic scope holder: initial clinical
experience and preliminary results using instrument tracking. IEEE/ASME Trans Mechatron 2010;
15(6): 879-6.
[http://dx.doi.org/10.1109/TMECH.2010.2080683]

[27]   Lieberman IH, Togawa D, Kayanja MM, *et al.* Bone-mounted miniature robotic guidance for pedicle
screw and translaminar facet screw placement: Part I--Technical development and a test case result.
Neurosurgery 2006; 59(3): 641-50.
[http://dx.doi.org/10.1227/01.NEU.0000229055.00829.5B] [PMID: 16955046]

[28]   Lang S, Mattheis S, Hasskamp P, *et al.* A european multicenter study evaluating the flex robotic
system in transoral robotic surgery. Laryngoscope 2017; 127(2): 391-5.
[http://dx.doi.org/10.1002/lary.26358] [PMID: 27783427]

[29]   Herry Y, Batailler C, Lording T, Servien E, Neyret P, Lustig S. Improved joint-line restitution in
unicompartmental knee arthroplasty using a robotic-assisted surgical technique. Int Orthop 2017;
41(11): 2265-71.

[http://dx.doi.org/10.1007/s00264-017-3633-9] [PMID: 28913557]

[30] Subramanian P, Wainwright TW, Bahadori S, Middleton RG. A review of the evolution of robotic-assisted total hip arthroplasty. Hip Int 2019; 29(3): 232-8.
[http://dx.doi.org/10.1177/1120700019828286] [PMID: 30963802]

[31] Weinstein GS, Quon H, Newman HJ, *et al.* Transoral robotic surgery alone for oropharyngeal cancer: an analysis of local control. Arch Otolaryngol Head Neck Surg 2012; 138(7): 628-34.
[http://dx.doi.org/10.1001/archoto.2012.1166] [PMID: 22801885]

[32] Kayhan FT, Kaya H, Yazici ZM. Transoral robotic surgery for tongue-base adenoid cystic carcinoma. J Oral Maxillofac Surg 2011; 69(11): 2904-8.
[http://dx.doi.org/10.1016/j.joms.2011.01.049] [PMID: 21549484]

[33] Olivetto M, Bettoni J, Testelin S, Lefranc M. Zygomatic implant placement using a robot-assisted flapless protocol: proof of concept. Int J Oral Maxillofac Surg 2023; 52(6): 710-5.
[http://dx.doi.org/10.1016/j.ijom.2022.12.002] [PMID: 36517307]

[34] Li C, Wang M, Deng H, *et al.* Autonomous robotic surgery for zygomatic implant placement and immediately loaded implant-supported full-arch prosthesis: a preliminary research. Int J Implant Dent 2023; 9(1): 12.
[http://dx.doi.org/10.1186/s40729-023-00474-2] [PMID: 37204483]

[35] Liu HH, Li LJ, Shi B, Xu CW, Luo E. Robotic surgical systems in maxillofacial surgery: a review. Int J Oral Sci 2017; 9(2): 63-73.
[http://dx.doi.org/10.1038/ijos.2017.24] [PMID: 28660906]

[36] Kwoh YS, Hou J, Jonckheere EA, Hayati S. A robot with improved absolute positioning accuracy for CT guided stereotactic brain surgery. IEEE Trans Biomed Eng 1988; 35(2): 153-60.
[http://dx.doi.org/10.1109/10.1354] [PMID: 3280462]

[37] Yang GZ, Cambias J, Cleary K, *et al.* Medical robotics—Regulatory, ethical, and legal considerations for increasing levels of autonomy. Sci Robot 2017; 2(4): eaam8638.
[http://dx.doi.org/10.1126/scirobotics.aam8638] [PMID: 33157870]

[38] Troccaz J, Dagnino G, Yang GZ. Frontiers of medical robotics: from concept to systems to clinical translation. Annu Rev Biomed Eng 2019; 21(1): 193-218.
[http://dx.doi.org/10.1146/annurev-bioeng-060418-052502] [PMID: 30822100]

[39] Dupont PE, Nelson BJ, Goldfarb M, *et al.* A decade retrospective of medical robotics research from 2010 to 2020. Sci Robot 2021; 6(60): eabi8017.
[http://dx.doi.org/10.1126/scirobotics.abi8017] [PMID: 34757801]

[40] Yip M, Salcudean S, Goldberg K, *et al.* Artificial intelligence meets medical robotics. Science 2023; 381(6654): 141-6.
[http://dx.doi.org/10.1126/science.adj3312] [PMID: 37440630]

[41] Winchester P, McColl R, Querry R, *et al.* Changes in supraspinal activation patterns following robotic locomotor therapy in motor-incomplete spinal cord injury. Neurorehabil Neural Repair 2005; 19(4): 313-24.
[http://dx.doi.org/10.1177/1545968305281515] [PMID: 16263963]

[42] Alashram AR, Annino G, Padua E. Robot-assisted gait training in individuals with spinal cord injury: A systematic review for the clinical effectiveness of Lokomat. J Clin Neurosci 2021; 91: 260-9.
[http://dx.doi.org/10.1016/j.jocn.2021.07.019] [PMID: 34373038]

[43] Topping M. An overview of the development of Handy 1, a rehabilitation robot to assist the severely disabled. Artif Life Robot 2000; 4(4): 188-92.
[http://dx.doi.org/10.1007/BF02481173]

[44] Ma Y, Wu X, Yi J, Wang C, Chen C. A review on human–exoskeleton coordination towards lower limb robotic exoskeleton systems. Int J Robot Autom 2019; 34(4): 431-51.
[http://dx.doi.org/10.2316/J.2019.206-0193]

[45] Ezaki S, Kadone H, Kubota S, *et al.* Analysis of gait motion changes by intervention using robot suit hybrid assistive limb (HAL) in myelopathy patients after decompression surgery for ossification of the posterior longitudinal ligament. Front Neurorobot 2021; 15: 650118.
[http://dx.doi.org/10.3389/fnbot.2021.650118] [PMID: 33867965]

[46] Taylor RH, Menciassi A, Fichtinger G, Dario P. Medical robotics and computer-integrated surgery. In: Siciliano B, Khatib O, Eds. Springer Handbook of Robotics. Berlin, Heidelberg: Springer 2008; pp. 1199-222.
[http://dx.doi.org/10.1007/978-3-540-30301-5_53]

[47] Dario P, Hannaford B, Menciassi A. Smart surgical tools and augmenting devices. IEEE Trans Robot Autom 2003; 19(5): 782-92.
[http://dx.doi.org/10.1109/TRA.2003.817071]

[48] Taylor RH, Lavelleé S, Burdea GC, Mösges R. Computer-integrated surgery. Technology and clinical applications. 1996. Clin Orthop Relat Res 1998; (354): 5-7.
[http://dx.doi.org/10.1097/00003086-199809000-00002] [PMID: 9755758]

[49] Kanade T, Davies B, Riviere CN. Special issue on medical robotics. Proc IEEE 2006; 94(9): 1649-51.
[http://dx.doi.org/10.1109/JPROC.2006.881292]

[50] Cleary K, Anderson J, Brazaitis M, *et al.* Final report of the technical requirements for image-guided spine procedures Workshop, Maryland, USA. Comput Aided Surg 2000; 5(3): 180-215.
[http://dx.doi.org/10.1002/1097-0150(2000)5:3<180::AID-IGS6>3.0.CO;2-C] [PMID: 10964090]

[51] Graham S, Taylor RH, Vannier M. Needs assessment for computer-integrated surgery systems. 2000; p. 931–9.
[http://dx.doi.org/10.1007/978-3-540-40899-4_96]

[52] Dupont PE, Simaan N, Choset H, Rucker C. Continuum robots for medical interventions. Proc IEEE Inst Electr Electron Eng 2022; 847-70.

[53] Shen D, Lao Z, Zeng J, Herskovits EH, Fichtinger G, Davatzikos C. Statistically optimized biopsy strategy for the diagnosis of prostate cancer. Proceedings 14th IEEE Symposium on Computer-Based Medical Systems CBMS 2001; 433-8.
[http://dx.doi.org/10.1109/CBMS.2001.941758]

[54] Dinggang Shen , Yiqiang Zhan , Davatzikos C. Segmentation of prostate boundaries from ultrasound images using statistical shape model. IEEE Trans Med Imaging 2003; 22(4): 539-51.
[http://dx.doi.org/10.1109/TMI.2003.809057] [PMID: 12774900]

[55] Tomazevic D, Likar B, Slivnik T, Pernus F. 3-D/2-D registration of CT and MR to X-ray images. IEEE Trans Med Imaging 2003; 22(11): 1407-16.
[http://dx.doi.org/10.1109/TMI.2003.819277] [PMID: 14606674]

[56] Sadowsky O, Ramamurthi K, Ellingsen LM, Chintalapani G, Prince JL, Taylor RH. Atlas-assisted tomography: Registration of a deformable atlas to compensate for limited-angle cone-beam trajectory. 3rd IEEE International Symposium on Biomedical Imaging: Macro to Nano 2006; 1244-7.
[http://dx.doi.org/10.1109/ISBI.2006.1625150]

[57] Blendea S, Eckman K, Jaramaz B, Levison TJ, DiGioia AM III. Measurements of acetabular cup position and pelvic spatial orientation after total hip arthroplasty using computed tomography/radiography matching. Comput Aided Surg 2005; 10(1): 37-43.
[http://dx.doi.org/10.3109/10929080500178032] [PMID: 16199380]

[58] Wan Z, Malik A, Jaramaz B, Chao L, Dorr LD. Imaging and navigation measurement of acetabular component position in THA. Clin Orthop Relat Res 2009; 467(1): 32-42.
[http://dx.doi.org/10.1007/s11999-008-0597-5] [PMID: 18979147]

[59] Drake JM, Joy M, Goldenberg A, Kreindler D. Computer- and robot-assisted resection of thalamic astrocytomas in children. Neurosurgery 1991; 29(1): 27-33.
[http://dx.doi.org/10.1227/00006123-199107000-00005] [PMID: 1870684]

[60]   Tombropoulos RZ, Adler JR, Latombe JC. CARABEAMER: a treatment planner for a robotic radiosurgical system with general kinematics. Med Image Anal 1999; 3(3): 237-64.
[http://dx.doi.org/10.1016/S1361-8415(99)80022-X] [PMID: 10710294]

[61]   Bernsmann K, Rosenthal A, Sati M, Ansari B, Wiese M. Anwendung eines CAS-Systems in der Arthroskopischen Kreuzbandchirurgie - Adaption und Applikation in der klinischen Praxis. Z Orthop Ihre Grenzgeb 2001; 139(4): 346-51.
[http://dx.doi.org/10.1055/s-2001-16922] [PMID: 11558054]

[62]   Nezhat C, Saberi NS, Shahmohamady B, Nezhat F. Robotic-assisted laparoscopy in gynecological surgery. JSLS 2006; 10(3): 317-20.
[PMID: 17212887]

[63]   Reichenspurner H, Damiano RJ, Mack M, *et al.* Use of the voice-controlled and computer-assisted surgical system zeus for endoscopic coronary artery bypass grafting. J Thorac Cardiovasc Surg 1999; 118(1): 11-6.
[http://dx.doi.org/10.1016/S0022-5223(99)70134-0] [PMID: 10384178]

[64]   Misra S, Ramesh KT, Okamura AM. Modeling of Tool-Tissue Interactions for Computer-Based Surgical Simulation: A Literature Review. Presence (Camb Mass) 2008; 17(5): 463-91.
[http://dx.doi.org/10.1162/pres.17.5.463] [PMID: 20119508]

[65]   Troccaz J, Grimson E, Mösges R, Eds. CVRMed-MRCAS'97. Proceedings of the First Joint Conference on Computer Vision, Virtual Reality and Robotics in Medicine and Medical Robotics and Computer-Assisted Surgery. Grenoble, France. Berlin, Heidelberg. Springer 1997.

[66]   Phee L, Menciassi A, Gorini S, Pernorio G, Arena A, Dario P. An innovative locomotion principle for minirobots moving in the gastrointestinal tract. Proceedings IEEE International Conference on Robotics and Automation (Cat No02CH37292) 2002; 1125-30.
[http://dx.doi.org/10.1109/ROBOT.2002.1014694]

[67]   Ota T, Patronik NA, Schwartzman D, Riviere CN, Zenati MA. Minimally invasive epicardial injections using a novel semiautonomous robotic device. Circulation 2008; 118 (Suppl.): S115-20.
[http://dx.doi.org/10.1161/CIRCULATIONAHA.107.756049] [PMID: 18824742]

[68]   Masia L, Krebs HI, Cappa P, Hogan N. Whole-Arm Rehabilitation Following Stroke: Hand Module. The First IEEE/RAS-EMBS International Conference on Biomedical Robotics and Biomechatronics 2006; 1085-9.
[http://dx.doi.org/10.1109/BIOROB.2006.1639236]

[69]   Chen CT, Lien WY, Chen CT, Wu YC. Implementation of an upper-limb exoskeleton robot driven by pneumatic muscle actuators for rehabilitation. Actuators 2020; 9(4): 106.
[http://dx.doi.org/10.3390/act9040106]

[70]   Morris B. Robotic surgery: applications, limitations, and impact on surgical education. MedGenMed 2005; 7(3): 72.
[PMID: 16369298]

[71]   Goradia TM, Taylor RH, Auer LM. Robot-assisted minimally invasive neurosurgical procedures: First experimental experience. In: Troccaz J, Grimson E, Mösges R, Eds. Proceedings of the 1st Joint Conference on Computer Vision, Virtual Reality and Robotics in Medicine and Medical Robotics and Computer-Assisted Surgery. Grenoble, France. Springer 1997; p. 319-22.

[72]   Taylor R, Jensen P, Whitcomb L, *et al.* A Steady-Hand Robotic System for Microsurgical Augmentation. Int J Robot Res 1999; 18(12): 1201-10.
[http://dx.doi.org/10.1177/02783649922067807]

[73]   Jakopec M, Harris SJ, Rodriguez y Baena F, Gomes P, Cobb J, Davies BL. The first clinical application of a "hands-on" robotic knee surgery system. Comput Aided Surg 2001; 6(6): 329-39.
[http://dx.doi.org/10.3109/10929080109146302] [PMID: 11954064]

[74]   Cadeddu JA, Stoianovici D, Kavoussi LR. Robotics in urologic surgery. Urology 1997; 49(4): 501-7.

[http://dx.doi.org/10.1016/S0090-4295(96)00561-4] [PMID: 9111617]

[75]　Davies BL, Hibberd RD, Ng WS, Timoney AG, Wickham JEA. The development of a surgeon robot for prostatectomies. Proc Inst Mech Eng H 1991; 205(1): 35-8.
[http://dx.doi.org/10.1243/PIME_PROC_1991_205_259_02] [PMID: 1670073]

[76]　Troccaz J, Peshkin M, Davies B. The use of localizers, robots, and synergistic devices in CAS. 1997.
[http://dx.doi.org/10.1007/BFb0029298]

[77]　Yang GZ, Mylonas GP, Kwok KW, Chung A. Perceptual docking for robotic control. In: Dohi T, Sakuma I, Liao H, Eds. Medical Imaging and Augmented Reality. Proceedings of MIAR 2008. Tokyo, Japan. Springer 2008; pp. 21-30.

[78]　Park S, Howe RD, Torchiana DF. Virtual fixtures for robotic cardiac surgery. In: Niessen WJ, Viergever MA, Eds. Medical Image Computing and Computer-Assisted Intervention – MICCAI 2001. Springer, Berlin, Heidelberg. 2001; pp. 1419-1420.
[http://dx.doi.org/10.1007/3-540-45468-3_252]

[79]　Li M, Okamura AM. Recognition of operator motions for real-time assistance using virtual fixtures. 11th Symposium on Haptic Interfaces for Virtual Environment and Teleoperator Systems 2003; 125-31.

[80]　Du G, Zhang P. A novel flexible virtual fixtures for teleoperation. ScientificWorldJournal 2014; 2014: 1-10.
[http://dx.doi.org/10.1155/2014/897242] [PMID: 24693252]

[81]　Li M, Taylor RH. Spatial motion constraints in a medical robot using virtual fixtures generated by anatomy. Proceedings of the 2004 IEEE International Conference on Robotics and Automation. New Orleans, LA. IEEE 2004; pp. 1270-75.

[82]　Knoll A, Mayer H, Staub C, Bauernschmitt R. Selective automation and skill transfer in medical robotics: a demonstration on surgical knot-tying. Int J Med Robot 2012; 8(4): 384-97.
[http://dx.doi.org/10.1002/rcs.1419] [PMID: 22605676]

[83]　Kragic D, Marayong P, Li M, Okamura AM, Hager GD. Human-machine collaborative systems for microsurgical applications. Int J Robot Res 2005; 24(9): 731-41.
[http://dx.doi.org/10.1177/0278364905057059]

[84]　Fei B, Ng WS, Chauhan S, Kwoh CK. The safety issues of medical robotics. Reliab Eng Syst Saf 2001; 73(2): 183-92.
[http://dx.doi.org/10.1016/S0951-8320(01)00037-0]

[85]　Taylor RH. A perspective on medical robotics. Proc IEEE. 2006 Sep; 94(9): 1652-64.
[http://dx.doi.org/10.1109/JPROC.2006.880669]

[86]　Roessler K, Ungersboeck K, Dietrich W, *et al.* Frameless stereotactic guided neurosurgery: Clinical experience with an infrared based pointer device navigation system. Acta Neurochir (Wien) 1997; 139(6): 551-9.
[http://dx.doi.org/10.1007/BF02750999] [PMID: 9248590]

[87]　Shen W, Gu J, Milios E. Robotic neurosurgery and clinical applications. Proceeding of the 2004 International Conference on Intelligent Mechatronics and Automation 2004; 114-9.

[88]　Boddu SP, Moore ML, Rodgers BM, Brinkman JC, Verhey JT, Bingham JS. A bibliometric analysis of the top 100 most influential studies on robotic arthroplasty. Arthroplast Today 2023; 22: 101153.
[http://dx.doi.org/10.1016/j.artd.2023.101153] [PMID: 37342364]

[89]　Monfaredi R, Concepcion-Gonzalez A, Acosta Julbe J, *et al.* Automatic path-planning techniques for minimally invasive stereotactic neurosurgical procedures—A systematic review. Sensors (Basel) 2024; 24(16): 5238.
[http://dx.doi.org/10.3390/s24165238] [PMID: 39204935]

[90]　Bro-Nielsen M, Gramkow C, Kreiborg S. Non-rigid image registration using a bone growth model. In:

Ayache N, Ed. CVRMed-MRCAS'97. Proceedings of the First Joint Conference: Computer Vision, Virtual Reality and Robotics in Medicine and Medical Robotics and Computer-Assisted Surgery. Grenoble, France. Berlin, Heidelberg: Springer 1997; p. 1-12.
[http://dx.doi.org/10.1007/BFb0029219]

[91]   McInerney T, Terzopoulos D. Deformable models in medical image analysis: a survey. Med Image Anal 1996; 1(2): 91-108.
[http://dx.doi.org/10.1016/S1361-8415(96)80007-7] [PMID: 9873923]

[92]   Wells WM, Grimson WEL, Kikinis R, Jolesz FA. Adaptive segmentation of MRI data. IEEE Trans Med Imaging 1996; 15(4): 429-42.
[http://dx.doi.org/10.1109/42.511747] [PMID: 18215925]

[93]   Fadda M, Bertelli D, Martelli S, Marcacci M, Dario P, Paggetti C, *et al.* Computer-assisted planning for total knee arthroplasty. In: Wells WM, Colchester A, Delp S, Eds Proceedings of Computer Assisted Surgery. 1997; pp. 617-28.
[http://dx.doi.org/10.1007/BFb0029287]

[94]   Patriciu A, Muntener M, Kavossi L, Stoianovici D. Image-guided robotic-assisted interventions. Imaging in Oncological Urology. 365-71.

[95]   Frangi AF, Niessen WJ, Vincken KL, Viergever MA. Multiscale vessel enhancement filtering. Proceedings of Medical Image Computing and Computer-Assisted Intervention. 1998; pp. 130-7.
[http://dx.doi.org/10.1007/BFb0056195]

[96]   Duong L, Mac-Thiong JM, Labelle H. Real time noninvasive assessment of external trunk geometry during surgical correction of adolescent idiopathic scoliosis. Scoliosis 2009; 4(1): 5.
[http://dx.doi.org/10.1186/1748-7161-4-5] [PMID: 19239713]

[97]   Himpens J, Leman G, Cadiere GB. Telesurgical laparoscopic cholecystectomy. Surg Endosc 1998; 12(8): 1091-1.
[http://dx.doi.org/10.1007/s004649900788] [PMID: 9685550]

[98]   Cuschieri A, Buess G, Périssat J, Eds. Operative Manual of Endoscopic Surgery. Berlin, Heidelberg: Springer Berlin Heidelberg 1992.
[http://dx.doi.org/10.1007/978-3-662-22257-7]

[99]   Egorov V, Sarvazyan AP. Mechanical imaging of the breast. IEEE Trans Med Imaging 2008; 27(9): 1275-87.
[http://dx.doi.org/10.1109/TMI.2008.922192] [PMID: 18753043]

[100]   Tendick F, Jennings RW, Tharp G, Stark L. Sensing and manipulation problems in endoscopic surgery: Experiment, analysis, and observation. Presence (Camb Mass) 1993; 2(1): 66-81.
[http://dx.doi.org/10.1162/pres.1993.2.1.66]

[101]   Cohn MB, Crawford LS, Wendlandt JM, Sastry SS. Surgical applications of milli-robots. J Robot Syst 1995; 12(6): 401-16.
[http://dx.doi.org/10.1002/rob.4620120606]

[102]   Hills JW, Jensen JF. Telepresence technology in medicine: principles and applications. Proc IEEE 1998; 86(3): 569-80.
[http://dx.doi.org/10.1109/5.662880]

[103]   Ottensmeyer MP, Hu J, Thompson JM, Ren J, Sheridan TB. Investigations into the performance of minimally invasive telesurgery with feedback time delays. Presence (Camb Mass) 2000; 9(4): 369-82.
[http://dx.doi.org/10.1162/105474600566871]

[104]   Giorgi C, Eisenberg H, Costi G, Gallo E, Garibotto G, Casolino DS. Robot-assisted microscope for neurosurgery. J Image Guid Surg 1995; 1(3): 158-63.
[http://dx.doi.org/10.1002/(SICI)1522-712X(1995)1:3<158::AID-IGS5>3.0.CO;2-9]   [PMID: 9079441]

[105]   Burckhardt CW, Flury P, Glauser D. Stereotactic brain surgery. IEEE Eng Med Biol Mag 1995; 14(3):

314-7.
[http://dx.doi.org/10.1109/51.391771]

[106] Eljamel MS. Validation of the PathFinder ™ neurosurgical robot using a phantom. Int J Med Robot 2007; 3(4): 372-7.
[http://dx.doi.org/10.1002/rcs.153] [PMID: 17914750]

[107] Chan F, Kassim I, Lo C, *et al.* Image-guided robotic neurosurgery—an *in vitro* and *in vivo* point accuracy evaluation experimental study. Surg Neurol 2009; 71(6): 640-7.
[http://dx.doi.org/10.1016/j.surneu.2008.06.008] [PMID: 19329150]

[108] Muacevic A, Wowra B, Reiser M. CyberKnife: review of first 1,000 cases at a dedicated therapy center. Int J CARS 2008; 3(5): 447-56.
[http://dx.doi.org/10.1007/s11548-008-0246-1]

[109] Nathoo N, Pesek T, Barnett GH. Robotics and neurosurgery. Surg Clin North Am 2003; 83(6): 1339-50.
[http://dx.doi.org/10.1016/S0039-6109(03)00157-9] [PMID: 14712870]

[110] Mettler L, Ibrahim M, Jonat W. One year of experience working with the aid of a robotic assistant (the voice-controlled optic holder AESOP) in gynaecological endoscopic surgery. Hum Reprod 1998; 13(10): 2748-50.
[http://dx.doi.org/10.1093/humrep/13.10.2748] [PMID: 9804224]

[111] Marescaux J, Rubino F. The ZEUS robotic system: experimental and clinical applications. Surg Clin North Am 2003; 83(6): 1305-15.
[http://dx.doi.org/10.1016/S0039-6109(03)00169-5] [PMID: 14712867]

[112] Falcone T, Goldberg JM, Margossian H, Stevens L. Robotic-assisted laparoscopic microsurgical tubal anastomosis: a human pilot study. Fertil Steril 2000; 73(5): 1040-2.
[http://dx.doi.org/10.1016/S0015-0282(00)00423-4] [PMID: 10785235]

[113] Ballantyne GH, Moll F. The da Vinci telerobotic surgical system: the virtual operative field and telepresence surgery. Surg Clin North Am 2003; 83(6): 1293-304.
[http://dx.doi.org/10.1016/S0039-6109(03)00164-6] [PMID: 14712866]

[114] Degueldre M, Vandromme J, Huong PT, Cadière GB. Robotically assisted laparoscopic microsurgical tubal reanastomosis: a feasibility study. Fertil Steril 2000; 74(5): 1020-3.
[http://dx.doi.org/10.1016/S0015-0282(00)01543-0] [PMID: 11056252]

[115] Box GN, Gong M. Multispecialty applications of robotic technology. In: Patel VR, Ed. Robotic urologic surgery. London: Springer; 2007; pp. 15-22.

[116] Camarillo DB, Krummel TM, Salisbury JK Jr. Robotic technology in surgery: Past, present, and future. Am J Surg 2004; 188(4) (Suppl.): 2-15.
[http://dx.doi.org/10.1016/j.amjsurg.2004.08.025] [PMID: 15476646]

[117] Nishihara S, Sugano N, Nishii T, Miki H, Nakamura N, Yoshikawa H. Comparison between hand rasping and robotic milling for stem implantation in cementless total hip arthroplasty. J Arthroplasty 2006; 21(7): 957-66.
[http://dx.doi.org/10.1016/j.arth.2006.01.001] [PMID: 17027537]

[118] Park SE, Lee CT. Comparison of robotic-assisted and conventional manual implantation of a primary total knee arthroplasty. J Arthroplasty 2007; 22(7): 1054-9.
[http://dx.doi.org/10.1016/j.arth.2007.05.036] [PMID: 17920481]

[119] Huynh LM, Kim YH. A computer-aided and robot-assisted surgical system for reconstruction of anterior cruciate ligament. Int J Precis Eng Manuf 2013; 14(1): 49-54.
[http://dx.doi.org/10.1007/s12541-013-0008-z]

[120] Stoianovici D. Robotic surgery. World J Urol 2000; 18(4): 289-95.
[http://dx.doi.org/10.1007/PL00007078] [PMID: 11000313]

[121] Davies BL, Hibberd RD, Coptcoat MJ, Wickham JEA. A surgeon robot prostatectomy—a laboratory evaluation. J Med Eng Technol 1989; 13(6): 273-7.
[http://dx.doi.org/10.3109/03091908909016201] [PMID: 2614807]

[122] Bzostek A, Schreiner S, Barnes AC, Cadeddu JA, Roberts WW, Anderson JH, *et al.* An automated system for precise percutaneous access of the renal collecting system. Proceedings 1997; pp. 299-308.
[http://dx.doi.org/10.1007/BFb0029249]

[123] Das H, Zak H, Johnson J, Crouch J, Frambach D. Evaluation of a telerobotic system to assist surgeons in microsurgery. Comput Aided Surg 1999; 4(1): 15-25.
[http://dx.doi.org/10.3109/10929089909148155] [PMID: 10417827]

[124] Hunter IW, Jones LA, Sagar MA, Lafontaine SR, Hunter PJ. Ophthalmic microsurgical robot and associated virtual environment. Comput Biol Med 1995; 25(2): 173-82.
[http://dx.doi.org/10.1016/0010-4825(94)00042-O] [PMID: 7554835]

[125] Reitz BA. What's new in cardiac surgery. J Am Coll Surg 2004; 198(5): 784-97.
[http://dx.doi.org/10.1016/j.jamcollsurg.2004.02.012] [PMID: 15110813]

[126] Woo YJ, Seeburger J, Mohr FW. Minimally invasive valve surgery. Semin Thorac Cardiovasc Surg 2007; 19(4): 289-98.
[http://dx.doi.org/10.1053/j.semtcvs.2007.10.005] [PMID: 18395627]

[127] Rosen M, Ponsky J. Minimally invasive surgery. Endoscopy 2001; 33(4): 358-66.
[http://dx.doi.org/10.1055/s-2001-13689] [PMID: 11315900]

[128] Cremer J, Mügge A, Wittwer T, *et al.* Early angiographic results after revascularization by minimally invasive direct coronary artery bypass (MIDCAB)1. Eur J Cardiothorac Surg 1999; 15(4): 383-8.
[http://dx.doi.org/10.1016/S1010-7940(99)00040-8] [PMID: 10371109]

[129] Modi P, Hassan A, Chitwood WR Jr. Minimally invasive mitral valve surgery: a systematic review and meta-analysis. Eur J Cardiothorac Surg 2008; 34(5): 943-52.
[http://dx.doi.org/10.1016/j.ejcts.2008.07.057] [PMID: 18829343]

[130] Nio D, Diks J, Bemelman WA, Wisselink W, Legemate DA. Laparoscopic vascular surgery: a systematic review. Eur J Vasc Endovasc Surg 2007; 33(3): 263-71.
[http://dx.doi.org/10.1016/j.ejvs.2006.10.004] [PMID: 17127084]

[131] Mack MJ, Magovern JA, Acuff TA, *et al.* Results of graft patency by immediate angiography in minimally invasive coronary artery surgery. Ann Thorac Surg 1999; 68(2): 383-9.
[http://dx.doi.org/10.1016/S0003-4975(99)00648-7] [PMID: 10475401]

[132] Carpentier A, Loulmet D, Aupècle B, *et al.* Chirurgie à cœur ouvert assistée par ordinateur. Premier cas opéré avec succès. C R Acad Sci III 1998; 321(5): 437-42.
[http://dx.doi.org/10.1016/S0764-4469(98)80309-0] [PMID: 9766192]

[133] Diodato MD Jr, Damiano RJ Jr. Robotic cardiac surgery: overview. Surg Clin North Am 2003; 83(6): 1351-67.
[http://dx.doi.org/10.1016/S0039-6109(03)00166-X] [PMID: 14712871]

[134] Cleary K, Nguyen C. State of the art in surgical robotics: clinical applications and technology challenges. Comput Aided Surg 2001; 6(6): 312-28.
[http://dx.doi.org/10.3109/10929080109146301] [PMID: 11954063]

[135] Kypson AP, Nifong LW, Chitwood WR Jr. Robotic cardiac surgery. J Long Term Eff Med Implants 2003; 13(6): 14.
[http://dx.doi.org/10.1615/JLongTermEffMedImplants.v13.i6.30] [PMID: 15056064]

[136] Sutherland GR, Latour I, Greer AD, Fielding T, Feil G, Newhook P. An image-guided magnetic resonance-compatible surgical robot. Neurosurgery 2008; 62(2): 286-93.
[http://dx.doi.org/10.1227/01.neu.0000315996.73269.18] [PMID: 18382307]

[137] Cadiere GB, Himpens J, Vertruyen M, Favretti F. A surgeon performed the world's first obesity

surgery at a distance. Obes Surg 1999; 9(2): 206-9.
[http://dx.doi.org/10.1381/096089299765553539] [PMID: 10340781]

[138] Cadière GB, Himpens J, Germay O, *et al.* Feasibility of robotic laparoscopic surgery: 146 cases. World J Surg 2001; 25(11): 1467-77.
[http://dx.doi.org/10.1007/s00268-001-0132-2] [PMID: 11760751]

[139] Cadière GB, Himpens J, Vertruyen M, *et al.* Evaluation of telesurgical (robotic) NISSEN fundoplication. Surg Endosc 2001; 15(9): 918-23.
[http://dx.doi.org/10.1007/s004640000217] [PMID: 11605106]

[140] Melvin WS, Needleman BJ, Krause KR, Schneider C, Ellison EC. Computer-enhanced vs. standard laparoscopic antireflux surgery. J Gastrointest Surg 2002; 6(1): 11-6.
[http://dx.doi.org/10.1016/S1091-255X(01)00032-4] [PMID: 11986012]

[141] Hashizume M, Sugimachi K. Robot-assisted gastric surgery. Surg Clin North Am 2003; 83(6): 1429-44.
[http://dx.doi.org/10.1016/S0039-6109(03)00158-0] [PMID: 14712877]

[142] Wang L, Yu Y, Wang J, Li S, Jiang T. Evaluation of the learning curve for robotic single-anastomosis duodenal–ileal bypass with sleeve gastrectomy. Front Surg 2022; 9: 969418.
[http://dx.doi.org/10.3389/fsurg.2022.969418] [PMID: 35937606]

[143] Law S. Minimally invasive techniques for oesophageal cancer surgery. Best Pract Res Clin Gastroenterol 2006; 20(5): 925-40.
[http://dx.doi.org/10.1016/j.bpg.2006.03.011] [PMID: 16997170]

[144] Jacobsen G, Elli F, Horgan S. Robotic surgery update. Surg Endosc 2004; 18(8): 1186-91.
[http://dx.doi.org/10.1007/s00464-003-8281-z] [PMID: 15095084]

[145] Rockall TA, Darzi A. Robot-assisted laparoscopic colorectal surgery. Surg Clin North Am 2003; 83(6): 1463-8.
[http://dx.doi.org/10.1016/S0039-6109(03)00156-7] [PMID: 14712879]

[146] Islam M, Atputharuban DA, Ramesh R, Ren H. Real-time instrument segmentation in robotic surgery using auxiliary supervised deep adversarial learning. IEEE Robot Autom Lett 2019; 4(2): 2188-95.
[http://dx.doi.org/10.1109/LRA.2019.2900854]

[147] Madhavan K, Kolcun JPG, Chieng LO, Wang MY. Augmented-reality integrated robotics in neurosurgery: are we there yet? Neurosurg Focus 2017; 42(5): E3.
[http://dx.doi.org/10.3171/2017.2.FOCUS177] [PMID: 28463612]

[148] Taylor RH, Menciassi A, Fichtinger G, Fiorini P, Dario P. Medical robotics and computer-integrated surgery. In: Siciliano B, Khatib O, Eds. Springer Handbook of Robotics. Springer, Cham 2016; pp. 1657-84.
[http://dx.doi.org/10.1007/978-3-319-32552-1_63]

[149] Hiller J, Landstorfer P, Marx P, Herbst M. Evaluation of the impact of faulty scanning trajectories in robot-based x-ray computed tomography. Meas Sci Technol 2021; 32(1): 15401.
[http://dx.doi.org/10.1088/1361-6501/abaf2a]

[150] Bai L, Yang J, Chen X, Sun Y, Li X. Medical robotics in bone fracture reduction surgery: a review. Sensors (Basel) 2019; 19(16): 3593.
[http://dx.doi.org/10.3390/s19163593] [PMID: 31426577]

[151] Karas CS, Chiocca EA. Neurosurgical robotics: a review of brain and spine applications. J Robot Surg 2007; 1(1): 39-43.
[http://dx.doi.org/10.1007/s11701-006-0006-6] [PMID: 25484937]

[152] Mao JZ, Agyei JO, Khan A, *et al.* Technologic evolution of navigation and robotics in spine surgery: a historical perspective. World Neurosurg 2021; 145: 159-67.
[http://dx.doi.org/10.1016/j.wneu.2020.08.224] [PMID: 32916361]

[153]   Fiani B, Quadri SA, Farooqui M, *et al.* Impact of robot-assisted spine surgery on health care quality and neurosurgical economics: A systemic review. Neurosurg Rev 2020; 43(1): 17-25.
[http://dx.doi.org/10.1007/s10143-018-0971-z] [PMID: 29611081]

[154]   Saniotis A, Henneberg M. Neurosurgical robots and ethical challenges to medicine. Ethics Sci Environ Polit 2021; 21: 25-30.
[http://dx.doi.org/10.3354/esep00197]

[155]   Moro C, Štromberga Z, Raikos A, Stirling A. The effectiveness of virtual and augmented reality in health sciences and medical anatomy. Anat Sci Educ 2017; 10(6): 549-59.
[http://dx.doi.org/10.1002/ase.1696] [PMID: 28419750]

[156]   Simaan N, Yasin RM, Wang L. Medical technologies and challenges of robot-assisted minimally invasive intervention and diagnostics. Annu Rev Control Robot Auton Syst 2018; 1(1): 465-90.
[http://dx.doi.org/10.1146/annurev-control-060117-104956]

[157]   Hogaboam L, Daim T. Technology adoption potential of medical devices: The case of wearable sensor products for pervasive care in neurosurgery and orthopedics. Health Policy Technol 2018; 7(4): 409-19.
[http://dx.doi.org/10.1016/j.hlpt.2018.10.011]

[158]   Parsley BS. Robotics in orthopedics: a brave new world. J Arthroplasty 2018; 33(8): 2355-7.
[http://dx.doi.org/10.1016/j.arth.2018.02.032] [PMID: 29605151]

[159]   Rivero-Moreno Y, Rodriguez M, Losada-Muñoz P, *et al.* Autonomous robotic surgery: has the future arrived? Cureus 2024; 16(1): e52243.
[http://dx.doi.org/10.7759/cureus.52243] [PMID: 38352080]

CHAPTER 4

Genomic Medicine and Personalized Healthcare

Sunita[1], Akhil Sharma[1], Akanksha Sharma[1], Shekhar Singh[2] and Shaweta Sharma[3],*

[1] *R. J. College of Pharmacy, Raipur, Uttar Pradesh-202165, India*

[2] *Faculty of Pharmacy, Babu Banarasi Das Northern India Institute of Technology, Lucknow, Uttar Pradesh-226028, India*

[3] *Department of Pharmacy, School of Medical and Allied Sciences, Galgotias University, Greater Noida, Uttar Pradesh-201310, India*

Abstract: Genomic medicine and personalized healthcare are important innovations in modern medicine that aim to customize healthcare based on individual differences in genetic profile. This chapter provides a brief overview of the developing field of genomic medicine, starting with the basics of human genome sequencing and the importance of genetics in disease prevention. Also, the chapter focuses on important technologies, including NGS, CRISPR gene editing, WGS, and genomic data types such as SNPs. The chapter discusses the importance of targeted medicine, illustrating how it outperforms classical methods through targeted therapy, decreased side effects, and individualized prevention. It also encompasses particular applications in oncology, pharmacogenomics, rare genetic conditions, and infectious diseases. The rapid growth of some technological advances, such as AI, ML, and big data implementation, plays a crucial role in genomics data analysis and interpretation. The challenges in genomic medicine, such as data privacy, ethical dilemmas, and lack of accessibility, are discussed. The chapter concludes by discussing the future of genomic medicine, referring to it as "the patient-centered solutions of the future".

Keywords: Data privacy, DNA sequencing, Genomic medicine, Personalized healthcare, Pharmacogenomics, Precision medicine.

INTRODUCTION

Genomic medicine is a novel approach to patient care that uses information about a person's genome to guide diagnosis, prevention, and treatment. Genomic medicine aims to identify the genomic foundations of diseases by analysing patterns in DNA, RNA, and proteins to provide personalized treatment options.

* **Corresponding author Shaweta Sharma**: Department of Pharmacy, School of Medical and Allied Sciences, Galgotias University, Greater Noida, Uttar Pradesh-201310, India; E-mail: shawetasharma@galgotiasuniversity.edu.in

Shaweta Sharma, Akhil Sharma, Shivkanya Fuloria & Anurag Singh (Eds.)
All rights reserved-© 2025 Bentham Science Publishers

Personalized healthcare uses this approach but adds information about the individual (including genetic, environmental, corporate, and lifestyle factors) to create a custom healthcare solution. Collectively, these paradigms are moving from a one-size-fits-all model to a precision model and improving patient clinical outcomes. Genomic medicine is a fourth revolution in the field of healthcare, possibly in the future as a main modality impacting other specialties such as oncology, pharmacogenomics, rare genetic disorders, infectious diseases, *etc.* It also assists in the detection of the predisposition to disease and increases the therapeutic effect while preventing the side effects [1, 2].

Importance in Modern Healthcare

Integrating genomic medicine into current healthcare offers the promise of significant paradigm shifts in critical areas of disease prevention, diagnosis, and treatment. This allows for preventive measures and personalized lifestyle modifications based on genetic susceptibilities. In the field of oncology, genomic profiling permits the selection of targeted therapies that boost efficiency and decrease adverse effects. It also helps healthcare providers to give medications based on a patient's genetic composition with the best possible dose and minimum adverse drug reaction–some of the significant benefits of pharmacogenomics. It contributes to a paradigm shift in the sense of preventive care that alleviates the economic burden imposed on the healthcare system by slowing down the progression of chronic diseases. In addition, genomic medicine provides patients with useful information about their health, which enables shared decision-making. The reason for its significance in present healthcare is its accuracy, and it could be a stepping stone for equal and efficient healthcare [3 - 5].

Role of Technology in Advancing Genomics

Technological developments have played a key role in bringing genomic medicine to the forefront of healthcare. Typical next-generation sequencing (NGS) technologies have revolutionized genetic analysis because they have successfully launched whole-genome sequencing into fast, more accurate, and cheaper approaches. The integration of big data analytics and machine learning tools has been instrumental in indicating patterns, analyzing large genomic datasets, and predicting disease risk. AI simplifies analysis of complex genetic interactions and can aid drug discovery by revealing novel therapeutic targets. In addition, partly due to the ease of keeping and exchanging genomic data, cloud computing provides the potential for collaborative research and speeding up innovations. Digital healthcare tools, alongside genomic data, such as wearables, can capture health metrics in real time, thus getting a comprehensive view of patients' health. In order to alleviate privacy challenges, secure and transparent genomic data sharing will be facilitated *via* the use of blockchain technology. Together, these technologies have moved genomics from the periphery to the center of precision medicine, enabling innovations in personalized medicine [6, 7].

UNDERSTANDING GENOMIC MEDICINE

Basics of Human Genome and DNA Sequencing

The entirety of human genetic information, over 3 billion base pairs of DNA, is known as the human genome, which describes the complete set of instructions for our development, function, and reproduction. This information is stored as sequences of four nucleotides: adenine (A), thymine (T), cytosine (C), and guanine (G). The genome consists of 23 pairs of chromosomes and harbors approximately 20,000-25,000 protein-coding genes and large non-coding regions responsible for regulating gene expression and function. The sequencing of our genome has been one of the most important achievements in biology and medicine, facilitated primarily by the advent of DNA sequencing technologies [8].

The same goes for DNA sequencing, which is basically just a form of determining the detailed order of nucleotides in a DNA molecule, which has changed a lot from its early beginnings. Foundation-level traditional methods, such as Sanger sequencing, were expensive and time-consuming. Next-generation sequencing (NGS) has changed the landscape, allowing the rapid, high-throughput analysis of whole genomes at a fraction of the cost. NGS platforms break DNA into little pieces, sequence them in parallel, and subsequently reassemble the data computationally. Novel technologies, such as third-generation sequencing, which already analyze larger fragments of DNA in real time, further enhance precision and reduce the time from sequencing to results [9].

The sequencing of the human genome, initially performed in 2003 as a result of the Human Genome Project, has provided unprecedented opportunities for understanding genetic variation, evolution, and susceptibility to diseases. It showed that even though humans share 99.9% of their DNA, the remaining 0.1% explains individuality and differences between us all, including the likelihood of the disease. These variations, such as single-nucleotide polymorphisms (SNPs) and structural changes, are often studied to understand genetic influences on health and disease.

The knowledge gleaned from DNA sequencing has broad applications. This allows us to find the mutations related to genetic diseases, come up with targeted therapies, and participate in pharmacogenomics, such as customizing the treatment based on an individual's genetics. In addition, innovation in sequencing has driven precision medicine and the use of genetic information to make diagnostic and therapeutic decisions, which has revolutionized the delivery of health care [10].

The Genome and its Role in Disease Prevention

The genome is an essential component of disease prevention through the knowledge of psychological predispositions, which allows for primary interventions and lifestyle changes. Genomic and omics database show that the interplay between genetics and disease is quite complicated, driven largely by inherited mutations but dependent in complex ways on the interactions that those mutations have with other genetic and environmental exposures. This knowledge underlies much of predictive and preventive medicine, in which genomic analysis identifies which individuals are likely to develop particular conditions [11].

Genomic discoveries related to genetic variants associated with the disease represent one of the most substantial contributions of the field. An example of this is the BRCA1 and BRCA2 genetic mutations that drastically increase the likelihood of developing breast and ovarian cancers. Suppose one has those variants, which can be found through genetic testing. In that case, physicians can prevent that disease through more rigorous screening and lifestyle changes, and at times, through preventive surgeries. In a similar vein, genome-wide association studies (GWAS) have established associations between certain genetic markers and diseases like diabetes, cardiovascular diseases, and autoimmune diseases, allowing for targeted preventative measures against possible future diseases [12].

Epigenetics is the science that explores how gene expression can change without modifications to the DNA sequence, further emphasizing how the genome can act as a protector against disease. Gene activity in a disease can be activated or silenced from hundreds of thousands of other genes purely through epigenetic modifications, which are often influenced by lifestyle habits like diet and stress, exposure to toxins, and other environmental factors. Clearly spelling out these mechanisms paves the way for strategies that can reduce risk, underlining the importance of risk-based prevention in a personalized manner [13].

A subset of genomics, pharmacogenomics aims to prevent diseases by optimizing drug therapy. Polymorphisms in genes involved in drug metabolism may cause response variations and/or adverse effects/therapeutic failures in patients. Clinicians can then prescribe medication based on the findings of the genomic screening to ensure that they can safely take it.

Genomic data are used to inform population-level strategies for infectious disease prevention and control in the field of public health. Genomic surveillance of infectious agents, including viruses such as SARS-CoV-2 and bacteria, gives us important clues in designing targeted vaccines and antimicrobial therapies. In addition, these large-scale genomic studies have the potential to inform health policies by identifying genetic determinants of trait measurements responsible for the susceptibility of certain populations to certain diseases, thus addressing health disparities.

Genomic insights, along with bioinformatics and data analytics innovations, are expected to enhance disease prevention at high levels of resolution and in a more proactive manner in the future. The genome serves as a blueprint for personalized and population-wide health interventions, transforming the approach to maintaining health and mitigating the burden of disease [14].

KEY TECHNOLOGIES OF GENOMIC MEDICINE

Genomic medicine integrates advanced technologies like Next-Generation Sequencing (NGS), CRISPR and gene editing, and Whole Genome Sequencing (WGS) to enable personalized healthcare. These tools revolutionize disease prediction, prevention, and treatment by unlocking the potential of genetic data [15]. Fig. (**1**) represents the various technologies of genomic medicine.

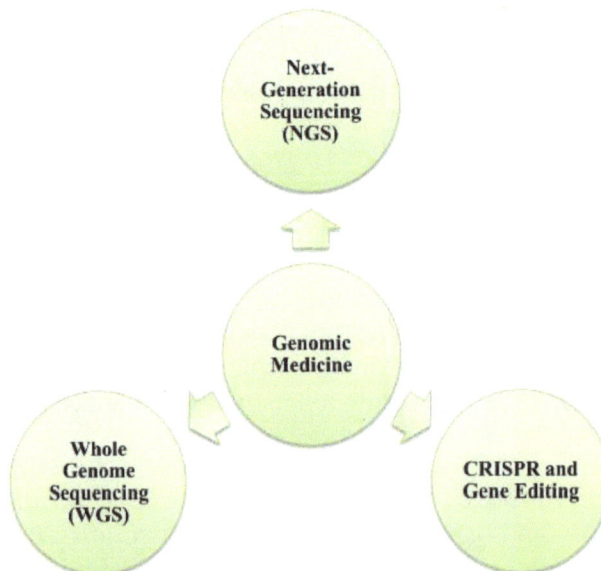

Fig. (1). Key technologies of genomic medicine.

Next-Generation Sequencing (NGS)

Next-generation sequencing (NGS) continues to serve as a revolutionary research and medical tool that drives rapid, in-depth, and cost-effective sequencing and analysis of complete genomes, exomes, or other extended/targeted regions of DNA and RNA. Sanger sequencing, as an example of the traditional sequencing approach, can identify only one DNA fragment (1 DNA molecule) at a time. At the same time, NGS enables massively parallel sequencing, in which millions of DNA molecules can be sequenced simultaneously. Such scalability has made NGS a key enabling technology in all fields of biological research, from oncology and infectious disease to personalized medicine [16].

In tumorigenesis, NGS can be used in cancer research to identify genetic mutations, translocations, and copy number variations. Molecular classification of breast cancers based on tumour molecular profiling enables the development of personalised treatment plans with the use of targeted therapies and predictive biomarkers. For example, the identification of mutations in genes such as BRCA1/2 or EGFR *via* NGS can inform treatment management for breast cancer and lung cancer [17].

Infectious disease diagnosis has also progressed rapidly with the advent of NGS. This technology enables pathogen identification, detection of antimicrobial resistance genes, and tracking of outbreaks through the sequencing of microbial genomes. It played a crucial role in characterizing SARS-CoV-2 during the COVID-19 pandemic, providing a comprehensive understanding of its evolution over time to inform public health measures.

Apart from diagnostics, NGS is a pillar of pharmacogenomics; knowledge of a patient's genotype helps inform drug choice and/or dosage in order to support its optimal efficacy and avoid side effects. Distantly, sequencing of RNA transcripts in a sample of isolated cells (RNA-Seq) provides information on the levels of gene expression patterns, facilitating insights into the mechanisms of the disease and potential targets for therapies [18].

CRISPR and Gene Editing

CRISPR (Clustered Regularly Interspaced Short Palindromic Repeat) offers a relatively rapid, precise, and inexpensive gene-editing tool, revolutionizing the field of gene editing. At the core of this revolutionary tech is an RNA-guided endonuclease, mainly Cas9, that can locate and modify specific DNA sequences While scientists have been able to replicate viral genes in bacteria for decades, CRISPR gave them a tool to utilize the natural mechanism that bacteria make use of to fight viruses to make specific cuts in the genome, like deletions and insertions, or to correct genetic mutations.

CRISPR is capable of doing much more than basic gene editing. It is mostly used for functional genomics, such as gene function, disease modeling, and epigenetic modifications. CRISPR-based tools, such as CRISPRi (Instrumentation of CRISPR Interference) and CRISPRa (Instrumentation of CRISPR Activation), can be utilized to silence and boost gene expression without any DNA coding sequence changes, offering an unparalleled platform to reveal gene regulation [19].

CRISPR has great potential when it comes to medical applications. This approach has been used in treating genetic conditions like sickle cell anemia and beta-thalassemia by targeting defective genes. Additionally, CRISPR-based therapies are also under investigation for use in treating cancer, especially for modifying immune cells, such as T cells, to better attack tumors. Even outside of human health, its use in the production of disease-resistant crops and livestock shows its promise.

CRISPR, in contrast, offers transformative potential but is also fraught with ethical and technical dilemmas. Its clinical application is hampered by off-target effects, which are genetic modifications produced outside the target site. Germline editing presents its ethical dilemmas since germline modifications are heritable, and questions arise over the long-term impact on human genetics [20].

Newer approaches also aim to address these problems. So-called high-fidelity variants of Cas9, including Cas12a and engineered Cas9 proteins, enhance specificity while decreasing off-target effects. The technology is further optimized *via* base and prime editing, which allows for highly specific, single-base modifications and precise insertions in the target without double-strand break induction, enabling safer and more precise genome editing.

The seamless integration of CRISPR is clearly evidenced by other technologies such as Next Generation Sequencing and bioinformatics that can rapidly bring about the advances needed for a personalized medicine revolution. This enables precise genetics to inform CRISPR-based, customized therapy. While the field continues to mature, CRISPR and gene editing will inevitably be at the heart of genomic medicine, providing potential cures for genetic diseases, attacking cancer repertoire, and driving therapeutic innovations [21].

Whole Genome Sequencing (WGS)

Whole-genome sequencing (WGS) is a game-changing technology that determines the complete DNA sequence of an organism. It includes the full complement of genes, as well as non-coding regions. WGS has transformed genomics by creating a sequential map of almost all of a person's genetic material. It has found utility in a vast majority of fields, from personalized medicine to rare disease diagnosis to cancer genomics to evolutionary biology.

Whole-genome sequencing (WGS) allows the identification of genetic variants that lead to particular diseases, and consequently aids in the design of personalized medicine. It identifies, for instance, the mutations in genes associated with drug metabolism, and recommends the best and safest medications for them. WGS enables the identification of somatic mutations in cancer, which can aid in the development of directed therapies in oncology [22].

WGS is important in the diagnosis of rare genetic disorders. Conventional diagnostics often fail to identify the genetic basis of complex disorders. Whole-genome sequencing (WGS) not only has the potential to identify pathogenic variants in novel genomic locations but also carries a diagnostic yield of up to 50% in selected cohorts. This has important implications for kids with undiagnosed illnesses.

Within the research field, WGS sheds light on genetic variation, population genetics, and evolutionary processes. It is essential for the discovery of new genes and regulatory elements, which supplements the understanding of biological systems. In addition, WGS contributes to infection surveillance by providing a genomic characterization of pathogens to precisely trace the sources of outbreaks and the mechanisms of antimicrobial resistance [23].

Whole genome sequencing (WGS) has great potential for clinical implementation, but some hurdles and challenges prevent its clinical implementation. The massive data output requires bioinformatics tools and high-volume data storage systems. The ethical issues of privacy, consent, and data sharing also needed to be addressed . These challenges aside, the continued development of advancing sequencing approaches, including nanopore and single-molecule sequencing, promise to bring further improvements in speed, precision, and price/performance for WGS [24].

TYPES AND USES OF GENOMIC DATA

Genomic data includes DNA sequences, gene expression profiles, and epigenetic markers, which are essential for personalized medicine, disease prediction, drug development, and understanding genetic disorders. It enables precision treatments and accelerates scientific discoveries in genetics and healthcare [25].

Genomic Variants

Genomic variants are genetic differences that occur naturally among individuals. Variants can be classified into single-nucleotide polymorphisms (SNPs), insertions, deletions, copy number variations, or structural variants. Genomic variants impact human health in numerous ways, including susceptibility to diseases, response to medications or environmental stresses, and even physical traits.

SNPs, the most common type of genomic variation, occur when a single base pair in the DNA sequence is altered. Nonetheless, other forms of variants, such as insertion and deletion, have the potential to create greater changes in the genetic material. Such structural changes can affect the function or regulation of a gene. For example, a deletion in a gene may render it unable to function, which may lead to genetic disorders [26].

Genomic variants, importantly, are being researched for their importance in many conditions, including cancer, cardiovascular, and autoimmune diseases. In clinical practice, knowledge of genomic variants facilitates genetic disorder diagnosis, disease risk prediction, and targeted treatment based on individual genetic profiles. These variants can be identified and characterized by technologies such as whole-genome sequencing and exome sequencing. More genomic variants are being discovered as research evolves, enabling better and more targeted clinical interventions [27].

SNPs (Single Nucleotide Polymorphisms)

Single-nucleotide polymorphisms, or SNPs, are the most common type of genetic variations between individuals. They happen when one of the nucleotides in the genome is replaced by another. SNPs may be present in non-coding or coding regions, with variable downstream effects on the expression or function of the gene in which they occur.

SNPs located in coding regions can occasionally lead to an amino acid substitution of the protein, which can affect protein structure and function. Consequently, this can lead to diseases or traits, including genetic disorders, modified responses to drugs, or the inclination to develop certain diseases, such as diabetes or cardiovascular disease. SNPs can also play a role in gene regulation in non-coding regions and will change how and when genes are expressed [28].

Single-nucleotide polymorphisms (SNPs) are the most common form of genetic variations among people, making them an attractive target for discovery and new research. The recent development of high-throughput sequencing methods has enabled high-throughput SNP association studies to examine SNPs associated with different diseases, traits, and drug responses. These types of studies have resulted in the identification of many genetic loci for diseases, such as breast cancer, Alzheimer's, and multiple sclerosis.

It is important to identify SNPs due to the concept in pharmacogenomics that tries to establish how gene variation among humans affects drug response. Based on genetic variation predicted by SNPs, scientists will be able to determine the efficacy of various types of drugs, the dose of the drug, and adverse reactions, and develop personalized medicine for better treatment. SNP analysis is also a critical part of population genetics, which is used to track migration pathways in the human genome and some evolutionary processes. Consequently, SNPs are important clinical and research tools that we will utilize to better understand the genetics behind human health and diseases [29].

PERSONALIZED HEALTHCARE AND ITS SIGNIFICANCE

Personalized, or Precision medicine, is a part of medicine that involves treatment tailored to the individual characteristics of each patient. It takes into account biological, environmental, and lifestyle factors to risk-stratify, devise personalized treatment, and improve therapeutic response. While traditional medicine employs a one-size-fits-all model, personalized medicine tailors an approach to the individual by collecting and analyzing comprehensive patient-specific information to make decisions about prevention, diagnosis, and treatment. This field has progressed rapidly due to the advances in genomics, big data analytics, and biomarker identification, enabling healthcare providers to facilitate more precise, efficient, and effective care at lower costs. Personalized medicine represents a paradigm shift, supporting proactive and patient-centered health care [30, 31].

Benefits Over Traditional Medicine

Precision Treatment Plans

Conventional medicine is based on protocols and standards that certainly do not work the same way for all, since our genetic and physiological uniqueness. Such variations in patients have been the basis of research on personalized medicine, which is a form of medicine that develops specific treatment methods through genomic and molecular data. For example, genomic profiling is used to reveal mutations that drive tumor growth in targeted drugs, such as tyrosine kinase inhibitors, for specific cancer therapies. Pharmacogenomics can also be used to determine how well patients metabolize certain drugs, allowing for prescriptions that are tailored to the individual and minimizing the need for trial-and-error dosing. A precision treatment will result in less unnecessary treatment, leading to a higher therapeutic success rate and, consequently, a better patient outcome [32, 33].

Reduced Adverse Drug Reactions

ADRs are an important topic in traditional medicine and occur due to differences in the individual metabolism of drugs. Pharmacogenomic testing is a critical step in personalized medicine whereby genetic variants that inform drug response are identified. Patients with specific polymorphisms of the CYP450 enzyme will process medicines such as warfarin or antidepressants differently, bringing the danger of the medicine being toxic or never functioning. Using such genetic information to stratify drug choice and dosing minimizes this risk. Moreover, real-world studies show that these personalized approaches significantly reduced hospitalization due to adverse drug reactions, indicating a strong potential for safer, patient-specific pharmacotherapy [34].

Tailored Preventive Measures

Conventional preventive healthcare follows generalized protocols that do not accountfor specific risk factors of a given individual. Instead, personalized medicine flips this on its head, revealing the opportunity for tailored prevention based on genetic screening, analysis of family history, and lifestyle data. For example, when a person undergoes BRCA1/2 gene testing and is found to be at a high risk of breast and ovarian cancers, they may decide to take actions like surveillance and preventive surgeries. Likewise, customized risk assessments for chronic illnesses, such as diabetes or cardiovascular disease, enable patients to make specific lifestyle lifestyle modifications or begin early treatments. Such a dedicated and patient-specific method considerably increases the prevention of disease and the promotion of health in the long run [35].

APPLICATION OF PERSONALIZED HEALTHCARE

Personalized healthcare tailors medical treatment based on individual genetic, environmental, and lifestyle factors, improving outcomes and precision. Fig. (**2**) describes the application of personalized healthcare.

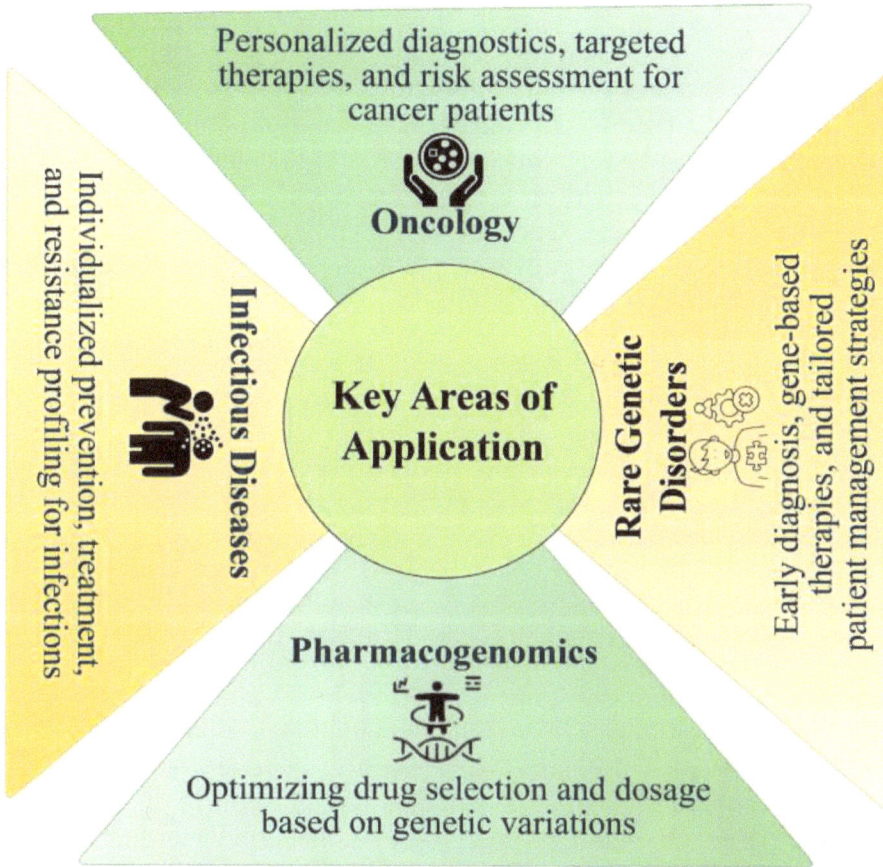

Fig. (2). Application of personalized healthcare.

Application in Oncology

Cancer genomics is a crucial component of personalized healthcare, transforming the way we diagnose, treat, and prevent cancer. Genomic profiling enables doctors to identify the specific DNA mutations that drive a particular cancer and to tailor treatment to target these mutations. This gives them a much better patient response than traditional treatment, such as chemotherapy, which is not effective for all patients and has numerous side effects . Both non-small cell lung cancer and breast cancer have specific mutations, like EGFR, BRCA, or KRAS, that oncologists use to target therapies (like tyrosine kinase inhibitors or PARP inhibitors), which have improved efficacy and lower side effects [36].

In addition, by identifying potential treatment options for individual patients, genomic profiling can help streamline drug selection for clinicians and avoid the trial-and-error process often seen with cancer drug use. For instance, a lung cancer patient who possesses a mutation in the EGFR gene may respond favourably to EGFR inhibitors (such as erlotinib). In contrast, another patient with the same cancer type and without such mutations will not derive benefit from that same treatment. Many of the specifics of cancer genomics also pertain to early detection and prevention. Genetic testing can identify individuals at an increased risk for specific cancers, allowing them to take preventive measures or intervene early, potentially saving human lives. Once the risk is known, for example, women with BRCA mutations may choose preventive surgeries, including mastectomies, to lower breast cancer risk.

Cancer genomics is also an important aspect of the idea of liquid biopsy (blood tests for circulating tumor DNA). This non-invasive approach allows for monitoring treatment response and potential recurrences, which is a key component of managing cancer long-term. This precision-driven approach marks a shift towards more personalized, patient-centered care, offering a better prognosis, minimizing unnecessary treatments, and improving the overall quality of life for cancer patients [37].

Application in Pharmacogenomics (Drug Response)

Pharmacogenomics, which studies genetic differences that impact individual drug responses, is a key component of personalized medicine. Pharmacogenomics is a field of research that associates the specific genetic variations affecting metabolism or response to the drug in a patient with the course of treatment that is safe and effective for that patient. Such individualisation accordingly minimises the prevalence of ADRs, among the main causes of hospitalisation and death globally. Genetic polymorphisms affecting the CYP450 family of enzymes may affect the metabolism of drugs, *e.g*, warfarin, clopidogrel, and some antidepressants. Specific genetic variants may necessitate higher doses, lower doses, or potentially another medication altogether to elicit a therapeutic effect, depending on the gene and the drug dosage [38].

In addition, pharmacogenomics improves the accuracy of cancer treatment. Some chemotherapeutic agents, such as 5-fluorouracil, may not be effective in patients with certain genetic profiles and may even become directly toxic. Other medications can be used for these people, thus avoiding side effects. For example, pharmacogenomic testing in psychiatry may help inform choices of antidepressants or antipsychotics as part of the patient-centered approach to reduce the historical trial-and-error paradigm.

In addition, pharmacogenomics appears to have a bright future in cardiovascular medicine. For example, patients with specific genetic signatures may be more responsive to statins, a type of medication used to treat high cholesterol. In contrast, others may have adverse reactions to statins or be non-responsive. While still in its early stages, the growth of pharmacogenomic testing in routine clinical care, in which genetic predisposition is factored into prescribing medications for a range of conditions, including cardiovascular diseases and autoimmune disorders, will undoubtedly contribute to the overall quality of life for patients by enhancing therapeutic efficacy and mitigating adverse effects [39].

Application in Rare Genetic Disorders

Personalized medicine is gradually bringing about fast and effective approaches that would help solve genetic disorders, which have traditionally been overlooked in generic healthcare models. While the associated genetic mutations for many rare genetic conditions have been identified, the advent of genomic sequencing technologies has moved the field toward discovering the causative mutations. Such discoveries have led to therapies and interventions that are being developed and have the potential to be tailored to the unique metabolic structure of the affected individual. On the other hand, rare diseases such as cystic fibrosis, Duchenne muscular dystrophy, and Tay-Sachs disease, previously deemed untreatable, have specific treatments based on genetic information. Cystic fibrosis (CF) due to CFTR mutations may be modulated by drugs such as Ivacaftor, which acts on the defective protein and can significantly improve symptoms such as sweating in patients with specific CFTR mutations [40].

Along with targeted therapies, genetic counseling has also emerged as a key component in the management of rare genetic disorders. Healthcare professionals can then analyze family history and genetic data to estimate the probability of such genetic conditions being inherited and provide preventive alternatives, such as prenatal screening or preimplantation genetic assessment (PGA). Additionally, an emerging branch of personalized medicine, gene therapy, may allow for the correction of DNA-level mutation, potentially curing things once thought impossible to treat [41].

Personalized health care is also vital for the early diagnosis of uncommon genetic disorders and subsequent treatment. Genomic sequencing identifies the genetic basis for previously undiagnosable symptoms, and clinicians can tailor treatments for patients more effectively. With the increase of understanding of the genetic underpinnings of rare diseases, precision therapy is only going to refine over time, giving patients the best opportunity of controlling or curing a once-thought-to-be moribund condition [42].

Application in Infectious Diseases

Personalized healthcare is not only sweeping the whole field of infectious disease, where the genetics of the microbe and the genetic characteristics of the host both influence the disease outcome and treatment response. Due to a combination of developments in genomic science, researchers have been able to detect unique paths that either enhance the virulence of the pathogen or boost its ability to resist drugs like the increasingly common antibiotic-resistant bacteria. Doctors can examine the genome of a pathogen to determine which antibiotics or antiviral drugs will be the most effective, with a lower likelihood of resistance and a more efficient treatment [43].

Though not discussed here, host genomics are equally important in the context of infectious diseases and complement the genomics of pathogens. The immune system also contains genetic variations that can affect how an individual responds to infections. For example, certain genetic backgrounds predispose individuals to disease susceptibility (*e.g.*, tuberculosis, HIV), while others may exhibit a more robust immune response. The knowledge of this genetic variation can help in the personalisation of preventive measures, such as vaccines or antiviral drugs, and tailoring treatment strategies to the individual [44].

Precision vaccines are one of the most promising trends in personalized healthcare for infectious diseases. Research on the role of genetic factors in vaccine responses could inspire personalized vaccination approaches. This means developing a booster shot for people with channels set up in their genome to be exposed to a particular vaccine, enabling them to take the anticipated vaccine in cases of disease, such as an outbreak, flu, or COVID-19, in a more potent or differently formulated way. In addition, it can also identify those at increased risk of such severe infections that they could benefit from other measures aimed at prevention, like early treatment or improved monitoring. Personalized healthcare enables a more specific, strategic, and operationally sound approach to addressing infectious diseases. Faster diagnosis leads to better care and reduces the spread of resistance. The integration of genomic sequencing into infection diagnosis/ treatment would certainly facilitate this process, moving us toward a more personalized model of care [45].

TECHNOLOGICAL ADVANCES DRIVING GENOMIC MEDICINE

Technological advancements, including AI, ML, big data, and cloud computing, are revolutionizing genomic medicine by enhancing data analysis, improving diagnostics, and enabling personalized treatments, thus accelerating healthcare innovations [46]. Fig. (**3**) illustrates the advancements in technology driving genomic medicine.

Technological Advancements Driving Genomic Medicine

Big Data and Cloud Computing for Genomic Data Storage and Processing

Artificial Intelligence (AI) and Machine Learning (ML) in Genomics

Bioinformatics and Data Interpretation

Blockchain for Secure and Transparent Data Sharing

Data Analysis and Pattern Recognition
AI-Powered Diagnostic Tools

Integrating Genomic Data with Electronic Health Records (EHR)

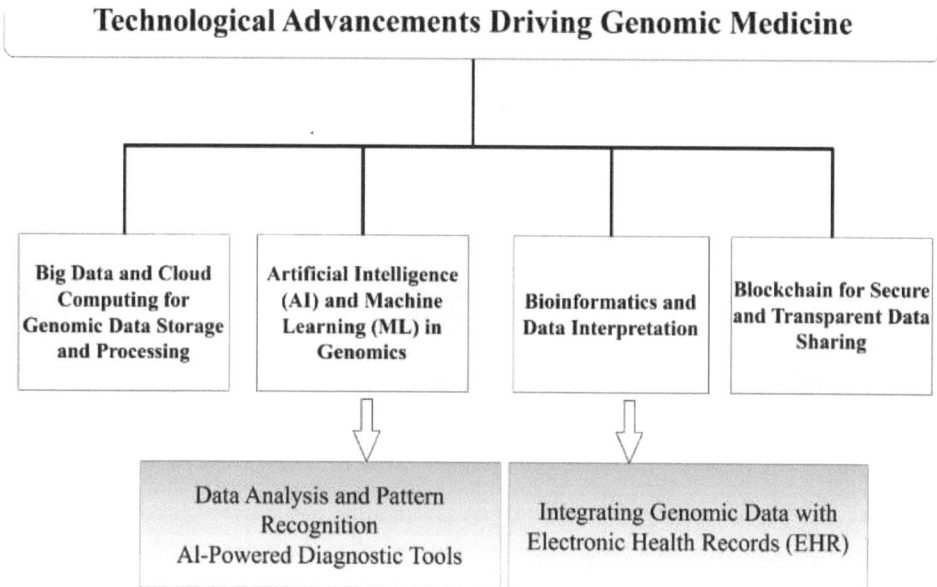

Fig. (3). Technological advancements driving genomic medicine.

Artificial Intelligence (AI) and Machine Learning (ML) in Genomics

AI and ML are transforming genomics by automating complex data analysis, uncovering patterns, and providing deeper insights into genetic variations, enabling personalized treatments and more accurate predictions of health outcomes [47].

Data Analysis and Pattern Recognition

Advancements in genomic data analysis can be attributed to AI and ML algorithms, which researchers are now applying to handle extensive amounts of genetic information with greater efficiency. They assist in identifying non-obvious patterns between DNA sequences that can reveal information about the disease, drug response, and genetic mutations that may provide the foundation of personalized medicine. AI and ML enable researchers to predict the effect of specific gene mutations on diseases, and identify rare genetic disorders, and possible therapeutic targets. The use of more sophisticated machine learning methods like deep learning can enhance the capability to learn complex genetic patterns, which are difficult for traditional methods to detect. It also helps analyze the extensive genomic data among various populations, thus increasing the knowledge of genetic diversity, as well as how this affects health. Automating all of these processes with AI increases the speed of genomic discoveries while minimizing human error and providing better predictions. As a result, there lies a great promise in applying AI to analyze data and observe patterns for making medical treatments and interventions better suited to the individual characteristics of each patient, paving the way to precision medicine [48].

AI-Powered Diagnostic Tools

Genomic diagnostics: AI-powered genomic diagnostic tools are changing the healthcare industry by providing a rapid, accurate, and non-invasive way of identifying genetic disorders. These tools employ sophisticated ML algorithms to process genetic data, identifying mutations, variants, and abnormalities that could signal genetic diseases. With remarkable precision, AI models can analyze and understand massive genomic datasets, decreasing the time and cost of diagnosing conditions such as cancer, neurological disorders, and rare genetic syndromes. Moreover, AI-based diagnostic tools are cross-functional and continue to learn from novel data over time, increasing their accuracy and effectiveness. That is, in the context of genomic medicine, these tools can be embedded as part of the clinical workflow to help healthcare providers make decisions on how best to treat patients. This, in turn, allows AI genomics to predict whether an individual will develop a certain disease, and what phenotype or response to a certain treatment, making AI a critical approach to personalized medicine. In addition, the use of these diagnostic tools may help limit diagnostic errors, simplify workflow, and enhance patient outcomes. These AI-powered tools will have a tremendous impact on the efficient diagnosis of genetic diseases and pave the way towards a future that sees timely and more accurate diagnoses, enabling more effective and personalized treatment [49, 50].

Big Data and Cloud Computing for Genomic Data Storage and Processing

The vast amounts of data generated by genomic sequencing require innovative solutions for storage, processing, and analysis. In genomic medicine, big data and cloud computing have evolved into essential tools that offer a scalable infrastructure to handle massive amounts of genetic data. The genomic datasets are stored on a preference for cloud computing, which is further facilitated by remote servers, allowing for the retrieval of genomic data from anywhere. This eliminates the need for local implementation and expensive storage solutions. They provide the necessary computational power for rapid and efficient processing of genomic data. Research scientists have been able to upload vast amounts of data, run complex algorithms, and analyze genomic variations without on-site infrastructure. Furthermore, cloud computing enables sharing and collaboration across global research teams, as well as data sharing and collaboration. The integration of heterogeneous data sources, such as electronic health records, clinical information, and environmental data, is made possible through the use of big data tools. The synergy of big data and cloud computing accelerates genomic discoveries, underpins personalized medicine, and ensures that genomic data can be accessed and processed efficiently with the scaling process of data sizes and complexities [51, 52].

Bioinformatics and Data Interpretation

Bioinformatics combines biology, computer science, and statistics to analyze and interpret genomic data. It enables the extraction of meaningful insights from complex genetic sequences, facilitating better healthcare decisions [53].

Integrating Genomic Data with Electronic Health Records (EHR)

Integrating genomic information with Electronic Health Records (EHR) is a necessary step to achieve personalized medicine. EHRs are the digital equivalent of patient records and generally include both clinical data and patient history, diagnosis, treatment, and other health related information. Having genomic data in EHRs allows healthcare providers better insight into a patient's health and helps drive informed decisions on treatment, preventative care, and personalized medicine. By combining these data, clinicians can gain insights into how genetic variations may affect a patient's risk for disease, their response to a medication, and the course of the disease. In addition, it increases the accuracy of diagnoses as physicians can now evaluate both environmental and genetic components to determine a given patient's health condition. Combining genomic data with EHRs not only enables clinical decision support but also allows seamless communication between providers, which is especially helpful in coordinating care for complex genetic disorders. Moreover, it provides data-driven insights to facilitate predictive analytics and reach at-risk patients with timely care interventions. However, for this integration to be successful, concerns about privacy and security must be addressed, and patient data must be kept private while allowing genomic data to effectively contribute to the practice of medicine [54, 55].

Blockchain for Secure and Transparent Data Sharing

Blockchain technology offers a promising opportunity to provide secure and transparent sharing of genomic data, which will address genomic privacy, genomic data integrity, and patients' consent issues. Blockchain offers a decentralized ledger that tracks each transaction or data exchange, which makes genomic data immutable and accountable. Through the use of blockchain, patients can be empowered to maintain access to their genetic data. Still, it also allows certain researchers or healthcare providers access on a permissioned basis, so they are the only parties that have proper access to their data. Furthermore, blockchain ensures that data exchanges are securely recorded in a transparent manner, which minimizes the risk of data breaches or unauthorized access. Such a responsibility is particularly critical in genomic medicine, where data sharing is a prerequisite for practice and research, but where this data sharing must be done responsibly. Also, blockchain enables the generation of smart contracts that automatically enforce data-sharing agreements, streamlining the consent process and lowering the administrative burden. Blockchain technology enables the secure, efficient, and transparent sharing of genomic data, leading to more collaborative research and faster progress in genomic medicine [56].

CHALLENGES AND ETHICAL CONSIDERATIONS

Table **1** highlights the challenges and corresponding ethical issues that must be navigated when implementing genomic medicine and personalized healthcare.

Table 1. Challenges and ethical considerations associated with genomic medicine and personalized healthcare.

S. No.	Challenges	Ethical Considerations
1	**Data Privacy and Security:** Risks associated with data privacy violations, unauthorized access, and misuse of sensitive genetic data range from management difficulties to entire government laws [57].	**Informed Consent:** In providing genetic data, patients need to be aware of the inherent risks, benefits, and possible consequences [62].
2	**Access and Equity:** Limited access to genomic technologies in underprivileged or rural areas can create disparities in healthcare [58].	**Discrimination & Stigmatization** These include the potential for genetic information to be used to discriminate against individuals in areas such as employment or insurance [63].
3	**Data Interpretation and Accuracy:** The complexity of genomic data makes it impossible to reliably interpret genetic variants and predict risks for diseases [59].	**Ownership of Genetic Data:** Ethical dilemmas arise over who owns and controls genetic data, whether it's the individual or the healthcare provider/researcher [64].
4	**Ownership of Genetic Data:** This brings about ethical dilemmas of whether genetic data is owned and controlled by the individual or the healthcare provider/researcher [60].	**Autonomy and Genetic Counseling:** The ethical issues come with the need to guarantee access to genetic counseling and rational patient decision-making [65].

(Table 1) cont.....

S. No.	Challenges	Ethical Considerations
5	**Incorporation into Clinical Practice:** Genomic medicine will be continuously translated into routine clinical practice, which will necessitate widespread training, standardization, and infrastructure [61].	**Equity in Access to Personalized Healthcare:** There is a risk that personalized treatments may only be available to wealthier individuals, exacerbating health inequalities [66].

FUTURE PROSPECTS

The future of medicine lies in genomic medicine and personalized healthcare with unparalleled precision, effective, and individualized treatment. The rapid momentum of genomics will eventually allow the integration of genomic information into routine clinical practice, guiding our understanding of genetic susceptibility to disease, earlier detection, and precise interventions. Drug effects will be improved, and side effects will be reduced, leading towards precision therapies for cancer, cardiovascular diseases, and neurological disorders, enabled by tailored therapies informed by the genetic makeup of an individual. The increasing access to genome sequencing technologies and improvements in bioinformatics and data analytics, in turn, will enable the provision of continuous health information for everybody in the future to mitigate human health management from reactive to proactive health management [67].

Gene editing tools like CRISPR have the potential to repair genetic mutations and prevent hereditary diseases, a remarkable move as we shift towards curative therapy. With genomics being melded with artificial intelligence and big data analytics, healthcare systems will be able to identify disease outbreaks, tailor treatment regimens, and develop tailored health plans based on continuous data streams from wearables and electronic health records. However, with these advancements, the ethical questions of genetic privacy, data safety, and the potential for genetic discrimination must be solved to ensure equitable access to genomic medicine and trust in genomics. Basically, genomic medicine has been changing how healthcare is delivered, making it more interactive, personal, and efficient [68].

CONCLUSION

Genomic medicine and personalized healthcare are revolutionizing the way we understand and manage health and disease. Utilizing the advances in the field of genomics, such as next-generation sequencing, gene editing, and whole-genome sequencing, it is now possible to provide more accurate and personalized treatments to patients, leading to higher efficacies and fewer side effects. Personalized medicine has the potential to transform multiple aspects of medicine, including oncology, pharmacogenomics, and the treatment of rare genetic diseases. Artificial intelligence, machine learning, big data, and bioinformatics are all key to the interpretation of complicated genomic data, aiding in diagnosis and enabling individualized treatment plans. To fully leverage these innovations, challenges related to data privacy, ethical issues surrounding genomic changes, and equity surrounding the delivery of genomic healthcare must be addressed. In the future, robust systems must be established to foster trust in genomic medicine, particularly in terms of data security, informed patient consent, and access. Healthcare will pivot around the personalization of treatment, all based on the genetic makeup of an individual, allowing for the prevention and treatment of the disease to be more timely and efficient. As research and technology continue to improve, genomic medicine could transform the healthcare system into a more affordable, equal, and effective provision for everyone.

REFERENCES

[1]   Pattan V, Kashyap R, Bansal V, Candula N, Koritala T, Surani S. Genomics in medicine: A new era in medicine. World J Methodol 2021; 11(5): 231-42.
        [http://dx.doi.org/10.5662/wjm.v11.i5.231] [PMID: 34631481]

[2]   Aggarwal S, Phadke SR. Medical genetics and genomic medicine in India: current status and opportunities ahead. Mol Genet Genomic Med 2015; 3(3): 160-71.
        [http://dx.doi.org/10.1002/mgg3.150] [PMID: 26029702]

[3]   Adapa CS. Eliminating duplicate medical records: How modern solutions are revolutionizing healthcare data management. J Comp Sci Tech Stud 2025; 7(2): 496-505.

[4]   Wickramasinghe N. The role for knowledge management in modern healthcare delivery. Int J Healthc Deliv Reform Initiatives 2010; 2(2): 1-9.
        [http://dx.doi.org/10.4018/jhdri.2010040101]

[5]   Xia M. Features of the modern healthcare management system. Public Administration and Regional Development 2024; 25(25): 900-20.
        [http://dx.doi.org/10.34132/pard2024.25.09]

[6]   Linder JE, Bastarache L, Hughey JJ, Peterson JF. The role of electronic health records in advancing genomic medicine. Annu Rev Genomics Hum Genet 2021; 22(1): 219-38.
        [http://dx.doi.org/10.1146/annurev-genom-121120-125204] [PMID: 34038146]

[7]   Prabhod KJ. The role of machine learning in genomic medicine: advancements in disease prediction and treatment. J Deep Learn Genomic Data Anal 2022; 2(1): 1-52.

[8]   Schuler GD, Boguski MS, Stewart EA, *et al.* A gene map of the human genome. Science 1996; 274(5287): 540-6.
        [http://dx.doi.org/10.1126/science.274.5287.540] [PMID: 8849440]

[9]   Nurk S, Koren S, Rhie A, *et al.* The complete sequence of a human genome. Science 2022; 376(6588): 44-53.
        [http://dx.doi.org/10.1126/science.abj6987] [PMID: 35357919]

[10]   Finishing the euchromatic sequence of the human genome. Nature 2004; 431(7011): 931-45.
        [http://dx.doi.org/10.1038/nature03001] [PMID: 15496913]

[11]   Jain N, Nagaich U, Pandey M, Chellappan DK, Dua K. Predictive genomic tools in disease stratification and targeted prevention: a recent update in personalized therapy advancements. EPMA J 2022; 13(4): 561-80.

[http://dx.doi.org/10.1007/s13167-022-00304-2] [PMID: 36505888]

[12]   Motsinger-Reif AA, Reif DM, Akhtari FS, *et al.* Gene-environment interactions within a precision environmental health framework. Cell Genomics 2024; 4(7): 100591.
[http://dx.doi.org/10.1016/j.xgen.2024.100591] [PMID: 38925123]

[13]   Cleeren E, Van der Heyden J, Brand A, Van Oyen H. Public health in the genomic era: will Public Health Genomics contribute to major changes in the prevention of common diseases? Arch Public Health 2011; 69(1): 8.
[http://dx.doi.org/10.1186/0778-7367-69-8] [PMID: 22958637]

[14]   Zimmern RL, Khoury MJ. The impact of genomics on public health practice: the case for change. Public Health Genomics 2012; 15(3-4): 118-24.
[http://dx.doi.org/10.1159/000334840] [PMID: 22488453]

[15]   Doble B, Schofield DJ, Roscioli T, Mattick JS. Prioritising the application of genomic medicine. NPJ Genom Med 2017; 2(1): 35.
[http://dx.doi.org/10.1038/s41525-017-0037-0] [PMID: 29263844]

[16]   Scott RH, Fowler TA, Caulfield M. Genomic medicine: time for health-care transformation. Lancet 2019; 394(10197): 454-6.
[http://dx.doi.org/10.1016/S0140-6736(19)31796-9] [PMID: 31395438]

[17]   Vincent AT, Derome N, Boyle B, Culley AI, Charette SJ. Next-generation sequencing (NGS) in the microbiological world: How to make the most of your money. J Microbiol Methods 2017; 138: 60-71.
[http://dx.doi.org/10.1016/j.mimet.2016.02.016] [PMID: 26995332]

[18]   Grada A, Weinbrecht K. Next-generation sequencing: methodology and application. J Invest Dermatol 2013; 133(8): 1-4.
[http://dx.doi.org/10.1038/jid.2013.248] [PMID: 23856935]

[19]   Adli M. The CRISPR tool kit for genome editing and beyond. Nat Commun 2018; 9(1): 1911.
[http://dx.doi.org/10.1038/s41467-018-04252-2] [PMID: 29765029]

[20]   Liu H, Wei Z, Dominguez A, Li Y, Wang X, Qi LS. CRISPR-ERA: a comprehensive design tool for CRISPR-mediated gene editing, repression and activation. Bioinformatics 2015; 31(22): 3676-8.
[http://dx.doi.org/10.1093/bioinformatics/btv423] [PMID: 26209430]

[21]   Xie X, Ma X, Zhu Q, Zeng D, Li G, Liu YG. CRISPR-GE: a convenient software toolkit for CRISPR-based genome editing. Mol Plant 2017; 10(9): 1246-9.
[http://dx.doi.org/10.1016/j.molp.2017.06.004] [PMID: 28624544]

[22]   Balloux F, Brønstad Brynildsrud O, van Dorp L, *et al.* From theory to practice: translating whole-genome sequencing (WGS) into the clinic. Trends Microbiol 2018; 26(12): 1035-48.
[http://dx.doi.org/10.1016/j.tim.2018.08.004] [PMID: 30193960]

[23]   Brlek P, Bulić L, Bračić M, *et al.* Implementing whole genome sequencing (WGS) in clinical practice: advantages, challenges, and future perspectives. Cells 2024; 13(6): 504.
[http://dx.doi.org/10.3390/cells13060504] [PMID: 38534348]

[24]   Carattoli A, Hasman H. PlasmidFinder and in silico pMLST: identification and typing of plasmid replicons in whole-genome sequencing (WGS). Horiz Gene Transf Methods Protoc 2020; pp. 285-94.

[25]   Greenbaum D, Luscombe NM, Jansen R, Qian J, Gerstein M. Interrelating different types of genomic data, from proteome to secretome: 'oming in on function. Genome Res 2001; 11(9): 1463-8.
[http://dx.doi.org/10.1101/gr.207401] [PMID: 11544189]

[26]   Naj AC, Schellenberg GD. Genomic variants, genes, and pathways of Alzheimer's disease: An overview. Am J Med Genet B Neuropsychiatr Genet 2017; 174(1): 5-26.
[http://dx.doi.org/10.1002/ajmg.b.32499] [PMID: 27943641]

[27]   Abecasis GR, Altshuler D, Auton A, *et al.* A map of human genome variation from population-scale sequencing. Nature 2010; 467(7319): 1061-73.

[http://dx.doi.org/10.1038/nature09534] [PMID: 20981092]

[28]   Rafalski A. Applications of single nucleotide polymorphisms in crop genetics. Curr Opin Plant Biol 2002; 5(2): 94-100.
[http://dx.doi.org/10.1016/S1369-5266(02)00240-6] [PMID: 11856602]

[29]   Gupta PK, Roy JK, Prasad M. Single nucleotide polymorphisms: a new paradigm for molecular marker technology and DNA polymorphism detection with emphasis on their use in plants. Curr Sci 2001; 524-35.

[30]   Tiryaki EU. The significance of personalized medicine in healthcare services of the 21st century: a brief literature review. Eur Respir J 2024; 10(6): 1-8.

[31]   Yuan B. What personalized medicine humans need and way to it—also on the practical significance and scientific limitations of precision medicine. Pharmacogenomics Pers Med 2022; 927-42.

[32]   Brown AE. The place of intellectual property under the BBNJ Agreement. In: Decoding Marine Genetic Resource Governance Under the BBNJ Agreement. Cham: Springer Nature Switzerland 2025; pp. 213-224.
[http://dx.doi.org/10.1007/978-3-031-72100-7_9]

[33]   Strianese O, Rizzo F, Ciccarelli M, *et al.* Precision and personalized medicine: how genomic approach improves the management of cardiovascular and neurodegenerative disease. Genes (Basel) 2020; 11(7): 747.
[http://dx.doi.org/10.3390/genes11070747] [PMID: 32640513]

[34]   Micaglio E, Locati ET, Monasky MM, Romani F, Heilbron F, Pappone C. Role of pharmacogenetics in adverse drug reactions: an update towards personalized medicine. Front Pharmacol 2021; 12: 651720.
[http://dx.doi.org/10.3389/fphar.2021.651720] [PMID: 33995067]

[35]   Recharla M, Chakilam C, Kannan S, Nuka ST, Suura SR. Harnessing AI and Machine Learning for Precision Medicine: Advancements in Genomic Research, Disease Detection, and Personalized Healthcare. Amer J Psych Rehab. 2025 Apr 9;28(1):112-23.

[36]   Hodgson DR, Wellings R, Harbron C. Practical perspectives of personalized healthcare in oncology. N Biotechnol 2012; 29(6): 656-64.
[http://dx.doi.org/10.1016/j.nbt.2012.03.001] [PMID: 22426411]

[37]   Butts C, Kamel-Reid S, Batist G, *et al.* Benefits, issues, and recommendations for personalized medicine in oncology in Canada. Curr Oncol 2013; 20(5): 475-83.
[http://dx.doi.org/10.3747/co.20.1253] [PMID: 24155644]

[38]   Weinshilboum RM, Wang L. Pharmacogenomics: precision medicine and drug response. Mayo Clin Proc 2017; 92(11): 1711-22.
[http://dx.doi.org/10.1016/j.mayocp.2017.09.001] [PMID: 29101939]

[39]   Hassan R, Allali I, Agamah FE, *et al.* Drug response in association with pharmacogenomics and pharmacomicrobiomics: towards a better personalized medicine. Brief Bioinform 2021; 22(4): bbaa292.
[http://dx.doi.org/10.1093/bib/bbaa292] [PMID: 33253350]

[40]   Sun W, Zheng W, Simeonov A. Drug discovery and development for rare genetic disorders. Am J Med Genet A 2017; 173(9): 2307-22.
[http://dx.doi.org/10.1002/ajmg.a.38326] [PMID: 28731526]

[41]   Kruer MC, Steiner RD. The role of evidence□based medicine and clinical trials in rare genetic disorders. Clin Genet 2008; 74(3): 197-207.
[http://dx.doi.org/10.1111/j.1399-0004.2008.01041.x] [PMID: 18657147]

[42]   Koch PJ, Koster MI. Rare genetic disorders: novel treatment strategies and insights into human biology. Front Genet 2021; 12: 714764.
[http://dx.doi.org/10.3389/fgene.2021.714764] [PMID: 34422015]

[43] Casanova JL, Abel L. Human genetics of infectious diseases: Unique insights into immunological redundancy. Semin Immunol 2018; 36: 1-12.
[http://dx.doi.org/10.1016/j.smim.2017.12.008] [PMID: 29254755]

[44] Burton H, Jackson C, Abubakar I. The impact of genomics on public health practice. Br Med Bull 2014; 112(1): 37-46.
[http://dx.doi.org/10.1093/bmb/ldu032] [PMID: 25368375]

[45] Chapman SJ, Hill AVS. Human genetic susceptibility to infectious disease. Nat Rev Genet 2012; 13(3): 175-88.
[http://dx.doi.org/10.1038/nrg3114] [PMID: 22310894]

[46] Florea GP. Bench and Bedside Medicine: A One-Way Contamination. In: Metacognition and Medical Humanities in Medical Education: The Missing Link in Medical Thinking. Cham: Springer Nature Switzerland 2025; pp. 41-56.
[http://dx.doi.org/10.1007/978-3-032-01070-4_4]

[47] Wei L, Niraula D, Gates EDH, *et al.* Artificial intelligence (AI) and machine learning (ML) in precision oncology: a review on enhancing discoverability through multiomics integration. Br J Radiol 2023; 96(1150): 20230211.
[http://dx.doi.org/10.1259/bjr.20230211] [PMID: 37660402]

[48] Valafar F. Pattern recognition techniques in microarray data analysis: a survey. Ann N Y Acad Sci 2002; 980(1): 41-64.
[http://dx.doi.org/10.1111/j.1749-6632.2002.tb04888.x] [PMID: 12594081]

[49] Dias R, Torkamani A. Artificial intelligence in clinical and genomic diagnostics. Genome Med 2019; 11(1): 70.
[http://dx.doi.org/10.1186/s13073-019-0689-8] [PMID: 31744524]

[50] Dlamini Z, Skepu A, Kim N, *et al.* AI and precision oncology in clinical cancer genomics: From prevention to targeted cancer therapies-an outcomes based patient care. Inform Med Unlocked 2022; 31: 100965.
[http://dx.doi.org/10.1016/j.imu.2022.100965]

[51] O'Driscoll A, Daugelaite J, Sleator RD. 'Big data', Hadoop and cloud computing in genomics. J Biomed Inform 2013; 46(5): 774-81.
[http://dx.doi.org/10.1016/j.jbi.2013.07.001] [PMID: 23872175]

[52] Yang J. Cloud computing for storing and analyzing petabytes of genomic data. J Ind Inf Integr 2019; 15: 50-7.
[http://dx.doi.org/10.1016/j.jii.2019.04.005]

[53] Calderón-González KG, Hernández-Monge J, Herrera-Aguirre ME, Luna-Arias JP. Bioinformatics tools for proteomics data interpretation. Adv Exp Med Biol 2016; 919: 281-341.

[54] Lau-Min KS, McKenna D, Asher SB, *et al.* Impact of integrating genomic data into the electronic health record on genetics care delivery. Genet Med 2022; 24(11): 2338-50.
[http://dx.doi.org/10.1016/j.gim.2022.08.009] [PMID: 36107166]

[55] Warner JL, Jain SK, Levy MA. Integrating cancer genomic data into electronic health records. Genome Med 2016; 8(1): 113.
[http://dx.doi.org/10.1186/s13073-016-0371-3] [PMID: 27784327]

[56] Tatineni S. Blockchain and data science integration for secure and transparent data sharing. Int J Adv Res Eng Technol 2019; 10(3): 470-80.

[57] Bonomi L, Huang Y, Ohno-Machado L. Privacy challenges and research opportunities for genomic data sharing. Nat Genet 2020; 52(7): 646-54.
[http://dx.doi.org/10.1038/s41588-020-0651-0] [PMID: 32601475]

[58] Simon R. Interpretation of genomic data: questions and answers. Semin Hematol 2008; 45(3): 196-

204.
[http://dx.doi.org/10.1053/j.seminhematol.2008.04.008] [PMID: 18582627]

[59]   Sayitoğlu M. Clinical interpretation of genomic variations. Turk J Haematol 2016; 33(3): 172-9.
[http://dx.doi.org/10.4274/tjh.2016.0149] [PMID: 27507302]

[60]   Piasecki J, Cheah PY. Ownership of individual-level health data, data sharing, and data governance.
BMC Med Ethics 2022; 23(1): 104.
[http://dx.doi.org/10.1186/s12910-022-00848-y] [PMID: 36309719]

[61]   Riess O, Sturm M, Menden B, *et al.* Genomes in clinical care. NPJ Genom Med 2024; 9(1): 20.
[http://dx.doi.org/10.1038/s41525-024-00402-2] [PMID: 38485733]

[62]   McGuire AL, Beskow LM. Informed consent in genomics and genetic research. Annu Rev Genomics
Hum Genet 2010; 11(1): 361-81.
[http://dx.doi.org/10.1146/annurev-genom-082509-141711] [PMID: 20477535]

[63]   Crumb SI. An evaluation framework to assess educational genetic websites: Are they meeting public
needs? [Master's thesis]. Seattle (WA): University of Washington 2013.

[64]   Malakar Y, Lacey J, Twine NA, McCrea R, Bauer DC. Balancing the safeguarding of privacy and data
sharing: perceptions of genomic professionals on patient genomic data ownership in Australia. Eur J
Hum Genet 2024; 32(5): 506-12.
[http://dx.doi.org/10.1038/s41431-022-01273-w] [PMID: 36631540]

[65]   El-Hazmi MAF. Ethics of genetic counseling—basic concepts and relevance to Islamic communities.
Ann Saudi Med 2004; 24(2): 84-92.
[http://dx.doi.org/10.5144/0256-4947.2004.84] [PMID: 15323267]

[66]   Hazin R, Brothers KB, Malin BA, *et al.* Ethical, legal, and social implications of incorporating
genomic information into electronic health records. Genet Med 2013; 15(10): 810-6.
[http://dx.doi.org/10.1038/gim.2013.117] [PMID: 24030434]

[67]   Johnson KB, Wei WQ, Weeraratne D, *et al.* Precision medicine, AI, and the future of personalized
health care. Clin Transl Sci 2021; 14(1): 86-93.
[http://dx.doi.org/10.1111/cts.12884] [PMID: 32961010]

[68]   Potter BK, Avard D, Graham ID, *et al.* Guidance for considering ethical, legal, and social issues in
health technology assessment: Application to genetic screening. Int J Technol Assess Health Care
2008; 24(4): 412-22.
[http://dx.doi.org/10.1017/S0266462308080549] [PMID: 18828935]

CHAPTER 5

Telehealth and Virtual Consultations

Jyoti Pandey[1,*], **Ganna Rajan**[2], **Gunjan**[1] and **Shaweta Sharma**[1]

[1] *Department of Pharmacy, School of Medical and Allied Sciences, Galgotias University, Greater Noida, Uttar Pradesh-201310, India*

[2] *Department of Pharmacy, SGRR University, Dehradun, Uttarkhand-248001, India*

Abstract: In the present scenario, with the advancement in technology, a new feature called Telemedicine has been introduced. Telemedicine is a blend of information and communication technologies (ICTs) with medical science. The virtual consultation is a part of telemedicine. The primary difference between a virtual consultation and a typical one is that it enables you to obtain a medical opinion without physically meeting the physician. Online consultations also allow doctors to communicate with other physicians and access various electronic medical records to support patient care. In the past two years, during the COVID-19 pandemic, we have seen that people prefer telemedicine over face-to-face interaction because it is considered safer. Fortunately, telemedicine and virtual consultations *via* video conferencing or other digital platforms can reduce the number of doctor visits and relieve patients of the time and expenses associated with traveling. Hence, telemedicine is fruitful in reducing treatment costs and saving time for patients and healthcare practitioners. Additionally, due to its quick and useful features, it helps improve hospital and clinic workflow. It would be simpler to monitor discharged patients and oversee their recovery with the help of this revolutionary technology. The primary goal of telemedicine and virtual consultation is to deliver high-quality healthcare services throughout India. This involves making healthcare more accessible to both affluent and impoverished communities, offering quicker, less expensive, and better communication for treatment, expert follow-up, and record storage. Geographical barriers to healthcare are lessened, particularly when it comes to reaching remote locations with inadequate transportation connections. Therefore, it can be concluded that telemedicine offers mutual benefits for both patients and healthcare providers. However, achieving its full potential is fraught with difficulties. This chapter explores several key legal and ethical issues relevant to the practice of telemedicine and virtual consultations, including the doctor-patient relationship, informed consent, patient rights, treatment workflow, malpractice, and confidentiality standards.

Keywords: Healthcare, Medical care, Telemedicine, Virtual consultation, Virtual technologies.

---

* Corresponding author Jyoti Pandey: Department of Pharmacy, School of Medical and Allied Sciences, Galgotias University, Greater Noida, Uttar Pradesh-201310, India; E-mail: jpandey1112@gmail.com

Shaweta Sharma, Akhil Sharma, Shivkanya Fuloria & Anurag Singh (Eds.)
All rights reserved-© 2025 Bentham Science Publishers

INTRODUCTION

Improved healthcare and greater accessibility for more people are made possible by cutting-edge technology and high-quality network services. One especially helpful tool that helps people maintain their long-term health and access preventive treatment is telemedicine. This is particularly beneficial for individuals who struggle to access high-quality healthcare due to budgetary or geographical limitations. The efficiency, organization, and accessibility of healthcare could all be enhanced by telehealth. This is a relatively new field of study, but it is growing rapidly. For instance, treating people with heart problems over the phone and remotely monitoring their vital signs has improved their overall quality of life while reducing their risk of hospitalization and mortality. People seek a diagnosis or rehabilitation plan for a variety of compelling reasons. As a result, patients may feel more assured that they are receiving the best possible care. Since telemedicine eliminates some of the obstacles that prevent patients from accessing this crucial kind of therapy, it is an excellent choice for treating mental health issues [1 - 3].

Patients can receive safe medical care *via* telemedicine at a mutually convenient time. This eliminates the need to take time off work or arrange childcare. When visiting a doctor's office, sitting close to other people increases the risk of infection, particularly for individuals with weakened immune systems or those with long-term medical conditions. Telemedicine lowers the risk of hospital-acquired infections. Additionally, doctors can earn more money by treating more patients online, and telemedicine companies can incur lower operational expenses. Patients are likely to be happier since they do not have to drive to the office, wait for treatment, or risk contracting an illness in the hospital, while caregivers are shielded from any infections from patients [4, 5].

The ability of medical professionals to treat multiple patients virtually has improved due to telemedicine. Telemedicine is likely to remain a viable option for a while, now that its worth has been established. Many physicians were first exposed to telehealth through video conferencing, but emerging telemedicine technology will deliver much more. For example, specialists can contribute remotely during crises, and clinicians can utilize natural language processing to automatically take notes during patient sessions. An Internet of Things (IoT) cloud platform may receive data gathered from medical equipment and organize it for use in patient care [6 - 8].

Patients in remote locations can greatly benefit from telemedicine, particularly in countries with limited or no healthcare services. Secure technology and software are necessary for both patients and physicians to maintain accurate medical information. When an in-person visit is not required, some clinics allow patients to continue receiving treatment from their normal physician by offering virtual meetings with doctors *via* online video conversations. Online consultations with a physician or nurse practitioner are an additional choice. These days, many large businesses incorporate automated health kiosks into their healthcare offerings. There are also nursing call centers where nurses provide home care guidance through question-and-answer sessions [9 - 11]. Prescription refills, taking blood pressure medication, and remembering appointments are all made possible by this technology, which supports health management. Additionally, patients may self-test, participate in specialized training programs for their condition, and consult physicians regarding their symptoms. In general, electronic health technology facilitates the management of chronic conditions by providing patients with access to treatment *via* smartphones and monitoring applications [12, 13].

Many believe that technology-assisted consultations help address many of the challenges in delivering healthcare to an aging and increasingly diverse population. Long-term results for major disorders like cancer are improving, and more individuals feel comfortable taking charge of their health, despite the health system's struggles with growing rates of long-term illness and reliance. According to the UK's National Information Board, to successfully address these health and demographic changes, a new type of healthcare system is required — one that reduces the prevalence of typical outpatient visits, for instance [14].

In addition to providing patients with advantages such as reduced travel expenses and discomfort, remote consultations can also be more economical for the healthcare system. Nonetheless, there are concerns that they could pose clinical hazards or be less palatable to staff and patients, as they can present logistical, technological, and legal difficulties. Research on remote consultations *via* video technology, such as Skype, is still in its infancy but is beginning to expand [15 - 17]. Specifically, a recent analysis identified 27 published studies on Skype's usage in clinical care, all but one of which not advantages [17].

Some of these studies involved as few as five patients, while the majority were brief descriptions of modest, early-stage programs. This evaluation includes a few more current studies as well as the higher-quality primary publications from Arnfield and colleagues that are relevant to our research. A study on family-based behavioral support for adolescents with poorly managed type 1 diabetes mellitus focused on the "working alliance," or the strength of the relationship between patients, caregivers, and medical professionals [18]. The authors found that ten Skype meetings were equally effective as ten in-person meetings in maintaining the working relationship [19].

The in-person and Skype groups showed similar levels of medication adherence and glucose control [20]. However, there were notable follow-up losses: follow-up data were accessible for just 32 out of 47 (out of 92) randomly assigned to Skype. Skype has been used to treat several chronic illnesses. Participants who got Skype treatment, however, had noticeably higher outcomes than those who attended in-person sessions at the 36-week follow-up. The authors hypothesised that these long-term advantages may have resulted from the increased attention paid to Skype sessions. A second explanation is offered by another study on Skype-enabled older persons that examined increased social interaction: Skype could be a useful tool for boosting social integration, which in turn could improve mental health [21, 22].

The use of Skype for orthopaedic follow-up treatment was investigated in a 2014 study [23]. Following complete joint replacement surgery, 78 individuals were eligible for the program. In addition to their routine follow-up sessions, participants were asked to have Skype consultations with their surgeon at five different intervals: one, three, four, six, and nine weeks. Of the 78 participants in the trial, 34 participated in at least one Skype consultation; however, 44 could not access the program due to insufficient equipment or internet connectivity. Although the study may not have been adequately powered to detect such a difference, no significant difference in clinical outcomes was observed between users and non-users. Those who were contacted by Skype, however, made fewer impromptu in-clinic visits or phoned the workplace to seek medical guidance. Postoperative satisfaction was greater among those who had a Skype consultation than among those who did not. The authors of a follow-up study on 228 participants, which included the initial sample, discovered that the Skype group had reduced patient-borne expenses and consultation time [24]. According to a related economic analysis, the Skype group also had much reduced service costs [25]. Although no patient had an "issue missed," a note accompanying it suggested that remote evaluation might not be as secure [26].

What is Virtual Consultation and Telemedicine?

The term "telemedicine" literally translates to "healing from a distance." In order to improve the health of individuals and communities, the World Health Organization defines it as the provision of healthcare services, where distance is a major factor, by medical professionals using information and communication technologies to share precise information for the diagnosis, treatment, and prevention of illnesses and injuries, as well as for research and evaluations and continuing education for healthcare providers [27]. The primary difference between a virtual consultation and a traditional medical consultation is that it enables you to obtain a medical opinion without physically seeing the physician

[28]. To review different electronic medical records, a doctor can also initiate a chat session with another doctor using virtual consultations [29]. Providing high-quality healthcare services throughout India is the main objective of telemedicine and virtual consultations. This entails enhancing access to healthcare for both affluent and impoverished populations by providing quicker, more economical, and improved communication for treatment, professional follow-ups, and record-keeping. Geographical obstacles are lessened by it, especially in isolated areas with limited transit options.

Why is Telemedicine Necessary for the Healthcare System?

Due to rising healthcare costs and patients' increasing demand for better care, more institutions are exploring the benefits of telemedicine. They aim to improve communication between doctors and patients who live far away and optimize the use of healthcare resources. Enhancing connectivity through telemedicine reduces hospital readmissions and improves patient adherence to treatment plans. Given that telemedicine enables physicians to establish support systems, share expertise, and deliver superior medical care, the advantages of increased communication also extend to doctor-to-doctor relationships. Telemedicine is a useful means of providing medical treatment online, typically through video conferencing, which enhances the patient experience, despite still encountering technological issues and detractors [30 - 32].

DATA EXTRACTION AND EVALUATION OF BIAS RISK

After testing and refining the data abstraction forms using a small number of studies, two team members independently retrieved data on study characteristics, demographics, interventions, and outcomes. They also assessed the risk of bias for the included studies using the ROBINS-I tool [33], which is used for non-randomized research, and the Cochrane Risk of Bias Tool, Version 2 for randomized controlled trials (RCTs) [34]. The team members reached a resolution to settle any disputes regarding the possibility of bias. The danger of bias was not screened for or evaluated by the study's authors.

Medicolegal Issues

(Fig. **1**) illustrates the various medicolegal issues associated with data extraction.

Doctor-Patient Relationship

When seeking therapy, patients trust and confide in medical professionals. One perceived obstacle to the proper doctor-patient relationship is the lack of in-person interaction in certain telemedicine modalities [35]. Maintaining the patient's confidence is crucial to fulfilling legal obligations. It is the responsibility of healthcare practitioners to build positive doctor-patient interactions [36].

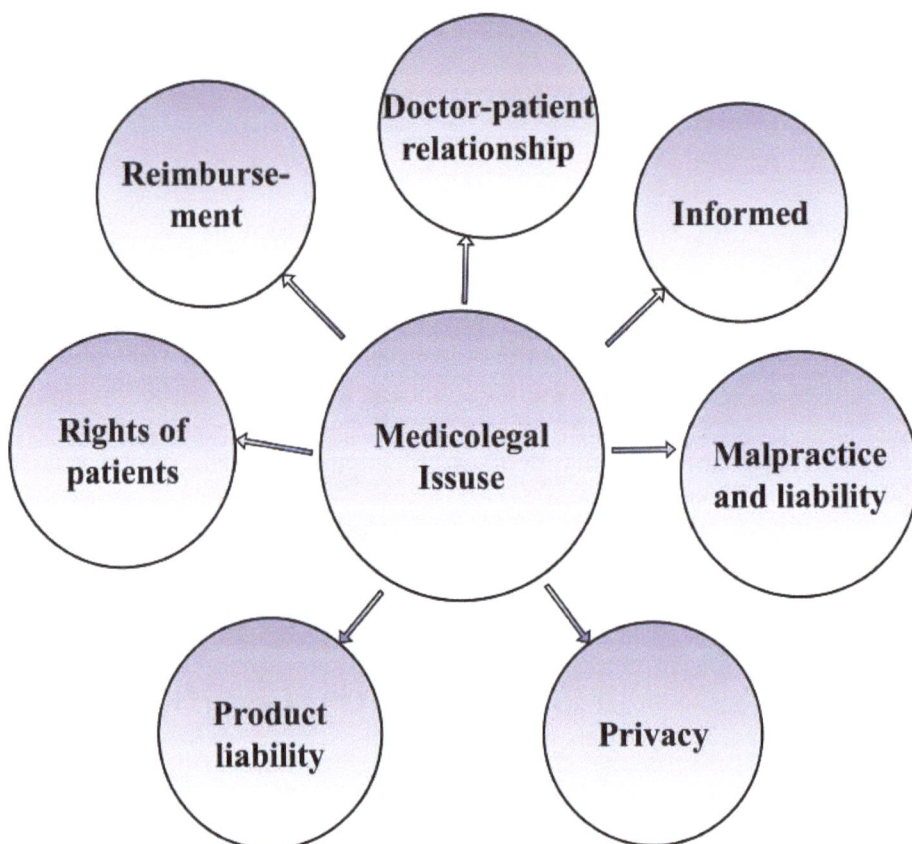

Fig. (1). Medicolegal issues

Informed Consent

When treating a patient, informed consent is a crucial medicolegal necessity; failing to obtain it is a crime and a tort [36]. Any medical engagement, whether it occurs in person or virtually through telemedicine or virtual consultation, should require informed consent [37]. Data transfer, therapy, monitoring, consultations, and telemedicine interactions all require consent. Determining whether the medicolegal importance of informed consent *via* telemedicine is similar to or different from that in conventional in-person encounters is also crucial [38]. There is sufficient proof that video conferences and other virtual consultations are therapeutically equivalent to in-person consultations in many specialties [39 - 41]. It is possible to obtain informed consent and document it properly. The 2009 Guiding Principles Regarding the Implementation of Telemedicine in Healthcare, issued by the World Medical Association, highlight this. Malaysia, France, the United Kingdom, South Africa, and California, USA, all need informed consent for telemedicine [37].

Malpractice and Liability

Following the establishment of the doctor–patient relationship, the doctor must treat the patient with the care and attention expected from a professional under similar circumstances [38]. It is important to consider whether medical indemnity insurance covers doctors for telemedicine and virtual consultations, including protection against potential claims of medical misconduct [35]. Every telemedicine encounter must include a "duty of care" defining the responsibilities of the patient or caregiver and all participating healthcare professionals. In relation to the various aspects and scope of treatment, healthcare providers should clearly define their duties and responsibilities.

Privacy

Since Hippocrates' time, the principle of autonomy has been a cornerstone of medical ethics, and regulations, such as the International Code of Medical Ethics, protect it [42]. It mandates that medical professionals maintain the privacy of patient data even after the patient has died. Everyone has the right to privacy, including when it comes to telemedicine [43]. Electronic patient records may be potentially compromised. Protecting this information is the medical professional's obligation [44]. Secure transmission of information is required. Maintaining password security is crucial to prevent unauthorized access to sensitive data. However, using telemedicine does not ensure privacy [39, 45, 46].

Product Liability

If a faulty product causes injury to a patient, the manufacturer is responsible. This implies that the manufacturer, which includes those who create the telemedicine computer systems, accompanying software, telemedicine-related accessories, the network provider, the healthcare service provider utilizing the technology, and the service provider in charge of maintaining the complete telemedicine system, bears the duty of care [36].

Rights of Patients

Patients have acknowledged rights in conventional medical practice, such as the freedom to accept or decline treatment, to choose and switch doctors while receiving treatment, to seek compensation, to maintain confidentiality, to retain dignity, to submit grievances, to obtain information, and to refuse treatment.

These rights likewise cover virtual consultations and telemedicine. Patients have the right to recognize the authorization or registration status of the service provider, the standards and safety guidelines, the electronic format of their medical records, and the complaint procedures they can use if they are harmed during a consultation [46].

Reimbursement

Medical insurance reimbursement is not yet available for telemedicine practices. Another requirement for compensation is whether or not telemedicine was necessary in the particular circumstance [35].

TELEMEDICINE'S CHARACTERISTICS AND CAPABILITIES WHEN INTEGRATED INTO A HEALTHCARE MANAGEMENT SYSTEM

The concept of telemedicine and the services that accompany it are now widely accepted and have been demonstrated to benefit society. The various characteristics and services offered by telemedicine, particularly in the healthcare industry, are illustrated in (Fig. **2**). Ultimately, it enhances the healthcare and medical professions by supporting remote services, promoting prescription adherence, facilitating chronic health management, and providing treatment for patients with serious and critical conditions. Furthermore, telemedicine encompasses a variety of wearable technologies that aid in patient treatment and offer continuous health updates [47, 48].

One cutting-edge technology that is frequently referred to as a disruptive innovation is telemedicine. Telemedicine utilizes a range of electronic communication techniques, including remote patient monitoring, teleconferencing, and image exchange, to connect with patients who reside far away. Moreover, physicians can utilize automation to deliver high-quality care. They must also enhance IT support systems and develop new file management strategies. For instance, primary care physicians can use virtual visits to consult experts when they have concerns about a patient's health or treatment plan. The specialist can respond online and schedule a virtual consultation with the doctor after examining test results, medical history, findings, X-rays, and other images. These virtual consultations can reduce unnecessary travel, shorten wait times for feedback, and do away with the need for unnecessary expert referrals. When a physician can remotely assess a patient, make a diagnosis, and document that encounter, the disease can be effectively managed [49 - 55]. The various features of telemedicine are described in (Fig. **2**)

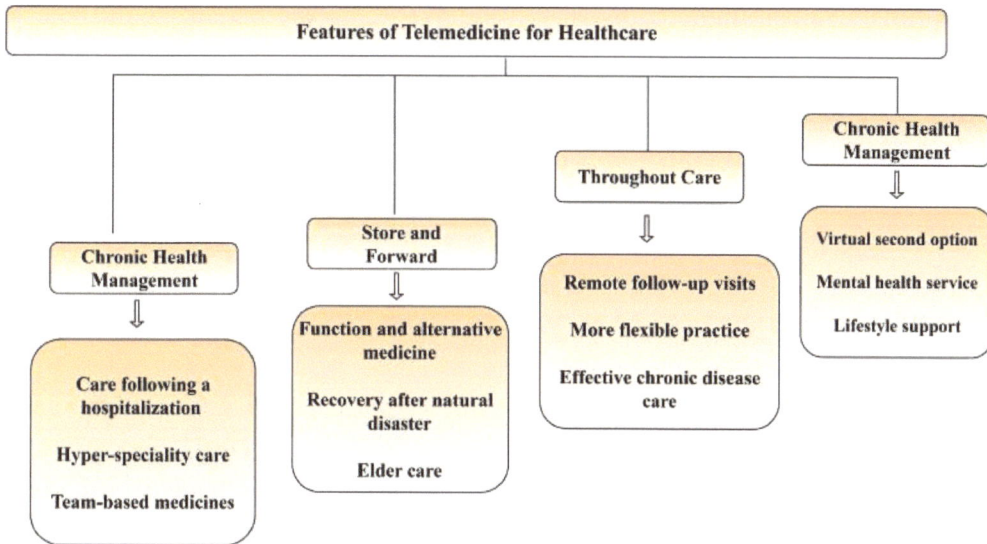

Fig. (2). Several telemedicine features and capabilities for the healthcare industry.

Physicians will greatly benefit from telemedicine options. However, when combined with artificial intelligence (AI), it can be far more effective. Simple activities can be made easier by reducing physician workloads and increasing job satisfaction. The application sends data in a timely and high-quality manner to ensure a smooth appointment. Medical personnel would be able to conduct more comprehensive examinations and search for any abnormalities. Viewing a doctor's open (available) time slots, upcoming appointments, and the ability to postpone them is advised. Healthcare analytics are often used to engage with the gathered data through a user interface. Better utilization of time and money is suggested by long-term storage and forward strategies. A range of electronic gadgets that deliver patient data directly to the analytical interface form the basis of telemonitoring [56, 57].

The medical and telemedicine industries have found this technology to be both beneficial and essential across multiple areas. Notably, it is transforming surgery, medical education, and clinical training. Patients should receive confirmation promptly once the doctor approves the requested appointment. Their accounts may include internal information such as reviews, updates, and critical hospital notifications. Doctors can manage their schedules to set up appointments at their convenience. Scheduling and rescheduling are frequent features of contemporary telemedicine software. When doctors are informed of an appointment, they can access the patient's medical record and other information to deliver accurate consultations and diagnoses [58, 59].Virtual reality (VR) technology has enabled more immersive communication uses for telemedicine equipment. Physicians and their colleagues can now view a 3D display in virtual reality during surgery. Using video conferencing, surgeons and other medical specialists can perform surgery on patients thousands of kilometers away. This enables medical teams on different continents to collaborate and hold video conferences on complex and urgent cases. To achieve this, the population of rural patients will benefit from increased financing for local healthcare, thanks to this technology. Furthermore, this technology may enable all patients to stay with friends and family [60 - 62].

METHOD OF TREATMENT AS IT APPLIES TO TELEMEDICINE CARE

A flowchart depicting the process for implementing culture-based telemedicine therapy in healthcare services is illustrated in (Fig. **2**). It offers state-of-the-art facilities and care at each stage of its implementation. The telehealth supportive care unit is the next step after the patient submits their complete information. This phase also involves assigning the patient to a clinical assistant. Following diagnosis and appropriate therapy or treatment, the patient receives optimal care. (Fig. **3**) illustrates the therapy workflow supported by telemedicine [63, 64].

Telecommunication technologies, such as telemedicine, improve administrative and clinical procedures. This all-inclusive approach provides emergency care for both life-threatening and non-life-threatening situations. It is typically used to treat patients with chronic diseases. A hospital might compensate for telemedicine, though, provided it has the right ambulance crew or other employees. Additionally, the telemedicine system might be extended to incorporate additional elements such as therapy dynamics graphs, e-prescriptions, and the patient's medical history. Additionally, after a consultation, doctors may readily continue to call patients for follow-ups or further discoveries. As a result, text messages are crucial, as they allow doctors to communicate with patients promptly and directly without requiring a follow-up session. Additionally, doctors can share information and prescription drugs between offices [65 - 67].

Healthcare surveillance is essential in the contemporary environment to maintain the standard of healthcare. The usage of digital health tracking services and technology has enabled smart connectivity systems. This technique enables direct patient control and significantly enhances patient insight, all with just basic video conferencing. Using the doctor's catalog saves time for both the patient and the healthcare provider. It improves the accuracy of the doctor-patient therapeutic process. The appointment scheduling tool allows doctors to stay informed about the status of their appointments. Before meeting with a patient, doctors may review their schedules and patient profiles. This allows for the filtering of patient profiles and shows the patient queue. The doctor can now easily reschedule appointments at any time, especially in emergencies. Telemedicine enables cloud-based data storage, including patient records and consultation recordings [68 - 70].

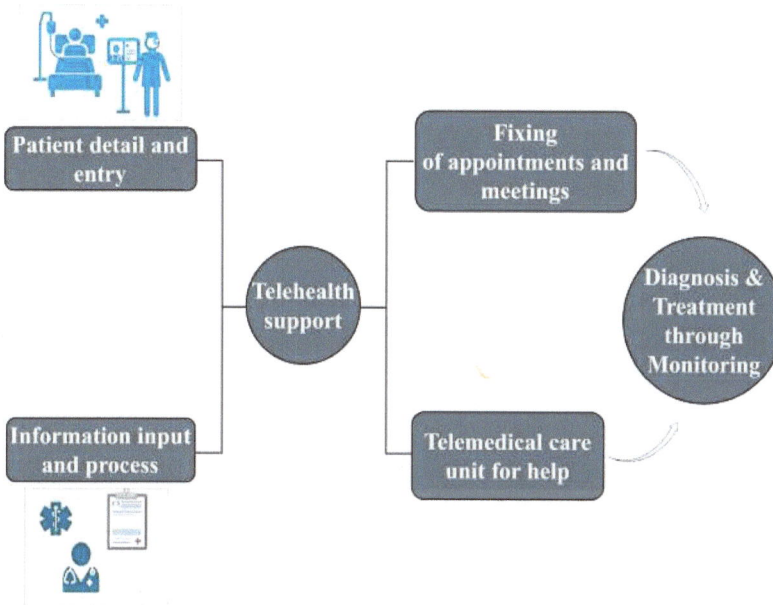

Fig. (3). Workflow therapy procedure with assistance from telemedicine.

The videos and photographs are taking the place of in-person evaluations. Businesses that supply telemedicine application software leverage cloud computing and app connections to enable real-time collaboration and remote patient diagnosis. Both patients and doctors save time by monitoring medical progress and doing the necessary examinations. The telehealth app ensures the easy collection and centralization of patient records. It expedites the delivery of healthcare services, benefiting pharmacies, consumers, and prescribing physicians. Doctors may prescribe and manage medications more accurately with the help of e-prescription functionality. In addition to enhancing communication and patient satisfaction, it also helps save time [71 - 74].

Telemedicine technology in healthcare enhances the quality of care for both patients and healthcare providers. The demand for telemedicine apps on smartphones is increasing and projected to grow further, fueling the industry's ongoing expansion. At electronically connected pharmacies, it enables doctors to access prescription insurance documentation and input relevant information. Mobile billing functionality should be included in all telemedicine applications.

The ability for patients to evaluate and compare healthcare providers is an essential part of any telemedicine program. Patient feedback is considered essential for quality management and professional development. Furthermore, it will help new patients choose the provider best suited to their needs [75, 76].

Telemedicine apps can expedite the treatment of various medical conditions [77, 78]. Technical equipment, such as a video platform and an internet connection, as well as portable equipment, can all help reduce the need for telemedicine technology. Comprehensive healthcare centers can facilitate telemedicine consultations using a scaled-down version of the same equipment. Equally important as hardware selection is the operational support required to run a telemedicine program. For any program to function properly, a compatible computer and technical support are necessary. Physicians always assess the needs based on available resources. The support staff will ensure reliable and secure internet connectivity. It also assists with logistical and technical issues that may arise during a clinic day, thereby avoiding interference with patient care [79 - 81].

Telemedicine has many benefits for medical professionals. Healthcare organizations utilize telemedicine in doctors' offices and skilled nursing facilities to deliver more effective care. When combined with telemedicine software, technology such as AI diagnostics, medical streaming apps, and electronic medical records can help physicians diagnose and treat patients more accurately. The doctors can now monitor patients in real-time and adjust treatment plans accordingly. By using telemedicine, doctors can treat more patients without expanding their workspace or hiring additional staff. However, many medical professionals and patients, particularly senior citizens, are struggling to adjust to telemedicine [82, 83].

KEY APPLICATION AREAS FOR TELEMEDICINE IN HEALTHCARE

Telemedicine technology enables a wide range of treatment options, including primary care consultations, physical therapy, psychotherapy, and many more. To administer treatment, it utilizes wireless devices such as computers and cell phones. Video conferencing is a common tool used in telemedicine. Some firms, however, decide to handle clients *via* phone calls or emails instead. Patients frequently work with their primary care provider in tandem with telemedicine. This technology can be particularly helpful when a patient needs to maintain physical distance or is unable to visit a medical facility. Without maintaining a physical office space, practitioners can offer weekend or extended-hour services. These practices are also increasingly appealing to the growing number of patients who use telemedicine as their primary care provider [84 - 86]. It offers a simple and cost-effective way to help individuals with serious illnesses manage their care, control symptoms, and prevent complications that could compromise their quality of life. The important uses of telemedicine in healthcare are listed in Table 1.

Table 1. Applications of telemedicine in the healthcare industry.

S. No.	Applications	Description	References
1.	Telehealth	Technological developments and innovative approaches in healthcare have greatly increased their relevance. When this technology is applied in healthcare, physicians, researchers, laboratory workers, and clinicians can all benefit from the concept of telehealth. The moment has arrived for medical organizations, hospital systems, and suppliers to incorporate telemedicine into their offerings. To make the process and implementation easier, Many companies also want to collaborate with telemedicine providers. Telemedicine is performed using a telemedicine device, which consists of a computer and portable medical equipment. Doctors also employ high-resolution imaging cameras to provide specialists with precise diagnostic images.	[87 - 90]
2.	Assist patients with disabilities.	Telemedicine improves service accessibility for patients with impairments. Other groups, including older people, those from culturally isolated backgrounds, and those who are jailed, also have easier access. Numerous medical conditions can be treated using telemedicine. It is effective when a patient is treated by a trained practitioner who gives them detailed information about their symptoms. Some publications claim that telemedicine patients save money by staying in the hospital for shorter periods of time. Additionally, shorter travel times may result in lower secondary costs, like gas.	[91 - 94]
3.	Treatment by remote	Virtual remote therapy has been demonstrated to be an effective method of preventing hospitalisation. Patients will avoid long commutes and opt for video visits if they want to see a clinician with highly specialized experience in a specific ailment. Each professional's skills and expertise can be utilized to their fullest potential. Healthcare may become a competitive sport when primary care and specialty doctors collaborate to deliver the best possible health outcomes to patients. Telemedicine, which permits safe remote communication between all medical experts and patients, makes this feasible.	[95 - 98]
4.	Treatments of schoolgoing children	The care of our growing aging population may benefit greatly from telemedicine. A child who becomes ill at school has two options: they can see a school nurse or have their parents get them and take them to an urgent care facility. Both options are typically inconvenient and perhaps unnecessary. Progressive schools and doctors may work together to conduct classroom video tours. In addition to advising or consoling parents, the provider may determine the necessary course of action. Furthermore, it has been demonstrated that having physicians available at all times, including weekends, is beneficial to patients who reside in assisted living facilities and are discharged from the hospital.	[99 - 102]

(Table 1) cont.....

S. No.	Applications	Description	References
5.	Effective for conditions that don't need laboratory testing	Any condition that does not need laboratory tests or a physical examination can benefit from telemedicine. Additionally, this technology offers ongoing therapy, such as psychotherapy. During the COVID-19 pandemic, patients who live far from a primary care institution might also receive better care. For patients who are unable to transport themselves, providers can broaden the scope of conditions they are prepared to treat. For illustration, a physician may prescribe medications *via* telemedicine to treat a potential illness.	[103 - 106]
6.	Virtual doctor's appointment	Millions of people anticipate virtual doctor's sessions in this era of social alienation. Telemedicine has reduced medical expenses while also enhancing patient medication adherence and overall quality of life. Telemedicine app growth is becoming a major focus for healthcare providers who want to offer customers online and distant healthcare services. For both patients and physicians, this technology enables the development of appropriate telemedicine applications. Additionally, when a strong authentication system is paired with a few details, patients perceive it as reliable and straightforward.	[107 - 110]
7.	Boost the overall effectiveness of the healthcare system.	The phrase "telehealth" refers to a wide range of tools and technologies used to treat patients and improve the overall functioning of the healthcare system. Telemedicine encompasses a greater range of online medical services. In addition to providing healthcare services, it is also utilized for non-clinical tasks, such as provider recruitment, administrative meetings, and continuing medical education. People can receive medical care even if they are unable to see a doctor in person. People who are unable to visit a doctor in person can get medical treatment through telemedicine, which employs assistive technology and mobile texting. Additionally, this technology can be used for follow-up appointments, the treatment of chronic illnesses, expert advice, medication monitoring, and a range of other remote health services accessible *via* secure audio and video connections.	[111 - 113]
8.	Enhance the coordination of patients.	Improved healthcare services and improved patient coordination are possible with telemedicine. Fragmented care can also lead to insufficient drug usage, treatment shortages, overuse of medical resources, and unnecessary or redundant care. The patient can quickly pay the minimal costs for telehealth services. This service can be provided comfortably, enhancing communication between the patient and the doctor. Patients benefit from fewer days away from work and lower travel costs. Alternatively, in terms of time, this approach offers less disruption to the duties of child or elder care, greater privacy, and the avoidance of close contact with potentially contagious patients.	[114 - 116]

(Table 1) cont.....

S. No.	Applications	Description	References
9.	Minimise the travel of patients.	Telehealth would significantly reduce the time allocated for visits. Patients will not have to travel to and wait in a hospital for hours. They can now use the app to travel to their meeting and make an online appointment. Furthermore, the cost of healthcare might be lower than it has ever been. Doctors can see patients in the convenience of their own homes. Those who require immediate medical treatment could also benefit from it. Physicians who have access to on-demand viewing must utilize an internal database with pre-installed queries. A variety of application programming interfaces and features can also provide quick and simple access.	[117 - 120]
10.	Teledentistry	This technology enhances dental treatment by enabling dentists to capture photos of teeth, dentures, and other dental components, as well as any relevant documentation, to assess and send to another professional for further evaluation. The ability to share information between dentists and dental experts to determine if a specific treatment is necessary for certain ailments is a crucial benefit of telemedicine in dentistry. To help patients avoid costly and complex procedures, specialists can also assist dentists in identifying problem areas and recommending preventive measures. People in rural or underprivileged areas who often lack access to medical professionals benefit from this relationship, just as they do from other telemedicine applications.	[121 - 124]
11.	Improved care for patients and clinicians	Telemedicine is expanding rapidly and offers several advantages for both patients and healthcare professionals. Better patient services are a priority for every healthcare professional, and telemedicine technologies will help doctors further develop and enhance their private practices in the process. Therefore, creating applications for medical video conferences within a medical facility is crucial for enhancing medical care. When implementing telemedicine technology in the healthcare industry, one significant factor is the barrier. This is because there is a severe global shortage of qualified healthcare professionals. This technology makes it easier to address the doctor shortage.	[125 - 128]
12.	Monitoring of digital health	AI and machine learning combined with digital health monitoring capabilities in telemedicine systems will provide more accurate diagnostic and treatment recommendations. Utilizing machine learning technology and video conferencing tools, with each patient's case in hand, the algorithm can be refined to provide a more accurate diagnosis for each individual. Telemedicine is the process of employing networking hardware to connect physicians in one place with patients in another. Transcript scheduling, review, and photo applications provide an alternative to in-person meetings. It ensures the safety of doctors and patients during a pandemic and facilitates the digital expansion of medical services.	[129 - 131]

(Table 1) cont.....

S. No.	Applications	Description	References
13.	Skincare	Patients can use a computer, tablet, or smartphone to communicate with their dermatologist using telemedicine. Dermatologists can evaluate patients with conditions such as psoriasis, bedsores, and eczema using high-resolution images and videos. This is especially beneficial for patients who are homebound. Dermatologists can use telemedicine technology to safely and reliably diagnose and treat skin conditions. Telemedicine may reduce the need for in-person visits while allowing patients to maintain their dignity. It also enhances communication between doctors and patients. Every healthcare professional has access to electronic patient management services.	[132 - 135]
14.	Monitor the patient's medication intake.	Telemedicine technology enables medical personnel to monitor their patients' medication schedules and habits. Doctors will now monitor their patients' health remotely using cutting-edge medical technologies. Through data transmission between systems, this technology enables the transmission of information, including blood pressure, glucose levels, pulse rhythm, and more. Telemedicine might be useful in this area because elderly patients are more prone to forgetting to take their medicines.	[136 - 140]
15.	Protect the patient from contagious illnesses.	Telemedicine contributes to a safer world for everyone. Patients who have a cold or the flu, for instance, should speak with their doctor before bringing germs to work. Providers are limited to infectious diseases when providing advice and monitoring patient progress. This comprehensive solution includes both controlled access rights management and robust network security features. By doing this, patient data transmitted *via* telemedicine devices may be safer. It is also a means of lowering the number of trips to the emergency room.	[141 - 144]
16.	Cost-effective	Telemedicine is a more economical method of administering healthcare than traditional methods. The fact that patients and doctors do not have to travel to visit each other makes this valid. Furthermore, video consultations are usually slightly more costly than in-person ones. Consultation reduces the expense of hospital setup and travel. Additionally, it saves money to add video conferencing and online booking to the healthcare system. This is especially helpful in areas where it may be difficult for patients to access a hospital for treatment. Telemedicine is also helping to broaden the scope of the medical sector. The research, knowledge, and development in this sector are now more widely accessible. Medical students' education and preparation are now more realistic thanks to video conferencing tools.	[145 - 147]

(Table 1) cont.....

S. No.	Applications	Description	References
17.	Minimise in-person meetings	Minimise in-person meetings. There are several practical uses for telemedicine. Face-to-face meetings are sometimes necessary, but they can often be arranged with the help of modern technology. This has several benefits that improve the general functioning of the facility. However, telemedicine enables medical professionals to monitor multiple patients simultaneously without needing to leave the medical facility. Telemedicine is utilized for visits and supervision in order to alleviate crowded emergency departments and treat patients in more urgent situations. With the use of telemedicine, hospitals can share medical information to provide care even more efficiently. Lastly, it helps lower the danger to general health by treating individuals who require supervision.	[148 - 150]

The engineering sector utilizes a range of cutting-edge technologies. Healthcare and related fields [151 - 154]. These aid in resolving several issues related to production, design, and creating a sustainable environment [155 - 157]. Telemedicine is frequently used to connect medical professionals treating patients in one location with specialists in another to provide telecommunication support. In rural or hard-to-reach locations where specialists are not readily available, this is particularly helpful. It is employed to conduct remote visits more cheaply and efficiently. The practice of telemedicine saw substantial advancements with the advent of the internet era.

As a substitute for visiting a physician for general and specialty care, remote healthcare can now be provided to patients at their homes, workplaces, or assisted living facilities, thanks to the development of smart technologies that support high-quality video streaming. Many claim that since the invention of the telephone, telemedicine has existed in one form or another. Instead of sending data over the phone, one may send pictures. In many nations, telemedicine is also a recognized part of the healthcare delivery system. It can be used for various purposes, such as assisting patients in setting up video follow-up meetings, enhancing compliance with aftercare visit guidelines, and alleviating stress for both patients and healthcare providers [158 - 160].

Modern mobile health apps enable telemedicine by connecting software to an interactive clinical interface. The treatment of patients with minor ailments, data exchange from studies, and imaging results are examples of noncritical events. Patients can also obtain prescriptions and purchase drugs through a customized application, with close cooperation with payment gateways. Real-time information transmission and analysis occur here. With the use of a single app, patients and physicians can easily communicate and share information, as these telemedicine systems are regularly connected. It is easy to gather patient data directly and send it to the appropriate doctor. A test result or a transcript of an appointment stored in a digital health record system folder might serve as this proof. Furthermore, it enables medical professionals to understand data after it has been gathered [161 - 163].

Confidential medical records are used extensively in telemedicine. It is employed to collect, store, and disseminate data, which helps in considering crucial factors in this field. A website that enables remote discussion with a doctor is known as telemedicine [164 - 166]. The gadget is connected to the hospital's internal infrastructure through mobile applications. Specialized modules might offer data visualizations, study comments, and cautions to support clinical judgments. This software utilizes a remote control to assist individuals with chronic and severe illnesses. Any patient who is admitted to the hospital and kept under surveillance throughout the operation occupies a valuable bed. Home health telemedicine can collect vital signs, facilitate video conferences, and trigger alarms at a nurse's station [167 - 170].

OBSTACLES TO UTILIZING TELEMEDICINE TECHNIQUES IN HEALTHCARE SERVICES

To help medical units and patients receive the best care possible, telemedicine care was successfully deployed despite numerous challenges, as shown in (Fig. **4**). Certain common and typical difficulties must be addressed when applying telehealth-related techniques to healthcare and related industries. It is imperative to avoid any form of privacy loss, confidential disclosure, fraud, abuse, and incorrect solutions, as these issues could demoralize people or exacerbate the situation from a health standpoint [171 - 173]. (Fig. **4**) shows common obstacles to using telemedicine to support healthcare.

When combined with other telehealth monitoring strategies, telemedicine can help patients and physicians better manage severe health conditions, such as diabetes and asthma. Additionally, physicians will follow up with patients at home after they are discharged from the hospital or recover from an injury. For doctors, patients' poor management is a significant source of concern. Device outages can still occur, despite advancements in medical technology that have made it easier to operate. Healthcare systems considering the implementation of telemedicine technologies, such as specialists, should meet industry standards. For professionals looking to integrate telemedicine into their medical centers, they offer a variety of practical options, facilitating the integration of telemedicine more smoothly [174, 175].

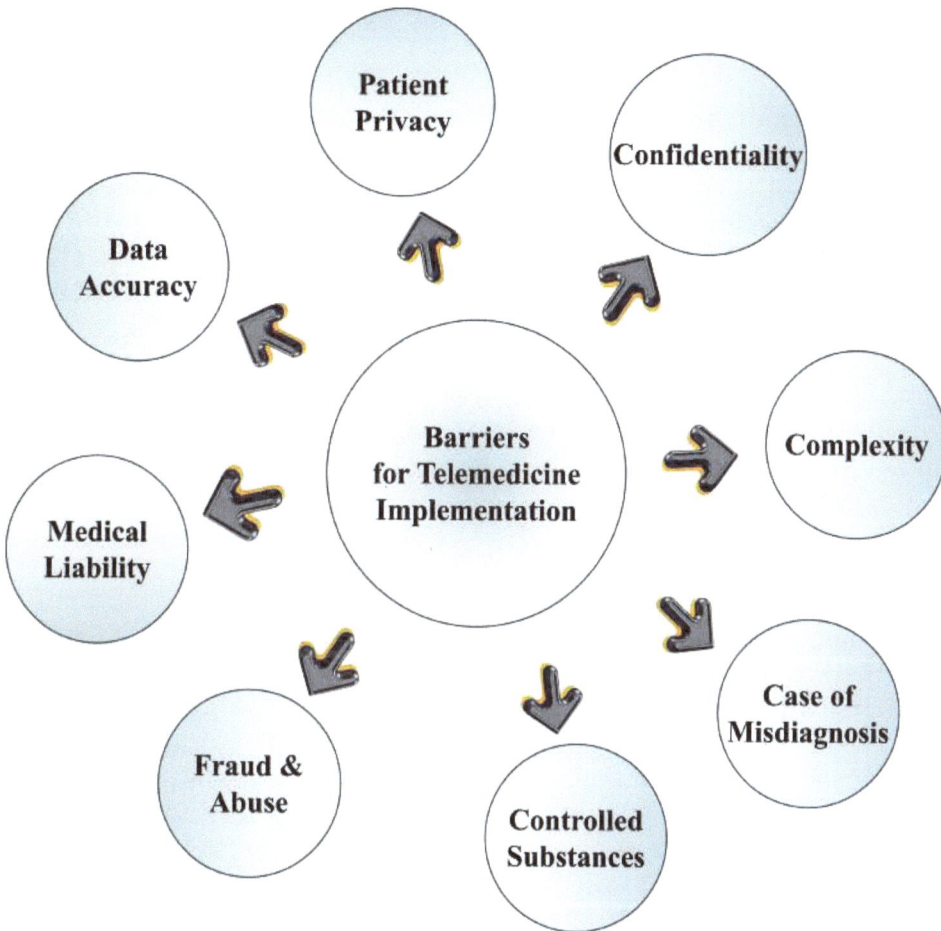

Fig. (4). Common obstacles to using telemedicine to help healthcare.

This telemedicine technique facilitates the sharing of patient information between doctors in different countries. Now, a primary care physician and a doctor may communicate without physically being in the same room by exchanging patient history and medical information. One practitioner can learn from the experiences of other practitioners because of the system's ability to convey data across long distances. As a result, there are fewer cases of redundant monitoring and inadequate drug management. Physicians may collect and disseminate information to their patients using patient portals. Health indicators and other data can be sent to doctors by medical devices, enabling them to modify therapy. Patients can now send biometric data to their physicians *via* wearable technologies or remote monitoring devices, such as pulse oximeters or blood pressure monitors. It can collect data, extract patient data from a dashboard or clinical decision support system, and display patient status in nearly real-time [176 - 178].

Long-distance patient information interchange is made possible *via* telemedicine, which is revolutionary. Accurate patient assessment is made possible by the real-time exchange of medical records, including imaging results, laboratory test results, and other relevant data. Telemedicine can help reduce ER overcrowding by requiring patients to first consult with a remote physician *via* video chat. A significant commitment of time and money is necessary for telemedicine, as healthcare networks that have adopted this technology can attest. To get the most out of the gadget, physicians, practice administrators, and other healthcare professionals need to know how to use it effectively. With more patients and fewer staff, telemedicine can eventually provide healthcare institutions with a strong return on investment, despite its initial high cost. Physicians can conduct clinical examinations and assess a patient's medical history and other information with this equipment [179 - 181].

Telemedicine services have enabled patients to access care from the comfort of their own homes. It is beneficial for those who require medical attention but cannot afford to travel hundreds of miles or endure lengthy wait times. Sharing the video will allow physicians at another hospital to view high-risk children in a matter of seconds. Additionally, this lessens the need to transfer infants to another hospital, which is costly and time-consuming. Patients may now visit a specialist without ever leaving their homes, unlike in the past when access to medical services was limited. When patients with contagious diseases avoid exposing themselves to others in crowded waiting areas, the spread of the disease is reduced. Additionally, people often schedule consultations during breaks from work or even after hours [182 - 184].

Telemedicine sets a new standard for technology-assisted treatment by facilitating better communication between patients and their caregivers, providing access to physicians and specialists, and encouraging patients and healthcare providers to avoid high-risk circumstances. Patients who abuse drugs can be treated using a variety of telemedicine strategies. Money is saved since treatment costs are frequently lower. As technology develops, the cost savings will become more noticeable. In terms of diagnosis and treatment, telemedicine is fantastic for both physicians and patients. It can serve as an excellent support system. This type of telemedicine technology is beneficial to medical professionals in providing patients with the correct medications and delivering effective patient care. Telemedicine can be more cost-effective for both patients and providers compared to traditional care. The healthcare professional would have telemedicine facilities on location to deliver appropriate therapy [185, 186].

Technology in telemedicine enables the provision of ongoing treatment to patients. This will aid in diagnosis and encourage appropriate self-care. Telemedicine services powered by AI will automatically analyze patient data and enable doctors to react quickly to emerging trends. By utilizing telemedicine technology, physicians will be able to care for a greater number of patients. Hospitals may be made smaller, and visits can be shortened. Having access to tele-urgent care might reduce the number of ER visits. In remote hospitals, it enables specialists to collaborate on cases. These live feeds include distant experts who are available for on-screen advice. The remote transfer of medical data from one place to another is known as telemedicine. The purpose of this is to increase an individual's level of fitness. It might not be easy to schedule a visit with a specialist or primary care physician. Data is being actively collected by this distant network and sent to other healthcare institutions for study. By utilizing this technology, mental health practices can continue to deliver high-quality care while serving a larger patient base. Better time management and more profitability are the outcomes. Parents will now cease taking their sick child out of the residence to consult a doctor [187 - 189].

The use of technology to transmit medical data from individuals in different geographic locations is known as telemonitoring. Using electronic devices, this type of monitoring enables doctors and primary caregivers to keep track of patients. Patients can also receive care at home thanks to telemonitoring technologies. As a result, they have more control over how their illnesses are treated and fewer hospital visits. Patients in remote areas are often unable to travel by air to hospitals or lack access to the cost-effective medical services that telemedicine offers. Working with other healthcare experts is one of their daily duties, which can be time-consuming. Telemedicine enables radiologists to collect high-quality images and receive commentary from anywhere. They can now operate more efficiently since they no longer need to be in the same area as the source when passing over the photographs. Practices in mental health, which are perhaps among the most popular telemedicine specialties, provide therapeutic sessions from any location [190 - 192].

CONCLUSION

Telemedicine has revolutionized healthcare delivery by offering accessible, efficient, and innovative solutions to address challenges faced by patients and healthcare providers. Its adoption in the healthcare system has led to improved patient outcomes, decreased costs, and made it easier for patients, particularly those living in remote or isolated areas. Telemedicine eliminates geographical and temporal obstacles, leading to timely medical interventions, better management of chronic diseases, and improved communication between patients and physicians.

Additionally, integrating faster technologies such as AI, IoT, and Cloud computing appears to boost telemedicine innovation through real-time monitoring, data-driven diagnosis, and healthcare division. In terms of patient management, virtual consultations, remote patient monitoring, e-prescriptions, and the transmission of medical data have streamlined the entire healthcare workflow, offering a better quality of care with a lower risk of infection or hospital-acquired illnesses. Telemedicine, despite several advantages, also faces barriers in technical, medicolegal, and logistical issues that need to be overcome for seamless implementation. Looking forward, the future of telemedicine is very promising . It can change the world around us by making the healthcare system more equitable and efficient, and promoting preventive care. As technology continues to advance and patients and providers conduct and accept telemedicine visits, the use of telemedicine will play a crucial role in developing a healthier world, with closer connections between patients and the healthcare system.

REFERENCES

[1]   Wilson LS, Maeder AJ. Recent directions in telemedicine: review of trends in research and practice. Healthc Inform Res 2015; 21(4): 213-22.
[http://dx.doi.org/10.4258/hir.2015.21.4.213] [PMID: 26618026]

[2]   Hajesmaeel-Gohari S, Bahaadinbeigy K. The most used questionnaires for evaluating telemedicine services. BMC Med Inform Decis Mak 2021; 21(1): 36.
[http://dx.doi.org/10.1186/s12911-021-01407-y] [PMID: 33531013]

[3]   Lupton D, Maslen S. Telemedicine and the senses: a review. Sociol Health Illn 2017; 39(8): 1557-71.
[http://dx.doi.org/10.1111/1467-9566.12617] [PMID: 29071731]

[4]   Sarhan F. Telemedicine in healthcare. 1: Exploring its uses, benefits and disadvantages. Nurs Times 2009; 105(42): 10-3.
[PMID: 19916354]

[5]   Moghadas A, Jamshidi M, Shaderam M. Telemedicine in healthcare system. 2008 World Automation Congress 2008; 1-6.

[6]   Chunara R, Zhao Y, Chen J, *et al.* Telemedicine and healthcare disparities: a cohort study in a large healthcare system in New York City during COVID-19. J Am Med Inform Assoc 2021; 28(1): 33-41.
[http://dx.doi.org/10.1093/jamia/ocaa217] [PMID: 32866264]

[7]   Flumignan CDQ, Rocha AP, Pinto ACPN, *et al.* What do Cochrane systematic reviews say about telemedicine for healthcare? Sao Paulo Med J 2019; 137(2): 184-92.
[http://dx.doi.org/10.1590/1516-3180.0177240419] [PMID: 31314879]

[8]   Kaspar BJ. Legislating for a new age in medicine: Defining the telemedicine standard of care to improve healthcare in Iowa. Iowa Law Rev 2013; 99: 839.

[9]   Rockwell KL, Gilroy AS. Incorporating telemedicine as part of COVID-19 outbreak response systems. Am J Manag Care 2020; 26(4): 147-8.
[http://dx.doi.org/10.37765/ajmc.2020.42784] [PMID: 32270980]

[10]   Bashshur R, Shannon G, Krupinski E, Grigsby J. The taxonomy of telemedicine. Telemed e-Health 2011; 17(6): 484-94.
[http://dx.doi.org/10.1089/tmj.2011.0103]

[11]   Funderskov KF, Boe Danbjørg D, Jess M, Munk L, Olsen Zwisler AD, Dieperink KB. Telemedicine in specialised palliative care: Healthcare professionals' and their perspectives on video

consultations—A qualitative study. J Clin Nurs 2019; 28(21-22): 3966-76.
[http://dx.doi.org/10.1111/jocn.15004] [PMID: 31328336]

[12] Lokkerbol J, Adema D, Cuijpers P, *et al.* Improving the cost-effectiveness of a healthcare system for depressive disorders by implementing telemedicine: a health economic modeling study. Am J Geriatr Psychiatry 2014; 22(3): 253-62.
[http://dx.doi.org/10.1016/j.jagp.2013.01.058] [PMID: 23759290]

[13] Charles BL. Telemedicine can lower costs and improve access. Healthc Financ Manage 2000; 54(4): 66-9.
[PMID: 10915354]

[14] Board NI. Personalised health and care 2020–using data and technology to transform outcomes for patients and citizens–a framework for action. London: HM Government 2014.

[15] Armfield NR, Gray LC, Smith AC. Clinical use of Skype: a review of the evidence base. J Telemed Telecare 2012; 18(3): 125-7.
[http://dx.doi.org/10.1258/jtt.2012.SFT101] [PMID: 22362829]

[16] Gentles SJ, Lokker C, McKibbon KA. Health information technology to facilitate communication involving health care providers, caregivers, and pediatric patients: a scoping review. J Med Internet Res 2010; 12(2): e22.
[http://dx.doi.org/10.2196/jmir.1390] [PMID: 20562092]

[17] Armfield NR, Bradford M, Bradford NK. The clinical use of Skype—For which patients, with which problems and in which settings? A snapshot review of the literature. Int J Med Inform 2015; 84(10): 737-42.
[http://dx.doi.org/10.1016/j.ijmedinf.2015.06.006] [PMID: 26183642]

[18] Horvath AO, Greenberg LS. Development and validation of the Working Alliance Inventory. J Couns Psychol 1989; 36(2): 223-33.
[http://dx.doi.org/10.1037/0022-0167.36.2.223]

[19] Freeman KA, Duke DC, Harris MA. Behavioral health care for adolescents with poorly controlled diabetes *via* Skype: does working alliance remain intact? J Diabetes Sci Technol 2013; 7(3): 727-35.
[http://dx.doi.org/10.1177/193229681300700318] [PMID: 23759406]

[20] Harris MA, Freeman KA, Duke DC. Seeing is believing: using Skype to improve diabetes outcomes in youth. Diabetes Care 2015; 38(8): 1427-34.
[http://dx.doi.org/10.2337/dc14-2469] [PMID: 26033508]

[21] Choi NG, Hegel MT, Marti CN, Marinucci ML, Sirrianni L, Bruce ML. Telehealth problem-solving therapy for depressed low-income homebound older adults. Am J Geriatr Psychiatry 2014; 22(3): 263-71.
[http://dx.doi.org/10.1016/j.jagp.2013.01.037] [PMID: 23567376]

[22] Jimison HB, Klein KA, Marcoe JL. A socialization intervention in remote health coaching for older adults in the home. 2013.
[http://dx.doi.org/10.1109/EMBC.2013.6611175]

[23] Sharareh B, Schwarzkopf R. Effectiveness of telemedical applications in postoperative follow-up after total joint arthroplasty. J Arthroplasty 2014; 29(5): 918-22.
[http://dx.doi.org/10.1016/j.arth.2013.09.019] [PMID: 24342278]

[24] Marsh JD, Bryant DM, MacDonald SJ, *et al.* Feasibility, effectiveness and costs associated with a web-based follow-up assessment following total joint arthroplasty. J Arthroplasty 2014; 29(9): 1723-8.
[http://dx.doi.org/10.1016/j.arth.2014.04.003] [PMID: 24881023]

[25] Marsh J, Hoch JS, Bryant D, *et al.* Economic evaluation of web-based compared with in-person follow-up after total joint arthroplasty. J Bone Joint Surg Am 2014; 96(22): 1910-6.
[http://dx.doi.org/10.2106/JBJS.M.01558] [PMID: 25410510]

[26] van Eck CF. Web-based follow-up after total joint arthroplasty proves to be cost-effective, but is it

safe? commentary on an article by Jacquelyn Marsh, PhD, *et al.*: "Economic evaluation of web-based compared with in-person follow-up after total joint arthroplasty". J Bone Joint Surg Am 2014; 96(22): e192.
[http://dx.doi.org/10.2106/JBJS.N.00829] [PMID: 25410520]

[27]   Telemedicine: opportunities and developments in member states: report on the second Global survey on eHealth. WHO 2010.

[28]   Raposo VL. Telemedicine: The legal framework (or the lack of it) in Europe. GMS Health Technol Assess 2016; 12: Doc03.
[PMID: 27579146]

[29]   Rosenkrantz AB, Sherwin J, Prithiani CP, Ostrow D, Recht MP. Technology-assisted virtual consultation for medical imaging. J Am Coll Radiol 2016; 13(8): 995-1002.
[http://dx.doi.org/10.1016/j.jacr.2016.02.029] [PMID: 27084068]

[30]   Albahri AS, Alwan JK, Taha ZK, *et al.* IoT-based telemedicine for disease prevention and health promotion: State-of-the-Art. J Netw Comput Appl 2021; 173: 102873.
[http://dx.doi.org/10.1016/j.jnca.2020.102873]

[31]   Bashshur RL, Shannon GW, Krupinski EA, Grigsby J, Kvedar JC, Weinstein RS, *et al.* National telemedicine initiatives: essential to healthcare reform. Telemed e-Health 2009; 15(6): 600-10.
[http://dx.doi.org/10.1089/tmj.2009.9960]

[32]   Manchanda S. Telemedicine–getting care to patients closer to home. Am J Respir Crit Care Med 2020; 201(12): P26-7.
[http://dx.doi.org/10.1164/rccm.2020C5] [PMID: 32271097]

[33]   Sterne JAC, Savović J, Page MJ, *et al.* RoB 2: a revised tool for assessing risk of bias in randomised trials. BMJ 2019; 366: l4898.
[http://dx.doi.org/10.1136/bmj.l4898] [PMID: 31462531]

[34]   Sterne JAC, Hernán MA, Reeves BC, *et al.* ROBINS-I: a tool for assessing risk of bias in non-randomised studies of interventions. BMJ 2016; 355: i4919.
[http://dx.doi.org/10.1136/bmj.i4919] [PMID: 27733354]

[35]   Silverman RD. Current legal and ethical concerns in telemedicine and e-medicine. London: SAGE Publications 2003.
[http://dx.doi.org/10.1258/135763303322196402]

[36]   Arné JL. [Ethical and legal aspects of telemedicine]. Bull Acad Natl Med 2014; 198(1): 119-30.
[PMID: 26259291]

[37]   Jack CL, Mars M. Informed consent for telemedicine in South Africa: A survey of consent practices among healthcare professionals in Durban, KwaZulu-Natal. S Afr J Bioeth Law 2013; 6(2): 55-9.
[http://dx.doi.org/10.7196/sajbl.287]

[38]   Siegal G. Telemedicine: licensing and other legal issues. Otolaryngol Clin North Am 2011; 44(6): 1375-84.
[http://dx.doi.org/10.1016/j.otc.2011.08.011] [PMID: 22032489]

[39]   Caryl CJ. Malpractice and other legal issues preventing the development of telemedicine. J Law Health 1997-1998; 12(1): 173-204.
[PMID: 10182029]

[40]   Sarhan F. Telemedicine in healthcare. 2: The legal and ethical aspects of using new technology. Nurs Times 2009; 105(43): 18-20.
[PMID: 19950459]

[41]   Bolcato V, Basile G, Bianco Prevot L, Fassina G, Rapuano S, Brizioli E, Tronconi LP. Telemedicine in Italy: Healthcare authorization profiles in the modern medico-legal reading. Int J Risk Safe Med. 2024 Nov;35(4):337-43.

[42]   Thakur KS, Sonwani NS. Telemedicine practice guidelines in India: Medico legal implications. J Ind Aca Foren Med. 2021 Dec;43(4):384-8.

[43]   Solimini R, Busardò FP, Gibelli F, Sirignano A, Ricci G. Ethical and Legal Challenges of Telemedicine in the Era of the COVID-19 Pandemic. Medicina. 2021 Nov 30;57(12):1314.

[44]   KV BM, Walarine MT. Technology-Assisted Early Disability Identification and Monitoring in Children: A Model for Middle-and Low Income Countries. Disability, CBR & Inclusive Development. 2023;34(3):183-91.

[45]   Surdu A, Foia CI, Luchian I, Trifan D, Budala DG, Scutariu MM, Ciupilan C, Puha B, Tatarciuc D. Telemedicine and Digital Tools in Dentistry: Enhancing Diagnosis and Remote Patient Care. Medicina. 2025 Apr 30;61(5):826.

[46]   D'Antonio G, Bolino G, Del Prete S, *et al.* Telemedical care for maritime workers: health care liability issues related to possible regulatory decoupl. Clin Ter 2025; 176(Suppl 1(2): 40-43.

[47]   El-Shafai W, Khallaf F, El-Rabaie ESM, El-Samie FEA. Robust medical image encryption based on DNA-chaos cryptosystem for secure telemedicine and healthcare applications. J Ambient Intell Humaniz Comput 2021; 12(10): 9007-35.
[http://dx.doi.org/10.1007/s12652-020-02597-5]

[48]   Kadir MA. Role of telemedicine in healthcare during COVID-19 pandemic in developing countries. Telehealth Med Today 2020; 5(2)

[49]   Mars M. Telemedicine and advances in urban and rural healthcare delivery in Africa. Prog Cardiovasc Dis 2013; 56(3): 326-35.
[http://dx.doi.org/10.1016/j.pcad.2013.10.006] [PMID: 24267440]

[50]   Chau PYK, Hu PJH. Investigating healthcare professionals' decisions to accept telemedicine technology: an empirical test of competing theories. Inf Manage 2002; 39(4): 297-311.
[http://dx.doi.org/10.1016/S0378-7206(01)00098-2]

[51]   Haleem A, Javaid M, Singh RP, Suman R. Telemedicine for healthcare: Capabilities, features, barriers, and applications. Sens Int 2021; 2: 100117.
[http://dx.doi.org/10.1016/j.sintl.2021.100117] [PMID: 34806053]

[52]   Kohnke A, Cole ML, Bush R. Incorporating UTAUT predictors for understanding home care patients' and clinician's acceptance of healthcare telemedicine equipment. J Technol Manag Innov 2014; 9(2): 29-41.
[http://dx.doi.org/10.4067/S0718-27242014000200003]

[53]   Bajowala SS, Shih J, Varshney P, Elliott T. The future of telehealth for allergic disease. J Allergy Clin Immunol Pract 2022; 10(10): 2514-23.
[http://dx.doi.org/10.1016/j.jaip.2022.08.022] [PMID: 36038132]

[54]   Lin JC, Kavousi Y, Sullivan B, Stevens C. Analysis of outpatient telemedicine reimbursement in an integrated healthcare system. Ann Vasc Surg 2020; 65: 100-6.
[http://dx.doi.org/10.1016/j.avsg.2019.10.069] [PMID: 31678131]

[55]   Javaid M, Haleem A, Pratap Singh R, Suman R. Significance of Quality 4.0 towards comprehensive enhancement in manufacturing sector. Sens Int 2021; 2: 100109.
[http://dx.doi.org/10.1016/j.sintl.2021.100109]

[56]   Ning AY, Cabrera CI, D'Anza B. Telemedicine in otolaryngology: a systematic review of image quality, diagnostic concordance, and patient and provider satisfaction. Ann Otol Rhinol Laryngol 2021; 130(2): 195-204.
[http://dx.doi.org/10.1177/0003489420939590] [PMID: 32659100]

[57]   Salehahmadi Z, Hajialiasghari F. Telemedicine in iran: chances and challenges. World J Plast Surg 2013; 2(1): 18-25.
[PMID: 25489500]

[58]   Von Wangenheim A, de Souza Nobre LF, Tognoli H, Nassar SM, Ho K. User satisfaction with asynchronous telemedicine: a study of users of Santa Catarina's system of telemedicine and telehealth. Telemed e-Health 2012; 18(5): 339-46.
[http://dx.doi.org/10.1089/tmj.2011.0197]

[59]   Ayatollahi H, Mirani N, Nazari F, Razavi N. Iranian healthcare professionals' perspectives about factors influencing the use of telemedicine in diabetes management. World J Diabetes 2018; 9(6): 92-8.
[http://dx.doi.org/10.4239/wjd.v9.i6.92] [PMID: 29988886]

[60]   Bahl S, Singh RP, Javaid M, Khan IH, Vaishya R, Suman R. Telemedicine technologies for confronting COVID-19 pandemic: a review. J Indus Integ Manag 2020; 5(4): 547-61.
[http://dx.doi.org/10.1142/S2424862220300057]

[61]   Whitten PS, Mair FS, Haycox A, May CR, Williams TL, Hellmich S. Systematic review of cost effectiveness studies of telemedicine interventions. BMJ 2002; 324(7351): 1434-7.
[http://dx.doi.org/10.1136/bmj.324.7351.1434] [PMID: 12065269]

[62]   Hooshmand M, Yao K. Challenges facing children with special healthcare needs and their families: telemedicine as a bridge to care. Telemed e-Health 2017; 23(1): 18-24.
[http://dx.doi.org/10.1089/tmj.2016.0055]

[63]   Blake KV. Telemedicine and adherence monitoring in children with asthma. Curr Opin Pulm Med 2021; 27(1): 37-44.
[http://dx.doi.org/10.1097/MCP.0000000000000739] [PMID: 33105234]

[64]   Persaud YK, Portnoy JM. Ten rules for implementation of a telemedicine program to care for patients with asthma. J Allergy Clin Immunol Pract 2021; 9(1): 13-21.
[http://dx.doi.org/10.1016/j.jaip.2020.10.005] [PMID: 33039648]

[65]   Mishra SK, Kapoor L, Singh IP. Telemedicine in India: current scenario and the future. Telemed e-Health 2009; 15(6): 568-75.
[http://dx.doi.org/10.1089/tmj.2009.0059]

[66]   Ly BA, Labonté R, Bourgeault IL, Niang MN. The individual and contextual determinants of the use of telemedicine: A descriptive study of the perceptions of Senegal's physicians and telemedicine projects managers. PLoS One 2017; 12(7): e0181070.
[http://dx.doi.org/10.1371/journal.pone.0181070] [PMID: 28732028]

[67]   Chatrath V, Attri J, Chatrath R. Telemedicine and anaesthesia. Indian J Anaesth 2010; 54(3): 199-204.
[http://dx.doi.org/10.4103/0019-5049.65357] [PMID: 20885864]

[68]   Dalley D, Rahman R, Ivaldi A. Health care professionals' and patients' management of the interactional practices in telemedicine videoconferencing: A conversation analytic and discursive systematic review. Qual Health Res 2021; 31(4): 804-14.
[http://dx.doi.org/10.1177/1049732320942346] [PMID: 32741261]

[69]   Martínez A, Villarroel V, Seoane J, Del Pozo F. Rural telemedicine for primary healthcare in developing countries. IEEE Technol Soc Mag 2004; 23(2): 13-22.
[http://dx.doi.org/10.1109/MTAS.2004.1304394]

[70]   Kyriacou E, Pavlopoulos S, Berler A, *et al.* Multi-purpose HealthCare Telemedicine Systems with mobile communication link support. Biomed Eng Online 2003; 2(1): 7.
[http://dx.doi.org/10.1186/1475-925X-2-7] [PMID: 12694629]

[71]   Yellowlees PM, Chorba K, Burke Parish M, Wynn-Jones H, Nafiz N. Telemedicine can make healthcare greener. Telemed e-Health 2010; 16(2): 229-32.
[http://dx.doi.org/10.1089/tmj.2009.0105]

[72]   Wernhart A, Gahbauer S, Haluza D. eHealth and telemedicine: Practices and beliefs among healthcare professionals and medical students at a medical university. PLoS One 2019; 14(2): e0213067.
[http://dx.doi.org/10.1371/journal.pone.0213067] [PMID: 30818348]

[73]   Javaid M, Haleem A, Singh RP, Suman R. Substantial capabilities of robotics in enhancing industry 4.0 implementation. Cognitive Robotics 2021; 1: 58-75.
[http://dx.doi.org/10.1016/j.cogr.2021.06.001]

[74]   Ahmad RW, Salah K, Jayaraman R, Yaqoob I, Ellahham S, Omar M. The role of blockchain technology in telehealth and telemedicine. Int J Med Inform 2021; 148: 104399.
[http://dx.doi.org/10.1016/j.ijmedinf.2021.104399] [PMID: 33540131]

[75]   Pooni R, Pageler NM, Sandborg C, Lee T. Pediatric subspecialty telemedicine use from the patient and provider perspective. Pediatr Res 2022; 91(1): 241-6.
[http://dx.doi.org/10.1038/s41390-021-01443-4] [PMID: 33753896]

[76]   Omboni S, McManus RJ, Bosworth HB, *et al.* Evidence and recommendations on the use of telemedicine for the management of arterial hypertension: an international expert position paper. Hypertension 2020; 76(5): 1368-83.
[http://dx.doi.org/10.1161/HYPERTENSIONAHA.120.15873] [PMID: 32921195]

[77]   Mihova P, Vinarova J, Petkov A, Penjurov I. Milestone before/after analysis of telemedicine implementation. Ukr J Telemed Med Telemat 2009; 7(1): 65-7.

[78]   Eisenstein E, Kopacek C, Cavalcante SS, Neves AC, Fraga GP, Messina LA. Telemedicine: a bridge over knowledge gaps in healthcare. Curr Pediatr Rep 2020; 8(3): 93-8.
[http://dx.doi.org/10.1007/s40124-020-00221-w] [PMID: 32837801]

[79]   Kruse CS, Bouffard S, Dougherty M, Parro JS. Telemedicine use in rural Native American communities in the era of the ACA: a systematic literature review. J Med Syst 2016; 40(6): 145.
[http://dx.doi.org/10.1007/s10916-016-0503-8] [PMID: 27118011]

[80]   Asiri A, AlBishi S, AlMadani W, ElMetwally A, Househ M. The use of telemedicine in surgical care: a systematic review. Acta Inform Med 2018; 26(2): 201-6.
[http://dx.doi.org/10.5455/aim.2018.26.201-206] [PMID: 30515013]

[81]   Parajuli R, Doneys P. Exploring the role of telemedicine in improving access to healthcare services by women and girls in rural Nepal. Telemat Inform 2017; 34(7): 1166-76.
[http://dx.doi.org/10.1016/j.tele.2017.05.006]

[82]   Rao B, Lombardi A II. Telemedicine: current status in developed and developing countries. J Drugs Dermatol 2009; 8(4): 371-5.
[PMID: 19363855]

[83]   Hailey DM, Crowe BL. Assessing the economic impact of telemedicine. Dis Manag Health Outcomes 2000; 7(4): 187-92.
[http://dx.doi.org/10.2165/00115677-200007040-00002]

[84]   Vasquez-Cevallos LA, Bobokova J, González-Granda PV, Iniesta JM, Gómez EJ, Hernando ME. Design and technical validation of a telemedicine service for rural healthcare in Ecuador Telemedicine and e-Health 2018; 24(7): 544-551.
[http://dx.doi.org/10.1089/tmj.2017.0130]

[85]   Kerleau M, Pelletier-Fleury N. Restructuring of the healthcare system and the diffusion of telemedicine. Eur J Health Econ 2002; 3(3): 207-14.
[http://dx.doi.org/10.1007/s10198-002-0131-8] [PMID: 15609145]

[86]   Ishfaq R, Raja U. Bridging the healthcare access divide: a strategic planning model for rural telemedicine network. Decis Sci 2015; 46(4): 755-90.
[http://dx.doi.org/10.1111/deci.12165]

[87]   de Figueiredo FAP, Cardoso FACM, Lopes RR, Miranda JP. On the application of massive MU-MIMO in the uplink of machine type communication systems. 2015 International Workshop on Telecommunications (IWT) IEEE 2015; 1-7.
[http://dx.doi.org/10.1109/IWT.2015.7224559]

[88]	Barbosa W, Zhou K, Waddell E, Myers T, Dorsey ER. Improving access to care: telemedicine across medical domains. Annu Rev Public Health 2021; 42(1): 463-81.
[http://dx.doi.org/10.1146/annurev-publhealth-090519-093711] [PMID: 33798406]

[89]	Gobburi RK, Olawade DB, Olatunji GD, Kokori E, Aderinto N, David-Olawade AC. Telemedicine use in rural areas of the United Kingdom to improve access to healthcare facilities: A review of current evidence. Informatics and Health 2025; 2(1): 41-8.
[http://dx.doi.org/10.1016/j.infoh.2025.01.003]

[90]	Moazzami B, Razavi-Khorasani N, Dooghaie Moghadam A, Farokhi E, Rezaei N. COVID-19 and telemedicine: Immediate action required for maintaining healthcare providers well-being. J Clin Virol 2020; 126: 104345.
[http://dx.doi.org/10.1016/j.jcv.2020.104345] [PMID: 32278298]

[91]	Haleem A, Javaid M, Singh RP, Suman R. Quality 4.0 technologies to enhance traditional Chinese medicine for overcoming healthcare challenges during COVID-19. Digit Chin Med 2021; 4(2): 71-80.
[http://dx.doi.org/10.1016/j.dcmed.2021.06.001]

[92]	Ng HS, Sim ML, Tan CM, Wong CC. Wireless technologies for telemedicine. BT Technol J 2006; 24(2): 130-7.
[http://dx.doi.org/10.1007/s10550-006-0050-9]

[93]	Al-Qirim N. Championing telemedicine adoption and utilization in healthcare organizations in New Zealand. Int J Med Inform 2007; 76(1): 42-54.
[http://dx.doi.org/10.1016/j.ijmedinf.2006.02.001] [PMID: 16621682]

[94]	Luciano E, Mahmood MA, Mansouri Rad P. Telemedicine adoption issues in the United States and Brazil: Perception of healthcare professionals. Health Informatics J 2020; 26(4): 2344-61.
[http://dx.doi.org/10.1177/1460458220902957] [PMID: 32072843]

[95]	Adewale OS. An internet-based telemedicine system in Nigeria. Int J Inf Manage 2004; 24(3): 221-34.
[http://dx.doi.org/10.1016/j.ijinfomgt.2003.12.014]

[96]	Stipa G, Gabbrielli F, Rabbito C, *et al.* The Italian technical/administrative recommendations for telemedicine in clinical neurophysiology. Neurol Sci 2021; 42(5): 1923-31.
[http://dx.doi.org/10.1007/s10072-020-04732-8] [PMID: 32974797]

[97]	Bokolo Anthony Jnr. Use of telemedicine and virtual care for remote treatment in response to COVID-19 pandemic. J Med Syst 2020; 44(7): 132.
[http://dx.doi.org/10.1007/s10916-020-01596-5] [PMID: 32542571]

[98]	Mathur P, Srivastava S, Lalchandani A, Mehta JL. Evolving role of telemedicine in health care delivery in India. Prim Health Care 2017; 7(1): 1079-2167.
[http://dx.doi.org/10.4172/2167-1079.1000260]

[99]	Hojabri R, Borousan E, Manafi M. Impact of using telemedicine on knowledge management in healthcare organizations: A case study. Afr J Bus Manag 2012; 6(4): 1604.

[100]	Krupinski EA, Weinstein RS. Telemedicine in an academic center—the Arizona Telemedicine Program Telemed e-Health 2013; 19(5): 349-56.

[101]	Haleem A, Javaid M, Singh RP, Suman R. Significant roles of 4D printing using smart materials in the field of manufacturing. Advanced Industrial and Engineering Polymer Research 2021; 4(4): 301-11.
[http://dx.doi.org/10.1016/j.aiepr.2021.05.001]

[102]	Iasbech PAB, Lavarda RAB. Strategy and practices. Int J Public Sector Management 2018; 31(3): 347-71.
[http://dx.doi.org/10.1108/IJPSM-12-2016-0207]

[103]	Pourmand A, Ghassemi M, Sumon K, Amini SB, Hood C, Sikka N. Lack of telemedicine training in academic medicine: are we preparing the next generation? Telemed e-Health 2021; 27(1): 62-7.
[http://dx.doi.org/10.1089/tmj.2019.0287]

[104] Chellaiyan V, Nirupama AY, Taneja N. Telemedicine in India: Where do we stand? J Family Med Prim Care 2019; 8(6): 1872-6.
[http://dx.doi.org/10.4103/jfmpc.jfmpc_264_19] [PMID: 31334148]

[105] Tasneem I, Ariz A, Bharti D, Haleem A, Javaid M, Bahl S. 3D printing technology and its significant applications in the context of healthcare education. J Indus Integ Manag 2023; 8(1): 113-30.
[http://dx.doi.org/10.1142/S2424862221500159]

[106] Shaikh A, Memon M, Memon N, Misbahuddin M. The role of service-oriented architecture in telemedicine healthcare system. 2009 International Conference on Complex, Intelligent and Software Intensive Systems 2009; 208-14.
[http://dx.doi.org/10.1109/CISIS.2009.181]

[107] Scalvini S, Vitacca M, Paletta L, Giordano A, Balbi B. Telemedicine: a new frontier for effective healthcare services. Monaldi Arch Chest Dis 2004; 61(4): 226-33.
[http://dx.doi.org/10.4081/monaldi.2004.686] [PMID: 15909613]

[108] Ito J, Edirippulige S, Aono T, Armfield NR. The use of telemedicine for delivering healthcare in Japan: Systematic review of literature published in Japanese and English languages. J Telemed Telecare 2017; 23(10): 828-34.
[http://dx.doi.org/10.1177/1357633X17732801] [PMID: 29081269]

[109] Xiong G, Greene NE, Lightsey HM IV, *et al.* Telemedicine use in orthopaedic surgery varies by race, ethnicity, primary language, and insurance status. Clin Orthop Relat Res 2021; 479(7): 1417-25.
[http://dx.doi.org/10.1097/CORR.0000000000001775] [PMID: 33982979]

[110] Sapci AH, Sapci HA. Digital continuous healthcare and disruptive medical technologies: m-Health and telemedicine skills training for data-driven healthcare. J Telemed Telecare 2019; 25(10): 623-35.
[http://dx.doi.org/10.1177/1357633X18793293] [PMID: 30134779]

[111] Magann EF, McKelvey SS, Hitt WC, Smith MV, Azam GA, Lowery CL. The use of telemedicine in obstetrics: a review of the literature. Obstet Gynecol Surv 2011; 66(3): 170-8.
[http://dx.doi.org/10.1097/OGX.0b013e3182219902] [PMID: 21689487]

[112] Palozzi G, Schettini I, Chirico A. Enhancing the sustainable goal of access to healthcare: findings from a literature review on telemedicine employment in rural areas. Sustainability (Basel) 2020; 12(8): 3318.
[http://dx.doi.org/10.3390/su12083318]

[113] de Moraes ERFL, Cirenza C, Lopes RD, *et al.* Prevalence of atrial fibrillation and stroke risk assessment based on telemedicine screening tools in a primary healthcare setting. Eur J Intern Med 2019; 67: 36-41.
[http://dx.doi.org/10.1016/j.ejim.2019.04.024] [PMID: 31320151]

[114] Drake C, Lian T, Cameron B, Medynskaya K, Bosworth HB, Shah K. Understanding telemedicine's "new normal": variations in telemedicine use by specialty line and patient demographics Telemed e-Health 2022; 28(1): 51-9.

[115] Brown EM. The Ontario telemedicine network: a case report Telemed e-Health 2013; 19(5): 373-6.
[http://dx.doi.org/10.1089/tmj.2012.0299]

[116] Pandian PS. An overview of telemedicine technologies for healthcare applications. Int J Biomed Clin Eng 2016; 5(2): 29-52.
[http://dx.doi.org/10.4018/IJBCE.2016070103]

[117] Ryu S. History of telemedicine: evolution, context, and transformation. Healthc Inform Res 2010; 16(1): 65-6.
[http://dx.doi.org/10.4258/hir.2010.16.1.65] [PMID: 22509475]

[118] O'Shea J, Berger R, Samra C, Van Durme D. Telemedicine in education: bridging the gap. Educ Health (Abingdon) 2015; 28(1): 64-7.
[http://dx.doi.org/10.4103/1357-6283.161897] [PMID: 26261117]

[119]   Sim R, Lee SWH. Patient preference and satisfaction with the use of telemedicine for glycemic control in patients with type 2 diabetes: a review. Patient Prefer Adherence 2021; 15: 283-98.
[http://dx.doi.org/10.2147/PPA.S271449] [PMID: 33603347]

[120]   Sharma R, Fleischut P, Barchi D. Telemedicine and its transformation of emergency care: a case study of one of the largest US integrated healthcare delivery systems. Int J Emerg Med 2017; 10(1): 21.
[http://dx.doi.org/10.1186/s12245-017-0146-7] [PMID: 28685213]

[121]   Nutalapati R, Jampani ND, Dontula BSK, Boyapati R. Applications of teledentistry: A literature review and update. J Int Soc Prev Community Dent 2011; 1(2): 37-44.
[http://dx.doi.org/10.4103/2231-0762.97695] [PMID: 24478952]

[122]   Chen JW, Hobdell MH, Dunn K, Johnson KA, Zhang J. Teledentistry and its use in dental education. J Am Dent Assoc 2003; 134(3): 342-6.
[http://dx.doi.org/10.14219/jada.archive.2003.0164] [PMID: 12699048]

[123]   Mariño R, Ghanim A. Teledentistry: a systematic review of the literature. J Telemed Telecare 2013; 19(4): 179-83.
[http://dx.doi.org/10.1177/1357633x13479704] [PMID: 23512650]

[124]   Daniel SJ, Kumar S. Teledentistry: a key component in access to care. J Evid Based Dent Pract 2014; 14 (Suppl.): 201-8.
[http://dx.doi.org/10.1016/j.jebdp.2014.02.008] [PMID: 24929605]

[125]   Khan SA, Omar H. Teledentistry in practice: literature review Telemed e-Health 2013; 19(7): 565-7.
[http://dx.doi.org/10.1089/tmj.2012.0200]

[126]   Fernández CE, Maturana CA, Coloma SI, Carrasco-Labra A, Giacaman RA. Teledentistry and mHealth for promotion and prevention of oral health: a systematic review and meta-analysis. J Dent Res 2021; 100(9): 914-27.
[http://dx.doi.org/10.1177/00220345211003828] [PMID: 33769123]

[127]   Sood S, Mbarika V, Jugoo S, Dookhy R, Doarn CR, Prakash N, *et al.* What is telemedicine? A collection of 104 peer-reviewed perspectives and theoretical underpinnings. Telemed e-Health 2007; 13(5): 573-90.

[128]   Armaignac DL, Saxena A, Rubens M, *et al.* Impact of telemedicine on mortality, length of stay, and cost among patients in progressive care units: experience from a large healthcare system. Crit Care Med 2018; 46(5): 728-35.
[http://dx.doi.org/10.1097/CCM.0000000000002994] [PMID: 29384782]

[129]   Schwalb P, Klecun E. The role of contradictions and norms in the design and use of telemedicine: healthcare professionals' perspective. AIS Trans Hum-Comput Interact 2019; 11(3): 117-35.
[http://dx.doi.org/10.17705/1thci.00116]

[130]   Abdellatif MM, Mohamed W. Telemedicine: An IoT Based Remote Healthcare System. Int J Online Biomed Eng 2020; 16(6)
[http://dx.doi.org/10.3991/ijoe.v16i06.13651]

[131]   Jin Z, Chen Y. Telemedicine in the cloud era: Prospects and challenges. IEEE Pervasive Comput 2015; 14(1): 54-61.
[http://dx.doi.org/10.1109/MPRV.2015.19]

[132]   Kamsu-Foguem B, Foguem C. Telemedicine and mobile health with integrative medicine in developing countries. Health Policy Technol 2014; 3(4): 264-71.
[http://dx.doi.org/10.1016/j.hlpt.2014.08.008]

[133]   Matusitz J, Breen GM. E-health: A new kind of telemedicine. Soc Work Public Health 2007; 23(1): 95-113.
[http://dx.doi.org/10.1300/J523v23n01_06]

[134]   Chih-Jen H. Telemedicine Information Monitoring System HealthCom 2008 - 10th International

Conference on e-Health Networking, Applications and Services; IEEE 2008; pp. 48-50.
[http://dx.doi.org/10.1109/HEALTH.2008.4600108]

[135] Shah AC, Badawy SM. Telemedicine in pediatrics: systematic review of randomized controlled trials. JMIR Pediatr Parent 2021; 4(1): e22696.
[http://dx.doi.org/10.2196/22696] [PMID: 33556030]

[136] Garai Á, Péntek I, Adamkó A. Revolutionizing healthcare with IoT and cognitive, cloud-based telemedicine. Acta Polytech Hung 2019; 16(2): 163-81.

[137] McConnochie KM, Ronis SD, Wood NE, Ng PK. Effectiveness and safety of acute care telemedicine for children with regular and special healthcare needs Telemed e-Health 2015; 21(8): 611-21.
[http://dx.doi.org/10.1089/tmj.2014.0175]

[138] Loeb AE, Rao SS, Ficke JR, Morris CD, Riley LH III, Levin AS. Departmental experience and lessons learned with accelerated introduction of telemedicine during the COVID-19 crisis. J Am Acad Orthop Surg 2020; 28(11): e469-76.
[http://dx.doi.org/10.5435/JAAOS-D-20-00380] [PMID: 32301818]

[139] Van Velsen L, Wildevuur S, Flierman I, Van Schooten B, Tabak M, Hermens H. Trust in telemedicine portals for rehabilitation care: an exploratory focus group study with patients and healthcare professionals. BMC Med Inform Decis Mak 2015; 16(1): 11.
[http://dx.doi.org/10.1186/s12911-016-0250-2] [PMID: 26818611]

[140] Das LT, Gonzalez CJ. Preparing telemedicine for the frontlines of healthcare equity. J Gen Intern Med 2020; 35(8): 2443-4.
[http://dx.doi.org/10.1007/s11606-020-05941-9] [PMID: 32495089]

[141] Dasgupta A, Deb S. Telemedicine: A new horizon in public health in India. Indian J Community Med 2008; 33(1): 3-8.
[http://dx.doi.org/10.4103/0970-0218.39234] [PMID: 19966987]

[142] Oborn E, Pilosof NP, Hinings B, Zimlichman E. Institutional logics and innovation in times of crisis: Telemedicine as digital 'PPE'. Inf Organ 2021; 31(1): 100340.
[http://dx.doi.org/10.1016/j.infoandorg.2021.100340]

[143] Waegemann CP. mHealth: the next generation of telemedicine? Telemed e-Health 2010; 16(1): 23-6.

[144] Djamasbi S, Fruhling A, Loiacono E. The influence of affect, attitude and usefulness in the acceptance of telemedicine systems. J Inf Technol Theory Appl 2009; 10(1): 4.

[145] Le LB, Rahal HK, Viramontes MR, Meneses KG, Dong TS, Saab S. Patient satisfaction and healthcare utilization using telemedicine in liver transplant recipients. Dig Dis Sci 2019; 64(5): 1150-7.
[http://dx.doi.org/10.1007/s10620-018-5397-5] [PMID: 30519848]

[146] Wechsler LR, Demaerschalk BM, Schwamm LH, *et al.* Telemedicine quality and outcomes in stroke: a scientific statement for healthcare professionals from the American Heart Association/American Stroke Association. Stroke 2017; 48(1): e3-e25.
[http://dx.doi.org/10.1161/STR.0000000000000114] [PMID: 27811332]

[147] Jennett P, Watanabe M. Healthcare and telemedicine: ongoing and evolving challenges. Dis Manag Health Outcomes 2006; 14 (Suppl. 1): 9-13.
[http://dx.doi.org/10.2165/00115677-200614001-00004]

[148] Shah MN, Gillespie SM, Wood N, *et al.* High-intensity telemedicine-enhanced acute care for older adults: an innovative healthcare delivery model. J Am Geriatr Soc 2013; 61(11): 2000-7.
[http://dx.doi.org/10.1111/jgs.12523] [PMID: 24164485]

[149] Mukhopadhyay A. QoS based telemedicine technologies for rural healthcare emergencies. 2017 IEEE Global Humanitarian Technology Conference (GHTC) San Jose, CA, USA, IEEE 2017; 1-7.
[http://dx.doi.org/10.1109/GHTC.2017.8239296]

[150] Javaid M, Khan IH. Virtual reality (VR) applications in cardiology: a review. J Indus Inte Manag 2022; 7(2): 183-202.
[http://dx.doi.org/10.1142/S2424862221300015]

[151] Javaid M, Khan IH, Vaishya R, Singh RP, Vaish A. Data analytics applications for COVID-19 pandemic. Curr Med Res Pract 2021; 11(2): 105-6.
[http://dx.doi.org/10.4103/cmrp.cmrp_82_20]

[152] Haleem A, Javaid M, Suman R, Singh RP. 3D printing applications for radiology: an overview. Indian J Radiol Imaging 2021; 31(1): 10-7.
[PMID: 34316106]

[153] Haleem A, Javaid M, Rab S. Impact of additive manufacturing in different areas of Industry 4.0. International Journal of Logistics Systems and Management 2020; 37(2): 239-51.
[http://dx.doi.org/10.1504/IJLSM.2020.110578]

[154] Suman R, Javaid M, Choudhary SK, *et al.* Impact of COVID-19 Pandemic on Particulate Matter (PM) concentration and harmful gaseous components on Indian metros. Sustainable Operations and Computers 2021; 2: 1-11.
[http://dx.doi.org/10.1016/j.susoc.2021.02.001]

[155] Gupta P, Haleem A, Javaid M. Designing of a carburettor body for ethanol blended fuel by using CFD analysis tool and 3D scanning technology J Sci Ind Res 2019; 78(7): 466-72.

[156] Javaid M, Babu S, Rab S, Vaishya R, Haleem A. Tribological review of medical implants manufactured by additive manufacturing. Tribology and Sustainability. Boca Raton: CRC Press 2021; pp. 379-95.
[http://dx.doi.org/10.1201/9781003092162-24]

[157] Larsen SB, Sørensen NS, Petersen MG, Kjeldsen GF. Towards a shared service centre for telemedicine: Telemedicine in Denmark, and a possible way forward. Health Informatics J 2016; 22(4): 815-27.
[http://dx.doi.org/10.1177/1460458215592042] [PMID: 26261216]

[158] Kidholm K, Ekeland AG, Jensen LK, *et al.* A model for assessment of telemedicine applications: mast. Int J Technol Assess Health Care 2012; 28(1): 44-51.
[http://dx.doi.org/10.1017/S0266462311000638] [PMID: 22617736]

[159] DeSilva S, Vaidya SS. The application of telemedicine to pediatric obesity: lessons from the past decade. Telemed J E Health 2021; 27(2): 159-66.
[http://dx.doi.org/10.1089/tmj.2019.0314] [PMID: 32293986]

[160] Philips R, Seim N, Matrka L, *et al.* Cost savings associated with an outpatient otolaryngology telemedicine clinic. Laryngoscope Investig Otolaryngol 2019; 4(2): 234-40.
[http://dx.doi.org/10.1002/lio2.244] [PMID: 31024993]

[161] Chen ET. Considerations of telemedicine in the delivery of modern healthcare. Am J Manag 2017; 17(3)

[162] Bashshur RL, Shannon GW, Smith BR, *et al.* The empirical foundations of telemedicine interventions for chronic disease management. Telemed J E Health 2014; 20(9): 769-800.
[http://dx.doi.org/10.1089/tmj.2014.9981] [PMID: 24968105]

[163] Justice EO. E-healthcare/telemedicine readiness assessment of some selected states in Western Nigeria. Int J Eng Technol 2012; 2(2): 195-201.

[164] Sohn S, Helms TM, Pelleter JT, Müller A, Kröttinger AI, Schöffski O. Costs and benefits of personalized healthcare for patients with chronic heart failure in the care and education program "Telemedicine for the Heart". Telemed J E Health 2012; 18(3): 198-204.
[http://dx.doi.org/10.1089/tmj.2011.0134] [PMID: 22356529]

[165] Mariani AW, Pêgo-Fernandes PM. Telemedicine: a technological revolution. Sao Paulo Med J 2012;

130(5): 277-8.
[http://dx.doi.org/10.1590/S1516-31802012000500001] [PMID: 23174864]

[166] Williams OE, Elghenzai S, Subbe C, Wyatt JC, Williams J. The use of telemedicine to enhance secondary care: some lessons from the front line. Future Healthc J 2017; 4(2): 109-14.
[http://dx.doi.org/10.7861/futurehosp.4-2-109] [PMID: 31098445]

[167] Javaid M, Haleem A, Pratap Singh R, Suman R. Industrial perspectives of 3D scanning: Features, roles and it's analytical applications. Sens Int 2021; 2: 100114.
[http://dx.doi.org/10.1016/j.sintl.2021.100114]

[168] Purohit B, Vernekar PR, Shetti NP, Chandra P. Biosensor nanoengineering: Design, operation, and implementation for biomolecular analysis. Sens Int 2020; 1: 100040.
[http://dx.doi.org/10.1016/j.sintl.2020.100040]

[169] Haleem A, Javaid M, Singh RP, Suman R, Rab S. Biosensors applications in medical field: A brief review. Sens Int 2021; 2: 100100.
[http://dx.doi.org/10.1016/j.sintl.2021.100100]

[170] Chandra P. Miniaturized label-free smartphone assisted electrochemical sensing approach for personalized COVID-19 diagnosis. Sens Int 2020; 1: 100019.
[http://dx.doi.org/10.1016/j.sintl.2020.100019] [PMID: 34766038]

[171] Acharya RV, Rai JJ. Evaluation of patient and doctor perception toward the use of telemedicine in Apollo Tele Health Services, India. J Family Med Prim Care 2016; 5(4): 798-803.
[http://dx.doi.org/10.4103/2249-4863.201174] [PMID: 28348994]

[172] Shamim-Uzzaman QA, Bae CJ, Ehsan Z, *et al.* The use of telemedicine for the diagnosis and treatment of sleep disorders: an American Academy of Sleep Medicine update. J Clin Sleep Med 2021; 17(5): 1103-7.
[http://dx.doi.org/10.5664/jcsm.9194] [PMID: 33599202]

[173] Ohinmaa A, Hailey D, Roine R. Elements for assessment of telemedicine applications. Int J Technol Assess Health Care 2001; 17(2): 190-202.
[http://dx.doi.org/10.1017/S0266462300105057] [PMID: 11446131]

[174] Zanaboni P, Knarvik U, Wootton R. Adoption of routine telemedicine in Norway: the current picture. Glob Health Action 2014; 7(1): 22801.
[http://dx.doi.org/10.3402/gha.v7.22801] [PMID: 24433942]

[175] Wootton R, Bahaadinbeigy K, Hailey D. Estimating travel reduction associated with the use of telemedicine by patients and healthcare professionals: proposal for quantitative synthesis in a systematic review. BMC Health Serv Res 2011; 11(1): 185.
[http://dx.doi.org/10.1186/1472-6963-11-185] [PMID: 21824388]

[176] Xue Y, Liang H, Mbarika V, Hauser R, Schwager P, Kassa Getahun M. Investigating the resistance to telemedicine in Ethiopia. Int J Med Inform 2015; 84(8): 537-47.
[http://dx.doi.org/10.1016/j.ijmedinf.2015.04.005] [PMID: 25991059]

[177] Khoong EC, Butler BA, Mesina O, *et al.* Patient interest in and barriers to telemedicine video visits in a multilingual urban safety-net system. J Am Med Inform Assoc 2021; 28(2): 349-53.
[http://dx.doi.org/10.1093/jamia/ocaa234] [PMID: 33164063]

[178] de Toledo P, Jiménez S, del Pozo F, Roca J, Alonso A, Hernandez C. Telemedicine experience for chronic care in COPD. IEEE Trans Inf Technol Biomed 2006; 10(3): 567-73.
[http://dx.doi.org/10.1109/TITB.2005.863877] [PMID: 16871726]

[179] Lin CF. Mobile telemedicine: a survey study. J Med Syst 2012; 36(2): 511-20.
[http://dx.doi.org/10.1007/s10916-010-9496-x] [PMID: 20703699]

[180] Whitten P. Telemedicine: communication technologies that revolutionize healthcare services. Generations 2006; 30(2): 20-4.

[181] Hu PJH. Evaluating telemedicine systems success: a revised model. Proceedings of the 36th Annual Hawaii International Conference on System Sciences. Big Island, HI, USA. EEE 2003; p. 8.

[182] Acheampong F, Vimarlund V. Business models for telemedicine services: a literature review. Health Syst (Basingstoke) 2015; 4(3): 189-203.
[http://dx.doi.org/10.1057/hs.2014.20]

[183] Kim YS. Telemedicine in the USA with focus on clinical applications and issues. Yonsei Med J 2004; 45(5): 761-75.
[http://dx.doi.org/10.3349/ymj.2004.45.5.761] [PMID: 15515185]

[184] Klaassen B, van Beijnum BJF, Hermens HJ. Usability in telemedicine systems—A literature survey. Int J Med Inform 2016; 93: 57-69.
[http://dx.doi.org/10.1016/j.ijmedinf.2016.06.004] [PMID: 27435948]

[185] Fox KC, Somes GW, Waters TM. Timeliness and access to healthcare services *via* telemedicine for adolescents in state correctional facilities. J Adolesc Health 2007; 41(2): 161-7.
[http://dx.doi.org/10.1016/j.jadohealth.2007.05.001] [PMID: 17659220]

[186] Coldebella B, Armfield NR, Bambling M, Hansen J, Edirippulige S. The use of telemedicine for delivering healthcare to bariatric surgery patients: A literature review. J Telemed Telecare 2018; 24(10): 651-60.
[http://dx.doi.org/10.1177/1357633X18795356] [PMID: 30343656]

[187] Xiao Y, Xuemin Shen , BO Sun , Lin Cai . Security and privacy in RFID and applications in telemedicine. IEEE Commun Mag 2006; 44(4): 64-72.
[http://dx.doi.org/10.1109/MCOM.2006.1632651]

[188] Hersh WR, Helfand M, Wallace J, *et al.* Clinical outcomes resulting from telemedicine interventions: a systematic review. BMC Med Inform Decis Mak 2001; 1(1): 5.
[http://dx.doi.org/10.1186/1472-6947-1-5] [PMID: 11737882]

[189] Al-Sofiani ME, Alyusuf EY, Alharthi S, Alguwaihes AM, Al-Khalifah R, Alfadda A. Rapid implementation of a diabetes telemedicine clinic during the coronavirus disease 2019 outbreak: our protocol, experience, and satisfaction reports in Saudi Arabia. J Diabetes Sci Technol 2021; 15(2): 329-38.
[http://dx.doi.org/10.1177/1932296820947094] [PMID: 32762362]

[190] Ateriya N, Saraf A, Meshram V, Setia P. Telemedicine and virtual consultation: The Indian perspective. Natl Med J India 2018; 31(4): 215-8.
[http://dx.doi.org/10.4103/0970-258X.258220] [PMID: 31134926]

[191] Leite H, Hodgkinson IR, Gruber T. New development: 'Healing at a distance'—telemedicine and COVID-19. Public Money Manag 2020; 40(6): 483-5.
[http://dx.doi.org/10.1080/09540962.2020.1748855]

[192] Constantinides P, Barrett M. Negotiating ICT development and use: The case of a telemedicine system in the healthcare region of Crete. Inf Organ 2006; 16(1): 27-55.
[http://dx.doi.org/10.1016/j.infoandorg.2005.07.001]

CHAPTER 6

Wearable Technology for Health Monitoring

Aryan Kumar[1]**, Shaweta Sharma**[1,*] **and Pushpak Singh**[1]

[1] *Department of Pharmacy, School of Medical and Allied Sciences, Galgotias University, Greater Noida, Uttar Pradesh-201310, India*

Abstract: Wearable technology in modern healthcare is an incredible tool for the provision of continuous monitoring, personalization, and better management of disease. With smartwatches, a fitness tracker, and sophisticated sensors, these gadgets collect and interpret data concerning heart rate, blood pressure, oxygen saturation, levels of glucose, and an electrocardiogram ECG. Progress in sensor technology, artificial intelligence, and networking has facilitated enhancements in patient outcomes and, in turn, contributed to the reduction of healthcare costs. Such advancements in wearables incorporate the use of AI in predictive analytics and anomaly detection to predict and intervene earlier in cases of arrhythmias, diabetes, and sleep apnea, among others. The advent of non-invasive biosensors has broadened their applications, facilitating continuous glucose monitoring and hydration status evaluation without the need for needles. These wearables, in conjunction with cloud-based platforms, enable seamless data interchange with healthcare professionals, hence improving remote patient monitoring and telemedicine applications. The COVID-19 pandemic expedited the utilisation of wearables for symptom tracking, recovery monitoring, and long-term effect identification. Furthermore, wearables are essential in clinical studies, as they provide real-world data on patient compliance and treatment effectiveness. Notwithstanding its potential, obstacles remain, encompassing concerns regarding data privacy, device precision, and the digital divide impacting accessibility. Emerging trends indicate the convergence of wearables with augmented reality (AR), 5G connectivity, and machine learning to enhance immersive and intelligent health solutions. As wearable technology advances, it is poised to transform patient-centered care, improving the accessibility, proactivity, and efficiency of health monitoring.

Keywords: Artificial intelligence in healthcare, Biosensors, Health monitoring, Remote patient monitoring, Wearable technology.

INTRODUCTION

In a rapidly evolving environment, almost all innovations must be interconnected, accessible from afar, and subject to analysis. To achieve this, we employ the Internet of Information.

---

[*] **Corresponding author Shaweta Sharma**: Department of Pharmacy, School of Medical and Allied Sciences, Galgotias University, Greater Noida, Uttar Pradesh-201310, India; E-mail: shawetasharma@galgotiasuniversity.edu.in

Shaweta Sharma, Akhil Sharma, Shivkanya Fuloria & Anurag Singh (Eds.)
All rights reserved-© 2025 Bentham Science Publishers

The Internet of Everything (IoE) enables objects to connect to the online world, thereby making them 'smart,' including devices like smartwatches and smart lights. The Internet of Things enhances human autonomy in interacting, contributing, and collaborating with objects [1]. The Internet of Things (IoT) has been implemented across various sectors, including agriculture, home automation, roadway management, transportation oversight, water supply management, vehicle management, electric power systems, and energy efficiency [2].

Wearable technology is rapidly becoming addictive due to its capacity to facilitate a level of self-awareness previously unattainable. The worldwide initiative for wearable technology in conjunction with medical devices has intensified in recent years, and numerous problems exist in integrating it with monitoring sensors. These wearable healthcare gadgets differ from the majority of medical devices in that they produce very extensive and intricate datasets, which is in contrast to conventional sensors. Intelligent wearable technology embodies the subsequent form factor of computational models, amalgamating features of a telephone, wristwatch, and fitness tracker, along with other biophysical sensors. We are in an era of mobile computing and networking for wireless and wearable technologies, as well as instruments for processing extensive health data resources [3, 4].

The technology of IoT-enabled portable gadgets with sensors is a swiftly growing field in medical treatment. As the healthcare sector advances, there is a demand for accessible diagnostics and effective data monitoring and administration. The ultimate objective is to integrate IoT into emergency services, connected residences, intelligent healthcare facilities, electronic health records, and similar domains [5]. The information gathered by intelligent devices and an advanced medical facility can track the signs of illness instantaneously. This can promote advancements regarding health care, medical procedures, drugs, and immunizations. The ultimate objective is to provide data security and accessibility for authorised individuals through cloud computing, fog computing, and similar technologies [6].

Coronavirus disease (COVID-19), which first arose in late 2019, resulted in over three million fatalities globally, significantly affecting patients' physical and mental health [7, 8]. It is crucial to monitor the physiological as well as hemodynamic characteristics of individuals, such as their body temperature, pulse, arterial pressure, as well as airflow, in order to evaluate their health status during treatment, especially for those with mild symptoms who are secluded at residence [9]. Furthermore, chronic conditions like cardiovascular disorders as well as hyperglycemia lead to a substantial number of annual deaths, including arteriosclerosis, diabetes, coronary heart disease, and hypertension, which can be successfully reduced with prompt identification and sustained constant surveillance [10 - 13]. However, the continuous monitoring of the above-described physiological indicators at home using traditional clinical procedures and instruments is challenging due to their limited practicality and high costs. Advancements in adaptable electronics, as well as nanotechnology, have led to the development of portable gadgets that demonstrate remarkable elasticity as well as skin-like conformity, making them significant contenders for healthcare applications [14 - 23]. Currently, various advanced medical devices have been developed for measuring blood pressure, body temperature, heartbeat, and glucose levels, utilizing piezoelectric effects, capacitance effects, and electrochemical principles [24 - 30]. These tracking devices can be easily integrated into smart clothing or watches for ongoing healthcare, enabling home-based telemedicine surveillance. This chapter aims to promote the evolution of ubiquitous health tracking devices, along with their healthcare implications, by focusing on recent breakthroughs in skin-like sensing technologies. It provides an extensive overview of health monitoring principles, device fabrication, potential clinical applications, and upcoming advancements [31, 32].

IOT AND HEALTHCARE

Health care constitutes one of the most respected sectors for IoT use. Through the Web of Things, clinicians can provide online assistance to individuals. Portable IoT-enabled wellness tracking gadgets can significantly reduce the gap between the person receiving treatment and the medical professional. The Internet of Things (IoT) enables personalised patient care by facilitating the assessment of health conditions and the formulation of tailored treatment strategies. Portable sensors would enable physicians to remotely monitor patients' health and respond instantly. Nonetheless, real-time metrics necessitate a continuous Internet connection. Despite the rapid advancement of IoT in healthcare, its implementation remains incomplete in many medical sectors [33]. The creation of suitable Internet applications for traditional medicine continues to encounter challenges. The substantial rise in medical research is likely to result in the Internet of Things garnering an increasing number of studies in the forthcoming years. Contemporary medical practitioners must gather extensive big data and analyse and interpret it to make informed and personalised recommendations. All of it requires substantial effort and time. Emerging IoT technology can expedite and streamline this process. The widespread implementation of electronic health registration has resulted in an increasing volume of digitised medical data. A comprehensive review and evaluation of all this information requires significant time. Moreover, it is essential to train medical personnel in AI-based technologies closely linked to IoT [34]. By leveraging the synergistic capabilities of digital innovations, such as the IoT and AI, physicians can more effectively customise treatments to meet patients' specific requirements. These technologies enable the management of a significantly larger volume of information for storage and analysis, facilitating the meticulous monitoring of the progression of a specific disease or process. Effectively integrating practical personal experience with innovative diagnostic, collecting, and analytical tools will result in beneficial transformations in healthcare management. The Internet of Things is profoundly transforming data generation, utilisation, and dissemination. Typical individuals often utilise these devices to monitor their dietary intake, sleep patterns, vital signs, physical activity, and other physiological conditions, while IoT technologies intermittently collect and analyse environmental data that influence personal health. This interoperability has initiated the development of innovative medicinal options [35]. The concept of IoT for healthcare is illustrated in Fig. (**1**)

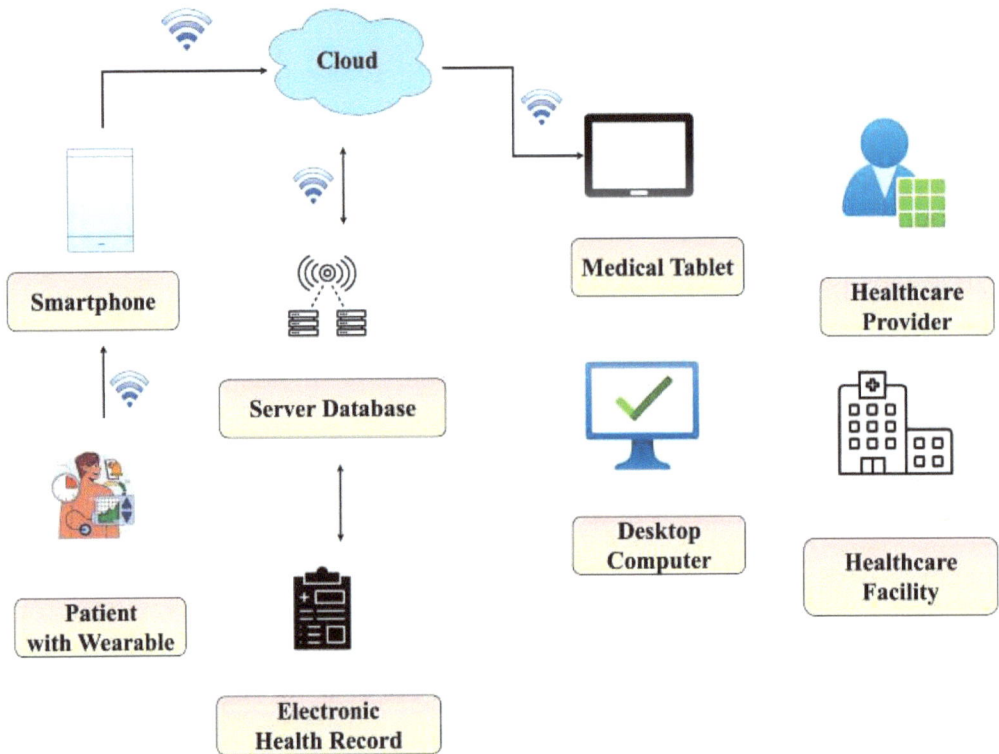

Fig. (1). The concept of IoT for healthcare.

ARCHITECTURE OF IOT-ENABLED PORTABLE SENSOR NETWORKS FOR HEALTH CARE SURVEILLANCE

A range of portable sensors is employed to create a wireless sensor network for remote patient monitoring. The essential structure of a Health Monitoring System

(HMS) is comprised mostly of wearable sensors. The sensor's information is transmitted to the data center using Zigbee, Bluetooth, or Wi-Fi. The information is subsequently transported over an interface channel to the information center for additional analysis. The same statistics are available in real-time to both the physician and the patient's caregivers, enabling them to detect any emergencies [36]. The analysis of IoT-enabled wearable sensor devices for health monitoring is presented in Fig. (2).

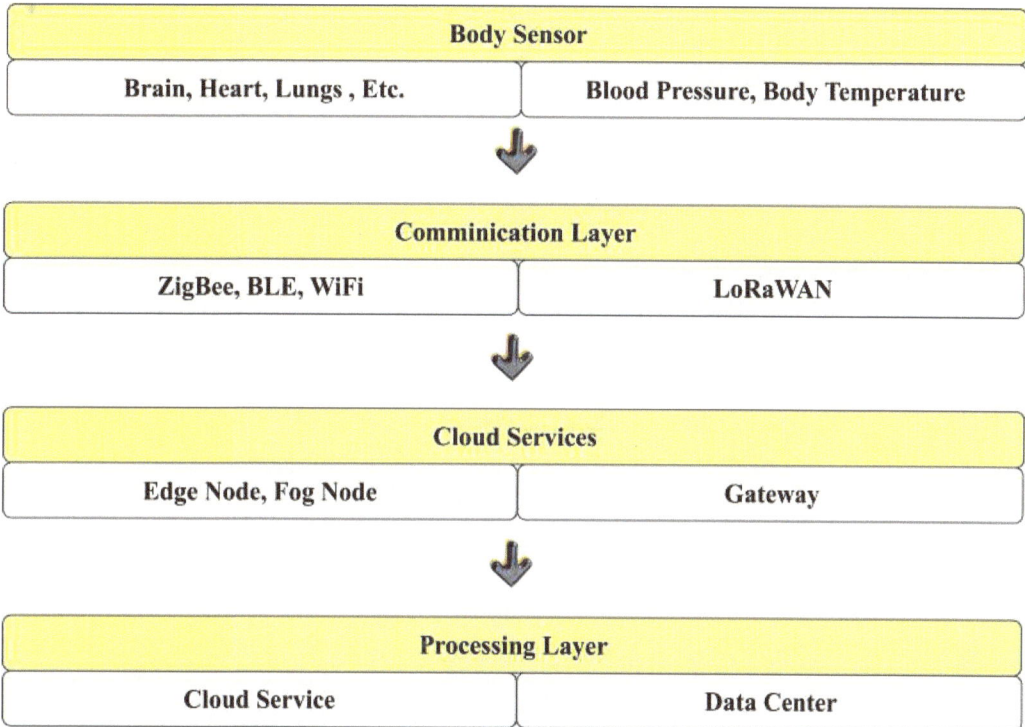

Body Sensor	
Brain, Heart, Lungs , Etc.	Blood Pressure, Body Temperature

⬇

Comminication Layer	
ZigBee, BLE, WiFi	LoRaWAN

⬇

Cloud Services	
Edge Node, Fog Node	Gateway

⬇

Processing Layer	
Cloud Service	Data Center

Fig. (2). Analysis of IoT-enabled wearable sensor devices for health monitoring.

Data Processing

In a device that collects information over a period, information is collected and then analyzed. The data are employed for preliminary processing, following which anomalies and erroneous items are removed. The information is then sent to computational frameworks, where it is processed using diverse machine learning methodologies. The data processing life cycle in healthcare is depicted in Fig. (3).

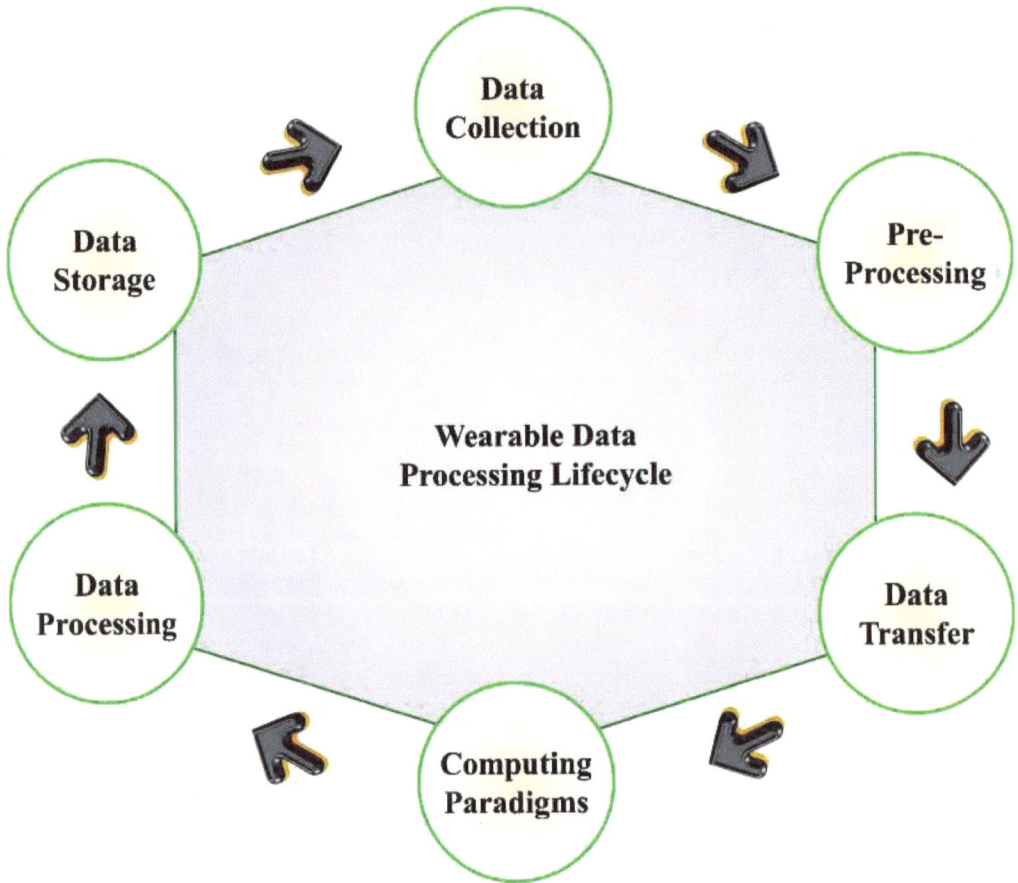

Fig. (3). Data processing life cycle in healthcare.

Data Transfer

The data transfer procedure is a standardised design for the transmission of information exchanged between two devices. In IoT-enabled healthcare systems, data processing is a multi-stage procedure that starts with the acquisition of physiological signals through wearable sensors. These sensors track diverse health parameters, including heart rate, blood pressure, and glucose levels, generating substantial amounts of raw data. This information is then forwarded to proximate gateways or edge devices using wireless communication protocols such as Bluetooth, Zigbee, or Wi-Fi. The initial processing of data on the edge tier involves noise reduction, signal conditioning, and feature extraction, ensuring that only relevant and high-quality information is passed forward. This approach reduces the volume of data sent to the central servers, and additionally, it enables real-time analysis with immediate feedback, which is necessary for prompt medical intervention. The data is then transferred to the cloud server for extensive analysis, long-term storage, and integration into electronic health records. Then, advanced analytics techniques and machine learning algorithms are used to extract patterns and predict health-related events, thereby supporting clinical decision-making processes. At the core of this structured data processing architecture lies an improvement of healthcare provision efficiency and effectiveness by exploiting the advantages of both edge and cloud computing resources [37]. The various categories of data transfer protocols are as follows:

File Transfer Protocol (FTP)

FTP is a conventional protocol utilized for the transmission of files between computers across a network. In healthcare, it is often employed to move large datasets, such as patient records or diagnostic images, between systems for processing and analysis. Its simplicity makes it suitable for non-real-time data exchange, but it lacks robust security features, requiring additional encryption layers for sensitive data.

Hypertext Transfer Protocol (HTTP) and HTTPS

HTTP is widely used in web-based healthcare applications for transmitting data between client devices and servers. HTTPS, the secure version, ensures encryption and authentication, making it essential for exchanging sensitive health information in applications like telemedicine or remote patient monitoring systems.

Message Queuing Telemetry Transport (MQTT)

MQTT is a lightweight protocol designed for resource-constrained IoT devices. It supports real-time data exchange with minimal bandwidth usage, making it ideal for transmitting health sensor data from wearable devices to central systems or cloud platforms [38].

LoRaWAN

The LoRaWAN Protocol is a broad, low-power, low-bitrate communication architecture designed for the Internet of Things (IoT). It is efficient for devices that run on batteries, especially in cases when conserving energy is critical. It features an extended range and low power consumption.

User Datagram Protocol (UDP)

UDP is a connectionless protocol that prioritizes speed over reliability, making it suitable for applications, such as real-time health data streaming. It is commonly used in scenarios where latency is critical, particularly in video conferencing for telemedicine.

Transmission Control Protocol/Internet Protocol (TCP/IP)

TCP/IP is the backbone of internet communication, ensuring reliable, error-checked, and ordered data transmission. It is widely used in healthcare for secure communication between systems, including electronic health record (EHR) exchanges [39].

Computing Paradigms

The computing paradigms employed in IoT-enabled healthcare systems are pivotal in managing the complex data flows and computational demands inherent in such environments. The concept of edge computing enables computation and data storage closer to the sources of data, including wearables and medical devices, thereby reducing latency and bandwidth consumption. It facilitates near-instant data processing and analysis, and is a prime requirement in applications that require real-time responses, such as continuous patient monitoring. Fog computing achieves this by creating a network of nodes that act as intermediaries between the edge and the cloud, providing additional computation and storage capabilities. This creates a layered architecture that facilitates better data handling and processing by distributing operations across the network according to unique requirements and priorities. On the other hand, cloud computing enables scalable and centralized resources, which are essential for massive data analysis, training of machine learning models, and long-term storage. Therefore, through these computing paradigms, healthcare systems in an IoT environment can easily find an equilibrium between the load across both local and centralized resources due to the timely processing of data, which is of great importance for delivering responsive, personalized healthcare services.

Communication Technologies

This section examines four key communication technologies commonly employed in IoT networks: Zigbee, LoRaWAN, Wi-Fi, and Bluetooth. Among these, ZigBee, Wi-Fi, and Bluetooth are short-range technologies, while LoRaWAN supports long-range communication. Although various wireless protocols are available, these four are considered the most suitable for the intended applications.

ZIGBEE

ZigBee operates based on the IEEE 802.15.4 standard and is designed for resource-constrained environments with low-power devices. It facilitates wireless personal area networking (WPAN) and was initially developed in 1998, with its standardization completed in 2003 [40]. ZigBee employs the Direct Sequence Spread Spectrum (DSSS) technique, offering a range of 10 to 100 meters with very low energy consumption. It supports various network topologies, including ad hoc, star, and mesh configurations. The technology provides a data transmission rate of 250 Kbps and utilizes a channel width of 5 MHz, making it highly cost-effective. The ZigBee network structure consists of three key components: the ZigBee coordinator (ZC), the ZigBee router (ZR), and the ZigBee end-device (ZED). The ZC acts as the central control unit, while the ZR functions as a dependable intermediary router within the network. The ZED is equipped with sensing functionalities and communicates with the primary network components [41].

LoRaWAN

LoRaWAN is a low-power wide-area network (LPWAN) technology that has garnered significant interest in recent years due to its applicability in Internet of Things (IoT) networks [42]. LoRaWAN is designed for low-power long-range IoT networks. While operating on unlicensed radio frequency bands, the range enjoyed by LoRaWAN cannot be rivaled: in rural settings, it reaches 15 km, and in urban areas, it reaches 5 km. This makes LoRaWAN applications appear in remote monitoring and rural health services. Regarding energy efficiency, LoRaWAN can go for years on a single battery. LoRaWAN relies on the transmission of small packets of data, such as vital health metrics and environmental measurements. The data rates vary from 250 bps up to 5.5 kbps. It easily allows the connection of large numbers of end nodes with gateways, significantly enhancing its scalability for large-scale IoT implementations. Despite its many advantages, LoRaWAN is unsuitable for high-bandwidth applications, such as video streaming or diagnostic imaging, due to its limited data transfer rate [43].

Wi-Fi

Wireless Fidelity is a wireless transmission technology founded on the IEEE 802.11 standard. Wi-Fi, based on the IEEE 802.11 standards, is a widely used technology for high-speed wireless internet connectivity. It is particularly effective in healthcare environments requiring high data transfer rates, such as hospitals and telemedicine systems. Wi-Fi offers data speeds of up to 6.75 Gbps with the latest Wi-Fi 6 standard, enabling the transmission of large files, such as medical imaging and diagnostic data. However, its high power consumption limits its suitability for battery-powered wearables. Wi-Fi's range, typically extending up to 50 meters indoors, enables seamless connectivity in controlled environments. While universally supported by most devices, Wi-Fi faces scalability challenges in IoT networks, as congestion and bandwidth sharing can lead to performance bottlenecks [44].

Bluetooth

Bluetooth is based on the IEEE 802.15.1 standard. It operates over a limited range and facilitates data sharing between both stationary and mobile devices. Bluetooth, particularly the Bluetooth Low Energy (BLE) variant, is a short-range wireless technology optimized for low-power IoT applications. With a range of 10–100 meters and data rates of up to 2 Mbps (BLE) or 24 Mbps (Bluetooth Classic), it is widely used in personal healthcare devices, such as fitness trackers, glucose monitors, and smartwatches. BLE's energy efficiency makes it ideal for wearable devices that require long battery life. The technology's secure and reliable data transfer capabilities ensure that sensitive health data is transmitted safely. Furthermore, Bluetooth's simple pairing process enhances user convenience. However, its short range and lower bandwidth compared to Wi-Fi or LoRaWAN limit its use to close-proximity healthcare applications, such as syncing data with mobile phones or tablets [45].

APPLICATION OF IOT-ASSISTED WEARABLE SENSOR FOR HEALTH CARE MONITORING

IoT-enabled wearables are currently prevalent. The user-friendliness of such devices has significantly enhanced their application across various fields. The impact of IoT on healthcare is substantial. Diverse technologies are associated with current technology that facilitates data generation for monitoring and analysis. Wearable sensors have numerous applications. For example, a fitness tracker is produced by multiple manufacturers. The primary objective is to track the individual's pulse, motions, and other metrics by utilising GPS and accelerometer data to ascertain the nature of the activity being performed. By inputting their weight, height, and age, the software may compute the calories expended, the altitudes reached, the steps ascended, the average heart rate, and many other metrics. Trackers provide a range of personalised services. Some of them have proposed estimating the SpO2 levels in the blood to address the ongoing pandemic. Furthermore, the measurements are quite precise. Consequently, even modest modifications to the design of wearables can enhance their effectiveness in capturing patients' vital signs. With the integration of Wi-Fi and other networking technologies discussed earlier, these devices can be transformed into cloud-based solutions.

Activity Recognition

Activity recognition is one of the most common applications of healthcare wearables today. Virtually every kind of fitness monitor executes this form of identification. Currently, fitness monitors are the primary technology used to assess an individual's activity. The majority are outfitted with a very accurate three-dimensional gyroscope that enables the sensor to calculate acceleration, with considerable speculation occurring concurrently. Furthermore, as a result of this methodical estimation, the wearable device determines if the user is walking, running, or sleeping. These wearables are equipped with integrated sensors, such as altimeters, that measure altitude above sea level. This allows them to track the number of flights of stairs climbed. The device typically works in tandem with a smartphone application, which manages operation and synchronizes data. During initial setup, the app usually collects personal information such as height, weight, age, gender, and other relevant data. This information is essential for accurately quantifying steps and distinguishing between different types of physical activity. Manufacturers also use aggregated user data to train algorithms that improve the device's ability to recognize movements, estimate metrics like BMI, and personalize activity tracking.

Stroke Rehabilitation

Cardiovascular illnesses are challenging to address without an effective management system for patient care. Uttara Gogate *et al.* utilised wireless sensor networks for cardiac patients. Numerous studies indicate that cardiovascular problems are common among elderly individuals. Their health may deteriorate at any moment. Patients with cardiac conditions necessitate ongoing surveillance; thus, this device can function as a live monitoring solution utilising WSN technology. This WSN comprises multiple medical-grade sensors and devices capable of monitoring heartbeat, pulse rate, body temperature, and blood pressure, while also ensuring continuous real-time ECG monitoring of the patient [46].

Blood Glucose Monitoring

The advancement of IoT devices for diabetic patients is commendable, leading to a significant improvement in the precision of blood glucose monitoring. The use of these vital signs to monitor patients during diabetic emergencies can be life-saving [47]. IoMT, or the Internet of Medical Things, is specifically tailored for the medical field. IoMT includes devices, such as glucometers, heart rate monitors, and endoscopic pills. These interconnected sensors, leveraging IoT technology, form a wireless body sensor network focused on diabetes. The outlined procedure is robust, adaptable, and cost-effective, utilizing medical-grade sensors and technology, making it more reliable than similar IoT-based systems. Several additional examples have been explored in the context of glucose monitoring applications [48]. One such system prioritizes the evaluation of critical whole-body vital signs, including blood glucose levels, through continuous health tracking. The data is transmitted sequentially to the cloud *via* an ESP8266 Wi-Fi module. A Cyber-Physical System (CPS) continuously monitors the patient's health metrics, including blood glucose (BG), blood pressure (BP), body temperature (BT), and heart rate (HR). A CPS framework has been proposed [49] where the primary characteristics of data storage are uniqueness and reliability, achieved through organized cloud data storage (OCDA). Additionally, an EMG sensor is used to analyze imbalances and discrepancies between neurons and muscles, with all collected data displayed on an LCD screen [50].

Respiration Monitoring

Various methods exist for monitoring the human respiratory system. Some researchers have employed specialized sensors to measure respiratory movements. Using a bioimpedance sensor can be particularly advantageous [51]. This multifunctional sensor emits a small electrical signal into the skin to comprehensively assess both respiratory motion and heart rate. The proposed system utilizes a customized respiratory detector that transmits analog data to the MCU. The sensor is attached to the patient's abdominal region. This highlights that wearables cannot accurately monitor respiration unless a medical-grade sensor is affixed to the abdomen [52].

Sleep Monitoring

A sleep tracking device helps individuals improve their sleeping habits and maintain a balanced lifestyle. It uses multiple sensors to monitor various physiological parameters. Many wearables frequently measure heart rate, pulse rate, SpO2 levels, and breathing patterns to assess sleep quality based on these indicators. These devices are typically multifunctional, incorporating GPS along with a combination of an altimeter and a three-axis accelerometer to evaluate an individual's sleep status. These features have made fitness bands an essential part of many people's daily lives.

An IoT gateway connects the physical layer (sensor nodes) to the server, enabling data collection and synchronization. This facilitates improved real-time communication between users and medical professionals. The findings of different studies support continuous monitoring of individuals during sleep, depicting the user under standard environmental conditions (ambient factors).

Although occasional noise spikes are detected, they are short-lived and do not cause significant interference. Parameters, such as heart rate, skin temperature, respiratory rate, and overall sleep squality, are illustrated and analysed in this chapter [53].

Blood Pressure Monitoring

Hypertension is so prevalent that approximately one in five individuals globally experiences elevated blood pressure. There are multiple methods to measure blood pressure, with the majority of physicians using a sphygmomanometer for this purpose. Additionally, wearables utilize heart rate monitoring technology to estimate blood pressure. By employing pulse wave analysis derived from pulse oximeter readings, these devices utilize specialized algorithms that incorporate criteria such as age, weight, and previously collected data to provide accurate blood pressure estimates. Heart disorders are common among the elderly, and their health can deteriorate suddenly, resulting in urgent and critical situations [54].

Wireless Sensor Network (WSN) systems can monitor various health parameters, including heart rate, pulse rate, body temperature, and blood pressure. For critically ill patients, medical-grade sensors enable real-time ECG monitoring for continuous health assessment. Efforts have also been made to design monitoring systems specifically for expectant mothers, which evaluate parameters, such as blood pressure, body temperature, heart rate, and fetal movements [55].

Advanced tissue differentiation is achieved using medical-grade ultrasonic sensors, enabling real-time imaging and monitoring of soft tissues. A proposed system utilizes a Raspberry Pi as the main processing unit, integrating various components, such as an LM35 temperature sensor for body temperature measurement and a blood pressure sensor for monitoring blood pressure. Additionally, heartbeat and ECG sensors are used to capture vital signs.

The system includes interfaces that connect all sensors to the Raspberry Pi, where the collected data is processed. This data is both stored locally on the Raspberry Pi and uploaded to the cloud for further analysis. Technologies like MATLAB and LabVIEW are employed for data visualization, allowing for a comprehensive understanding of the gathered health information [56].

Stress Monitoring

Stress monitoring involves assessing key vital signs and comparing them to baseline measurements taken during rest. In diabetic individuals, a drop in blood pressure or insulin levels, or the onset of sudden respiratory discomfort, can signal elevated stress levels. Wearable devices are capable of detecting these conditions and alerting the user to slow down or take corrective action. These alerts often serve as reminders to hydrate or provide motivational messages, offering reassurance or boosting the patient's morale.

Sweat gland activity plays a significant role in stress detection. In addition to perspiration, subtle changes in bodily fluids can also indicate that an individual is under stress. The Trier Social Stress Test (TSST) is a widely used method for assessing actual stress levels. Although this approach is not applicable to wearable devices, it remains a reliable tool for controlled stress evaluation [57].

Medical Adherence

Medical adherence, the extent to which patients follow prescribed treatments, including medication schedules, lifestyle modifications, and healthcare recommendations, is a critical factor in achieving positive health outcomes. Non-adherence can lead to reduced treatment efficacy, increased medical complications, and elevated healthcare costs.

IoT-assisted wearable sensors have emerged as innovative solutions to this challenge by enabling real-time monitoring, seamless data integration, and personalized interventions to enhance adherence. Wearable technology incorporates advanced components, such as accelerometers and physiological sensors. For instance, a smartwatch can monitor medication adherence by analyzing movement data from its accelerometer, helping ensure that patients follow their treatment plans.

These devices also offer real-time alerts. One notable example is the Embrace smartwatch, which records critical health events, such as seizures and immediately alerts caregivers or healthcare professionals. This ensures timely intervention and improved management of medical emergencies [58]. Wearable devices enable continuous data integration by collecting vital health metrics, such as heart rate, activity levels, and other physiological signals. This data is analyzed to assess adherence to treatment protocols, providing healthcare professionals with a deeper understanding of a patient's condition. As a result, therapies can be adjusted in a timely manner, ensuring that care remains both appropriate and effective. The benefits of IoT-assisted wearable sensors extend beyond adherence monitoring. These devices contribute to better patient outcomes by reducing the risk of complications and enhancing treatment effectiveness. Continuous monitoring also encourages greater patient engagement with their healthcare routines, empowering individuals to take an active role in managing their health [59].

Cancer Patient Monitoring

Cancer is a condition that lacks an effective treatment. The tumour must be excised solely through chemotherapy, resulting in the patient experiencing weakness and poor health. It is imperative to attend to the patient in this state, as they are susceptible to numerous complications. This paper presents the author's endeavor to establish an IoT-based framework and a layered architecture. Five layers have been delineated for this system, which include the Cancer Care Layer, Hospital Layer, Service Layer, Datacenter Layer, and Security Management Layer. Each layer is characterized by its respective name. This device utilizes medical-grade sensors that are capable of detecting tumor cells present in the patient. Cloud support and analytical capabilities help physicians make informed decisions in critical scenarios. The sensors are integrated with WSN technology and other intelligent devices to enable global data transmission. When compared to existing systems, the proposed model demonstrated enhanced robustness across nearly all evaluated aspects [60].

Asthma and Mental Health Management

Exacerbations make asthma a suitable candidate for IoT-based healthcare solutions. It affects hundreds of millions worldwide. Young and active, most patients are seeking reliable management options. Wristbands that monitor allergen levels and notify users of common triggers are essential for detecting and managing exacerbations. IoT-enabled inhalers can provide doctors with accurate data on patient adherence and device usage [61, 62].

Asthma, like mental health conditions, has a chronic aspect. In addition to the monitoring solutions described earlier, the Internet of Things can enhance patient support services. Furthermore, when combined with AI technologies, IoT may facilitate supportive interactions with diverse applications, ranging from identifying suicidal ideation to providing routine cognitive rehabilitation for individuals with dementia or mild cognitive impairment [63]. An overview of medical wearable devices is illustrated in Fig. (4).

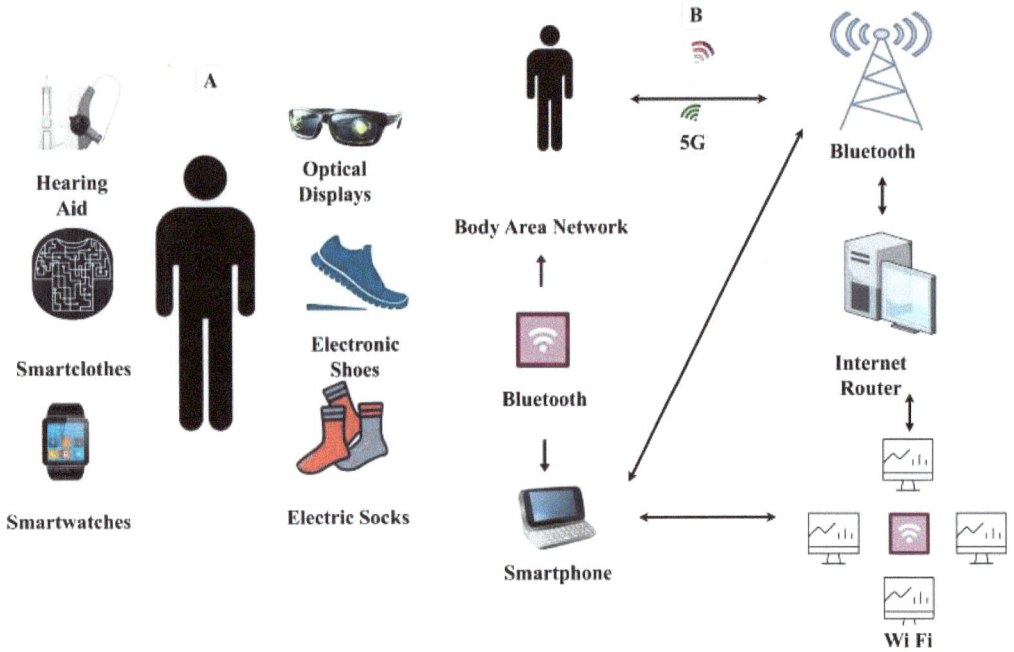

Fig. (4). Medical wearable devices.

WEARABLE DEVICE TYPES

Wearable devices are classified into two categories: Dermal and biofluidic-based wearable devices.

Dermal Wearable Devices

Skin, as a vital part of the human body, serves as an excellent medium for noninvasive healthcare wearables. Skin-integrated sensors support both physiological and psychological monitoring, assisting in the tracking of various medical conditions, including cardiovascular and neuromuscular disorders. Additionally, these devices enable the detection of numerous health issues by analyzing skin secretions, such as sweat, both qualitatively and quantitatively. Wearables for skin applications can be categorized into two main types based on their interaction with the skin: textile-based and epidermal-based. Textile-based wearables incorporate sensors into clothing, while epidermal-based devices adhere directly to the skin, resembling a tattoo, and are collectively known as electronic skin (e-skin) [64].

Biofluidic-based Wearable Device

These devices utilize biological fluids, such as sweat, saliva, tears, and urine, which contain crucial biomarkers for diagnostics and monitoring. Wearable healthcare devices can function independently or in conjunction with other systems. By incorporating microfluidic technology, valuable insights can be gained from various biofluids [65]. Wearable sensors are categorized based on their operational principles into mechanical sensors, electrical sensors, optical sensors, and chemical sensors [66].

Wearable Mechanical Sensor

A wearable mechanical sensor converts mechanical stimuli into electrical signals that can be analyzed and interpreted. These sensors are classified into four types: piezoresistive, piezoelectric, capacitive, and iontronic. Piezoresistive sensors operate based on the "piezoresistive effect," where the electrical properties of conductive materials change when they undergo mechanical deformation. Capacitive sensors detect changes in capacitance caused by mechanical forces, while iontronic sensors respond to pressure variations. Piezoelectric sensors utilize the piezoelectric effect, where certain materials generate electrical charges when subjected to external mechanical forces, pressure, or strain. Mechanical stress alters the electrical polarization within the piezoelectric material, resulting in changes in surface charge (voltage) due to this polarization shift [67].

Wearable Electrical Sensors

These devices detect variations in the skin's electrical resistance or changes in capacitive or conductive properties at the skin's surface by utilizing resistive or capacitive sensors. Circuits with high input impedance are commonly employed to capture the subtle fluctuations in electrical charge [68].

Wearable Optical Sensors

Wearable optical sensors respond to environmental changes induced by biological, chemical, or physical factors by generating optical signals [69]. Various types of optical sensor components are commonly used to assess chemical or biological variations in a given environment, including colorimetric, plasmonic, and fluorometric sensors. Colorimetric sensors detect changes in color when exposed to specific analytes, often resulting from biological or chemical interactions. Absorbance measurements are typically used to quantify these color changes [70]. By shining light on the sensor and collecting and analyzing the reflected or transmitted light, we can determine how the sensor responds.

Plasmonic sensors rely on nanostructures or metal-dielectric interfaces that exhibit optical resonance at specific wavelengths, which depend on the geometry of the structure. Interaction with a particular biological or chemical target can shift the resonance wavelength of the plasmonic sensor [71, 72].

Fluorometric sensors rely on fluorescent materials, such as organic dyes, fluorescent proteins, or quantum dots, to detect environmental changes [73]. These fluorescent molecules require an excitation light source to elevate electrons to a higher energy level, causing them to emit light at a specific wavelength upon returning to the ground state. The intensity or temporal variations of the fluorescent signal are typically correlated with the concentration of the analyte. Due to the separation provided by optical filters, fluorometric sensors can more effectively detect weaker emission signals by reducing interference from the excitation light, which occurs at different wavelengths within the optical spectrum [74].

Wearable Chemical Sensor

In most cases, a chemical or biological sensor consists of two parts: a receptor for recognition and a transducer for signal conversion [75]. Effective integration of a wearable chemical sensor with biofluids enables the translation of chemical signals into electrical or optical formats. Colorimetric signal detection is frequently applied to convert chemical signals into optical signals, similar to the technique used in urine-based pregnancy tests. Chemical-to-optical sensing offers two significant advantages [76]: exceptionally low cost and simplicity achieved by eliminating the need for localized electronics, sensors, and supplementary components; and the ability to utilize elements from the extensive repository of colorimetric or fluorometric assays employed in traditional benchtop biofluid studies.

Electrochemical sensors, which convert chemical signals into electrical signals, are commonly used in wearable chemical sensors for several reasons: these sensors require no user intervention to monitor or document data; in some cases, they reduce the necessary technology by eliminating the need for light sources, optics, or detectors; and many sensors are reagent- and label-free, allowing them to function immediately upon contact with the biofluid [77]. The benefits of wearable sensors are presented in Fig. (5).

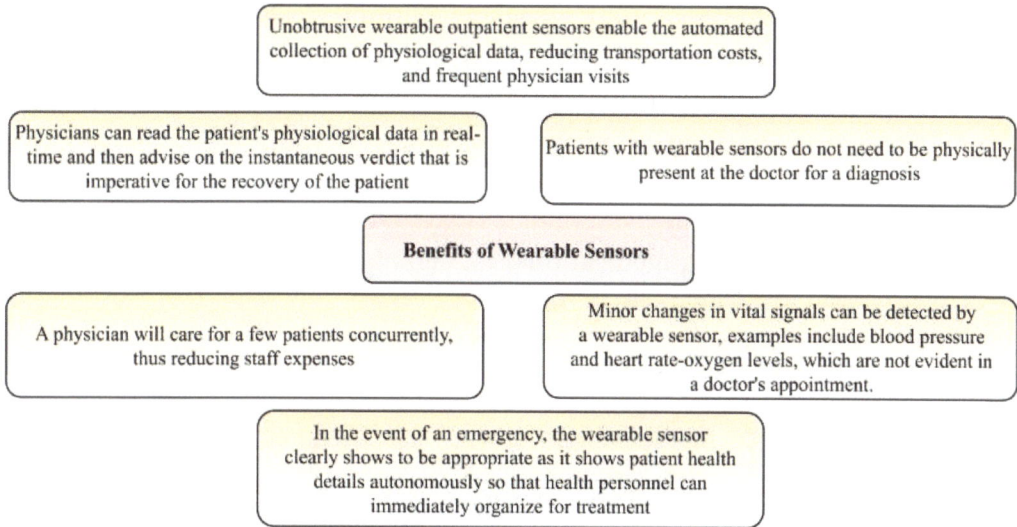

Fig. (5). Benefits of wearable sensors.

INTERNET-ENABLED HEALTHCARE MANAGEMENT FOR THE GLOBAL COVID-19 PANDEMIC

COVID-19 was a global pandemic caused by the Severe Acute Respiratory Syndrome Coronavirus 2 (SARS-CoV-2), affecting over 215 countries. By June 1, 2020, the World Health Organization (WHO) reported 6,057,853 confirmed cases and more than 371,166 deaths [78]. The first outbreak of the virus was traced to the Wuhan seafood market in Hubei province, China, in late December 2019. On January 9, 2020, the WHO officially declared it a public health emergency of international concern. Symptoms may manifest up to 14 days post-exposure and include fever or chills, cough, dyspnea, fatigue, myalgia, headache, anosmia or ageusia, pharyngitis, rhinorrhea, nausea, vomiting, and diarrhea. The absence of adequate medicinal treatments or vaccines initially resulted in significant global loss of life and economic decline [79].

Prediction and Diagnosis of Diseases

The prediction and diagnosis of diseases through the Internet of Things (IoT) and artificial intelligence (AI) represent significant advancements in modern healthcare. IoT devices, such as wearable sensors, medical imaging systems, and smart diagnostic tools, collect vast amounts of patient data, including vital signs, movement patterns, and environmental factors. This real-time data is transmitted to cloud platforms or edge computing devices, where AI algorithms analyze it to identify abnormalities, patterns, and trends indicative of potential health issues [80]. Predictive healthcare utilizes AI-based systems that analyze patient data both historically and in real-time through machine learning. These systems can detect subtle markers of disease that may elude human observation, such as variations in heart rate patterns indicative of early-stage arrhythmias or changes in glucose levels signaling prediabetes. Predictive models can assess a patient's risk of developing cardiovascular diseases, diabetes, or certain cancers based on lifestyle factors, genetic predispositions, and physiological data. AI-powered diagnostic tools, especially deep learning models like convolutional neural networks (CNNs), excel at analyzing medical images, demonstrating exceptional accuracy in detecting diseases such as lung cancer, breast tumors, and neurological conditions from X-rays, CT scans, and MRIs. These systems not only reduce diagnostic errors but also accelerate the diagnostic process, enabling healthcare providers to detect and treat diseases at earlier stages. The integration of IoT with AI brings personalized medicine into reality, as diagnostic systems adapt to a patient's unique profile. For example, an AI-based system analyzing data from wearable devices can offer tailored advice to help manage chronic conditions such as hypertension or asthma. It can even predict flare-ups and recommend preventive measures to improve patients' quality of life [81]. This capability is especially valuable in critical epidemiological applications, facilitating the prompt recognition of infectious disease outbreaks. The integrated data from wearable sensors and health records supports the development of predictive models for disease propagation, enabling timely and effective interventions [82].

Healthcare Management

The integration of IoT technologies into healthcare management has revolutionized patient care and resource optimization, especially during the COVID-19 pandemic. Remote patient monitoring has become a central component of health management solutions, enabling providers to continuously track patients' vital signs, symptoms, and overall health from a distance. IoT devices, including wearable sensors and smart monitoring tools, transmit real-time data to healthcare professionals, facilitating remote intervention without the need for in-person visits. This approach enhances safety by protecting patients from potential exposure and ensures uninterrupted care for both chronic patients and those recovering from infections.

Beyond remote monitoring, resource optimization through IoT has been crucial in enhancing efficiencies within healthcare operations. With IoT devices in place, frontline medical workers no longer need to spend excessive time on manual processing, as many screening tasks are automated. Contactless temperature scanners, wearable health monitors, and automated patient check-in systems have become essential tools for making initial screenings both efficient and safe. IoT systems help reduce infection exposure among healthcare workers, shorten patient flow cycles, and free up resources for critical care by automating routine processes.

Another important aspect of IoT-enabled healthcare management is the management of the cold chain for transporting and storing vaccines and sensitive medications. Sensors integrated with IoT devices continuously monitor temperature and humidity in real-time during transport and storage. If these conditions deviate from required thresholds, immediate alerts are triggered to ensure that medical supplies maintain their integrity and efficacy. This application was particularly valuable during the global COVID-19 vaccination campaigns, where precise storage conditions were critical to preserving vaccine potency.

Overall, IoT technologies have significantly enhanced healthcare management by providing innovative solutions for remote patient care, optimizing operational efficiency, and ensuring quality control. This foundation supports the development of healthier, more effective, and patient-centered healthcare systems, addressing not only the acute challenges posed by global health emergencies like COVID-19 but also long-term healthcare needs. An example of combining data-driven methods with wearable devices for healthcare applications is illustrated in Table **1**.

Table 1. Example of combining data-driven methods with wearables for healthcare applications.

Application	Device Type	Measured Parameters	Environment Type	Outcome Metric	Accuracy/Performance	Ref.
Glucose-level prediction	Dexcom G6+	Interstitial glucose levels, electrodermal response, dermal temperature, and physical activity	At home	Accurate glucose prediction	92% sensitivity	[83]
-	Dexcom C4, Dexcom C7 plus, Medtronic iPro2	Glucose concentration	Clinical and home visits	Predictive capabilities for glucose spikes	88% accuracy	[84]
-	Abbott FreeStyle Libre	Glucose concentration	At home	Continuous glucose monitoring	90% RMSE reduction	[85]
Epilepsy management	Empatica E4	Motor seizures	Controlled environment	Seizure detection	85% F1-score	[86]
Fatigue/drowsiness	Eyeglass platform	Facial action detection, blinks, percentage of eye closure	Controlled environment	Real-time fatigue monitoring	80% specificity	[87, 88]

(Table 1) cont.....

Application	Device Type	Measured Parameters	Environment Type	Outcome Metric	Accuracy/Performance	Ref.
Parkinson disease	Six Opal IMU sensors	Balance and gait features	Clinical setting	Differentiation between Parkinson's and tremors	87% sensitivity	[89]
-	Great Lakes NeuroTechnologies	Free movement gyroscope data	Controlled environment	Precise tracking of mobility decline	88% AUC	[90]
Mood disorder	Mi Band 2 + App Support	Daily phone usage, sleep data, step count data, and mood scores	Home and follow-ups	Detection of mood trends	83% accuracy	[91]
Respiratory disorders	Non-commercial chest wearables	Respiratory behaviours	Controlled environment	Early detection of respiratory irregularities	81% sensitivity	[92]
SARS-CoV-2 detection	Fitbit	Heart rate, activity data	At home	COVID-19 pre-symptomatic detection	76% specificity	[93]
-	Everion Biofourmis	Heart rate, heart rate variability, respiration rate, oxygen saturation, blood pulse wave, skin temperature, and actigraphy	Controlled environment	Continuous monitoring for COVID-19 progression	82% accuracy	[94]

CHALLENGES AND FUTURE ASPECTS

The wearables are equipped with sensors that capture patient data and transmit it to host devices *via* Bluetooth or Zigbee. A multitude of issues require resolution. The unresolved problems in IoT-enabled wearable sensor systems for healthcare are highlighted in Fig. (**6**).

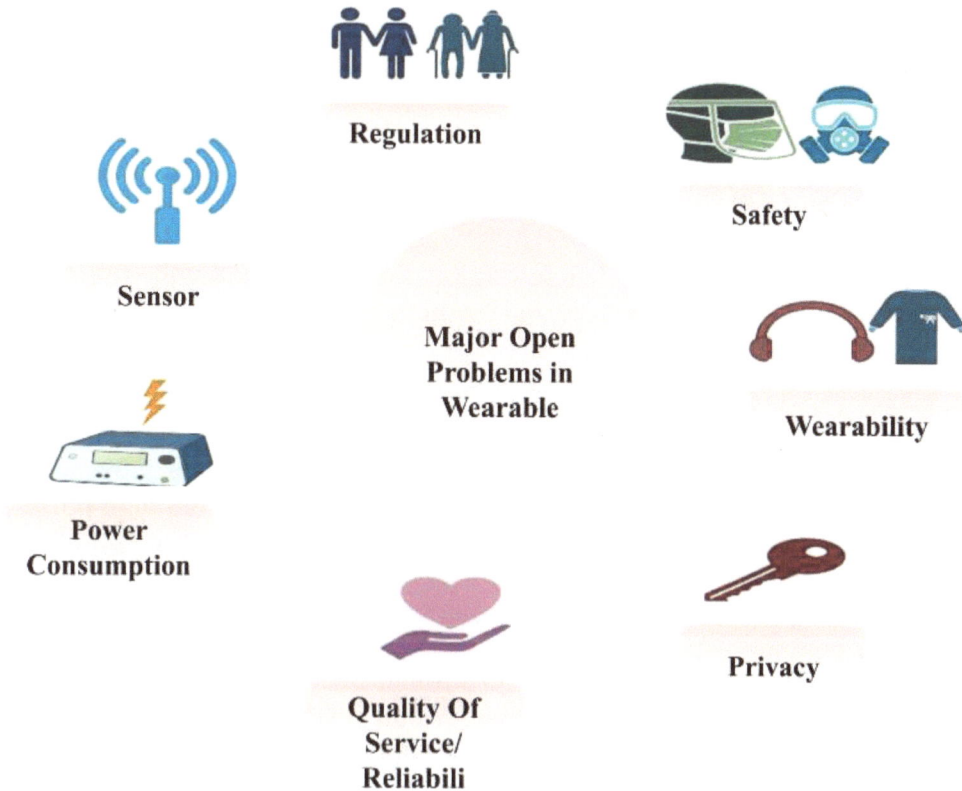

Fig. (6). Unresolved issues in IoT-enabled wearable sensor systems for healthcare.

Data Resolution

One of the biggest challenges in wearable healthcare technology is the resolution of data, as miniaturized sensors often struggle to achieve high accuracy. These sensors need to be as small and lightweight as possible to ensure comfort and practicality, but this frequently comes at the expense of data accuracy and reliability. The issue is further complicated by variability in sensor quality, data collection methods, and processing algorithms across different devices. For example, the same health parameter, such as heart rate or oxygen saturation, may yield different readings depending on the device used, the placement of sensors, or how the data is interpreted.

Wider standardization of data collection practices, combined with the application of advanced algorithms, would enhance the reliability and accuracy of wearable data. Regulatory measures should also be implemented to ensure that wearables used for critical health monitoring or clinical decision-making meet clinical-grade standards of data quality. The context in which data is used also affects quality expectations; for example, fitness tracking may tolerate some inaccuracies, but clinical applications require high precision to prevent misdiagnosis or unnecessary anxiety for patients.

The integration of wearable data into healthcare systems further highlights the need for standardized protocols and robust data processing frameworks. Efforts to enhance sensor technologies and establish universal standards can help mitigate the challenges associated with data resolution, thereby unlocking the full potential of wearable devices in personalized and predictive healthcare.

Power Consumption

The extensive use of wearables presents a challenge in fuelling the gadgets. According to the principle of miniaturisation, smaller machines consume less power; nonetheless, they are at an increased risk of damage from high power. In the realm of wearables, a reliable power source is important. The simultaneous usage of numerous sensors escalates power requirements, exacerbating the situation. The primary challenge lies in accommodating all sensors with a sufficiently durable battery that lasts a minimum of one to two days. The current power constraint is primarily addressed through the use of lithium-ion polymer batteries and a micro-PCB protection circuit to improve device charging efficiency. In a sensitive setting, power consumption must be handled with utmost vigilance.

Privacy

The Internet of Things poses significant risks to privacy. Numerous privacy concerns related to healthcare IoT have emerged globally, with multiple network attacks causing prolonged service disruptions and substantial financial losses. However, in healthcare, these risks are even more critical compared to commercial IoT systems. Healthcare data is especially vulnerable to exploitation, making it highly sensitive and perilous. For instance, data collected from sensors on a smartwatch can reveal sleep patterns, dietary habits, daily routines, and other personal information. Therefore, safeguarding user data privacy and protecting individual identities is essential.

Wearability

Wearability is a significant challenge in healthcare wearables, emphasizing user comfort, practicality, and long-term usability. To be effective, wearable devices must strike a balance between advanced functionality and ergonomic design. Key considerations include lightweight materials, flexibility, skin compatibility, and water resistance. Devices should seamlessly integrate into daily life without causing discomfort or irritation, even during prolonged use or physical activities.

Many wearable devices suffer from overheating, uncomfortable fits, and excessive bulk, leading most users to eventually discard them. Their designs often fail to meet users' needs, especially considering the diversity in body shapes and sensitivities. Additionally, the lack of durability and water resistance diminishes wearability for those who use these devices outdoors or during athletic activities. Wearables must be both rugged and comfortable to support long-term use. Another important aspect of wearability lies in the user experience. Difficult interfaces and insufficient training can result in low adoption rates, as users often find devices unintuitive or hard to operate. Enhancing user education about device functionality and providing accessible support systems can help overcome these barriers, ultimately promoting better engagement and improved health outcomes.

Incorporating these elements effectively into wearables will enhance their practicality, improve patient adherence, and maximize their potential in healthcare monitoring and management.

Safety

The sensors utilised must prioritize user safety above all else. Both the sensors and the device need to be safe to wear, causing no adverse effects during use or long-term harm to the body. Wearables should be designed to protect the wearer as well as those around them. Although these devices are not cheap or unregulated, they remain widely available in the market, and many consumers purchase them due to their affordability. However, the use of malfunctioning or low-quality devices can pose risks to both the user and people nearby.

Artificial Intelligence and Decision Support

Artificial intelligence (AI) methodologies, including machine learning, expert systems, and knowledge representation techniques, are extensively utilized in medical diagnosis, prognosis, and medical education [95]. AI healthcare systems primarily focus on the manipulation and transformation of data and knowledge. Expert or knowledge-based systems contain medical information specific to narrowly defined tasks. They analyze patient data to derive reasoned conclusions based on established rules and logical inference. When sufficient knowledge is unavailable, machine learning methods can be applied to examine collections of clinical cases to characterize the status of a particular patient or disease.

Sensor Robustness

The sensors employed can be enhanced for greater durability and used dynamically to partially identify diseases or other health metrics. For example, a pulse sensor not only measures pulse rate but also assists in heart rate detection. Consequently, heart rate can be estimated using the pulse rate sensor; however, precise heart rate detection is not achieved in this context. This calculation relies on monitoring blood flow, which can sometimes lead to inaccuracies. To improve reliability, the limitations of these sensors must be addressed. Therefore, it is essential to develop future systems that integrate multiple sensors to obtain more accurate measurements, enabling the detection of heart abnormalities through pulse sensing [91 - 95].

CONCLUSION

This chapter stresses the transformative potential of wearable technology in healthcare, focusing on its role in continuous monitoring, disease management, and personalized care. Advanced sensors are integrated into Internet of Things (IoT) frameworks to capture real-time physiological data, such as heart rate, blood pressure, and glucose levels effectively. Wearable technology leverages advances in artificial intelligence to enable predictive analytics and early intervention for chronic conditions like diabetes, cardiovascular disease, and sleep apnea, thereby reducing healthcare costs and improving patient outcomes. During the COVID-19 pandemic, wearable devices gained prominence for tracking symptoms, monitoring recovery, and supporting remote healthcare services. Equipped with non-invasive biosensors, these devices facilitate seamless sharing of health data with professionals *via* cloud platforms, advancing telemedicine. Beyond individual monitoring, wearables have also proven valuable in clinical research by providing real-world data on treatment adherence and effectiveness. Despite the pros offered by wearable technologies, data privacy concerns, accuracy limits, and digital divides continue to influence access. These issues will have to be addressed to popularize and integrate wearable technologies equally in society. Emerging trends, such as merging wearables with augmented reality, 5G, and machine learning, have the potential to further enhance the functionality of immersive solutions in healthcare. The article covers a wide range of applications, from fitness tracking to disease-specific monitoring, and further underlines their utility in chronic cases of asthma and diabetes. Other innovations in sensor technology, such as biofluidic sensors, e-skin, and graphene-based sensors, are expanding diagnostic capabilities. However, technical challenges, such as sensor resolution, power consumption, and user comfort, demand constant innovation to improve reliability and user experience. Wearable technology is revolutionizing healthcare by filling the gap between traditional medical practices and digital solutions. With strategic advancements and the resolution of existing challenges, wearables are poised to become indispensable tools in preventive and precision medicine, ensuring accessible and efficient healthcare for all.

REFERENCES

[1]   Jagadeeswari V, Subramaniyaswamy V, Logesh R, Vijayakumar V. A study on medical Internet of Things and Big Data in personalized healthcare system. Health Inf Sci Syst 2018; 6(1): 14.
[http://dx.doi.org/10.1007/s13755-018-0049-x] [PMID: 30279984]

[2]   Kaur P, Kumar R, Kumar M. A healthcare monitoring system using random forest and internet of things (IoT). Multimedia Tools Appl 2019; 78(14): 19905-16.
[http://dx.doi.org/10.1007/s11042-019-7327-8]

[3]   Lu L, Zhang J, Xie Y, *et al*. Wearable health devices in health care: narrative systematic review. JMIR Mhealth Uhealth 2020; 8(11): e18907.
[http://dx.doi.org/10.2196/18907] [PMID: 33164904]

[4]   Mamdiwar SD, R A, Shakruwala Z, Chadha U, Srinivasan K, Chang CY. Recent advances on IoT-assisted wearable sensor systems for healthcare monitoring. Biosensors (Basel) 2021; 11(10): 372.
[http://dx.doi.org/10.3390/bios11100372] [PMID: 34677328]

[5]   Rashmi IR, Sahana MK, Sangeetha R, Shruthi KS. IoT-based patient health monitoring system for remote doctors uses embedded technology. Int J Eng Res Technol (Ahmedabad) 2020; 8: 230-3.

[6]   Vahdati M, Gholizadeh HamlAbadi K, Saghiri AM. IoT-based healthcare monitoring using blockchain. In: Namasudra S, Deka C, Eds. Applications of Blockchain in Healthcare. Springer, Singapore 2021; pp. 141-70.

[7]   Sastimoglu Z, Subramaniam S, Faisal AI, Jiang W, Ye A, Deen MJ. Wearable PPG-based BP estimation methods: A systematic review and meta-analysis. IEEE J Biomed Health Inform 2025; 29(4): 2439-2452.
[PMID: 40030275]

[8]   Broza YY, Haick H. Biodiagnostics in an era of global pandemics—From biosensing materials to data management. VIEW 2022; 3(2): 20200164.
[http://dx.doi.org/10.1002/VIW.20200164] [PMID: 34766159]

[9]   Xu Q, Fang Y, Jing Q, *et al*. A portable triboelectric spirometer for wireless pulmonary function monitoring. Biosens Bioelectron 2021; 187: 113329.
[http://dx.doi.org/10.1016/j.bios.2021.113329] [PMID: 34020223]

[10]   Popescu M, Ungureanu C. Green nanomaterials for smart textiles dedicated to environmental and biomedical applications. Materials. 2023;16(11):4075.Chen G, Xiao X, Zhao X, Tat T, Bick M, Chen J. Electronic textiles for wearable point-of-care systems. Chem Rev 2021; 122(3): 3259-91.
[PMID: 34939791]

[11]   Zhou Y, Zhao X, Xu J, *et al*. Giant magnetoelastic effect in soft systems for bioelectronics. Nat Mater 2021; 20(12): 1670-6.
[http://dx.doi.org/10.1038/s41563-021-01093-1] [PMID: 34594013]

[12]   Zhao X, Zhou Y, Xu J, *et al*. Soft fibers with magnetoelasticity for wearable electronics. Nat Commun 2021; 12(1): 6755.
[http://dx.doi.org/10.1038/s41467-021-27066-1] [PMID: 34799591]

[13]   Ruan L, Wang Y, Zhao X, Li F, Liu C, Tao W, Liang H, Zhang X, Yang W. Magnetic Functional Materials for Haptic Interfaces. Authorea. 2024;1:29.

[14]   Li A, Ho HH, Barman SR, Lee S, Gao F, Lin ZH. Self-powered antibacterial systems in environmental purification, wound healing, and tactile sensing applications. Nano Energy 2022; 93: 106826.
[http://dx.doi.org/10.1016/j.nanoen.2021.106826]

[15]   Ganesan S, Ramajayam K, Kokulnathan T, Palaniappan A. Recent advances in two-dimensional MXene-based electrochemical biosensors for sweat analysis. Molecules 2023; 28(12): 4617.
[http://dx.doi.org/10.3390/molecules28124617] [PMID: 37375172]

[16]   Nguyen N, Lin ZH, Barman SR, *et al.* Engineering an integrated electroactive dressing to accelerate wound healing and monitor noninvasively progress of healing. Nano Energy 2022; 99: 107393.
[http://dx.doi.org/10.1016/j.nanoen.2022.107393]

[17]   Wang Z, Zhang Y, Wang T, *et al.* Organic flux synthesis of covalent organic frameworks. Chem 2023; 9(8): 2178-93.
[http://dx.doi.org/10.1016/j.chempr.2023.03.026]

[18]   Safaei J, Gao Y, Hosseinpour M, *et al.* Vacancy engineering for high-efficiency nanofluidic osmotic energy generation. J Am Chem Soc 2023; 145(4): 2669-78.
[http://dx.doi.org/10.1021/jacs.2c12936] [PMID: 36651291]

[19]   Lin Z, Zhi C, Qu L. Nano Research Energy: An interdisciplinary journal centered on nanomaterials and nanotechnology for energy. Nano Research Energy 2022; 1(1): e9120005.
[http://dx.doi.org/10.26599/NRE.2022.9120005]

[20]   Gu J, Peng Y, Zhou T, Ma J, Pang H, Yamauchi Y. Porphyrin-based framework materials for energy conversion. Nano Research Energy 2022; 1: e9120009.
[http://dx.doi.org/10.26599/NRE.2022.9120009]

[21]   Zhou Z, Chen K, Li X, *et al.* Sign-to-speech translation using machine-learning-assisted stretchable sensor arrays. Nat Electron 2020; 3(9): 571-8.
[http://dx.doi.org/10.1038/s41928-020-0428-6]

[22]   Zhou Y, Mazur F, Fan Q, Chandrawati R. Synthetic nanoprobes for biological hydrogen sulfide detection and imaging. VIEW 2022; 3(4): 20210008.
[http://dx.doi.org/10.1002/VIW.20210008]

[23]   Gomey S, Guliani E, Choudhary K, Sengupta S, Chakraborty B, Raula M. Photoactive metal chalcogenides towards CO2 reduction–a review. Colloid Polym Sci 2024; 302(8): 1149-67.
[http://dx.doi.org/10.1007/s00396-024-05235-0]

[24]   Lin H, He M, Jing Q, *et al.* Angle-shaped triboelectric nanogenerator for harvesting environmental wind energy. Nano Energy 2019; 56: 269-76.
[http://dx.doi.org/10.1016/j.nanoen.2018.11.037]

[25]   Zheng Q, Peng M, Liu Z, *et al.* Dynamic real-time imaging of living cell traction force by piezo-phototronic light nano-antenna array. Sci Adv 2021; 7(22): eabe7738.
[http://dx.doi.org/10.1126/sciadv.abe7738] [PMID: 34039600]

[26]   Lin Z, Sun C, Liu W, *et al.* A self-powered and high-frequency vibration sensor with layer-powder-layer structure for structural health monitoring. Nano Energy 2021; 90: 106366.
[http://dx.doi.org/10.1016/j.nanoen.2021.106366]

[27]   Peng M, Li Z, Liu C, *et al.* High-resolution dynamic pressure sensor array based on piezo-phototronic effect tuned photoluminescence imaging. ACS Nano 2015; 9(3): 3143-50.
[http://dx.doi.org/10.1021/acsnano.5b00072] [PMID: 25712580]

[28]   Zhang J, Xu Q, Li H, *et al.* Self-powered electrodeposition system for sub-10-nm silver nanoparticles with high-efficiency antibacterial activity. J Phys Chem Lett 2022; 13(29): 6721-30.
[http://dx.doi.org/10.1021/acs.jpclett.2c01737] [PMID: 35849530]

[29]   Lin H, Liu Y, Chen S, *et al.* Seesaw structured triboelectric nanogenerator with enhanced output performance and its applications in self-powered motion sensing. Nano Energy 2019; 65: 103944.
[http://dx.doi.org/10.1016/j.nanoen.2019.103944]

[30]   Shi S, Jiang Y, Xu Q, *et al.* A self-powered triboelectric multi-information motion monitoring sensor and its application in wireless real-time control. Nano Energy 2022; 97: 107150.

[http://dx.doi.org/10.1016/j.nanoen.2022.107150]

[31]   He M, Lin YJ, Chiu CM, *et al.* A flexible photo-thermoelectric nanogenerator based on MoS₂/PU photothermal layer for infrared light harvesting. Nano Energy 2018; 49: 588-95.
[http://dx.doi.org/10.1016/j.nanoen.2018.04.072]

[32]   Sadoughi F, Behmanesh A, Sayfouri N. Internet of things in medicine: A systematic mapping study. J Biomed Inform 2020; 103: 103383.
[http://dx.doi.org/10.1016/j.jbi.2020.103383] [PMID: 32044417]

[33]   Paranjape K, Schinkel M, Nanayakkara P. Short keynote paper: Mainstreaming personalized healthcare—Transforming healthcare through a new era of artificial intelligence. IEEE J Biomed Health Inform 2020; 24(7): 1.
[http://dx.doi.org/10.1109/JBHI.2020.2970807] [PMID: 32054591]

[34]   Ergen O, Belcastro KD. AI-driven advanced Internet of Things (IoTx2): The future seems irreversibly connected in medicine. Anatol J Cardiol 2019; 22(2) (Suppl. 2): 15-7.
[http://dx.doi.org/10.14744/AnatolJCardiol.2019.73466] [PMID: 31670717]

[35]   Birje MN, Hanji SS. Internet of things based distributed healthcare systems: a review. Journal of Data, Information and Management 2020; 2(3): 149-65.
[http://dx.doi.org/10.1007/s42488-020-00027-x]

[36]   Tukade TM, Banakar R. Data transfer protocols in IoT—An overview. Int J Pure Appl Math 2018; 118(16): 121-38.

[37]   Wu T, Wu F, Qiu C, Redouté JM, Yuce MR. A rigid-flex wearable health monitoring sensor patch for IoT-connected healthcare applications. IEEE Internet Things J 2020; 7(8): 6932-45.
[http://dx.doi.org/10.1109/JIOT.2020.2977164]

[38]   Patel WD, Pandya S, Koyuncu B, Ramani B, Bhaskar S, Ghayvat H. NXTGeUH: LoRaWAN-based next-generation ubiquitous healthcare system for vital signs monitoring & falls detection In: 2018 IEEE Punecon. IEEE 2018; pp. 1-8.

[39]   Lounis K, Zulkernine M. Attacks and defenses in short-range wireless technologies for IoT. IEEE Access 2020; 8: 88892-932.
[http://dx.doi.org/10.1109/ACCESS.2020.2993553]

[40]   Mohammed MN, Desyansah SF, Al-Zubaidi S, Yusuf E. An Internet of Things-based smart homes and healthcare monitoring and management system. J Phys: Conf Ser. IOP Publishing 2020; p. 12079.
[http://dx.doi.org/10.1088/1742-6596/1450/1/012079]

[41]   Patel WD, Pandya S, Koyuncu B, Ramani B, Bhaskar S, Ghayvat H. NXTGeUH: LoRaWAN-based next-generation ubiquitous healthcare system for vital signs monitoring & falls detection . IEEE 2018; pp. 1-8.

[42]   Osorio A, Calle M, Soto JD, Candelo-Becerra JE. Routing in LoRaWAN: Overview and challenges. IEEE Commun Mag 2020; 58(6): 72-6.
[http://dx.doi.org/10.1109/MCOM.001.2000053]

[43]   Almotairi KH. Application of internet of things in healthcare domain. J Umm Al-Qura Uni Eng Arch. 2023 Mar;14(1):1-2.

[44]   Diffie W, Hellman M. New directions in cryptography. IEEE Trans Inf Theory 1976; 22(6): 644-54.
[http://dx.doi.org/10.1109/TIT.1976.1055638]

[45]   Gogate U, Bakal J. Healthcare monitoring system based on wireless sensor network for cardiac patients. Biomed Pharmacol J 2018; 11(3): 1681-8.
[http://dx.doi.org/10.13005/bpj/1537]

[46]   Adeniyi EA, Ogundokun RO, Awotunde JB. IoMT-based wearable body sensors network healthcare monitoring system. IoT in Healthcare and Ambient Assisted Living 2021; pp. 103-21.
[http://dx.doi.org/10.1007/978-981-15-9897-5_6]

[47]   Mhatre P, Shaikh A, Khanvilkar S. Non-invasive e-health care monitoring system using IoT. Int J Innov Res Technol 2020; 6: 307-11.

[48]   Monisha K, Babu MR. A novel framework for a healthcare monitoring system through IoT and personalized healthcare systems. In: Krishna PV, Gurumoorthy S, Obaidat MS. Internet of Things and Personalized Healthcare Systems. Springer, Singapore 2018; pp. 21-36.

[49]   Maduri PK, Dewangan Y, Yadav D, Chauhan S, Singh K. IoT-based patient health monitoring portable kit. 2nd International Conference on Advances in Computing, Communication, Control and Networking (ICACCCN). IEEE; 2020. p. 513–6.
[http://dx.doi.org/10.1109/ICACCCN51052.2020.9362985]

[50]   Talpur MSH, Bhuiyan MZA, Wang G. Energy-efficient healthcare monitoring with smartphones and IoT technologies. Int J High Perf Comp Net 2015; 8(2): 186-94.
[http://dx.doi.org/10.1504/IJHPCN.2015.070019]

[51]   Haghi M, Neubert S, Geissler A, *et al.* A flexible and pervasive IoT-based healthcare platform for physiological and environmental parameters monitoring. IEEE Internet Things J 2020; 7(6): 5628-47.
[http://dx.doi.org/10.1109/JIOT.2020.2980432]

[52]   Mamdiwar SD, R A, Shakruwala Z, Chadha U, Srinivasan K, Chang CY. Recent advances on IoT-assisted wearable sensor systems for healthcare monitoring. Biosensors. 2021 Oct 4;11(10):372.

[53]   Sankaran S, Murugan PR, Chandrasekaran D, Murugan V, Alaguramesh K, Britto PI, *et al.* Design of IoT-based healthcare monitoring systems using Raspberry Pi: A review of the latest technologies and limitations. 2020 International Conference on Communication and Signal Processing (ICCSP) 2020; 28-32.
[http://dx.doi.org/10.1109/ICCSP48568.2020.9182325]

[54]   Pardeshi V, Sagar S, Murmurwar S, Hage P. Health monitoring systems using IoT and Raspberry Pi—a review. 2017 International Conference on Innovative Mechanisms for Industry Applications (ICIMIA) 2017; 134-7.
[http://dx.doi.org/10.1109/ICIMIA.2017.7975587]

[55]   Gochhayat SP, Lal C, Sharma L, *et al.* Reliable and secure data transfer in IoT networks. Wirel Netw 2020; 26(8): 5689-702.
[http://dx.doi.org/10.1007/s11276-019-02036-0]

[56]   Kadhim KT, Alsahlany AM, Wadi SM, Kadhum HT. An overview of the patients' health status monitoring system based on the Internet of Things (IoT). Wirel Pers Commun 2020; 114(3): 2235-62.
[http://dx.doi.org/10.1007/s11277-020-07474-0]

[57]   Godi B, Viswanadham S, Muttipati AS, Samantray OP, Gadiraju SR. E-healthcare monitoring system using IoT with machine learning approaches. 2020 International Conference on Computer Science, Engineering and Applications (ICCSEA) 2020; 1-5.
[http://dx.doi.org/10.1109/ICCSEA49143.2020.9132937]

[58]   Onasanya A, Elshakankiri M. Smart integrated IoT healthcare system for cancer care. Wirel Netw 2021; 27(6): 4297-312.
[http://dx.doi.org/10.1007/s11276-018-01932-1]

[59]   Mittelstadt B. Ethics of the health-related internet of things: a narrative review. Ethics Inf Technol 2017; 19(3): 157-75.
[http://dx.doi.org/10.1007/s10676-017-9426-4]

[60]   Gomes BTP, Muniz LCM, Da Silva e Silva FJ, *et al.* A middleware with comprehensive quality of context support for Internet of Things applications. Sensors (Basel) 2017; 17(12): 2853.
[http://dx.doi.org/10.3390/s17122853] [PMID: 29292791]

[61]   Latif S, Qadir J, Farooq S, Imran M. How 5G wireless (and concomitant technologies) will revolutionize healthcare? Future Internet 2017; 9(4): 93.
[http://dx.doi.org/10.3390/fi9040093]

[62] Iqbal SMA, Mahgoub I, Du E, Leavitt MA, Asghar W. Advances in healthcare wearable devices. NPJ Flex Electron 2021; 5(1): 9.
[http://dx.doi.org/10.1038/s41528-021-00107-x]

[63] Li S, Ma Z, Cao Z, Pan L, Shi Y. Advanced wearable microfluidic sensors for healthcare monitoring. Small 2020; 16(9): 1903822.
[http://dx.doi.org/10.1002/smll.201903822] [PMID: 31617311]

[64] Heikenfeld J, Jajack A, Rogers J, *et al.* Wearable sensors: modalities, challenges, and prospects. Lab Chip 2018; 18(2): 217-48.
[http://dx.doi.org/10.1039/C7LC00914C] [PMID: 29182185]

[65] Park KI, Son JH, Hwang GT, *et al.* Highly-efficient, flexible piezoelectric PZT thin film nanogenerator on plastic substrates. Adv Mater 2014; 26(16): 2514-20.
[http://dx.doi.org/10.1002/adma.201305659] [PMID: 24523251]

[66] Bera TK, Bera S, Nagaraju J, Chakraborty B. Multiple inhomogeneity phantom imaging with a LabVIEW-based electrical impedance tomography (LV-EIT) system. In: Guha D, Chakraborty B, Dutta HS, Eds Computer, Communication, and Electrical Technology. CRC Press 2017; pp. 273-7.
[http://dx.doi.org/10.1201/9781315400624-52]

[67] Taffoni F, Formica D, Saccomandi P, Pino G, Schena E. Optical fiber-based MR-compatible sensors for medical applications: an overview. Sensors (Basel) 2013; 13(10): 14105-20.
[http://dx.doi.org/10.3390/s131014105] [PMID: 24145918]

[68] Kim HN, Ren WX, Kim JS, Yoon J. Fluorescent and colorimetric sensors for detection of lead, cadmium, and mercury ions. Chem Soc Rev 2012; 41(8): 3210-44.
[http://dx.doi.org/10.1039/C1CS15245A] [PMID: 22184584]

[69] Bhat MP, Vinayak S, Yu J, Jung HY, Kurkuri M. Colorimetric receptors for the detection of biologically important anions and their application in designing molecular logic gates. ChemistrySelect 2020; 5(42): 13135-43.
[http://dx.doi.org/10.1002/slct.202003147]

[70] Liu Y, Hu S, Gan N, Yu Z. Wearable patch biosensor through electrothermal film-stimulated sweat secretion for continuous sweat glucose analysis at rest. Anal Chem. 2024.

[71] Wu J, Liu W, Ge J, Zhang H, Wang P. New sensing mechanisms for design of fluorescent chemosensors emerging in recent years. Chem Soc Rev 2011; 40(7): 3483-95.
[http://dx.doi.org/10.1039/c0cs00224k] [PMID: 21445455]

[72] Heikenfeld J. Non-invasive analyte access and sensing through eccrine sweat: challenges and outlook circa 2016. Electroanalysis 2016; 28(6): 1242-9.
[http://dx.doi.org/10.1002/elan.201600018]

[73] Koh A, Kang D, Xue Y, *et al.* A soft, wearable microfluidic device for the capture, storage, and colorimetric sensing of sweat. Sci Transl Med 2016; 8(366): 366ra165.
[http://dx.doi.org/10.1126/scitranslmed.aaf2593] [PMID: 27881826]

[74] Bandodkar AJ, Wang J. Non-invasive wearable electrochemical sensors: a review. Trends Biotechnol 2014; 32(7): 363-71.
[http://dx.doi.org/10.1016/j.tibtech.2014.04.005] [PMID: 24853270]

[75] Narin A, Kaya C, Pamuk Z. Automatic detection of coronavirus disease (COVID-19) using X-ray images and deep convolutional neural networks. Pattern Anal Appl 2021; 24(3): 1207-20.
[http://dx.doi.org/10.1007/s10044-021-00984-y] [PMID: 33994847]

[76] Li Q, Guan X, Wu P, *et al.* Early transmission dynamics in Wuhan, China, of novel coronavirus–infected pneumonia. N Engl J Med 2020; 382(13): 1199-207.
[http://dx.doi.org/10.1056/NEJMoa2001316] [PMID: 31995857]

[77] McCall B. COVID-19 and artificial intelligence: protecting health-care workers and curbing the

spread. Lancet Digit Health 2020; 2(4): e166-7.
[http://dx.doi.org/10.1016/S2589-7500(20)30054-6] [PMID: 32289116]

[78] Bai L, Yang D, Wang X, Tong L, Zhu X, Zhong N, *et al.* Chinese experts' consensus on the Internet of Things-aided diagnosis and treatment of coronavirus disease 2019 (COVID-19). Clin eHealth 2020; 3: 7-15.

[79] Sanyaolu A, Okorie C, Hosein Z, *et al.* Global pandemicity of COVID-19: situation report as of June 9, 2020. Infect Dis (Auckl) 2021; 14: 1178633721991260.
[http://dx.doi.org/10.1177/1178633721991260] [PMID: 33597811]

[80] Bent B, Cho PJ, Henriquez M, *et al.* Engineering digital biomarkers of interstitial glucose from noninvasive smartwatches. NPJ Digit Med 2021; 4(1): 89.
[http://dx.doi.org/10.1038/s41746-021-00465-w] [PMID: 34079049]

[81] Cichosz SL, Jensen MH, Hejlesen O. Short-term prediction of future continuous glucose monitoring readings in type 1 diabetes: Development and validation of a neural network regression model. Int J Med Inform 2021; 151: 104472.
[http://dx.doi.org/10.1016/j.ijmedinf.2021.104472] [PMID: 33932763]

[82] Rodríguez-Rodríguez I, Chatzigiannakis I, Rodríguez JV, Maranghi M, Gentili M, Zamora-Izquierdo MÁ. Utility of big data in predicting short-term blood glucose levels in type 1 diabetes mellitus through machine learning techniques. Sensors (Basel) 2019; 19(20): 4482.
[http://dx.doi.org/10.3390/s19204482] [PMID: 31623111]

[83] Nasseri M, Pal Attia T, Joseph B, *et al.* Non-invasive wearable seizure detection using long–short-term memory networks with transfer learning. J Neural Eng 2021; 18(5): 056017.
[http://dx.doi.org/10.1088/1741-2552/abef8a] [PMID: 33730713]

[84] Rostaminia S, Lamson A, Maji S, Rahman T, Ganesan DW. NCE: eyewear solution for upper face action units monitoring. Proceedings of the 11th ACM Symposium on Eye Tracking Research & Applications 2019; 1-3.
[http://dx.doi.org/10.1145/3314111.3322501]

[85] Rostaminia S, Mayberry A, Ganesan D, Marlin B, Gummeson J. iLid: eyewear solution for low-power fatigue and drowsiness monitoring. Proceedings of the 11th ACM Symposium on Eye Tracking Research & Applications 2019; 1-3.
[http://dx.doi.org/10.1145/3314111.3322503]

[86] Moon S, Song HJ, Sharma VD, *et al.* Classification of Parkinson's disease and essential tremor based on balance and gait characteristics from wearable motion sensors *via* machine learning techniques: a data-driven approach. J Neuroeng Rehabil 2020; 17(1): 125.
[http://dx.doi.org/10.1186/s12984-020-00756-5] [PMID: 32917244]

[87] Hssayeni MD, Jimenez-Shahed J, Burack MA, Ghoraani B. Ensemble deep model for continuous estimation of Unified Parkinson's Disease Rating Scale III. Biomed Eng Online 2021; 20(1): 32.
[http://dx.doi.org/10.1186/s12938-021-00872-w] [PMID: 33789666]

[88] Bai R, Xiao L, Guo Y, *et al.* Tracking and monitoring mood stability of patients with major depressive disorder by machine learning models using passive digital data: prospective naturalistic multicenter study. JMIR Mhealth Uhealth 2021; 9(3): e24365.
[http://dx.doi.org/10.2196/24365] [PMID: 33683207]

[89] Chen A, Zhang J, Zhao L, *et al.* Machine-learning enabled wireless wearable sensors to study individuality of respiratory behaviors. Biosens Bioelectron 2021; 173: 112799.
[http://dx.doi.org/10.1016/j.bios.2020.112799] [PMID: 33190052]

[90] Bogu GK, Snyder MP. Deep learning-based detection of COVID-19 using wearables data. MedRxiv 2021.
[http://dx.doi.org/10.1101/2021.01.08.21249474]

[91] Acampora G, Cook DJ, Rashidi P, Vasilakos AV. A survey on ambient intelligence in healthcare. Proc

IEEE 2013; 101(12): 2470-94.
[http://dx.doi.org/10.1109/JPROC.2013.2262913] [PMID: 24431472]

[92]   Abuseta Y. Cook DJ, Rashidi P, Vasilakos AV. A Context-Aware Framework for IoT-Based Healthcare Monitoring Systems. A survey on ambient intelligence in healthcare. Proc IEEE. 2013; 101 (12): 2470–94.

[93]   Chiuchisan I, Costin HN, Geman O. Adopting the Internet of Things technologies in health care systems. 2014 International Conference and Exposition on Electrical and Power Engineering (EPE). IEEE 2014; pp. 532-5.
[http://dx.doi.org/10.1109/ICEPE.2014.6969965]

[94]   Rahaman A, Islam M, Islam M, Sadi M, Nooruddin S. Developing IoT-based smart health monitoring systems: A review. Revue d'Intelligence Artificielle 2019; 33(6): 435-40.
[http://dx.doi.org/10.18280/ria.330605]

[95]   Nandankar P, Thaker R, Mughal SN, Saidireddy M, Kostka JE, Nag A. An IoT-based healthcare data analytics using fog and cloud computing. Turk J Physiother Rehabil 2021; 3: 32.

CHAPTER 7

IoT and Connected Devices in Healthcare

Pushpak Singh[1]**, Shaweta Sharma**[1,*] **and Aryan Kumar**[1]

[1] *Department of Pharmacy, School of Medical and Allied Sciences, Galgotias University, Greater Noida, Uttar Pradesh-201310, India*

Abstract: The integration of IoT (Internet of Things) in healthcare is enhancing and revolutionising the methods by which healthcare providers provide patient care and measure health through continuous monitoring. IoT-enabled wearable devices and remote patient monitoring systems promote the constant and immediate collection of health data, enabling individuals to effectively manage chronic illnesses, such as cardiovascular diseases, diabetes, and respiratory disorders. Contemporary gadgets, such as smartwatches equipped with sensors for heart rate and ECG monitoring, alongside continuous glucose monitors for blood sugar level assessment, deliver personalised, real-time data that improves patient outcomes. Asthma and COPD sufferers can benefit from smart inhalers equipped with monitoring technology that checks drug adherence and warns of possible problems. Networked devices enhance cost efficiency by decreasing hospital readmissions and outpatient visits, facilitating effective patient self-management, and optimizing healthcare delivery. However, the widespread adoption of IoT faces challenges, like cybersecurity issues, data privacy violations, and a lack of interoperability between devices, which hinder integration with the existing healthcare systems. Regulatory barriers, primarily related to device approval and data protection laws, also hinder the full integration of IoT technologies into healthcare. This holds promising prospects for IoT in healthcare, especially with the anticipated introduction of 6G technology, which will enable faster data transfer and reduced latency, while allowing for better connectivity to increase the efficiency of real-time monitoring and telemedicine applications. The power of artificial intelligence would support predictive analytics and decision-making processes. Healthcare monitoring will benefit from high data capacity with minimal latency. This can be achieved through the practical application of IoT in smart beds, telemedicine platforms, and fall detection systems, thereby improving patient outcomes and operational efficiency. Achieving this will require addressing the aforementioned challenges as IoT technology continues to advance.

Keywords: AI, Cloud computing, Connected devices, Data analytics, Healthcare automation, Interoperability, IoT, Plockchain, Smart sensors, Telemedicine, Wearable technology.

---

[*] **Corresponding author Shaweta Sharma**: Department of Pharmacy, School of Medical and Allied Sciences, Galgotias University, Greater Noida, Uttar Pradesh-201310, India; E-mail: shawetasharma@galgotiasuniversity.edu.in

Shaweta Sharma, Akhil Sharma, Shivkanya Fuloria & Anurag Singh (Eds.)
All rights reserved-© 2025 Bentham Science Publishers

INTRODUCTION

The Internet of Things (IoT) refers to the concept of interconnecting everyday products with the Internet, enabling them to collect and exchange data. IoT encompasses devices, such as smart home appliances, wearables like fitness bands, and industrial sensors, *e.g.*, factory monitoring systems. They are widely used in various industries, including home automation, manufacturing, healthcare, and transportation. The primary objective is to enhance efficiency, offer real-time monitoring, and automate processes to conserve time and resources [1, 2].

The Internet of Medical Things (IoMT) is a specialized subset of IoT that incorporates IoT technology into the healthcare field, which is currently transforming the medical sector by introducing innovative services through the use of connected devices and sensors. Medical devices and applications connected to healthcare systems are used to enhance patient care and improve health management. Examples include wearable health devices (*e.g.* heart rate monitors, glucose meters), smart hospital equipment (*e.g.*, connected infusion pumps, ECG machines), hand hygiene monitoring systems, ingestible sensors, remote patient monitoring tools (*e.g.*, telehealth platforms, IoT-enabled sensors), depression or mood tracking, connected contact lenses, Parkinson's disease monitoring systems, connected inhalers. These technologies are all designed to continuously monitor vital health parameters, such as sleep quality, heart rate, and blood pressure. The Internet of Things in healthcare (H-IoT) comprises a network of medical devices integrated with sensors, software, and connectivity to gather, transmit, and analyse data, thereby enhancing patient care, optimising healthcare systems, and significantly improving a person's quality of life. These systems enable automated decision-making and facilitate seamless communication among patients, healthcare providers, and medical systems. By utilizing these devices, healthcare providers can remotely monitor patients, access vital patient information instantly, collect real-time data for analysis, and facilitate streamlined communication between medical professionals. This enables medical professionals to make quicker decisions and potentially implement life-saving interventions [3].

The healthcare industry's Internet of Things (IoT) market was worth $139.74 billion in 2023 and is expected to reach $822.54 billion by 2032, growing from $175.61 billion in 2024, with a compound annual growth rate (CAGR) of 21.3%. The Internet of Things in the healthcare market was dominated by the Asia Pacific region in 2023, accounting for 40.32% of the total market share [4]. In 2023, the size of the IoT market in India reached US$1.2 billion. The market is expected to reach US$3.3 billion by 2032, with a CAGR of 12.17% from 2024 to 2032, according to IMARC Group [5]. Furthermore, these devices can mitigate the likelihood of prescription errors by offering alerts and reminders for both healthcare practitioners and patients. The objective is to provide a more interconnected and personalised healthcare approach that advantages both patients and providers. The incorporation of IoT devices in healthcare can transform this sector and significantly enhance the quality of patient care [6].

Function of IoT in Healthcare

IoT technology in healthcare assists patients, physicians, hospitals, carers, and insurance companies. Patients may utilise wearables, such as fitness bands and wireless devices, to track their physical activity and inform health-related decisions [6]. IoT devices, encompassing wearables and implanted sensors, gather essential physiological data, such as blood pressure, glucose levels, body temperature, respiration rate, heart rate, and rhythm. This data is transmitted using communication protocols, including Bluetooth, Wi-Fi, and specific IoT protocols, to healthcare servers or cloud-based systems [7]. In the healthcare sector, IoT technologies are currently being applied to offer new possibilities for remote monitoring, enhancing patient care, customised treatment strategies, improving patient outcomes, and streamlining healthcare delivery [8]. The IoT in healthcare notably enhances patient care while also significantly lowering healthcare costs by optimizing processes, automating routine tasks, facilitating simultaneous data acquisition and monitoring, and reducing the need for costly interventions [9].

IoT platforms enhance healthcare operations by automating administrative tasks, improving efficiency, and reducing the need for a large administrative workforce, resulting in cost savings. Furthermore, common duties, such as monitoring vital signs and recording medication administration, can be automated, thereby reducing the likelihood of errors and decreasing labor expenses. Primarily, the prompt detection and concurrent monitoring capabilities of IoT assist in preventing costly medical complications, minimizing hospitalizations, and alleviating the need for costly therapies, thereby substantially reducing healthcare costs. Wearable sensors are employed in healthcare applications to gather physiological data from patients, including body temperature, blood pressure, heart rate, rhythm, electrocardiogram (ECG), and electroencephalogram (EEG). It also helps in augmenting the engagement of a patient [10].

Empowering patients with more autonomy in healthcare involves motivating them to track their health information and interact more effectively with healthcare professionals. Additionally, environmental data may be collected, including temperature, humidity, time, and date, which are stored in a log [11].

Although IoT technology offers significant benefits for healthcare providers in terms of vital information, it also presents challenges, including privacy and security risks associated with the dissemination of sensitive health information through connected devices. Additionally, not all individuals may have access to or the resources to pay for these advanced technologies, which could lead to disparities in healthcare access and quality. A robust IT infrastructure is also necessary to manage the substantial data volumes produced by connected devices.

Potential of IoT in Healthcare

Healthcare practitioners and regulators must address these concerns to ensure equitable access to the benefits of IoT technology in healthcare management for all individuals. By implementing appropriate security protocols and providing assistance to those lacking access to these devices, the healthcare system can enhance the overall outcome for individuals managing persistent health conditions, such as diabetes. Although this technology has the potential to reshape chronic disease management, it is vital that it is deployed in a manner that ensures its use is inclusive and protects patient confidentiality [12].

Addressing the issues caused by the Internet of Things (IoT) in healthcare requires close cooperation among healthcare professionals, technology developers, healthcare industries, legislators, and patients. By establishing clear regulations and guidelines for data protection and privacy, we can mitigate potential risks and ensure that patient information remains secure. Additionally, investing in cybersecurity measures and training for healthcare professionals can help prevent data breaches and unauthorized access to personal health information. Ultimately, by collaborating on these concerns, we can fully leverage the advantages of IoT technology in healthcare and improve the overall quality of patient care [13, 14]. (Fig. **1**) illustrates the conceptual framework of IoT in healthcare.

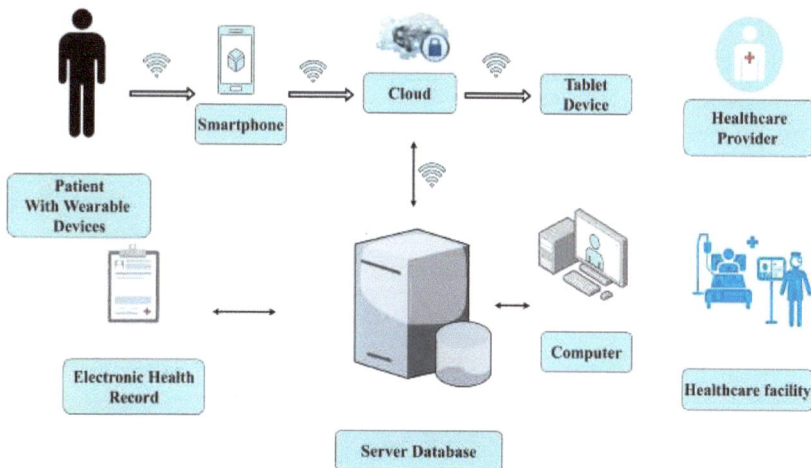

Fig. (1). Conceptual diagram of IoT in healthcare.

This will not only lead to better patient outcomes but also foster trust between healthcare providers and patients. Collaboration between government agencies, technology companies, and healthcare organizations is crucial in creating a safe and efficient IoT ecosystem in healthcare. By staying proactive in addressing cybersecurity threats, we can pave the way for a more connected healthcare system that prioritizes patient safety and privacy. Stakeholders must work together to establish standards and regulations that protect patient data and ensure secure transmission of information. Clear guidelines and protocols for IoT devices in healthcare will help mitigate risks and prevent potential breaches. For example, implementing encryption and authentication measures on IoT devices in hospitals will safeguard sensitive patient information from cyberattacks. Regular security audits and staff training on cybersecurity best practices will further prevent unauthorized access to connected medical devices.

DATA MANAGEMENT AND CONNECTIVITY IN IOT

The healthcare sector has adopted many IoT technologies, reshaping conventional medical practices into creative, data-centric processes. By leveraging interconnected devices, sensors, and real-time analytics, these technologies improve patient outcomes, boost operational performance, and promote preventative healthcare approaches.

Foundational Elements of Healthcare IoT Technology

IoT Sensor Technologies

Sensors constitute a fundamental element of IoT devices. Sensors play a vital role in capturing and transmitting data from a range of sources that include blood glucose levels, thermal patterns, stress levels, SpO2 levels, and other health metrics. They can be incorporated into medical devices, wearable tech, and even embedded in the body. Thermograph sensors detect temperature fluctuations on surfaces, aiding in the identification of abnormalities, such as early-stage tumours. They are frequently utilised in medical diagnostics, such as breast cancer diagnosis, by observing localised temperature elevations linked to neoplastic growth [15]. Table **1** summarizes the various medical sensors and their applications, highlighting their roles in monitoring and diagnostics across healthcare settings.

Table 1. Medical Sensors and their Applications.

Sensor Type	Measurement	Clinical Application(s)	Ref.
Electrocardiogram (ECG)	Cardiac electrical activity	Detecting arrhythmias, heart disease	[10]

(Table 1) cont.....

Sensor Type	Measurement	Clinical Application(s)	Ref.
Glucose Meter	Glucose concentrations within the blood or interstitial fluid	Monitoring diabetes	[12]
Respiratory Rate Monitor	The rhythm and rate of breathing	Monitoring of respiratory diseases, such as sleep apnoea	[16]
Galvanic Skin Response (GSR)	Skin conductance	Monitoring stress and emotional states; wearable mental health applications	[17]
pH Sensors	Acid-base balance	Sweat analysis for fitness, hydration, or metabolic monitoring	[18]
Bioimpedance Sensors *e.g.* MedStorm™ PainSensor	Electrical impedance of body tissues Measure pain intensity	Body composition analysis for fitness and heart failure monitoring	[19]
Infrared Thermography	Thermal patterns	Fever or inflammation detection; public health screening	[15]
Wearable Sweat Sensors	Electrolytes, hydration, and glucose	IoT-enabled dashboards for athletes or chronic disease patients	[20]

Connectivity in IoT

In Healthcare IoT (H-IoT), key technologies for remote patient monitoring, including IoT devices, wearable tech, and telemedicine services, comprise near field communication, Wi-Fi, radio frequency identification, ultra-wideband, Bluetooth, IEEE 802.15.4, long-term evolution, Z-wave, and 5G. They are critical for healthcare practitioners to obtain crucial patient information based on geographic location. Collectively, they rely on a robust network that facilitates instant communication and expedited decision-making processes. However, data security and patient privacy are major concerns when using such technologies [21].

Wi-fi

Wi-Fi technology for data transmission has advanced, incorporating new standards, such as Wi-Fi 6 and Wi-Fi 6E [21]. Wi-Fi offers higher capacity, quicker speeds, and lower latency, facilitating the development of novel applications and services. However, it is constrained by a range of 100 meters. It can be utilised effectively for data transmission between heterogeneous entities without the need for a router in a mobile ad-hoc environment. Given these beneficial advancements in Wi-Fi, it is expected to assume a progressively significant role in the healthcare sector, as well as other sectors that require reliable and rapid wireless network access [22].

Bluetooth

Bluetooth technology, invented in 1994 as a wireless communication method, is extensively utilised in IoT devices, such as smartphones, smartwatches, and fitness bands, employing frequency-hopping spread spectrum (FHSS) [23]. To prevent interference from other wireless devices functioning within the same frequency spectrum, it works in the range of 2.4–2.4835 GHz. This technology operates within the unlicensed frequency bands designated for industrial, scientific, and medical use [24].

RFID

RFID (Radio Frequency Identification), established on the concept of machine-to-machine (M2M) communication, involves the use of RF identification and comprises an RFID reader and its associated RFID tags. RFID readers identify RF tags by detecting signals reflected from them and transmit the retrieved information to a database within the radio range, typically between 10 cm and 100 m [25].

Zigbee

Zigbee is a wireless technology designed for economical, low-latency, low-data-rate, and low-power IoT data networks and applications requiring extended battery life, such as remote patient monitoring devices. The implementation of sleep modes allows devices to deactivate their radios and minimise power consumption when not engaged in data transmission or reception. Zigbee employs a collision avoidance technique known as CSMA-CA (Carrier-Sense Multiple Access with Collision Avoidance) to diminish the probability of data collisions, retries, and acknowledgments, hence enhancing robustness [26].

Near Field Communication (NFC)

NFC is a contactless communication technology based on RFID technology, which relies on electromagnetic fields to facilitate data transfer between two devices with an emphasis on short-range communication. NFC technology facilitates several applications, including personal identification, access control, payment processing, and data sharing between devices [27].

LTE (4G) and WiMAX

LTE (Long-Term Evolution) is a crucial technology for facilitating reliable, high-speed data transmission in healthcare systems, particularly for mobile and remote healthcare services. WiMAX represents a notable long-range technology utilised for data transfer between local servers and base stations in smart healthcare systems. Additionally, LTE-M (LTE for Machines) is regarded as an improvement in supporting IoT. LTE enables patients to engage in virtual consultations with physicians *via* video calls, thereby diminishing wait times and enhancing healthcare accessibility, especially in underserved areas. Nevertheless, 3GPP must enhance coverage, battery longevity, and device intricacy [28].

5G Network

5G networks, M2M communication, and the IoT are considered fundamental components of intelligent healthcare. The implementation of 5G, characterized by high transmission speeds, ultra-low latency, boosted mobile broadband, and stronger network capacity than 4G, would facilitate innovation in healthcare [29]. As an example, ultra-low-latency connectivity enables an ambulance to facilitate remote diagnostic operations [30]. Furthermore, smart healthcare is projected to expand substantially by 12.5% by 2025 [31]. It possesses the capability to transfer and handle extensive medical data, facilitate interactive video, and enable real-time remote device control [32]. For example, large X-ray (XR) image files, including magnetic resonance images, may be transmitted by patients to specialists for evaluation [33]. (Fig. **2**) illustrates the IoT healthcare network architecture.

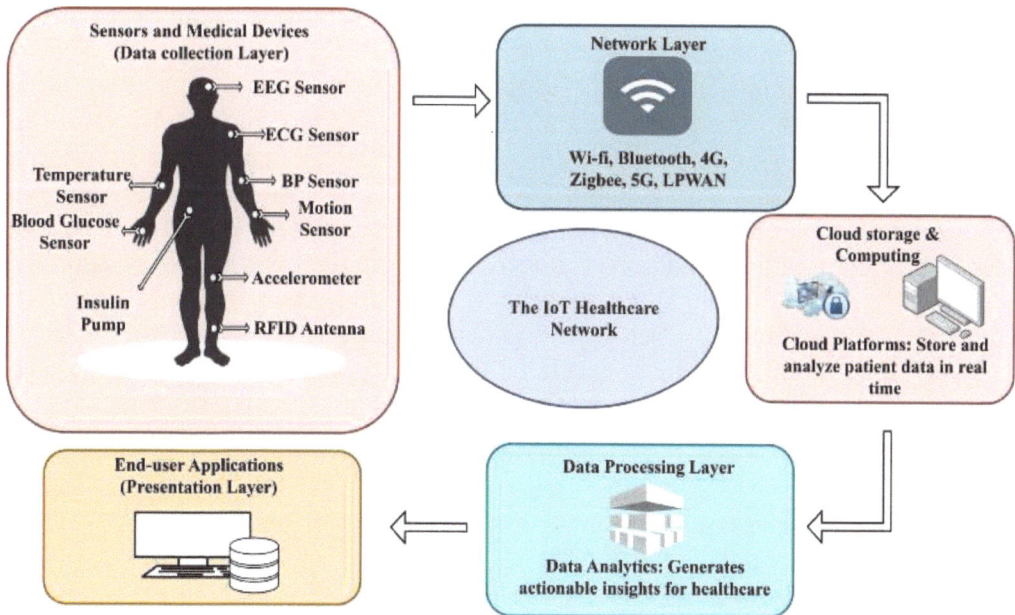

Fig. (2). IoT healthcare network architecture.

STORAGE AND DATA PROCESSING IN IOT

Cloud Storage

Cloud storage serves as the principal solution for handling the substantial volumes of data produced by IoT devices. It also offers data redundancy and disaster recovery functionality, assuring that patient data remains accessible and secure. Cloud provides a framework for storage and management [34]. Devices, such as wearables, sensors, and medical equipment, constantly gather health-related data, which depends on secure storage, processing, and real-time access. IoT healthcare devices frequently utilise cloud-based storage solutions to securely store acquired data. To ensure the accessibility of patient health data from anywhere while maintaining data integrity and confidentiality, cloud storage enables scalable and affordable data management [35]. Amazon Web Services (AWS) provides customised solutions for healthcare data, ensuring secure, HIPAA-compliant storage for patient records, test results, and sensor data [36].

Edge Computing

Edge computing is a distributed computing framework that was developed to extend cloud computing by processing data locally at the "edge" of the network. It brings computation and data storage closer to the data source instead of relying on a centralized data-processing server in the cloud. The intermediate nodes possess computing and storage capacities. Edge computing provides cloud computing functionalities within the Radio Area Network (RAN) to dramatically minimise latency and deepen understanding of context. It lacks centralised computing resources, hence minimising data overload. Critical information, including personal identification details and sensitive information, can be analysed without transmitting data to the cloud server, hence enhancing data security since sensitive data is processed locally. Edge computing has numerous benefits, including reduced response times by relocating processing from the cloud to the edge. However, it encounters challenges related to security and privacy. It shares some security concerns with cloud computing. Nevertheless, the security mechanisms presented within the cloud framework do not apply to the edge framework [37].

Fog Computing

Fog computing enriches the cloud computing model by relocating data processing, storage, and transmission closer to the devices and sensors that produce data. Fog computing enables physicians to make informed decisions during emergencies and enhances the protection of confidential information with ultra-reduced latency as compared to cloud-based applications. Processing power, networking resources, and end-user capabilities are all provided by fog and cloud computing. The fog nodes are closer to the network edge in fog computing, which reduces latency compared to cloud computing. Fog nodes handle limited computing tasks, necessitating the usage of routers, access points, signal repeaters, modems, IoT gateways, smartphones, and similar devices. Fog facilitates real-time analysis by enforcing storage and computation in proximity to the end devices [38].

The IoT-fog computing-based healthcare architecture comprises three layers: device, fog, and cloud computing. At the device layer, IoT-enabled sensors and monitors adhered to patients gather real-time health data, transmitting it to the fog layer through Wi-Fi or mobile networks. The fog layer processes and analyses data locally, providing real-time insights and minimizing latency. It links the device and cloud layer, enhancing resource allocation efficiency. The cloud layer manages extensive storage, processing, and sophisticated analytics for data, surpassing the fog layer's capabilities, hence ensuring complete patient records and facilitating future healthcare initiatives [39].

Semantic Computing

The process involves extracting information from multiple IoT devices and providing tailored services to users. This involves recognising proper information, employing it efficiently, and structuring it for certain uses. In a smart healthcare system, IoT devices like wearable sensors gather patient health data, which is subsequently analysed to deliver personalised suggestions or alerts to patients and healthcare providers. The procedure involves decision analysis to ascertain the suitable data extraction strategy, ensuring the service aligns accurately with user requirements. Instruments like the Web Ontology Language (OWL) and the Resource Description Framework (RDF) are essential for meeting these resource requirements [40].

APPLICATIONS OF IOT TECHNOLOGY IN HEALTHCARE (H-IOT)

Wearable Devices

The significance of wearables lies in the utility they provide, helping not only patients but also healthcare providers by managing health concerns at a low cost. These devices are equipped with sensors and accessories, such as smartwatches, smartphones, pendants, and dental sensors, that collect data on the patient's health and their surrounding environment. Upon collection, that information is communicated through servers, where it is accessible *via* a smartphone. Mobile applications connected to IoT wearables amplify the computational capabilities of the devices [41].

Smart Glasses

These glasses have been developed for the monitoring of vital signs and activity tracking, frequently incorporating functions, such as heart rate monitoring and activity measurement. They are equipped with gyroscopes, microphones, accelerometers, and image sensors. The user interface is user-friendly and supports voice commands. Examples comprise Google Glass for Enterprise, Vuzix Blade, JINS MEME, and ReconJet [42, 43].

Smart Contact Lenses

They strengthen vision, measure glucose levels through tears, and track glaucoma progression by evaluating eye lens curvature. Elevated intraocular pressure (IOP), a critical element in glaucoma, may result in permanent blindness if not treated. IOP-monitoring lenses facilitate the prevention of illness onset and advancement by early diagnosis and therapy [44].

Smart Watches and Wearable Pendants

Smartwatches often feature sophisticated capabilities, including a heart rate monitor. These advanced devices employ a method known as photo-plethysmography to precisely assess the individual's heart rate. Specialised sensors and light beams on the smartwatch enable precise quantification of variations in blood volume in the wrist. This technique produces a PPG (Photoplethysmogram) waveform that yields essential data utilized to determine the heart rate of an individual [45, 46]. Wearable pendants worn by patients can detect falls, abrupt movements, or prolonged inactivity following sudden changes. As a result, an alert is sent to emergency services along with the patient's location. The application was especially helpful during the COVID-19 pandemic, when numerous families were unable to visit elderly relatives, ensuring their safety [47]. (Fig. **3**) highlights key IoT applications in healthcare, including wearable devices, disease prediction systems, and smart-enabled medical technologies for enhanced patient monitoring and care.

DISEASE PREDICTION AND HEALTHCARE NETWORK

Internet-assisted disease prediction is a rapidly evolving concept for detection, monitoring, and expedited treatment procedures utilising software applications and artificial intelligence-trained models or electronic devices to foster next-generation healthcare advancements. Currently, the medical sector is predominantly reliant on and interconnected through the utilisation of IoT and electronic networks for healthcare services.

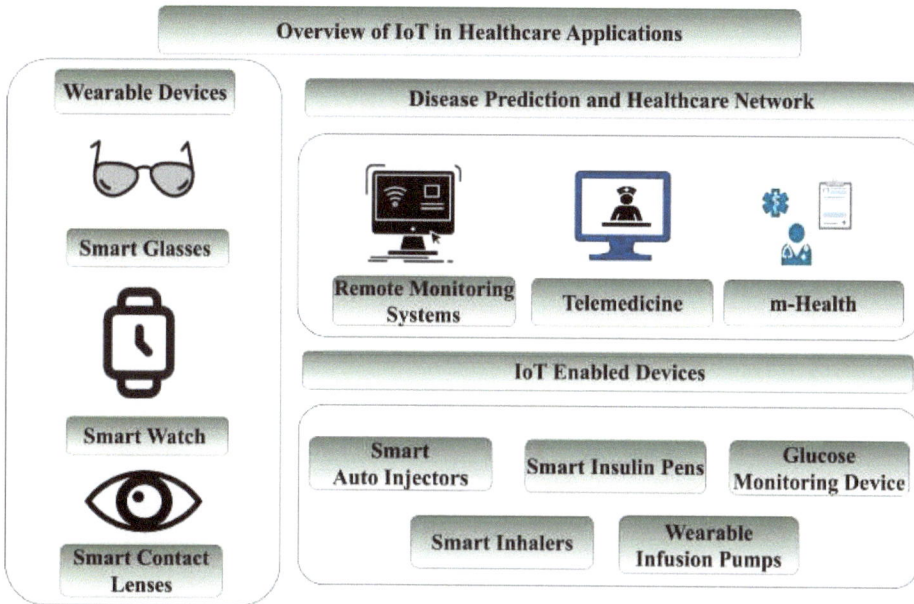

Fig. (3). IoT applications in healthcare: wearables, disease prediction, and enabled devices.

Examples include Comarch Healthcare, which provides a range of healthcare technology solutions, such as hospital IT systems, radiology software, remote medical care, and electronic health record (EHR) administration. Table **2** provides an overview of telehealth products, including their descriptions, highlighting their functionalities and applications in remote healthcare.

Table 2. Telehealth Products and their Descriptions.

Product	Description	Ref.
Comarch Diagnostic Point	A strategy for healthcare institutions to enhance operational efficiency. It comprises devices and software for assessing critical parameters, gathering data *via* Bluetooth, and relaying it to the Remote Care Centre utilising a tablet application.	[48]
Comarch Life Wristband	A waterproof device designed for durability, featuring an extended battery life and an SOS button. It identifies loss of consciousness, immediately notifies telecare centres, and grants medical personnel access to electronic health records and emergency information.	[49]
Comarch CardioVest	A gadget for cardiac monitoring that captures and transmits ECG data to a telemedicine platform for analysis. It facilitates prompt detection and comprehensive cardiac evaluations.	[50]

REMOTE HEALTHCARE SYSTEM

Remote Patient Monitoring, or RPM, uses advancements in technology like wearable devices, sensors, and communications tools to monitor patients' health conditions, collect all essential health information, and facilitate virtual consultations between the patient and the healthcare providers. This approach enables continuous monitoring of health metrics, such as respiratory rate, blood pressure, and heart rate, symptoms like fever or shortness of breath, and other health indicators, such as glucose levels, oxygen saturation, and physical activity, eliminating the need for regular in-person consultations, especially in rural or remote areas [51].

For paralysed patients or patients with mobility impairments, remote patient monitoring offers essential healthcare access by monitoring physiological data of cardiovascular and respiratory information. All such data collected is securely passed to healthcare providers for reviewing the information, offering timely medical interventions, ensuring ongoing monitoring, enabling early detection of potential health issues, and reducing the risk of complications and unnecessary hospital readmissions. Additionally, RPM can support personalised care plans, improve medication management, and enhance the overall quality of life for patients with limited mobility [52].

Mobile-Health (M-Health)

The application of m-health in healthcare encompasses education and awareness, disease diagnosis, outbreak monitoring, remote data gathering, remote monitoring, personal digital assistance, telehealth or telemedicine, and support in disease management. Key features of various healthcare systems, highlighting their structural, operational, and patient-care differences, are summarized in Table 3.

Table 3. Healthcare Systems and their Key Features.

System Name	Purpose	Key Features/Functionality	Ref.
AirStrip, AirStripOB/Cardiology	Synchronize data across many devices	Monitors cardiovascular problems *via* smartphones, tablets, and laptops; consolidates data from electronic health records and clinical solutions across diverse care environments.	[53]
PatientSafe, PatientTouch System	Enhance communication and care coordination within the healthcare sector	Integrates diverse medical devices to improve communication and care efficacy.	[54]

(Table 3) cont.....

System Name	Purpose	Key Features/Functionality	Ref.
AIIMS-WHO CCENBC	Assist nursing personnel and neonatologists in resource-constrained environments.	Helps nurses and neonatologists at smaller hospitals with limited resources.	[54]

Telemedicine

Telemedicine has been shown to be effective in managing chronic illnesses, such as diabetes and hypertension, *via* remote monitoring and virtual consultations, enhancing patient outcomes and convenience [55]. In mental health, telepsychiatry enhances accessibility to care, diminishes stigma, and provides prompt assistance. Its use in emergency treatment has demonstrated the potential to decrease hospital admissions and improve triage procedures [56].

McGinley *et al.* assessed telemedicine for multiple sclerosis (MS) over 24 months in the realm of long-term illness treatment, demonstrating comparable clinical outcomes to in-clinic therapy, with enhanced accessibility, economic benefits, and elevated patient satisfaction. Mobile applications like MDLIVE enhance telemedicine by linking users with licensed physicians for non-emergency consultations, providing rapid support with wait times under 15 minutes, and broadening access to behavioral and psychiatric therapy [57].

IOT-ENABLED DEVICES

Smart Insulin Pens

Smart insulin pens utilise IoT technology to monitor and regulate insulin administration for diabetic individuals. Smart insulin pens facilitate accurate drug dosing depending on glucose levels, ensuring timely administration and preventing health issues. They transmit precise dosage and scheduling information wirelessly, facilitating treatment monitoring. By monitoring dosages and glucose levels, users can identify patterns and obtain personalised treatment and lifestyle adjustment advice using the associated smartphone application. For instance, the InPen, developed by Companion Medical, facilitates insulin dosage calculation using an integrated diabetes management application [58]. The Tempo Pen, built by Lilly, records the time and dosage of each injection and syncs the data with the corresponding diabetes management application [59].

Glucose Monitoring Devices

Patients with diabetes may suffer from multiple metabolic disorders, including prolonged hyperglycemia. Monitoring blood sugar levels reveals fluctuations in glucose levels and aids in daily activities, such as eating habits, water intake, and medication administration. An optical-based approach is proposed. A light beam is directed toward human tissue to measure glucose levels in real time [60].

The concentration of glucose is then determined by analysing the energy that is absorbed, reflected, or scattered. Data is uploaded to a server and subsequently transmitted to designated physicians for additional analysis [61]. The sensors remain continuously connected to the Internet Protocol Version 6 (IPv6) for seamless data sharing with the corresponding healthcare service provider. IoT enables data transfer between the patient and the service provider. An identical methodology was employed to identify and prevent the COVID-19 pandemic. Furthermore, alternative technologies like transdermal sensors require extensive calibration and are more vulnerable to uncontrolled environments [62]. Despite this, other factors influence glucose estimation, including perspiration, skin texture, ambient temperature, and atmospheric pressure. Consequently, the pursuit of novel and more precise non-invasive methods remains underway [63].

Yao *et al.* developed a wireless health-monitoring contact lens for non-invasive, continuous glucose assessment in tears [64]. The lens features enzyme-based electrochemical glucose sensors that utilise glucose oxidase to catalyse reactions between glucose and oxygen, resulting in the formation of hydrogen peroxide and gluconolactone. Electrodes subsequently detect hydrogen peroxide, ensuring great selectivity and efficiency [65]. As presented in Table **4**, innovative wearable infusion pumps are emerging as promising tools for glucose monitoring.

Wearable infusion pumps administer medication through a subcutaneous catheter. Their small size, portability, and ability to provide precise doses at predetermined intervals ensure that patients receive continuous treatment all day long. Wearable infusion pumps reduce the potential for infection at the infusion site by minimizing disruptions to the infusion site and allowing for more flexible and adaptable medication administration. For more tailored care, wearable infusion pumps can assess glucose levels in real time and modify medicine dosage accordingly. The Medtronic SynchroMed™ II Infusion System is a programmable implanted pump intended for spinal medication administration, frequently utilised for pain and spasticity management. Nonetheless, it involves implant surgery, has a limited battery lifespan, and may result in complications [68].

Table 4. Innovative Wearable Infusion Pumps for Glucose Monitoring.

Device Name	Technology Used	Key Features	Challenges	Ref.
GlucoTrack	Ultrasonic and thermal technology	Determines glucose concentrations from the earlobe; minimally invasive; requires individual calibration.	Calibration dependency.	[66]

(Table 4) cont.....

Device Name	Technology Used	Key Features	Challenges	Ref.
FreeStyle Libre	Flash glucose monitoring system	Measures glucose levels in humans; facilitates continuous glucose monitoring without the need for finger-pricking.	High false positive rate for hypoglycemia.	[66]
SugarBEAT	Disposable skin patch with transmitter	Non-invasively measures glucose with a dermal patch; wirelessly links to a transmitter.	Still under development.	[67]
GlucoWise	Low-power radio waves	Quantifies glucose levels *via* the earlobe using non-invasive technologies.	Still under development.	[67]

Smart Inhalers

Smart inhalers are a kind of wearable medication delivery device that can help individuals with asthma and chronic obstructive pulmonary disease (COPD) control their symptoms. These devices can assess a patient's treatment compliance over time and remind them to take their medication as prescribed for medication adherence. Some high-tech inhalers can monitor lung function and provide doctors and patients with useful input. Smart inhalers can help improve patient outcomes, lower healthcare costs, and tailor treatment plans with the data they collect.

For instance, the Teva Pharmaceuticals ProAir® Digihaler™ is a digital inhaler that monitors usage data and automates dosing for the management of asthma and COPD using albuterol. It has age restrictions, limited emergency use, and requires maintenance [69].

Smart Auto-Injectors

Medication can be precisely administered with the use of smart auto-injectors, which are programmable medical devices. They can communicate with other devices or networks and share data in real-time because they are built with IoT technology. Insulin, epinephrine, and other drugs are administered *via* smart auto-injectors that are Internet of Things (IoT) enabled. They can be preset to provide medication at scheduled intervals or upon the detection of specific physiological parameters, such as glucose levels in diabetic individuals. For example, the Amgen Neulasta Onpro Kit is an intelligent auto-injector designed to manage neutropenia during chemotherapy, featuring companion smartphone control for pegfilgrastim administration. Its constraints encompass exclusive subcutaneous administration, high expense, and reliability concerns [70].

IMPLANTABLE SMART DRUG DELIVERY DEVICES

Implantable Drug-Eluting Stents

Drug-eluting stents are placed in blood vessels to administer drugs, such as anti-inflammatory or antiproliferative agents, directly to the targeted area. Healthcare providers can easily modify the supply rate of the stents using a smartphone or other wireless device. The Abbott Xience Sierra™ is a drug-coated implanted stent intended for remote monitoring in the management of coronary artery disease. It administers everolimus, an immunosuppressive agent, to prevent restenosis subsequent to coronary artery angioplasty. Despite this, problems may occur, necessitating re-treatment for certain patients [71].

Implantable Infusion Pumps

Implantable pumps deliver drugs, like analgesics or chemotherapeutic agents, directly to specific locations and can be electronically managed using a smartphone or other devices, enabling healthcare professionals to modify the administration rate. These sensor-driven pumps, commonly utilised for insulin or chronic pain management, are surgically implanted and have sensors that monitor the patient's state, modulating medicine supply as required. The Abbott Infinity™ Deep Brain Stimulation (DBS) device is an implanted infusion pump designed for deep brain stimulation treatment in patients with Parkinson's disease. It administers drugs like levodopa to alleviate symptoms. Nonetheless, it entails an invasive treatment, poses the danger of neurological side effects, and necessitates regular follow-up [72].

Ingestible Smart Drug Delivery Devices

Ingestible smart drug delivery systems powered by IoT technology are rapidly gaining traction in the healthcare sector. These devices employ IoT, which enables real-time monitoring and precise medication distribution, thereby improving the accuracy, effectiveness, and overall efficiency of the delivery process. Abilify MyCite® by Proteus Digital Health is an ingestible tablet with a sensor that collaborates with a wearable patch to monitor medication adherence and collect health data. It administers aripiprazole, an antipsychotic utilised for the treatment of schizophrenia and bipolar disorder. Notwithstanding its prospective advantages, the device encounters constraints like restricted availability, privacy concerns, and high costs [73].

SMART HOSPITAL INFRASTRUCTURE

Smart Wheelchair

The smart wheelchair model features sophisticated GPS-based location tracking and obstacle recognition technology. These technologies provide immediate adjustments to climatic circumstances, such as deploying an umbrella or head covering during precipitation or excessive temperatures. Moreover, mood-responsive features improve user comfort and engagement with the surroundings. This represents a substantial advancement in tackling the difficulties encountered by those with limited mobility, promoting a more liberated and dignified living [74].

Smart Robots

Throughout the COVID-19 pandemic, IoT-enabled robots played a crucial role in hospital environments. These robots, integrated with IoT technology, were utilised for functions like the disposal of infectious materials, object transportation, cleaning, and room disinfection. Germ-eliminating robots utilise UV light for ongoing, automated sanitation in medical facilities. This technology has subsequently proliferated to various public venues, such as train stations, universities, grocery stores, movie theatres, and residences, establishing a novel benchmark for sanitation and safety across sectors [75].

Smart Beds

IoT-enabled smart beds, utilising technologies, such as LoRaWAN, facilitate real-time monitoring of patient activities, including alterations in bed rail position, which is transmitted wirelessly to a dashboard at the nurse's station. This enables carers to enhance the monitoring of patient mobility and ensures prompt responses during emergencies. Furthermore, these beds may be operated remotely to modify patient comfort and support, providing individualised treatment. When combined with other healthcare devices, such as oxygen monitors and infusion pumps, smart beds optimise patient management, improving overall care efficiency [76].

ADVANCED APPLICATIONS

Augmented Reality (AR)

In the modern context of Industry 4.0, augmented reality is an important tool in the development, instruction, and progress of newer technologies. The inclusion of information technology in the health sector is highly innovative. Healthcare providers can benefit from augmented reality (AR) in several ways, including better surgical outcomes, enhanced remote monitoring, and improved learning and teaching. AR played an important role in training and raising awareness about hand hygiene to curb COVID-19 and other illnesses [77].

Personalized Medicine

The goal of personalised medicine is to provide more accurate and efficient healthcare by customising treatment plans for each patient based on their unique genetic, environmental, and lifestyle factors. A study employing the Latent Dirichlet Allocation (LDA) model aims to forecast future treatment regimens for diabetes, illustrating the significance of data-driven insights in improving patient outcomes [78]. A separate study focuses on pediatric patients with type 1 diabetes, incorporating IoT and mHealth technology to assess the influence of physical exercise on blood glucose levels. This facilitates tailored meal advice, highlighting the promise of personalised healthcare in the management of chronic conditions in children. Such developments represent substantial progress in utilising technology for personalised medical care [79].

CHALLENGES IN IMPLEMENTING H-IOT

The numerous performance-related obstacles of the H-IoT, including security, latency, reliability, and efficiency, pose significant challenges to the advancement of H-IoT. An enhanced H-IoT system must exhibit minimal latency, extraordinary reliability, energy efficiency, and robust security. (Fig. **4**) presents the key challenges in IoT healthcare technology.

Low Latency and Energy Consumption

The major challenge of H-IoT is the real-time data transmission and analysis, due to data delay in processing or transmission, since data delay may deprive health practitioners of capacity to make timely and informed medical decisions in emergency response systems, predictive health analytics, remote patient monitoring, telemedicine, medication adherence monitoring, and early disease detection. Low latency is crucial for timely responses and informed decision-making; nevertheless, attaining this necessitates specialised hardware, optimised network infrastructure, and sophisticated software solutions. Edge and fog computing frameworks, augmented by AI, diminish latency by processing data nearer to the source, hence ensuring efficiency in time-sensitive H-IoT systems [80]. Despite the numerous advantages, issues about latency, response time, and energy usage remain. Unlike wearable H-IoT devices, which can be recharged regularly, implantable devices necessitate sustainable energy solutions for long-term operation. To tackle these challenges, the Energy-Efficient Internet of

Medical Things to Fog Interoperability of Task Scheduling (EEIoMT) architecture has been introduced to enhance task scheduling to prioritise essential jobs while regulating energy consumption [81].

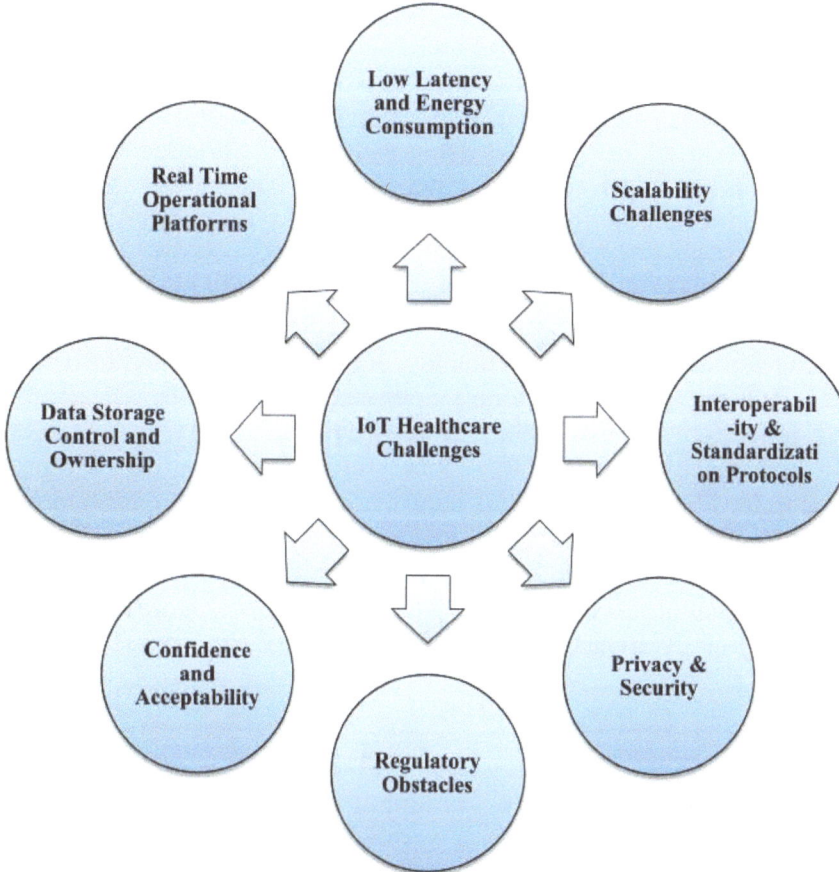

Fig. (4). Challenges in IoT healthcare technology.

Real-Time Operational Platforms

The health status of an individual can be more thoroughly assessed by data gathered from multiple sensors. Nonetheless, the significant amount of data produced needs specialised processing techniques for the extraction of valuable information. Numerous current algorithms struggle to efficiently process all data, necessitating real-time data handling techniques. Although deep learning has the aptitude to manage extensive real-time datasets, it is essential to extract relevant and non-redundant features for precise analysis and decision-making [82].

Challenges in Privacy and Security

H-IoT deals with highly sensitive information regarding patients. Hence, security is of the utmost concern. With the growing interconnection of devices and systems, the risk of cyberattacks and data breaches increases, as cybercriminals often target medical information for identity theft, falsification of health records, creation of fake medical records, and other illicit purposes. A security breach might result in major consequences, such as the exposure of personal medical data or the manipulation of medical devices, potentially endangering patients. To alleviate these dangers, H-IoT systems necessitate stringent security protocols to guarantee the confidentiality, integrity, and availability of patient data, along with the safety of medical devices. Nonetheless, H-IoT systems are limited in resources, complicating the implementation of lightweight algorithms that ensure energy economy. To tackle these issues, energy-efficient machine learning or deep learning algorithms that can manage lightweight cryptography have been suggested. However, computational complexities persist. The fog model, employing federated systems proximate to devices, might enhance security by mitigating risks linked to centralised processing and augmenting data protection. Moreover, the IoMT raises additional security concerns, including vulnerability to man-in-the-middle attacks and a lack of security knowledge among users [13, 14]. To tackle these challenges, the RECC-VC security enhancement approach has been suggested, integrating K-anonymity, optimised neural networks, and blockchain technology to boost precision and security in IoMT systems [83].

Data Storage, Control, and Ownership

Transparency regarding data storage, control, and ownership is crucial for the progression of IoT-based healthcare. Essential factors encompass identifying the location of centralised cloud data storage, ownership rights, and user control over data, including the ability to request deletion. The exchange of data among states, territories, and worldwide poses issues regarding privacy, security, and secrecy. These matters have to be regulated by federally enforced standards; yet, multinational providers may not comply with these codes. Consequently, strategic planning and explicit guidelines are essential for developing resilience rules and frameworks for IoT healthcare systems [82].

Interoperability and Standardization Protocols

Interoperability and standardisation challenges provide substantial obstacles to the extensive implementation of IoT in healthcare. The absence of standardised communication protocols and machine-to-machine agreements hinders seamless integration across various devices and systems. This fragmentation, resulting from each manufacturer developing distinct architectures and protocols, leads to vertical silos that obstruct data transfer and system interaction without significant alterations. Attaining semantic interoperability is essential for facilitating big data analytics and decision-making in healthcare. As the IoT ecosystem expands, it is crucial to solve interoperability concerns through established frameworks to fully realise the potential of IoT-enabled healthcare, therefore boosting safety, productivity, and user satisfaction for physicians and patients alike [84].

Scalability Challenges

Scalability issues need to be addressed in order to facilitate the extensive deployment of H-IoT systems. At the same time, it is necessary to maintain dependable data transmission through efficient access mechanisms to prevent packet loss. Current routing protocols frequently encounter difficulties because of the dynamic characteristics of H-IoT networks. Localization, coverage, and the standardization of wearable and implantable sensors are also crucial for seamless connectivity. Furthermore, data traffic must be managed without incurring additional expenses or processing lags. Network calibration poses a challenge due to the incessant alteration of nodes, while mobility difficulties further impair performance as sensors on the human body influence network availability during user relocation [85].

Regulatory Obstacles in Healthcare Internet of Things

IoT-enabled healthcare devices are governed by frameworks, such as the FDA's Software as a Medical Device (SaMD) guidelines, mandating robust validation processes, cybersecurity protocols, and post-market monitoring. The incorporation of IoT in healthcare raises concerns about patient privacy and data security, particularly with devices that can capture and store sensitive information. Adherence to rules, such as HIPAA (Health Insurance Portability and Accountability Act), is essential for safeguarding electronic health information (ePHI) [86].

Confidence and Acceptability

The public's inadequate awareness of the security of health data held on cloud servers, which are often located in unknown or foreign locations, constitutes a substantial obstacle to the implementation of H-IoT. Although the potential of IoT is evident, many individuals may not entirely recognise its advantages or the value it offers in healthcare. Issues regarding data breaches and confidentiality risks endure; nevertheless, the anticipated benefits must surpass these issues to facilitate the wider adoption of IoT-enabled healthcare systems. The faith of healthcare professionals in IoT is essential. Their adoption is reliant upon elements like technological correctness, user-friendliness, compatibility with existing systems, individual attitudes, organisational readiness, and patient interactions [87].

CASE STUDIES ON IOT IN HEALTHCARE

Case Study: Internet of Things in Diabetes Management

An innovative case study examines the application of IoT and artificial intelligence to enhance diabetes management. The research combines Continuous Glucose Monitoring (CGM) devices with IoT and deep learning to forecast blood glucose levels in patients who are suffering from Type-1 Diabetes. Conventional continuous glucose monitoring devices notify consumers when glucose levels are above safe limits. Nonetheless, these systems frequently operate reactively, resulting in possible delays in intervention.

To tackle this issue, researchers devised an innovative methodology that integrates IoT-enabled wearable devices, cloud computing, and a deep learning model utilising cascaded recurrent neural networks and limited Boltzmann machines. This system predicts glucose levels up to 30 minutes ahead. The predictive capability facilitates prompt medical decisions, mitigating hazards, such as hyperglycemia and related sequelae, including neuropathy and cardiovascular disorders. The use of IoT for instantaneous data transfer and processing guarantees that patients obtain actionable insights *via* mobile applications, thereby strengthening self-management and improving outcomes [88].

Case Study: Smart Inhalers for Asthma Medication Adherence Management

This study analyzes the obstacles and enablers for the incorporation of smart inhalers into asthma management within the Dutch healthcare framework. Smart inhalers, featuring usage tracking, reminders, and personalised feedback, demonstrate the potential to enhance drug adherence, inhalation strategies, and asthma management. Focus groups, including patients (n=9) and healthcare professionals (n=7), along with interviews conducted with policymakers (n=4) and developers (n=4), yielded significant insights. Facilitators comprise user-centric designs, intuitive applications, customised features, minimum disruption to established habits, and the opportunity for a national platform to enhance implementation efficiency.

Obstacles encompass compatibility challenges with inhalers and electronic health records (EHRs), restricted consultation duration, elevated expenses, absence of reimbursement, and environmental considerations. Privacy concerns and ambiguous data utilisation policies impede uptake, alongside sluggish technology progress and opposition from conventional healthcare frameworks. This study emphasizes the necessity of engaging all stakeholders in the creation of user-friendly, secure, and evidence-based smart inhalers. Rectifying deficiencies in reimbursement structures, guaranteeing device interoperability, and modifying healthcare processes are essential for effective integration. Recommendations also encompass ways to mitigate environmental hazards and provide customised solutions for the effective execution of asthma care [89].

FUTURE PROSPECTS

The future potential of IoT-based devices and drug delivery systems is extensive and encouraging. Such systems have the potential to completely transform the healthcare sector and its services. Technological advancements and the increasing demand for personalized medicine establish IoT-based drug delivery as a tailored treatment approach, leading to improved patient care. With IoT devices integrated with drug delivery systems, patient health can be monitored in real-time, allowing healthcare providers to adjust the necessary treatments, thereby improving their outcomes. Additionally, drugs administered through an IoT platform can enhance the effectiveness of drug delivery, thereby reducing the chances of medication errors and increasing patient compliance.

Artificial Intelligence (AI)

Artificial Intelligence (AI) is transforming the Internet of Things (IoT) in healthcare by facilitating intelligent systems to execute intricate operations that usually necessitate human intelligence, like visual understanding, speech identification, and informed decision making. In the Internet of Medical Things applications, AI improves e-healthcare by facilitating precision medicine and providing immediate answers for diagnosis and treatment strategies based on historical and real-time data. AI-driven classifiers automate functions, such as collecting patient information, scheduling appointments, and recommending therapies. NLP extracts significant insights from unstructured data, including laboratory reports and clinical notes. Machine learning forecasts future health issues by examining historical data using supervised, unsupervised, or reinforcement learning, rendering IoMT systems proactive and adaptive for enhanced healthcare results. Machine learning models utilise supervised and unsupervised learning to forecast future health issues, establishing a comprehensive foundation for preventative healthcare. These AI-driven innovations establish IoMT as a crucial facilitator for real-time, data-informed healthcare solutions, enhancing decision-making and patient outcomes in the future.

Blockchain

The future of blockchain in healthcare systems will likely be influenced by its capacity to offer secure and decentralised access control. The complexity of integrating blockchain solutions, especially in transitioning from conventional systems, necessitates the growing significance of new architectures and frameworks. Future advancements may integrate blockchain with swarm intelligence algorithms, as examined in research on electronic health records (EHRs), enabling seamless data exchange between IoT devices, wearable technology, and healthcare providers. These advancements may facilitate safer and more efficient handling of health data, particularly in contexts where privacy and access control are critical. With scalability and security as primary factors, blockchain will persist in transforming healthcare, thus delivering more efficient, patient-centred treatment while minimising operational difficulties. This integration will enhance patient care by supplying healthcare practitioners with current, secure information, irrespective of location.

6G Network

The future of 6G in healthcare is set to transform the IoT landscape by meeting the increasing need for highly dynamic, autonomous, and intelligent services that 5G cannot adequately fulfil. As smart devices proliferate and new IoT applications emerge, like remote robotic surgery and driverless vehicles, 6G is anticipated to provide significant enhancements in data sensing, networking, and communication. Its ultra-low latency and capacity for extensive, seamless connectivity will augment the provision of IoT services and increase the overall user experience.

The capabilities of 6G will enhance healthcare applications, especially in telemedicine and remote care. The amalgamation of AI with 6G will provide immersive experiences, like 360-degree video streaming and holographic displays, thereby revolutionising remote diagnostics and medical education. This will be especially advantageous for virtual and augmented reality (VR/AR) applications, which are becoming increasingly essential in healthcare education, patient care, and rehabilitation. The superior Quality of Experience (QoE) that 6G ensures will be crucial for the efficacy of real-time medical applications, where accuracy and promptness are vital. This advanced network will facilitate the extensive use of novel healthcare technology, rendering remote, personalised care a global reality [85 - 89].

CONCLUSION

The incorporation of IoT in healthcare signifies a dramatic change, providing chances to enhance patient outcomes, transform healthcare delivery, and encourage innovative medical solutions. The crucial function of IoT-enabled medicine delivery systems is to offer accuracy, efficacy, and real-time monitoring. These technologies enhance adherence, reduce prescription errors, and provide personalised treatment regimens customised to particular patient requirements. Additionally, IoT-driven advancements in chronic disease management include devices like smart inhalers for asthma and sophisticated diabetes monitoring systems, which demonstrate how technology can bridge gaps in existing care models and empower both patients and healthcare professionals.

The challenges related to IoT in healthcare have been rigorously studied. Concerns regarding data security, privacy, and ownership are significant, necessitating the establishment of explicit legislative frameworks at both national and international levels to foster patient trust and system dependability. Interoperability and standardisation are essential; without them, the fragmented nature of IoT ecosystems would persistently hinder seamless data sharing and integration among devices and platforms. Furthermore, financial obstacles, including elevated development expenses and restricted reimbursement frameworks, pose additional challenges to widespread adoption. Overcoming these obstacles through cooperative policies and strategic investments is essential to realising IoT's complete promise in healthcare.

The future of IoT in healthcare is driven by advanced technologies, such as AI, blockchain, and 6G networks. AI enhances IoT functionalities *via* sophisticated data analysis, predictive modelling, and instantaneous decision-making, facilitating a transition from reactive to proactive care. Blockchain provides secure, decentralised systems for the management of sensitive health information, guaranteeing transparency and patient autonomy. The emergence of 6G networks offers exceptional connectivity, minimal latency, and facilitation of immersive applications, such as AR/VR, transforming healthcare, medical education, and remote diagnostics. Collectively, these breakthroughs signify the advent of a new epoch in personalised, efficient, and scalable healthcare solutions.

REFERENCES

[1]   Juma M, Alattar F, Touqan B. Securing big data integrity for industrial IoT in smart manufacturing based on the trusted consortium blockchain (TCB). IoT 2023; 4(1): 27-55.
[http://dx.doi.org/10.3390/iot4010002]

[2]   Krishankumar R, Ecer F. Selection of IoT service provider for sustainable transport using q-rung orthopair fuzzy CRADIS and unknown weights. Appl Soft Comput 2023; 132: 109870.
[http://dx.doi.org/10.1016/j.asoc.2022.109870]

[3]   Clemente-Lopez D, Rangel-Magdaleno JJ, Muñoz-Pacheco JM. A lightweight chaos-based encryption scheme for IoT healthcare systems. Internet of Things 2024; 25: 101032.
[http://dx.doi.org/10.1016/j.iot.2023.101032]

[4]   Abdalla M. Inclusive role of Internet of (Healthcare) Things in digital health: Challenges, methods, and future directions. In: Khamparia A, Gupta D, Eds. Generative Artificial Intelligence for Biomedical and Smart Health Informatics. Wiley 2024; pp. 239-58.
[http://dx.doi.org/10.1002/9781394280735.ch12]

[5]   Market Data Forecast. IoT healthcare market 2024. Available from: https://www.marketdataforecast.com/market-reports/iot-healthcare-market

[6]   Alraja MN, Barhamgi H, Rattrout A, Barhamgi M. An integrated framework for privacy protection in IoT — Applied to smart healthcare. Comput Electr Eng 2021; 91: 107060.
[http://dx.doi.org/10.1016/j.compeleceng.2021.107060]

[7]   Li C, Wang J, Wang S, Zhang Y. A review of IoT applications in healthcare. Neurocomputing 2024; 565: 127017.
[http://dx.doi.org/10.1016/j.neucom.2023.127017]

[8]   Mohammed BG, Hasan DS. Smart healthcare monitoring system using IoT. International Journal of Interactive Mobile Technologies (iJIM) 2023; 17(1): 141-52.
[http://dx.doi.org/10.3991/ijim.v17i01.34675]

[9]   Krishnamoorthy S, Dua A, Gupta S. Role of emerging technologies in future IoT-driven Healthcare 4.0 technologies: a survey, current challenges and future directions. J Ambient Intell Humaniz Comput 2023; 14(1): 361-407.
[http://dx.doi.org/10.1007/s12652-021-03302-w]

[10]   Bhatt V, Chakraborty S. Improving service engagement in healthcare through internet of things based healthcare systems. J Sci Tech Pol Manag 2023; 14(1): 53-73.
[http://dx.doi.org/10.1108/JSTPM-03-2021-0040]

[11]   Abd El-Aziz RM, Taloba AI, Alghamdi FA. Quantum computing optimization technique for IoT platform using modified deep residual approach. Alex Eng J 2022; 61(12): 12497-509.
[http://dx.doi.org/10.1016/j.aej.2022.06.029]

[12]   Inoue S, Egi M, Kotani J, Morita K. Accuracy of blood-glucose measurements using glucose meters and arterial blood gas analyzers in critically ill adult patients: systematic review. Crit Care 2013; 17(2): R48.
[http://dx.doi.org/10.1186/cc12567] [PMID: 23506841]

[13]   Kumar M, Kumar A. Botnet dynamics and measures for India. In: Chakraborty M, Jha RK, Balas VE, Sur SN, Kandar D, Eds. Trends in wireless communication and information security. Singapore: Springer 2021; pp. 301-9.

[14]   Akhtar MAK, Kumar M. Detection of DDoS attack using Naive Bayes classifier. In: Kumar A, Reddy SSS, Eds. Advancements in security and privacy initiatives for multimedia images. IGI Global Scientific Publishing 2021; pp. 214-25.https://www.igi-global.com/chapter/detection-of-ddos-attack-using-naive-bayes-classifier/262075 Internet
[http://dx.doi.org/10.4018/978-1-7998-2795-5.ch009]

[15]   Elouerghi A, Bellarbi L, Khomsi Z, Jbari A, Errachid A, Yaakoubi N. A flexible wearable thermography system based on a bioheat microsensors network for early breast cancer detection: IoT technology. J Electr Comput Eng 2022; 2022(1): 1-13.
[http://dx.doi.org/10.1155/2022/5921691]

[16]   De Fazio R, Stabile M, De Vittorio M, Velázquez R, Visconti P. An overview of wearable piezoresistive and inertial sensors for respiration rate monitoring. Electronics (Basel) 2021; 10(17): 2178.
[http://dx.doi.org/10.3390/electronics10172178]

[17] Yang X, McCoy E, Anaya-Boig E, *et al.* The effects of traveling in different transport modes on galvanic skin response (GSR) as a measure of stress: An observational study. Environ Int 2021; 156: 106764.
[http://dx.doi.org/10.1016/j.envint.2021.106764] [PMID: 34273874]

[18] Tang Y, Zhong L, Wang W, *et al.* Recent advances in wearable potentiometric pH sensors. Membranes (Basel) 2022; 12(5): 504.
[http://dx.doi.org/10.3390/membranes12050504] [PMID: 35629830]

[19] Ghita M, Neckebroek M, Juchem J, Copot D, Muresan CI, Ionescu CM. Bioimpedance sensor and methodology for acute pain monitoring. Sensors (Basel) 2020; 20(23): 6765.
[http://dx.doi.org/10.3390/s20236765] [PMID: 33256120]

[20] Min J, Tu J, Xu C, *et al.* Skin-interfaced wearable sweat sensors for precision medicine. Chem Rev 2023; 123(8): 5049-138.
[http://dx.doi.org/10.1021/acs.chemrev.2c00823] [PMID: 36971504]

[21] Jiang H, Yan N, Ma K, Wang Y. A wideband circularly polarized dielectric patch antenna with a modified air cavity for Wi-Fi 6 and Wi-Fi 6E applications. IEEE Antennas Wirel Propag Lett 2023; 22(1): 213-7.
[http://dx.doi.org/10.1109/LAWP.2022.3201077]

[22] George A, Mohammadi A, Marcel S. Prepended domain transformer: Heterogeneous face recognition without bells and whistles. IEEE Trans Inf Forensics Security 2023; 18: 133-46.
[http://dx.doi.org/10.1109/TIFS.2022.3217738]

[23] Ye J, Gharavi H, Hu B. Fast beam discovery and adaptive transmission under frequency selective attenuations in sub-terahertz bands. IEEE Trans Signal Process 2023; 71: 727-40.
[http://dx.doi.org/10.1109/TSP.2023.3236166]

[24] Chen CY, Cheng MH, Cheng M, Yang CF. Using iBeacon components to design and fabricate a low-energy and simple indoor positioning method. Sens Mater 2023; 35(3): 703.
[http://dx.doi.org/10.18494/SAM4109]

[25] Want R. Near field communication. IEEE Pervasive Comput 2011; 10(3): 4-7.
[http://dx.doi.org/10.1109/MPRV.2011.55]

[26] Cheng H, Li Y. New luminescent Cd(II) coordination polymer and its protective activity on Alzheimer's disease. Sci Adv Mater 2022; 14(3): 505-11.
[http://dx.doi.org/10.1166/sam.2022.4229]

[27] Ahammad SH, Nagajyothi D, Priya PP, *et al.* Defected ground–structured symmetric circular ring antenna for near-field scanning plasmonic applications. Plasmonics 2023; 18(2): 541-9.
[http://dx.doi.org/10.1007/s11468-022-01784-8]

[28] Mehmood Y, Ahmad F, Yaqoob I, Adnane A, Imran M, Guizani S. Internet-of-things-based smart cities: Recent advances and challenges. IEEE Commun Mag 2017; 55(9): 16-24.
[http://dx.doi.org/10.1109/MCOM.2017.1600514]

[29] Agiwal M, Saxena N, Roy A. Towards connected living: 5G enabled Internet of Things (IoT). IETE Tech Rev 2019; 36(2): 190-202.
[http://dx.doi.org/10.1080/02564602.2018.1444516]

[30] Dananjayan S, Raj GM. 5G in healthcare: how fast will be the transformation? Ir J Med Sci 2021; 190(2): 497-501.
[http://dx.doi.org/10.1007/s11845-020-02329-w] [PMID: 32737688]

[31] Vergütz A, G Prates N Jr, Henrique Schwengber B, Santos A, Nogueira M. An architecture for the performance management of smart healthcare applications. Sensors (Basel) 2020; 20(19): 5566.
[http://dx.doi.org/10.3390/s20195566] [PMID: 32998439]

[32] Soldani D, Fadini F, Rasanen H, Duran J, Niemela T, Chandramouli D. 5G mobile systems for

healthcare IEEE 85th Vehicular Technology Conference. VTC Spring 2017; pp. 1-5.https://ieeexplore.ieee.org/document/8108602
[http://dx.doi.org/10.1109/VTCSpring.2017.8108602]

[33]   Le TV, Hsu CL. An anonymous key distribution scheme for group healthcare services in 5 G-enabled multi-server environments. IEEE Access 2021; 9: 53408-22.
[http://dx.doi.org/10.1109/ACCESS.2021.3070641]

[34]   Kumar Sharma D, Sreenivasa Chakravarthi D, Ara Shaikh A, Al Ayub Ahmed A, Jaiswal S, Naved M. The aspect of vast data management problem in healthcare sector and implementation of cloud computing technique. Mater Today Proc 2023; 80: 3805-10.
[http://dx.doi.org/10.1016/j.matpr.2021.07.388]

[35]   Stergiou CL, Plageras AP, Memos VA, Koidou MP, Psannis KE. Secure monitoring system for IoT healthcare data in the cloud. Appl Sci (Basel) 2023; 14(1): 120.
[http://dx.doi.org/10.3390/app14010120]

[36]   Bouslama A, Laaziz Y, Tali A, Eddabbah M. AWS and IoT for real-time remote medical monitoring. International Journal of Intelligent Enterprise 2019; 6(2/3/4): 369.
[http://dx.doi.org/10.1504/IJIE.2019.101137]

[37]   Zhao Y, Wang W, Li Y, Colman Meixner C, Tornatore M, Zhang J. Edge computing and networking: A survey on infrastructures and applications. IEEE Access 2019; 7: 101213-30.
[http://dx.doi.org/10.1109/ACCESS.2019.2927538]

[38]   Elhadad A, Alanazi F, Taloba AI, Abozeid A. Fog computing service in the healthcare monitoring system for managing the real-time notification. J Healthc Eng 2022; 2022: 1-11.
[http://dx.doi.org/10.1155/2022/5337733] [PMID: 35340260]

[39]   Pareek K, Tiwari PK, Bhatnagar V. Fog computing in healthcare: A review. IOP Conf Ser Mater Sci Eng 2021; 1099(1): 12025.

[40]   Gigli M, Koo S. Internet of Things: Services and applications categorization. Advances in Internet of Things 2011; 1(2): 27-31.
[http://dx.doi.org/10.4236/ait.2011.12004]

[41]   Zhang Y, Cui J, Ma K, Chen H, Zhang J. A wristband device for detecting human pulse and motion based on the Internet of Things. Measurement 2020; 163: 108036.
[http://dx.doi.org/10.1016/j.measurement.2020.108036]

[42]   Poongodi T, Krishnamurthi R, Indrakumari R, Suresh P, Balusamy B. Wearable devices and IoT. In: Balas VE, Solanki VK, Kumar R, Ahad Md AR, Eds. A handbook of internet of things in biomedical and cyber physical systems. Cham: Springer International Publishing 2020; pp. 245-73.
[http://dx.doi.org/10.1007/978-3-030-23983-1_10]

[43]   Göken M, Başoğlu AN, Dabic M. Exploring adoption of smart glasses: applications in the medical industry In: 2016 Portland International Conference on Management of Engineering and Technology. PICMET 2016; pp. 3175-84.

[44]   Smart Contact Lenses in Ophthalmology: Innovations, Applications, and Future Prospects. 2024. Available from: https://www.mdpi.com/2072-666X/15/7/856

[45]   Dunn J, Kidzinski L, Runge R, *et al.* Wearable sensors enable personalized predictions of clinical laboratory measurements. Nat Med 2021; 27(6): 1105-12.
[http://dx.doi.org/10.1038/s41591-021-01339-0] [PMID: 34031607]

[46]   Isakadze N, Martin SS. How useful is the smartwatch ECG? Trends Cardiovasc Med 2020; 30(7): 442-8.
[http://dx.doi.org/10.1016/j.tcm.2019.10.010] [PMID: 31706789]

[47]   Reeder B, David A. Health at hand: A systematic review of smart watch uses for health and wellness. J Biomed Inform 2016; 63: 269-76.
[http://dx.doi.org/10.1016/j.jbi.2016.09.001] [PMID: 27612974]

[48] Comarch Diagnostic Point 2024. Available from: https://www.comarch.com/ healthcare/products/ remote-medical-care/comarch-diagnostic-point/

[49] Comarch - Global IT Business Products Provider 2024. Available from: https://www.comarch.com/ healthcare/products/remote-medical-care/ remote-care-services/wristband/

[50] Comarch - Global IT Business Products Provider 2024. Available from: https://www.comarch.com/ healthcare/products/remote-medical-care/remote-cardiac-care/

[51] Mohammadzadeh N, Rezayi S, Saeedi S. Telemedicine for patient management in remote areas and underserved populations. Disaster Med Public Health Prep 2023; 17: e167.
[http://dx.doi.org/10.1017/dmp.2022.76] [PMID: 35586911]

[52] Shaik T, Tao X, Higgins N, *et al.* Remote patient monitoring using artificial intelligence: Current state, applications, and challenges. Wiley Interdiscip Rev Data Min Knowl Discov 2023; 13(2): e1485.
[http://dx.doi.org/10.1002/widm.1485]

[53] AirStrip® | Products | Cardiology 2024. Available from: https://www.airstrip.com/products/cardiology

[54] Patra R, Bhattacharya M, Mukherjee S. IoT-based computational frameworks in disease prediction and healthcare management: strategies, challenges, and potential. In: Marques G, Bhoi AK, Albuquerque VHCd, KS H, Eds. IoT in healthcare and ambient assisted living. Singapore: Springer 2021; pp. 17–41.
[http://dx.doi.org/10.1007/978-981-15-9897-5_2]

[55] Ma Y, Zhao C, Zhao Y, *et al.* Telemedicine application in patients with chronic disease: a systematic review and meta-analysis. BMC Med Inform Decis Mak 2022; 22(1): 105.
[http://dx.doi.org/10.1186/s12911-022-01845-2] [PMID: 35440082]

[56] Sharifi Kia A, Rafizadeh M, Shahmoradi L. Telemedicine in the emergency department: an overview of systematic reviews. J Public Health (Berl) 2023; 31(8): 1193-207.
[http://dx.doi.org/10.1007/s10389-021-01684-x]

[57] McGinley M, Carlson JJ, Reihm J, *et al.* Virtual versus usual in-office care for multiple sclerosis: The VIRTUAL-MS multi-site randomized clinical trial study protocol. Contemp Clin Trials 2024; 142: 107544.
[http://dx.doi.org/10.1016/j.cct.2024.107544] [PMID: 38657731]

[58] InPenTM Smart Insulin Pen | Medtronic. 2024. Available from: 2021 https://www.medtronicdiabetes.com/products/inpen-smart-insulin-pen-system

[59] Lilly will begin the rollout of Tempo® Personalized Diabetes Management Platform | Eli Lilly and Company 2024. Available from: https://investor.lilly.com/news-releases/news-release-details/li-ly-begin-rollout-tempor-personalized-diabetes-management

[60] Alarcón-Paredes A, Francisco-García V, Guzmán-Guzmán I, Cantillo-Negrete J, Cuevas-Valencia R, Alonso-Silverio G. An IoT-based non-invasive glucose level monitoring system using Raspberry Pi. Appl Sci (Basel) 2019; 9(15): 3046.
[http://dx.doi.org/10.3390/app9153046]

[61] So CF, Choi KS, Wong TK, Chung JW. Recent advances in noninvasive glucose monitoring. Med Devices (Auckl) 2012; 5: 45-52.
[PMID: 23166457]

[62] Yadav J, Rani A, Singh V, Murari BM. Prospects and limitations of non-invasive blood glucose monitoring using near-infrared spectroscopy. Biomed Signal Process Control 2015; 18: 214-27.
[http://dx.doi.org/10.1016/j.bspc.2015.01.005]

[63] Ferrante do Amaral CE, Wolf B. Current development in non-invasive glucose monitoring. Med Eng Phys 2008; 30(5): 541-9.
[http://dx.doi.org/10.1016/j.medengphy.2007.06.003] [PMID: 17942360]

[64] Yao H, Shum AJ, Cowan M, Lähdesmäki I, Parviz BA. A contact lens with embedded sensor for

monitoring tear glucose level. Biosens Bioelectron 2011; 26(7): 3290-6.
[http://dx.doi.org/10.1016/j.bios.2010.12.042] [PMID: 21257302]

[65]   Heller A, Feldman B. Electrochemical glucose sensors and their applications in diabetes management. Chem Rev 2008; 108(7): 2482-505.
[http://dx.doi.org/10.1021/cr068069y] [PMID: 18465900]

[66]   Tamar L, Avner G, Yulia M, Keren H, Karnit B. Non-Invasive Glucose Monitoring: A Review of Challenges and Recent Advances. Curr Trends Biomedical Eng & Biosci. 2017; 6(5): 555696.
[http://dx.doi.org/10.19080/CTBEB.2017.06.555696]

[67]   Talib AJ, Alkahtani M, Jiang L, *et al.* Lanthanide ions doped in vanadium oxide for sensitive optical glucose detection. Opt Mater Express 2018; 8(11): 3277-87.
[http://dx.doi.org/10.1364/OME.8.003277]

[68]   Medtronic.   SynchroMed™   II   Intrathecal   Pump   2024.   Available   from: https://www.medtronic.com/en-us/healthcar-
-professionals/products/neurological/drug-infusion-systems/synchromed-ii-intrathecal-pump.html

[69]   Teva Pharmaceuticals. Teva announces availability of ProAir® Digihaler® (albuterol sulfate 117 mcg) inhalation   powder   for   patients   with   asthma   and   COPD   2024.   Available   from: https://www.tevapharm.com/news-and-media/latest-news/teva-annou-
ces-availability-of-proair-digihaler-albuterol-sulfate-117-mcg-inhalation-powder-for-patie/

[70]   Neulasta 2024. Available from: https://www.neulasta.com

[71]   Abbott.   XIENCE   Skypoint   Better   Expansion,   Deliverability   2024.   Available   from: https://www.cardiovascular.abbott/us/en/hcp/products/percutaneous-coronar-
-intervention/xience-family/xience-skypoint.html

[72]   Abbott. Parkinson's and Deep Brain Stimulation 2024. Available from: https://www.abbott.com/life-changing-tech/parkinsons-deep-brain-stimulation-dbs-infinity.html

[73]   U.S. Food and Drug Administration. FDA approves pill with sensor that digitally tracks if patients have ingested their medication. PR Newswire 2017. Available from: https://www.fda.gov/news-events/press-announcements/fda-approves-pill-sensor-digitally-tracks-if-patients-have-ing-
sted-their-medication

[74]   Kumar D, Malhotra R, Sharma SR. Design and construction of a smart wheelchair. Procedia Comput Sci 2020; 172: 302-7.
[http://dx.doi.org/10.1016/j.procs.2020.05.048]

[75]   Murphy RR, Gandudi VB, Adams J. Applications of robots for COVID-19 response. http://arxiv.org/abs/2008.06976 arXiv preprint arXiv:2008.06976 2020.

[76]   Ould S, Guertler M, Hanna P, Bennett NS. Internet-of-Things-enabled smart bed rail for application in hospital beds. Sensors (Basel) 2022; 22(15): 5526.
[http://dx.doi.org/10.3390/s22155526] [PMID: 35898030]

[77]   Gerup J, Soerensen CB, Dieckmann P. Augmented reality and mixed reality for healthcare education beyond surgery: an integrative review. Int J Med Educ 2020; 11: 1-18.
[http://dx.doi.org/10.5116/ijme.5e01.eb1a] [PMID: 31935130]

[78]   Ni Ki C, Hosseinian-Far A, Daneshkhah A, Salari N. Topic modelling in precision medicine with its applications in personalized diabetes management. Expert Syst 2022; 39(4): e12774.
[http://dx.doi.org/10.1111/exsy.12774]

[79]   Zholdas N, Mansurova M, Postolache O, Kalimoldayev M, Sarsembayeva T. A personalized mHealth monitoring system for children and adolescents with T1 diabetes by utilizing IoT sensors and assessing physical activities. Int J Comput Commun Control 2022; 17(3).
[http://dx.doi.org/10.15837/ijccc.2022.3.4558]

[80]   Lee G, Saad W, Bennis M. An online optimization framework for distributed fog network formation

with minimal latency. IEEE Trans Wirel Commun 2019; 18(4): 2244-58.
[http://dx.doi.org/10.1109/TWC.2019.2901850]

[81]   Kumar M, Kumar A, Verma S, *et al.* Healthcare Internet of Things (H-IoT): current trends, prospects, applications, challenges, and security issues. Electronics (Basel) 2023; 12(9): 2050.
[http://dx.doi.org/10.3390/electronics12092050]

[82]   Kelly JT, Campbell KL, Gong E, Scuffham P. The Internet of Things: impact and implications for health care delivery. J Med Internet Res 2020; 22(11): e20135.
[http://dx.doi.org/10.2196/20135] [PMID: 33170132]

[83]   Kumar M. Kavita, Verma S, Kumar A, Ijaz MF, Rawat DB. ANAF-IoMT: a novel architectural framework for IoMT-enabled smart healthcare systems by enhancing security based on RECC-VC. IEEE Trans Industr Inform 2022; 18(12): 8936-43.
[http://dx.doi.org/10.1109/TII.2022.3181614]

[84]   Rubí JNS, Gondim PRL. Interoperable internet of medical things platform for e-Health applications. Int J Distrib Sens Netw 2020; 16(1)
[http://dx.doi.org/10.1177/1550147719889591]

[85]   Ranjan R, Ch B. A comprehensive roadmap for transforming healthcare from hospital-centric to patient-centric through healthcare internet of things (IoT). Engineered Science. 2024 Jun 17;30:1175.

[86]   Mascarenhas M, Martins M, Ribeiro T, *et al.* Software as a medical device (SaMD) in digestive healthcare: regulatory challenges and ethical implications. Diagnostics (Basel) 2024; 14(18): 2100.
[http://dx.doi.org/10.3390/diagnostics14182100] [PMID: 39335779]

[87]   Lee H, Park YR, Kim HR, *et al.* Discrepancies in demand for Internet of Things services among older people and people with disabilities, their caregivers, and health care providers: face-to-face survey study. J Med Internet Res 2020; 22(4): e16614.
[http://dx.doi.org/10.2196/16614] [PMID: 32293575]

[88]   Nasser AR, Hasan AM, Humaidi AJ, *et al.* IoT and cloud computing in health care: a new wearable device and cloud-based deep learning algorithm for monitoring of diabetes. Electronics (Basel) 2021; 10(21): 2719.
[http://dx.doi.org/10.3390/electronics10212719]

[89]   van de Hei SJ, Stoker N, Flokstra-de Blok BMJ, *et al.* Anticipated barriers and facilitators for implementing smart inhalers in asthma medication adherence management. NPJ Prim Care Respir Med 2023; 33(1): 22.
[http://dx.doi.org/10.1038/s41533-023-00343-w] [PMID: 37208358]

CHAPTER 8

Blockchain Solutions for Secure and Efficient Health Data Management

Ashish Verma[1], Akhil Sharma[2], Shivkanya Fuloria[3], Shaikh Yahya[4], Anurag Singh[5] and Shaweta Sharma[6,*]

[1] *Department of Pharmacy, Mangalmay Pharmacy College, Greater Noida, Uttar Pradesh-201306, India*

[2] *R. J. College of Pharmacy, Raipur, Uttar Pradesh-202165, India*

[3] *Department of Pharmaceutical Chemistry, Faculty of Pharmacy, AIMST University, Jalan Bedong—Semeling 08100 Bedong, Kedah, Malaysia*

[4] *Department of Pharmaceutical Chemistry, School of Pharmaceutical Education and Research, Jamia Hamdard, New Delhi-110062, India*

[5] *School of Computing Science and Engineering, Galgotias University, Greater Noida, Uttar Pradesh-201310, Uttar Pradesh-201310, India*

[6] *Department of Pharmacy, School of Medical and Allied Sciences, Galgotias University, Greater Noida, Uttar Pradesh-201310, India*

Abstract: Challenges in health data management include difficulties with data security, privacy, and interoperability. When healthcare organizations store patient information in electronic formats, the need for systems to address these issues becomes even more vital. Innovative methods such as blockchain technology and big data analytics are emerging as promising solutions for these challenges. Blockchain is used to create a secure and decentralized structure that helps ensure the immutability, transparency, and privacy of health records. In contrast, big data is used to analyze large amounts of data to improve patient care, predict disease outbreaks, and even optimize healthcare operations. This chapter explains the integration of blockchain and big data in healthcare, providing insights into how blockchain security measures and big data inputs will assist in filling the existing gaps. Blockchain improves big data analytics by providing data integrity and traceability, allowing secure exchange between medical systems. Examples of this integrated approach can be seen in applications in EHRs, clinical trials, public health monitoring, and supply chain management. However, challenges such as scalability, privacy concerns, and regulatory limitations persist. This chapter concludes by evaluating the benefits of this integration over traditional systems, highlighting its potential to improve healthcare outcomes and enhance trust in health data management.

---

[*] **Corresponding author Shaweta Sharma**: Department of Pharmacy, School of Medical and Allied Sciences, Galgotias University, Greater Noida, Uttar Pradesh-201310, India; E-mail: shawetasharma@galgotiasuniversity.edu.in

Shaweta Sharma, Akhil Sharma, Shivkanya Fuloria & Anurag Singh (Eds.)
All rights reserved-© 2025 Bentham Science Publishers

Keywords: Big data analytics, Blockchain, Data privacy, Health data management, Healthcare operations, Healthcare security, Interoperability.

INTRODUCTION

The healthcare sector is dealing with major issues in managing data because of the huge volume and complexity of healthcare data, such as electronic health records (EHRs), medical imaging, lab results, and patient monitoring data. This data is typically siloed across multiple systems and platforms, leading to further difficulty for healthcare providers in sharing or accessing it in a timely manner. Moreover, healthcare institutions also face unique regulatory requirements regarding patient confidentiality and data security. They are pervasive issues, and data inconsistency caused by diverse formats and incomplete records can challenge data analysis and the ability of systems to interact effectively. In addition, more diverse data, such as clinical, administrative, and real-time patient data, need to be integrated into one system to make more informed decisions. Healthcare providers constantly deal with delayed information exchange, manual data entry errors, and security risks caused by growing cyber threats. As the healthcare landscape transitions to a more patient-centric, value-based care model, the need for effective healthcare data management has never been more crucial. These challenges are critical and call for novel solutions to make data more accessible, secure, and reliable, all while ensuring privacy and regulatory compliance [1, 2].

Health care is sensitive, and therefore, data security and privacy are paramount. Patient confidentiality and the integrity of medical records are at risk due to cyberattacks, data breaches, and unauthorized access. Protecting data privacy also involves the use of effective security protocols like cryptography, access restriction, and authentication measures to prevent data theft or misappropriation. In addition, healthcare data should be able to interoperate across multiple platforms and systems so that different healthcare providers, organizations, and other stakeholders can share information easily and securely. In the absence of interoperability, disparate data systems block the delivery of high-quality care and produce poor patient outcomes. The absence of standardized healthcare data formats adds an extra layer of complexity to interoperability initiatives. Technologies that standardize data-sharing protocol and technology to enable increased communication across various platforms will also be critical for data exchange and, ultimately, comprehensive patient care. Utilizing blockchain and big data analytics, problems such as poor data quality, high susceptibility to breaches, and time-consuming assessment/reporting procedures can be resolved. These technologies can work together to enable healthcare systems to be more transparent, trustworthy, and interconnected [3, 4].

Blockchain and Big Data Analytics have a significant impact on the healthcare field, as these technologies are transforming healthcare data management. Blockchain is a form of distributed ledger technology that allows secure, transparent, and tamper-resistant record-keeping in a decentralized manner. In healthcare, blockchain can be utilized for the storage of medical records, protecting them from data breaches and making sure there are no unauthorized changes to the data in any way. This enables a safe framework for exchanging patient data between various organizations, including healthcare providers, while controlling access and privacy. In addition to the characteristics above, Blockchain includes smart contracts that are capable of automating administrative procedures, minimizing human error, and boosting operational efficiency.

Big Data Analytics is transforming the healthcare industry by allowing for large-scale, structured, and unstructured data processing and analysis. With the help of advanced algorithms and machine learning techniques, it extracts actionable insights from patient data, including predictive analytics for early disease detection, personalized treatment plans, and operational enhancements. Healthcare providers can utilize Big Data Analytics to make data-driven decisions, optimize resource utilization, and enhance patient outcomes. When integrated with blockchain, Big Data Analytics can provide a more secure and efficient environment for data sharing, analysis, and decision-making. These two technologies, when combined, have the potential to significantly enhance the effectiveness, efficacy, security, and efficiency of healthcare systems, while also reducing costs and improving patient care quality [5, 6].

BLOCKCHAIN TECHNOLOGY IN HEALTHCARE

Blockchain is a revolutionary technology that facilitates secure, transparent, and decentralized transactions without requiring any central authority. Blockchain technology is a game-changer that allows safe, transparent, and decentralized transactions without needing a central authority. At its core, it is a distributed ledger system that records data over multiple computers in a manner that makes it virtually impossible to change or tamper with the data once it has been added to the system. The structure of blockchain provides data integrity and transparency, which makes it a perfect solution for industries like healthcare, where the exchange of accurate and secure data is imperative [7, 8]. Fig. (**1**) describes the use of blockchain technology in the healthcare industry.

Key Components of Blockchain

The foundational elements of blockchain include the decentralized ledger, consensus mechanisms, and cryptography. Blockchain technology is built on top of the decentralized ledger. Blockchain is data shared between a network of nodes (computers), each node contains a copy of the ledger, providing redundancy and security, unlike traditional databases, which store data under the management of a centralized server. By eliminating intermediaries, rent-seeking mediators are removed, thereby reducing the costs and risks associated with a single point of failure.

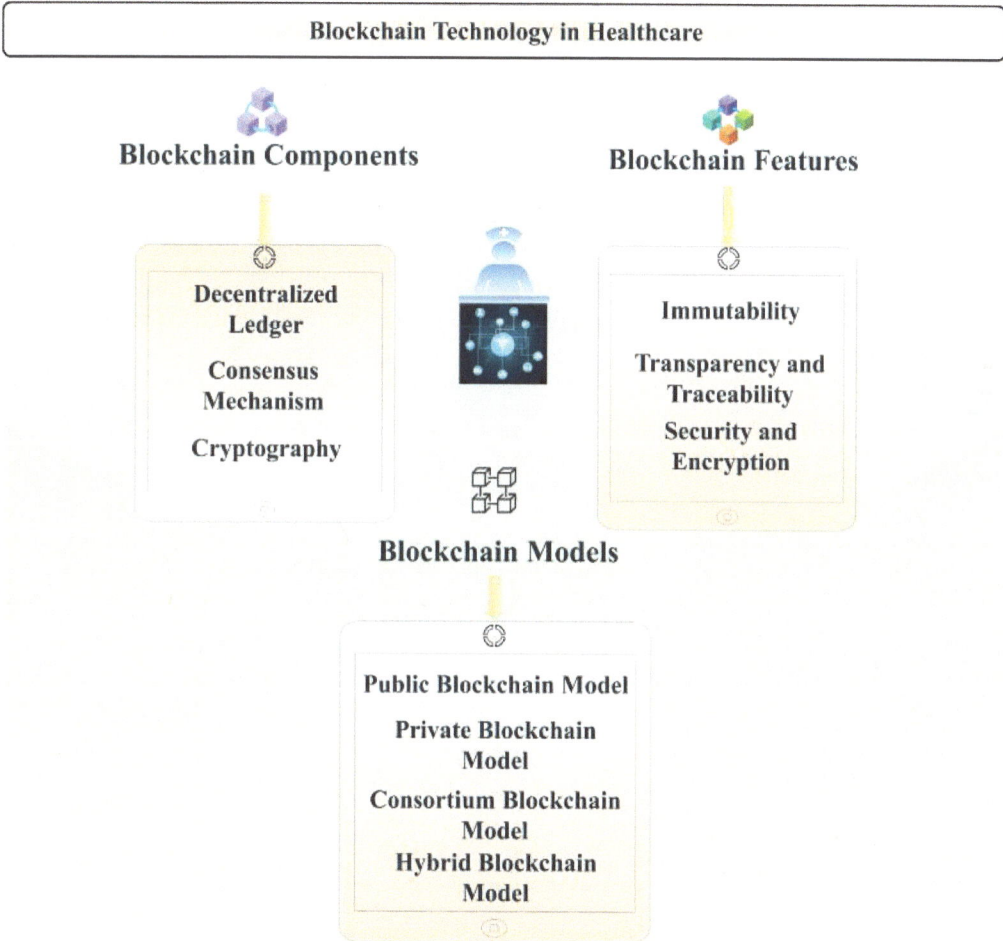

Fig. (1). Blockchain technology in the healthcare industry.

The consensus mechanism is the most popular and widely adopted protocol in the world of blockchain. Two widely utilized consensus algorithms are Proof of Work (PoW) and Proof of Stake (PoS), which enable network participants (miners or validators) to solve complex mathematical puzzles or prove their stake in the network to validate transactions. This system ensures that fraudulent transactions are never processed. Instead, only true and valid data is added to the blockchain [9].

Additionally, Cryptography is a crucial element in maintaining the security and privacy of data in blockchain systems. Blockchain uses public and private keys to encrypt each transaction so only authorized individuals can access or change data. Hash functions are used to enhance security, enabling a unique digital fingerprint for each data block, which makes tampering with stored information virtually undetectable. Collectively, these features create a strong and secure framework for managing data across numerous applications, including health care, where privacy, security, and accuracy are crucial [10].

Blockchain Features in Healthcare Data Management

Blockchain technology offers a robust framework for healthcare systems by ensuring data immutability, enhancing transparency and traceability, and providing top-notch security and encryption. These features collectively streamline data management, foster trust, and safeguard sensitive health information.

Immutability

Immutability in blockchain ensures that once data is added to the system, it cannot be altered or deleted. This feature is critical to healthcare as it ensures the authenticity and integrity of medical records, prescriptions, and patient history. For example, blockchain ensures the immutability of clinical trial data, which eliminates the threat of data alteration, while meeting regulatory requirements. This permanence fosters trust among stakeholders, as healthcare providers, researchers, and patients can access accurate and unaltered data. Moreover, immutability in a blockchain helps manage patient consent efficiently, *i.e.*, once a patient grants consent and the block is created, it cannot be undone or changed. Blockchain facilitates the auditing of medical records, litigation processes, and the verification of clinical research by offering an immutable register, establishing it as a foundation for trustworthy healthcare data management [11, 12].

Transparency and Traceability

Blockchain's important features of transparency and traceability greatly propel healthcare benefits. Blockchain allows for a single source of truth, accessible to all stakeholders, including patients, providers, and payers, through a distributed ledger system. For example, in pharmaceutical supply chains, the blockchain enables real-time tracking of drugs, from their manufacturing to their distribution, thus mitigating counterfeiting and quality assurance. In the context of health-related work, traceability enables the transfer of information more easily between different healthcare providers, thereby ensuring a consistent patient experience and reducing errors. Additionally, transparency means that all transactions are recorded and visible to authorized participants, promoting accountability and trust. Blockchain also empowers patients by providing them with access to their health records and the ability to track how their data is used. This visibility is consistent with modern healthcare's approach to patient-centered care, while simultaneously ensuring the trustworthiness of data handling processes [13, 14].

Security and Encryption

Blockchain employs advanced security measures, such as cryptographic techniques and decentralized architecture, to protect sensitive healthcare data. In contrast to traditional systems that rely on centralized servers, data is distributed across a network of nodes on the blockchain, thereby significantly reducing the risk of cyberattacks. Private key cryptography provides for the confidentiality of patient data in that it must be accessed or modified by someone with a similar private key. This feature is of critical importance regarding breaches, which pose a significant risk in connected medical devices. Blockchain can create secure identity management that allows patients to manage access to their health data. Blockchain's decentralization, encryption, and access control come together to form a protective framework that meets the challenges of securing healthcare data in the digital era [15, 16].

Blockchain Models for Healthcare

Blockchain models in healthcare facilitate secure, transparent, and efficient data management, enhancing privacy, data integrity, and interoperability while supporting various decentralized applications across the healthcare ecosystem [17].

Public Blockchain Model

In a public blockchain model, anyone can participate in the network without any restrictions. This approach guarantees that the healthcare data that is being stored on it is transparent, accountable, and immutable, which makes it a boon for healthcare applications. Public blockchains, such as Ethereum and Bitcoin, are open and trustless, meaning users do not need to rely on a central authority to verify transactions or access data. In the healthcare context, public blockchains have a scalability problem, often due to the time and computational power needed to process transactions. Public blockchains provide transparency and make it easier to keep track of healthcare data so that providers and organizations are responsible for their activities. While public blockchains have their advantages, the model does come with challenges, especially concerning privacy, which could hide sensitive health information from being displayed unless it is encrypted properly. To combat this, privacy-preserving methods such as zero-knowledge proofs and encryption are used [18, 19].

Private Blockchain Model

A private blockchain model is a permissioned network restricting unauthorized participants from joining and validating transactions. Private blockchains, on the other hand, have predetermined participants with an access control mechanism that restricts participants to trusted entities such as healthcare providers, pharmaceutical companies, or insurance firms. Private blockchains in healthcare allow sensitive data to be managed securely and efficiently, with a focus on maintaining patient privacy and confidentiality. As only authorized entities are able to access the blockchain, the system can achieve much higher scalability and faster processing of transactions, which is crucial for healthcare ecosystems where a real-time exchange of data is needed. Since fewer participants are involved in the consensus, these blockchains also have the advantage of requiring less energy compared to public blockchains. On the other hand, one of the disadvantages is the risk of decentralization, as a limited number of trusted entities govern the network. While this makes transactions more reliable and faster, it could compromise the decentralized ideology of blockchain technology. Even more, restricted access may limit the benefit of pervasive transparency and security offered by blockchains across a wide ecosystem. However, in this scenario, private blockchains are a perfect solution both regarding private healthcare data management and within the context of improving the workflow inside healthcare organizations [20, 21].

Consortium Blockchain Model

In collaboration with a group of trusted entities or organizations from the same industry and sector, a consortium blockchain is conducted and usually operated. This model brings a compromise between decentralization of a public blockchain and centralization of private blockchains. A typical example in the real world is how multiple hospitals, healthcare providers, research institutions, and insurers use consortium blockchain to share and manage patient data securely. The network's permissions are limited, but it is controlled by multiple parties, all of which have equal rights to validate transactions. Maintaining privacy and security, this structure reduces the risk of a single point of failure. These are some real benefits of consortium blockchains because they create an environment for larger organizations to efficiently share information amongst themselves while maintaining a system of trust and transparency. Because a consortium can create shared policies that all members adhere to, regulatory compliance becomes much easier, as they can be structured to follow healthcare regulations like HIPAA. Healthcare research and clinical trials benefit immensely from data-sharing, and the consortium model currently facilitates this information sharing, bringing incredibly powerful insights to the fore. Nevertheless, as in private blockchains, the consortium is still not fully decentralized, since the control is still in the hands of a restricted group of participants. Moreover, it could result in governance challenges since various parties with different objectives and interests can lead to disputes. In conclusion, despite these challenges, consortium blockchains provide a powerful layered solution for organizations seeking to improve data sharing and collaboration in healthcare without compromising privacy and security [22, 23].

Hybrid Blockchain Model

A hybrid blockchain model merges aspects of both public and private blockchains to provide a solution with advantages from both worlds. In the context of healthcare, hybrid blockchains are more commonly used, allowing sensitive patient data to be stored on a private blockchain while publicly sharing data types such as research findings, healthcare information, and non-sensitive patient information. This model is customizable, allowing organizations to determine which data should be made public and which data should remain private based on the needs of the healthcare ecosystem. Hybrid blockchains provide more flexibility by merging the benefits of the scalability, speed, and privacy of private blockchains with the transparency and trust that public blockchains provide. This is especially beneficial in healthcare applications where some data, like electronic health records (EHRs), is required to be confidential. Still, other types are open for research or policy-making purposes. The hybrid model also helps alleviate concerns about centralization, providing a controlled environment where participants can confirm transactions while preserving sensitive data from unauthorized access [24, 25].

Applications of Blockchain in Health Data

Blockchain enhances patient data control, facilitates real-time data sharing, and streamlines healthcare processes.

Interoperability Across Healthcare Systems

A critical issue in contemporary healthcare is interoperability, in which disparate systems can lead to poor data sharing between providers. Blockchain can provide a distributed solution that bridges this gap. Blockchain ensures that patient data is always accurate, timely, and readily available across diverse platforms, even when different healthcare institutions or organizations are involved, *via* its distributed ledger technology. Every participant on the network shares the same ledger, which is automatically updated when any changes are made, so everyone is working with the same information [26].

Blockchain adds standardized protocols for data formatting and transfer, leading to standardization in data sharing. This removes intermediaries, minimizing delays and administrative overhead. It also addresses data silos, where information becomes trapped in a single system and is unavailable across the network, and ensures the portability of data. This is especially relevant in cross-border healthcare settings, where care provided may involve multiple institutions using disparate systems.

Moreover, the cryptographic and security protocols of blockchains can protect patient data privacy, even when it is shared across various organizations. Blockchain adds more trust value by addressing the validity of access to data, thereby making clinical decision-making more effective. This sustainable technology opens up opportunities for every healthcare organization to have more flexible, efficient, and secure data sharing across different systems; thus, creating better care and improving the quality of patient outcomes [27].

Secure Sharing of Health Records

The secure sharing of health records has always been a critical challenge in healthcare, where privacy concerns and data breaches are prevalent. Traditional systems of sharing patient information often use centralized databases, which can be subject to hacking and unauthorized access. The decentralized and tamper-proof nature of blockchain technology presents an optimal solution to these problems. A distributed ledger means that health records are not under the control of any single entity, making it much harder to breach [28].

All transactions and updates to the health record on the blockchain are encrypted, time-stamped, and added to the ledger in a manner that is transparent but secure. This ensures that even if someone accesses patient data, it can be traced back and forms an immutable audit trail. The transparency offered by Blockchain facilitates the Identification and prevention of unauthorized access or tampering with health information. Furthermore, blockchain gives patients more control over their healthcare data. They keep records safe and control who has access to their valuable information and who can give permission by using private keys. This empowered user approach to data provides exceptional privacy and security.

Moreover, the decentralized nature of blockchain reduces the potential for data loss. This means patient data is safe and active even in the event of a failure in any component of the system. The blockchain serves as a decentralized backup that is highly resistant to failures, thus providing ease of access while maintaining the confidentiality of these records [29].

Smart Contracts for Healthcare Agreements

Smart contracts are self-executing contracts whose terms of agreement or conditions are written into code. In the realm of healthcare, they can be applied to automate administrative and legal processes within the compliance space, thus eliminating the need for intermediaries, while ensuring the timely and accurate execution of agreements. These benefits make blockchain-based smart contracts an excellent fit for healthcare contracts because they are built on transparency, efficiency, and security [30].

One of the primary applications of smart contracts in healthcare is in managing insurance claims. Smart contracts help automate the validation, processing, and payment of claims as per the conditions laid out in the insurance policy, where all parameters have to be fulfilled. The smart contract can use that information to automatically check that when a patient visits a healthcare provider and a claim is submitted, it complies with the predefined criteria. The contract executes the payment automatically when the conditions are met without human intervention. This reduces administrative burden, reduces errors, and expedites claim processing, leading to enhanced efficiency for both healthcare providers and patients. In the field of patient consent, smart contracts can also ensure that patients' healthcare data is only shared with authorized parties. For example, a patient can sign a smart contract that permits certain healthcare providers to access data for a limited time or purpose, ensuring that privacy preferences are respected [31].

BIG DATA ANALYTICS IN HEALTHCARE

Big Data Analytics is a term that refers to studying and deriving valuable insights from extensive, diverse, and rapidly growing datasets. In healthcare, data usually comes from EHRs, wearable devices, clinical trials, and patient monitoring systems. The aim is to identify trends, enhance patient outcomes, streamline processes, and anticipate potential health risks. Big Data Analytics uses advanced technologies like machine learning and artificial intelligence (AI) to work with and analyze these large amounts of data [32].

The key characteristics of Big Data, often referred to as the "four Vs," define the challenges and opportunities associated with it and are outlined in Table **1**. Fig. (**2**) illustrates the role of big data analytics in the healthcare industry.

Big Data Analytics in Healthcare

Volume

Veracity 4 Vs Variety

Velocity

Characteristics of Big Data Analytics

Machine Learning and
Artificial Intelligence (AI)

Data Mining and
Predictive Modelling

Genomic Data
Analysis

Techniques

Descriptive
Analytics

Natural Language
Processing (NLP) in
Health Data

Prescriptive
Analytics

**Techniques in Big Data Analytics for
Health Data Management**

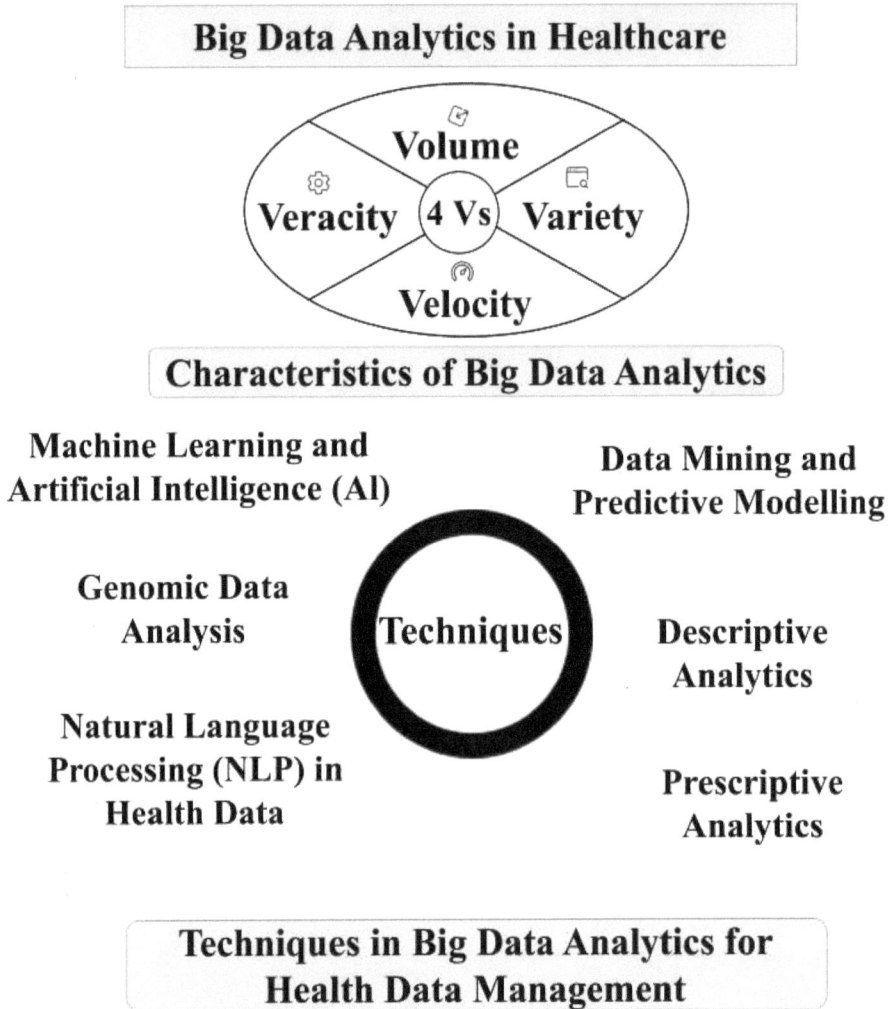

Fig. (2). Big data analytics in the healthcare industry.

Table 1. The key characteristics of big data.

S. No.	Characteristics of Big Data Analytics (Four Vs)	Description
1	Volume	A huge amount of data is produced, such as patient records, medical images, test results, and monitoring data. Needs scalable algorithms to analyze large sets of data [33].
2	Variety	Different types of healthcare data, such as structured (numeric test results) and unstructured data (medical images, doctors' notes), require systems that can process all data types [34].

(Table 1) cont.....

S. No.	Characteristics of Big Data Analytics (Four Vs)	Description
3	Velocity	The scale of the data being generated, for example, real-time data from wearables and patient monitoring systems, requires the ability to process near-real-time data or make decisions quickly.
4	Veracity	The accuracy and reliability of healthcare data can be somewhat incomplete or inconsistent. Big Data Analytics ensures the quality of data for accurate reports [35].

Role of Big Data in Healthcare Data Management

Big Data plays a crucial role in healthcare data management by enabling the processing and analysis of vast amounts of patient data to improve care delivery, enhance decision-making, and optimize healthcare operations.

Predictive Analytics for Patient Care

Healthcare predictive analytics is used to analyze Big Data that can provide information to enhance treatment plans, prevent hospital readmissions, and predict patient outcomes. Machine learning models are built by examining historical data sets, helping in the prediction of patient health trends, spotting patients at risk, and allowing proactive care by making data-driven predictions. Predictive models can analyze a patient's health history, lifestyle, genetic information, and real-time health data to forecast the risk of developing conditions like diabetes, heart disease, or sepsis. This can help healthcare providers tailor treatment approaches, provide timely interventions, and prevent avoidable hospital admissions. For instance, algorithms can identify patients at risk for deterioration and suggest early interventions like medication adjustments or additional monitoring, improving patient outcomes and reducing costs. Real-time data from wearables, EMRs, and patient-reported outcomes further improves prediction accuracy. The use of predictive analytics further extends into resource allocation, enabling healthcare organizations to identify and concentrate on high-risk patients and effectively allocate the appropriate staffing resources, thereby improving both care quality and operational efficiency [36, 37].

Disease Surveillance and Outbreak Prediction

The use of Big Data analytics has become an integral component of disease surveillance and outbreak prediction, helping healthcare systems detect infectious diseases, track their spread, and respond to outbreaks more effectively. Predictive health surveillance systems utilize machine learning techniques to analyze large datasets collected from diverse sources, including hospitals, community clinics, public health reports, social media, and environmental data, to identify patterns and warning signs of impending outbreaks. For example, real-time monitoring of influenza-like illness symptoms can provide early signals of an impending flu outbreak, enabling public health agencies to mobilize resources, implement preventive measures, and inform the public promptly. Big Data also enables more precise predictions on the spread of disease, allowing researchers to identify the geographic areas most susceptible to outbreaks, as well as their potential scope. Machine learning algorithms analyze historical outbreaks, predictive weather patterns, and demographic data to predict future occurrences, allowing a more targeted response that uses fewer resources. In addition, incorporating genomic data in surveillance systems can also enhance our ability to detect new pathogens, monitor the emergence of mutations, and assist clinicians in developing optimal therapies and vaccines. Prompt detection and control of outbreaks are essential for minimizing the human health consequences [38, 39].

Healthcare Operational Efficiency

Big Data is revolutionizing healthcare operational efficiency by optimizing resource allocation, reducing waste, and improving patient flow. Healthcare providers can eliminate these inefficiencies through the analysis of large datasets, which will inform data-driven solutions to enhance productivity. Predictive analytics, for instance, can accurately predict patient admission rates and allow hospitals to proactively manage bed capacity, staffing levels, and resource allocation. By identifying patterns in patient care delivery, including patient wait times, delays in treatments, or bottlenecks in diagnostic paths, health systems can become more efficient in delivering care, enhancing the patient experience, and lowering operational costs at the same time. Furthermore, Big Data enables supply chains to optimize themselves, predicting when a specific supply or medication will be required, and delivering it as necessary, thus coming at a minimum cost in terms of storage. Healthcare organizations can thereby use the data to predict when they will experience peak demand, and schedule human resources as needed, to ensure that the right number of healthcare professionals are available to tend to patients. It can also facilitate the establishment of quality management frameworks through Big Data by tracking KPIs, enabling healthcare providers to measure performance, identify areas for improvement, and refine service delivery over time. These data-driven strategies contribute to a more efficient, cost-effective healthcare system [40, 41].

Techniques Associated with Big Data Analytics for Health Data Management

Techniques of big data analytics in health data management involve machine learning, AI, data mining, predictive and prescriptive modeling, descriptive analytics, NLP, and genomic data analysis to enhance decision-making and improve patient outcomes.

Machine Learning and Artificial Intelligence (AI)

Machine learning (ML) and artificial intelligence (AI) are revolutionary tools of healthcare big data analytics. ML algorithms, such as supervised and unsupervised learning, identify features in intricate medical data, allowing them to predict patient results, treatment effectiveness, and disease advancement. AI systems, which typically use ML, can automate decision-making, offering personalized treatment recommendations by leveraging historical data. AI's deep learning models mathematically learn from large amounts of unstructured data, such as medical images and clinical notes, and achieve high levels of accuracy in diagnosing conditions such as cancer, heart disease, and neurological disorders. AI applications in healthcare help with predictive analytics that minimize risks to patients and also improve patient care, as well as the operational efficiency of the healthcare organization. AI tools are also enhancing drug discovery and designs for clinical trials by predicting the compounds that have the best chance of success. Overall, machine learning and AI contribute significantly to precision medicine and the transformation of healthcare delivery [42, 43].

Data Mining and Predictive Modeling

Data mining is the process of deriving meaningful insight, patterns, trends, and relations from large health datasets. In health care, it is used for detecting disease outbreaks, forecasting patient admissions, and revealing hidden risk factors. Predictive modeling, often used in line with data mining, involves analyzing historical data to predict future events. Techniques such as regression analysis, decision trees, and neural network models are used to analyze complex healthcare data to predict health risks, disease progression, and treatment responses. For instance, predictive models might assess a patient's risk for chronic conditions such as diabetes or heart disease based on their genetic, demographic, and lifestyle information. These models consider not only clinical data but also genomic and environmental factors, which lead to actionable insights that help healthcare providers make data-driven decisions. This aids in customizing treatments, effectively controlling hospital resources, and ultimately enhancing patient outcomes by identifying health hazards in the early stages [44, 45].

Descriptive Analytics

Descriptive analytics in healthcare refers to statistical methods to summarize and interpret past health-related data. It examines past health records, clinical outcomes, and demographics to reveal patterns, behaviors, and trends. Reanalysis like this is key to identifying problems such as above-average patient readmission rates or health disparities in particular population segments. Doctors and hospitals can leverage descriptive analytics to evaluate the success of treatments, monitor disease progression, and quantify outcomes over time. Descriptive analytics enable administrators and clinicians to make informed decisions based on past performance through dashboards, reports, and visualizations. For instance, hospitals may observe trends in either patient satisfaction or infection rates, allowing for better practices and improved quality of care. While descriptive analytics provides a foundation for decision-making, it does not predict future outcomes, but it plays a pivotal role in understanding what has happened and why [46, 47].

Prescriptive Analytics

Prescriptive analytics in health care uses advanced algorithms and optimization techniques to suggest actions that can deliver the best outcomes. It is more than predictive analytics; it helps derive actionable insights that inform healthcare decision-making. Prescriptive models might analyze a patient's personal medical history, genetic information, and lifestyle, and then recommend the best treatment approach for that person. These models typically use some combination of machine learning, simulation, and optimization tools to generate hypothetical scenarios to guide clinical evidence-based decisions. Furthermore, prescriptive analytics can improve the efficiency of hospital operations, including optimizing resource allocation and scheduling of staff and equipment. It can even help manage inventory better by predicting demand for medical supplies. Prescriptive analytics suggests possible options for how to handle a potential future scenario, allowing decision makers in healthcare to drive down costs, boost patient outcomes, and streamline operational efficiencies. Prescriptive analytics in clinical decision support systems is revolutionizing the operations of healthcare systems and aligning them more closely with patient needs and outcomes [48, 49].

Natural Language Processing (NLP) in Health Data

Natural Language Processing (NLP) is important in health data analytics as it allows the extraction and understanding of unstructured data (*e.g.*, Clinical notes, clinical records, and research articles). NLP enables computers to interpret human language in the medical domain. These techniques include entity recognition, sentiment analysis, and part-of-speech tagging. NLP assists in identifying key entities, such as symptoms, diagnoses, treatments, and outcomes, by processing large volumes of text data that can be analyzed with structured data. NLP could also help to enhance patient care by streamlining the documentation process, relieving some of the burden on healthcare providers, and reducing clinical note inaccuracies. In research, NLP is used to analyze medical literature, helping scientists track the latest developments in drug discovery and clinical trials. Moreover, NLP-based chatbots and virtual assistants can improve patient access and help streamline healthcare services in real-time [50, 51].

Genomic Data Analysis

The analysis of genomic data is one of the key tools of personalized medicine and allows the study of genetic variants and their effects on health. High-throughput sequencing technology can generate a large amount of genomic and transcriptomic information from patients to better understand diseases and gain insights into the genetic determinants of diseases, drug response, and treatment outcomes. These complex datasets require data analytics techniques, including bioinformatics algorithms, to process, analyze, and interpret the information. Researchers and clinicians can precisely define the predispositions to diseases, such as cancer, diabetes, and neurological disorders, by identifying the genetic mutations present in patients. Furthermore, genomic data analytics plays a critical role in the design of precision medicine, where treatments are personalized based on an individual's genetic constitution. This methodology ensures treatments are as effective as possible with the fewest negative side effects. Leveraging genomic data alongside EHRs adds even more potential value, allowing for precision medicine where clinicians develop interventions tailored to an individual based on their genetic profile, lifestyle choices, and environmental influences [52, 53].

INTEGRATING BLOCKCHAIN AND BIG DATA ANALYTICS FOR DATA MANAGEMENT

Integrating blockchain and big data analytics in healthcare ensures secure, transparent, and scalable data management, enhancing efficiency, data integrity, and improving decision-making processes through advanced analytics and real-time access [54].

How Blockchain Enhances Big Data Analytics in Healthcare?

Blockchain improves big data analytics by ensuring secure data transactions, enhancing data accuracy, and providing immutable records, which support reliable insights and decision-making in healthcare applications [55].

Data Security, Integrity, and Traceability

Blockchain improves the security, integrity, and traceability of healthcare data by maintaining immutable records and transparent transaction logs. In a healthcare setting, patient information is highly sensitive, and blockchain provides a decentralized ledger that prevents unauthorized access, fraud, and tampering. Each transaction on the blockchain is cryptographically secured, ensuring that data cannot be altered or erased without a trace, thereby guaranteeing its integrity. Blockchain can help big data analytics to keep the information in the healthcare system at a high-security level, but it can still analyze big data without jeopardizing patient privacy and data quality. This integration strengthens trust among stakeholders, reduces data breaches, and facilitates regulatory compliance, allowing healthcare professionals to access accurate, reliable data for improved decision-making and patient care [56].

Facilitating Secure Sharing of Health Data Across Organizations

Blockchain enables secure data sharing between organizations by providing a decentralized and immutable ledger that allows secure, permissioned access to sensitive medical information. This is a common data sharing method used in traditional systems where data is shared with central servers or intermediaries, leaving firm endpoints vulnerable to cyberattacks or unauthorized access. In contrast, blockchain distributes data across participants through validation *via* consensus mechanisms and allows direct utilization of data. It eliminates intermediaries, minimizes the potential for data breaches, and allows for secure real-time exchange of information between healthcare providers, insurance companies, and patients. This further enables the sharing of data with smart contracts on the blockchain, which automatically enforces privacy policies and access controls. This ensures that only authorized parties can access specific data, reducing the likelihood of data misuse. Moreover, blockchain's transparent nature enables participants to trace and validate the flow of data, mitigating the risk of tampering or misuse during the sharing process. By securely and efficiently sharing data, healthcare organizations can collaborate on patient care, leading to better health outcomes and coordinated care across multiple providers [57, 58].

Challenges in Integrating Blockchain and Big Data Analytics

The challenges that arise when integrating blockchain and big data analytics for healthcare data management are described in Table **2**.

Table 2. Obstacles in the Integration of Blockchain and Big Data Analytics in Data Management.

S. No.	Challenges	Description
1	Interoperability	Integrating various healthcare systems and databases with blockchain and big data analytics is difficult due to variations in data formats and protocols [59].

(Table 2) cont.....

S. No.	Challenges	Description
2	Data Quality and Accuracy	Large volumes of data come from heterogeneous sources in blockchain and big data systems, making the validation and accuracy of healthcare data a challenge.
3	Data Storage and Management	Efficient storage and management of large amounts of healthcare data on the blockchain pose a challenge since there is limited storage and efficient data processing [60].
4	Data Ownership and Access Control	Establishing clear guidelines for who owns and has access to healthcare data and how control is distributed across blockchain networks is often complicated.
5	Integration Complexity	The integration of blockchain and big data analytics requires advanced technical expertise, which may not be readily available in healthcare settings [61].

Benefits of Integration

The integration of blockchain with big data analytics enhances data security, promotes transparency, improves decision-making, and fosters trust across healthcare organizations and stakeholders.

Increased Trust and Data Authenticity

The combination of blockchain with big data analytics enhances trust and privacy by providing an immutable and transparent record of healthcare transactions. The decentralized nature of blockchain ensures that no single entity has authority over the data, guaranteeing equal access to all participants and confidence in the integrity of the information. When a transaction is recorded on the blockchain and tagged with a timestamp, it becomes impossible to change or delete, as it would be widely reported and tied to other transactions, such as a medical record update, an entry in a billing ledger, or a prescription. Healthcare systems utilize such data to ensure that all healthcare information accessed by healthcare professionals, patients, and insurers is trustworthy. This confidence is reinforced by big data analytics, which uses quickly accessible pools of data from thousands of accurate and verifiable sources in order to extract it and create measurable insights. Further, by ensuring data authenticity, stakeholders can trust decisions based on proven and untouchable records. This leads to fewer inconsistencies, less fraud, and better accountability across the healthcare value chain. Moreover, when patients have more control and transparency and share their data securely with healthcare providers, they can have more trust in the system and be more involved in managing their healthcare [62, 63].

Improved Healthcare Outcomes

Big data analytics and blockchain integration optimize healthcare outcomes by providing precise, timely, and secure access to a complete view of patient data, thereby enhancing decision-making and treatment efficiency. The blockchain allows for the sharing of data between different sectors of healthcare providers so that care teams have a single view of a patient's medical history, diagnoses, treatments, and outcomes. This holistic approach allows for more personalized care, as doctors can access complete and up-to-date information, reducing the risk of errors and redundant tests. Big data analytics further enhances this process by analyzing vast amounts of data to identify patterns, predict patient outcomes, and optimize treatment plans. By confirming the integrity and transparency of data using blockchain, healthcare providers can depend on the insights generated through big data analytics, resulting in improved decision-making and enhanced health management. Additionally, the integration enables early detection of health issues by catching trends in patient data that may go undetected. Thus, Blockchain and big data analytics complement one another well, leading to coordinated care, reduced treatment delays, higher patient satisfaction, and enhanced total healthcare delivery, and hence the marriage of those gears is often a frontier innovation for the health systems [64 - 66].

ADVANTAGES OF BLOCKCHAIN AND BIG DATA IN HEALTHCARE OVER THE CURRENT SYSTEM

Blockchain and big data offer enhanced data security, transparency, and efficiency in healthcare, allowing real-time insights, reducing fraud, and improving patient outcomes compared to traditional systems.

Clinical Trials

Blockchain technology is revolutionizing the clinical trial process by improving transparency, integrity of data, and real-time monitoring. Traditionally, clinical trials have struggled with data tampering, fraud, and inefficiencies in tracking patient outcomes. Blockchain addresses these concerns with an immutable ledger of all trial-related data, ensuring the impossibility of changing entered information. This process generates a transparent, auditable record of the progress of the trial, which enhances confidence among regulators, patients, and researchers. Also, the use of blockchain allows for the monitoring of valuable patient data in real-time, thereby ensuring timely access to information, including drug effectiveness, side effects, and patient progression. These can also help researchers quickly adapt trial protocols, minimizing delays and resulting in improved conduct of trials. The use of blockchain also accelerates the approval process by ensuring that data is reliable and traceable, which is particularly important when submitting findings to regulatory bodies. By providing enhanced data sharing, blockchain can also facilitate increased collaboration between institutions that, as a result, would accelerate the discovery of new treatments and therapies. This level of transparency and real-time monitoring increases accountability, decreases the likelihood of fraudulent activities, and enhances the quality and safety of clinical trials [67 - 71].

Public Health Monitoring

Blockchain and big data can be used to improve public health and disease monitoring during epidemics or outbreaks. Its use of blockchain technology ensures a trustworthy, impervious ledger for documenting and transmitting sensitive health information instantaneously. Public health authorities can access reliable, tamper-proof information from hospitals, research labs, and other health institutions, ensuring that the information is both accurate and trustworthy. This is particularly crucial in epidemic scenarios, where rapid decision-making is vital. Blockchain facilitates secure data sharing among global health organizations, enabling coordinated responses across borders, reducing delays, and improving the efficiency of containment efforts. Furthermore, through big data analytics, large-scale health data can be processed to identify emerging trends, predict outbreaks, and measure the effectiveness of public health interventions. Predictive analytics helps public health officials monitor the spread of infectious diseases, allocate resources better, and respond more proactively. Moreover, specifically, when it comes to sensitive health information, blockchain plays a critical role in helping to ensure data privacy and integrity. Integrating the strengths of blockchain security and big data analytics can make an immediate positive impact on the public health organization's ability to contain epidemics while saving lives and resources [72, 73].

Supply Chain Management

In the domain of healthcare logistics, blockchain paired with big data analytics in supply chain management is driving a revolution. The pharmaceutical and medical device industry has always placed a high priority on the importance of product tracking and traceability to both regulatory compliance and patient safety. Blockchain technology serves as a secure, tamper-proof ledger, recording every transaction in the supply chain, from the time a product is manufactured to the moment it is delivered. Analyzing blockchain-protected data with big data can drive mapping for inefficiencies, bottlenecks, and possible risks in the supply chain, enabling healthcare providers and distributors to act early. This not only results in optimized supply chain strategies but also provides real-time analysis to further improve aspects such as inventory management, demand forecasting, distribution strategies, *etc*. In addition, the transparency of the blockchain can ensure that the products can be tracked, allowing healthcare organizations to verify the authenticity and quality of medical products. This reduces the risk of counterfeiting, a growing concern in global health care. Blockchain technology helps share secure data between different stakeholders, such as manufacturers, distributors, healthcare providers, *etc*., and enables better communication and operations in the supply chain, enhancing patient safety. A more robust and reliable healthcare supply chain is thus supported by the integration of blockchain and big data analytics [74, 75].

CONCLUSION

The integration of blockchain and big data analytics in healthcare data management holds transformative potential, addressing significant challenges like data security, privacy, and interoperability. Blockchain technology ensures the integrity, transparency, and security of health data with an immutable and decentralized structure that can secure the sharing of health records and enable smart contracts. Meanwhile, big data analytics allows healthcare systems to utilize extensive data for predictive analytics, disease surveillance, and operational enhancement. When combined, blockchain enhances big data by providing data authenticity, privacy, and traceability, which creates trust in healthcare organizations and increases decision-making processes.

This unified method provides significant improvements over existing solutions, including more secure EHRs, improved transparency in clinical trials, and better surveillance reported for public health. Additionally, big data analysis of blockchain-logged transactions offers deeper insights into supply chain management, enhancing the efficiency and safety of healthcare operations. Even with blockchain and big data analytics being challenging to implement, the adoption has far-reaching consequences and can improve healthcare systems and their outcomes in innumerable ways. This convergence heralds a new era in healthcare technology, addressing challenges, strengthening cybersecurity, enhancing productivity, and providing better treatment by leveraging data.

REFERENCES

[1]   Gupta A. From data to insights: engineering the analytics engine in Salesforce CRM cloud to drive intelligence. ESP J Eng Technol Adv (ESP-JETA) 2024; 4(4): 43-55.

[2]   Raghupathi W, Raghupathi V. Big data analytics in healthcare: promise and potential. Health Inf Sci Syst 2014; 2(1): 3.
[http://dx.doi.org/10.1186/2047-2501-2-3] [PMID: 25825667]

[3]   Shojaei P, Vlahu-Gjorgievska E, Chow YW. Security and privacy of technologies in health information systems: a systematic literature review. Computers 2024; 13(2): 41.
[http://dx.doi.org/10.3390/computers13020041]

[4]   Quazi F, Khanna A, Gorrepati N. Data security & privacy in healthcare. SSRN 4942328. 2024; 24.

[5]   Angraal S, Krumholz HM, Schulz WL. Blockchain Technology. Circ Cardiovasc Qual Outcomes 2017; 10(9): e003800.
[http://dx.doi.org/10.1161/CIRCOUTCOMES.117.003800] [PMID: 28912202]

[6]   Agbo CC, Mahmoud QH, Eklund JM. Blockchain technology in healthcare: a systematic review. Healthcare (Basel) 2019; 7(2): 56.
[http://dx.doi.org/10.3390/healthcare7020056] [PMID: 30987333]

[7]   Khezr S, Moniruzzaman M, Yassine A, Benlamri R. Blockchain technology in healthcare: a comprehensive review and directions for future research. Appl Sci (Basel) 2019; 9(9): 1736.
[http://dx.doi.org/10.3390/app9091736]

[8]   Saeed H, Malik H, Bashir U, *et al.* Blockchain technology in healthcare: A systematic review. PLoS One 2022; 17(4): e0266462.
[http://dx.doi.org/10.1371/journal.pone.0266462] [PMID: 35404955]

[9]   Yaga D, Mell P, Roby N, Scarfone K. Blockchain technology overview. Natl Inst Stand Technol Intern Rep 8202. Gaithersburg (MD): National Institute of Standards and Technology 2019.

[10]   Li W, He M, Haiquan S. An overview of blockchain technology: applications, challenges, and future trends. Proceedings of the 2021 IEEE 11th International Conference on Electronics Information and Emergency Communication (ICEIEC) Beijing, China. IEEE 2021; p. 31-39.
[http://dx.doi.org/10.1109/ICEIEC51955.2021.9463842]

[11]   Yaqoob I, Salah K, Jayaraman R, Al-Hammadi Y. Blockchain for healthcare data management: opportunities, challenges, and future recommendations. Neural Comput Appl 2022; 34(14): 11475-90.
[http://dx.doi.org/10.1007/s00521-020-05519-w]

[12]   Hovorushchenko T, Moskalenko A, Osyadlyi V. Methods of medical data management based on blockchain technologies. J Reliab Intell Environ 2023; 9(1): 5-16.
[http://dx.doi.org/10.1007/s40860-022-00178-1] [PMID: 35646514]

[13]   Alzoubi MM. Investigating the synergy of blockchain and AI: enhancing security, efficiency, and transparency. J Cyber Secur Technol 2024; 6: 1-29.

[14]   Prisca Amajuoyi , Amajuoyi P, Adeusi KB, Scott AO. The role of IoT in boosting supply chain transparency and efficiency. Mag Sci Adv Res Rev 2024; 12(1): 178-97.
[http://dx.doi.org/10.30574/msarr.2024.11.1.0081]

[15]   Tatineni S. Blockchain and data science integration for secure and transparent data sharing. Int J Adv Res Eng Technol 2019; 10(3): 470-80.

[16]   Molli VL. Blockchain technology for secure and transparent health data management: opportunities and challenges. J Healthc AI ML 2023; 10(10): 1-5.

[17]   Zarour M, Ansari MTJ, Alenezi M, *et al.* Evaluating the impact of blockchain models for secure and trustworthy electronic healthcare records. IEEE Access 2020; 8: 157959-73.
[http://dx.doi.org/10.1109/ACCESS.2020.3019829]

[18]   Gul MJ, Subramanian B, Paul A, Kim J. Blockchain for public health care in smart society. Microprocess Microsyst 2021; 80: 103524.
[http://dx.doi.org/10.1016/j.micpro.2020.103524]

[19]   Chukwu E, Garg L. A systematic review of blockchain in healthcare: frameworks, prototypes, and implementations. IEEE Access 2020; 8: 21196-214.
[http://dx.doi.org/10.1109/ACCESS.2020.2969881]

[20]   Jayabalan J, Jeyanthi N. Scalable blockchain model using off-chain IPFS storage for healthcare data security and privacy. J Parallel Distrib Comput 2022; 164: 152-67.
[http://dx.doi.org/10.1016/j.jpdc.2022.03.009]

[21] Rahmadika S, Rhee KH. Blockchain technology for providing an architecture model of decentralized personal health information. Int J Eng Bus Manag 2018; 10: 1847979018790589.
[http://dx.doi.org/10.1177/1847979018790589]

[22] Dib O, Brousmiche KL, Durand A, Thea E, Hamida EB. Consortium blockchains: overview, applications, and challenges. Int J Adv Telecommun 2018; 11(1): 51-64.

[23] Chen X, He S, Sun L, Zheng Y, Wu CQ. A survey of consortium blockchain and its applications. Cryptography 2024; 8(2): 12.
[http://dx.doi.org/10.3390/cryptography8020012]

[24] Liu J, Yan L, Wang D. A hybrid blockchain model for trusted data of supply chain finance. Wirel Pers Commun 2022; 127(2): 919-43.
[http://dx.doi.org/10.1007/s11277-021-08451-x] [PMID: 33850344]

[25] Polge J, Ghatpande S, Kubler S, Robert J, Le Traon Y. Blockperf: a hybrid blockchain emulator/simulator framework. IEEE Access 2021; 9: 107858-72.
[http://dx.doi.org/10.1109/ACCESS.2021.3101044]

[26] Sharma A, Malviya R, Sundram S. Role of deep learning, blockchain and Internet of Things in patient care. In: Malviya R, Ghinea G, Dhanaraj RK, Balusamy B, Sundram S, Eds. Deep learning for targeted treatments: transformation in healthcare. 1st ed. Hoboken (NJ): John Wiley & Sons; 2022. p. 39-75.

[27] Elangovan D, Long CS, Bakrin FS, *et al.* The use of blockchain technology in the health care sector: systematic review. JMIR Med Inform 2022; 10(1): e17278.
[http://dx.doi.org/10.2196/17278] [PMID: 35049516]

[28] Butt GQ, Sayed TA, Riaz R, Rizvi SS, Paul A. Secure healthcare record sharing mechanism with blockchain. Appl Sci (Basel) 2022; 12(5): 2307.
[http://dx.doi.org/10.3390/app12052307]

[29] Chen Y, Ding S, Xu Z, Zheng H, Yang S. Blockchain-based medical records secure storage and medical service framework. J Med Syst 2019; 43(1): 5.
[http://dx.doi.org/10.1007/s10916-018-1121-4] [PMID: 30467604]

[30] Khatoon A. A blockchain-based smart contract system for healthcare management. Electronics (Basel) 2020; 9(1): 94.
[http://dx.doi.org/10.3390/electronics9010094]

[31] Nishi FK, Shams-E-Mofiz M, Khan MM, Alsufyani A, Bourouis S, Gupta P, *et al.* [Retracted] Electronic healthcare data record security using blockchain and smart contract. J Sens 2022; 2022(1): 7299185.

[32] Belle A, Thiagarajan R, Soroushmehr SM, Navidi F, Beard DA, Najarian K. Big data analytics in healthcare. BioMed Res Int 2015; 2015(1): 370194.
[PMID: 26229957]

[33] Dash S, Shakyawar SK, Sharma M, Kaushik S. Big data in healthcare: management, analysis and future prospects. J Big Data 2019; 6(1): 54.
[http://dx.doi.org/10.1186/s40537-019-0217-0]

[34] Lee CH, Yoon HJ. Medical big data: promise and challenges. Kidney Res Clin Pract 2017; 36(1): 3-11.
[http://dx.doi.org/10.23876/j.krcp.2017.36.1.3] [PMID: 28392994]

[35] Ghasemaghaei M. Understanding the impact of big data on firm performance: The necessity of conceptually differentiating among big data characteristics. Int J Inf Manage 2021; 57: 102055.
[http://dx.doi.org/10.1016/j.ijinfomgt.2019.102055]

[36] Sa S, Rai BK, Meshram AA, Gunasekaran A, Chandrakumarmangalam S. Big data in healthcare management: a review of literature. Am J Theor Appl Bus 2018; 4(2): 57-69.

[http://dx.doi.org/10.11648/j.ajtab.20180402.14]

[37]   El aboudi N, Benhlima L. Big data management for healthcare systems: architecture, requirements, and implementation. Adv Bioinforma 2018; 2018(1): 1-10.
[http://dx.doi.org/10.1155/2018/4059018] [PMID: 30034468]

[38]   Dattangire R, Biradar D. Leveraging big data for disease surveillance and public health interventions. Int J Glob Innov Solut (IJGIS) 2024; 72024: 11.

[39]   Waldner C. Big data for infectious diseases surveillance and the potential contribution to the investigation of foodborne disease in Canada. Winnipeg, Canada: National Collaborating Centre for Infectious Diseases 2017.

[40]   Alghamdi A, Alsubait T, Baz A, Alhakami H. Healthcare analytics: a comprehensive review. Engineering, Technology & Applied Science Research 2021; 11(1): 6650-5.
[http://dx.doi.org/10.48084/etasr.3965]

[41]   Keikhosrokiani P, Ed. Big data analytics for healthcare: datasets, techniques, life cycles, management, and applications. Academic Press 2022.

[42]   Mehta N, Pandit A, Shukla S. Transforming healthcare with big data analytics and artificial intelligence: A systematic mapping study. J Biomed Inform 2019; 100: 103311.
[http://dx.doi.org/10.1016/j.jbi.2019.103311] [PMID: 31629922]

[43]   Anand G, Vashisht P. Predictive and descriptive analytics in healthcare. In: Data-Driven Analytics for Healthcare. Apple Academic Press 2025; pp. 1-14.
[http://dx.doi.org/10.1201/9781003558743]

[44]   Sharma AK, Sharma DM, Purohit N, Rout SK, Sharma SA. Analytics techniques: descriptive analytics, predictive analytics, and prescriptive analytics. In: Jeyanthi PM, Choudhury T, Hack-Polay D, Singh TP, Abujar S, Eds. Decision intelligence analytics and the implementation of strategic business management. Cham: Springer 2022; p. 1-14.
[http://dx.doi.org/10.1007/978-3-030-82763-2_1]

[45]   El Morr C, Ali-Hassan H. In: Analytics in Healthcare. Springer, Cham 2019; pp. 57-70.
[http://dx.doi.org/10.1007/978-3-030-04506-7_4]

[46]   Lone K, Sofi SA. Descriptive, predictive, and prescriptive analytics in healthcare.In: Singh H, Bhatt R, Thakral P, Verma DC, Eds. Data Science for Effective Healthcare Systems. Chapman and Hall/CRC 2022; pp. 89-103.
[http://dx.doi.org/10.1201/9781003215981-9]

[47]   Muneeswaran V, Nagaraj P, Dhannushree U, Ishwarya Lakshmi S, Aishwarya R, Sunethra B. A framework for data analytics-based healthcare systems. In: Raj JS, Iliyasu AM, Bestak R, Baig ZA, Eds. Innovative data communication technologies and application. Singapore: Springer 2021; pp. 83-96.
[http://dx.doi.org/10.1007/978-981-15-9651-3_7]

[48]   Anand G, Vashisht P. Predictive and descriptive analytics in healthcare. In: Sharma M, Vashisht P, Senthil Kumar AV, Singh C, Amine A, Eds. Data-driven analytics for healthcare. 1st ed. Waretown (NJ): Apple Academic Press 2025; p. 14.

[49]   Van Calster B, Wynants L, Timmerman D, Steyerberg EW, Collins GS. Predictive analytics in health care: how can we know it works? J Am Med Inform Assoc 2019; 26(12): 1651-4.
[http://dx.doi.org/10.1093/jamia/ocz130] [PMID: 31373357]

[50]   Fanni SC, Febi M, Aghakhanyan G, Neri E. Natural language processing. In: Klontzas ME, Fanni SC, Neri E, Eds. Introduction to Artificial Intelligence. Cham: Springer International Publishing 2023; pp. 87-99.
[http://dx.doi.org/10.1007/978-3-031-25928-9_5]

[51]   Jones KS. Natural language processing: a historical review. In: Zampolli A, Calzolari N, Palmer M, Eds. Current issues in computational linguistics: in honour of Don Walker. Dordrecht: Springer 1994;

p. 3-16.
[http://dx.doi.org/10.1007/978-0-585-35958-8_1]

[52]   Hassan M, Awan FM, Naz A, *et al.* Innovations in genomics and big data analytics for personalized medicine and health care: a review. Int J Mol Sci 2022; 23(9): 4645.
[http://dx.doi.org/10.3390/ijms23094645] [PMID: 35563034]

[53]   Khan M. Bioinformatics and machine learning: analyzing genomic data for personalized medicine
[http://dx.doi.org/10.31219/osf.io/93584]

[54]   Vo HT, Kundu A, Mohania MK. Research directions in blockchain data management and analytics. EDBT 2018; pp. 445-8.

[55]   Bhuiyan MZ, Zaman A, Wang T, Wang G, Tao H, Hassan MM. Blockchain and big data to transform healthcare. Proceedings of the International Conference on Data Processing and Applications 2018; 62-8.
[http://dx.doi.org/10.1145/3224207.3224220]

[56]   Khatri S, Alzahrani FA, Ansari MTJ, Agrawal A, Kumar R, Khan RA. A systematic analysis on blockchain integration with the healthcare domain: scope and challenges. IEEE Access 2021; 9: 84666-87.
[http://dx.doi.org/10.1109/ACCESS.2021.3087608]

[57]   Tanwar S, Parekh K, Evans R. Blockchain-based electronic healthcare record system for healthcare 4.0 applications. J Inform Sec App 2020; 50: 102407.
[http://dx.doi.org/10.1016/j.jisa.2019.102407]

[58]   Chenthara S, Ahmed K, Wang H, Whittaker F, Chen Z. Healthchain: A novel framework on privacy preservation of electronic health records using blockchain technology. PLoS One 2020; 15(12): e0243043.
[http://dx.doi.org/10.1371/journal.pone.0243043] [PMID: 33296379]

[59]   Rozony FZ, Aktar MNA, Ashrafuzzaman M, Islam A. A systematic review of big data integration challenges and solutions for heterogeneous data sources. Acad J Bus Adm Innov Sust 2024; 4(4): 1-18.
[http://dx.doi.org/10.69593/ajbais.v4i04.111]

[60]   Chen H, Hailey D, Wang N, Yu P. A review of data quality assessment methods for public health information systems. Int J Environ Res Public Health 2014; 11(5): 5170-207.
[http://dx.doi.org/10.3390/ijerph110505170] [PMID: 24830450]

[61]   Ghadi YY, Mazhar T, Shahzad T, *et al.* The role of blockchain to secure internet of medical things. Sci Rep 2024; 14(1): 18422.
[http://dx.doi.org/10.1038/s41598-024-68529-x] [PMID: 39117650]

[62]   Velmovitsky PE, Bublitz FM, Fadrique LX, Morita PP. Blockchain applications in health care and public health: increased transparency. JMIR Med Inform 2021; 9(6): e20713.
[http://dx.doi.org/10.2196/20713] [PMID: 34100768]

[63]   Majnarić LT, Babič F, O'Sullivan S, Holzinger A. AI and big data in healthcare: towards a more comprehensive research framework for multimorbidity. J Clin Med 2021; 10(4): 766.
[http://dx.doi.org/10.3390/jcm10040766] [PMID: 33672914]

[64]   Jayasri NP, Aruna R. Big data analytics in health care by data mining and classification techniques. ICT Express 2022; 8(2): 250-7.
[http://dx.doi.org/10.1016/j.icte.2021.07.001]

[65]   Akila A, Parameswari R, Jayakumari C. Big data in healthcare: management, analysis, and future prospects. In: Jaya A, Kalaiselvi K, Goyal D, Al-Jumeily D, Eds. Handbook of Intelligent Healthcare Analytics. Knowledge Engineering with Big Data Analytics 2022; pp. 309-26.
[http://dx.doi.org/10.1002/9781119792550.ch14]

[66]   Zhang X, Wang Y. RETRACTED ARTICLE: Research on intelligent medical big data system based

on Hadoop and blockchain. EURASIP J Wirel Commun Netw 2021; 2021(1): 7.
[http://dx.doi.org/10.1186/s13638-020-01858-3]

[67]   Seymour T, Frantsvog D, Graeber T. Electronic health records (EHR). Am J Health Sci 2012; 3(3): 201-10.
[http://dx.doi.org/10.19030/ajhs.v3i3.7139]

[68]   Mantey EA, Zhou C, Srividhya SR, Jain SK, Sundaravadivazhagan B. Integrated blockchain-deep learning approach for analyzing the electronic health records recommender system. Front Public Health 2022; 10: 905265.
[http://dx.doi.org/10.3389/fpubh.2022.905265] [PMID: 35602165]

[69]   Das SR, Jhanjhi NZ, Asirvatham D, Rizwan F, Javed D. Securing AI-based healthcare systems using blockchain technology. AI Techniques for Securing Medical and Business Practices. IGI Global 2025; pp. 333-56.

[70]   Singh A, Verma A, Sharma A, Malviya R, Sekar M. Use of artificial intelligence and robotics: Making the drug development process easier. In: Pharmaceutical industry 4.0: Future, Challenges & Application. River Publishers 2023; pp. 145-185.
[http://dx.doi.org/10.1201/9781003442493]

[71]   Singh B, Kaunert C, Jermsittiparsert K. Managing health data landscapes and blockchain framework for precision medicine, clinical trials, and genomic biomarker discovery. In: Digitalization and the Transformation of the Healthcare Sector. IGI Global Scientific Publishing 2025; pp. 283-310.
[http://dx.doi.org/10.4018/979-8-3693-9641-4.ch010]

[72]   Maina KA. The effects of blockchain on improving the governance of public healthcare information in Kenya [doctoral dissertation]. University of Johannesburg (South Africa) 2022.

[73]   Datta S, Sinha D. BSEIFFS: Blockchain-secured edge-intelligent forest fire surveillance. Future Gener Comput Syst 2023; 147: 59-76.
[http://dx.doi.org/10.1016/j.future.2023.04.015]

[74]   Gurtu A, Johny J. Potential of blockchain technology in supply chain management: a literature review. Int J Phys Distrib Logist Manag 2019; 49(9): 881-900.
[http://dx.doi.org/10.1108/IJPDLM-11-2018-0371]

[75]   Blossey G, Eisenhardt J, Hahn G. Blockchain technology in supply chain management: an application perspective. Proceedings of the 52nd Hawaii International Conference on System Sciences. HI, USA. Honolulu (HI) 2019; p. 6885-94.
[http://dx.doi.org/10.24251/HICSS.2019.824]

CHAPTER 9

Human-Centered Design in Health Tech Innovations

Akanksha Sharma[1], Shaweta Sharma[2], Ashish Verma[3], Sunita[1], Shilpa Thukral[4] and Akhil Sharma[1,*]

[1] *R.J College of Pharmacy, Raipur, Uttar Pradesh-202165, India*

[2] *Department of Pharmacy, School of Medical and Allied Sciences, Galgotias University, Greater Noida, Uttar Pradesh-201310, India*

[3] *Department of Pharmacy, Mangalmay Pharmacy College, Greater Noida, Uttar Pradesh-201306, India*

[4] *Dnyan Ganga College of Pharmacy, Thane, Maharashtra-400615, India*

Abstract: Human-Centered Design (HCD) plays a pivotal role in transforming health technology by focusing on the needs, preferences, and experiences of end-users, such as patients and healthcare providers. This chapter describes HCDs while emphasizing their role in addressing challenges in traditional health tech design and meeting the growing demand for user-friendly healthcare solutions. Core HCD principles, such as user-centric approaches, empathy-driven research, and iterative feedback loops, are detailed, along with techniques, such as user personas, journey mapping, and prototyping. HCD is being applied in health tech innovations, not only in medical devices but also in mobile health (mHealth) applications. Practical examples of this include the variety of wearable health monitors, telemedicine platforms, and simplified clinician interfaces. The value of HCD is multifaceted, leading to better patient outcomes from designs that make patients feel at home in familiar environments. Clinicians also see increased efficiency due to less cognitive load and less resistance to technology adoption, as a result of tools that seamlessly integrate into their workflows. Additionally, when new technologies, such as AI, IoT, and data analytics, are integrated into HCD frameworks, personalized and continually evolving healthcare experiences are created. These include difficulties in finding the right balance between usability and technological sophistication, navigating regulatory and ethical hurdles, and encouraging interdisciplinary collaboration that continues to hinder effective deployment. This discussion serves as positive reinforcement for a collaborative, hands-on approach to health tech design, where innovation meets user needs and results in technologies for healthcare that empower patients, support clinicians, and streamline the delivery of care.

* **Corresponding author Akhil Sharma**: R.J College of Pharmacy, Raipur, Uttar Pradesh-202165, India; E-mail: xs2akhil@gmail.com

Shaweta Sharma, Akhil Sharma, Shivkanya Fuloria & Anurag Singh (Eds.)
All rights reserved-© 2025 Bentham Science Publishers

Keywords: Electronic health records, Healthcare, Human-centered design, Medical devices, Mobile health (mHealth) applications, Prototyping, User-centric approaches.

INTRODUCTION

Human-Centered Design (HCD) is a design method that focuses on the user's needs, behaviors, and interests during the design process. Grounded in empathy and collaboration, HCD entails engaging with end-users firsthand to guarantee that the product or solution meets the users' expectations and addresses their pain points. This is in contrast to traditional design, which, in some cases, had more focus on being technically feasible or delivering a business goal, even if the usability of the product was compromised, where the process was involved [1, 2].

In health technology, the HCD is a multidisciplinary process taking into consideration diverse areas, such as engineering, design, psychology, and healthcare. It requires multiple loops of creating prototypes, testing them, and making adjustments based on user input to guarantee effective solutions that also support the user journey. The fundamental aspects of HCD are to observe the user environment, iteratively engage with users in the design process, and design solutions that can meet varying demands [3].

Importance of HCD in Health Tech

The healthcare field itself is complex, with multiple actors like patients, service providers, administrators, and regulators. Each has different needs, wants, and pain points, so a user-centered approach is critical for creating viable health tech products. The importance of HCD in health technology lies in its ability to address these complexities while delivering meaningful and practical innovations.

One of the major benefits of HCD in health tech is its ability to improve patient engagement. HCD focuses on making technologies that are easier to understand and utilize, thus empowering patients to take an active role in managing their health. Wearable devices that monitor vital signs or mobile applications aiding chronic disease management are more effective if they are intuitive and easy to use, as they promote regular use and adherence to treatment plans [4].

Healthcare providers often face significant cognitive and operational burdens, particularly when interacting with cumbersome or poorly designed technologies. By focusing on user-centered design principles, HCD can create tailored solutions that meet the needs of clinicians while maintaining the integrity of their workflow, ultimately helping to ease their cognitive burden in their day-to-day practices. Emerging technologies in healthcare, especially telemedicine, artificial intelligence (AI), and IoT-enabled devices, have greatly enhanced the potential.

However, their usage can rely heavily on user experience. One of the key barriers to adopting new technology is overcoming resistance from users. HCD seeks to manage these concerns through the reduction of learning curves and ensuring new solutions fit seamlessly into the workstream. HCD can accelerate the widespread adoption of innovative health technologies. The design of health technologies without a focus on the needs of a diverse user team may result in excluding certain populations, such as older adults, people with disabilities, or people with limited digital literacy. HCD involves designing for diverse audiences to ensure accessibility and availability for all people. It helps cover the digital divide gap and empowers equal access for all to avail the healthcare solution [5, 6].

Overview of Challenges in Traditional Health Tech Design

Although health technology has transformed healthcare delivery, conventional design practices often fail to consider user needs, resulting in poor adoption, inefficiency, and user dissatisfaction. Throughout history, health technologies have often been developed with a focus on capabilities and organizational objectives instead of user needs. This has resulted in products that may be functional but are often difficult to use, leading to frustration among patients and healthcare providers alike [7].

Technological innovation is essential to health tech, but there can be an overemphasis on new features, and this may come at the expense of usability. Technological overkill can lead to unwieldy user interfaces with too many features to learn when the focus is more on showcasing technical chops than solving users' problems. Such an approach often leads to technologies that are left unused or fall by the wayside altogether. Traditional health tech designs typically neglect the need for accessibility to meet the diverse needs of users, including those with disabilities, older adults, or people with low health or digital literacy. For example, a mobile health application with a complicated interface or small text size may be difficult for older adults to use, thereby limiting its effectiveness and dissemination [8].

Another significant challenge in traditional health tech design is the lack of interoperability and integration across healthcare systems. The isolated development of technologies leads to silos of information, making seamless communication and coordination among healthcare providers a challenge. These silos not only affect care quality but also create a burden for users who have to deal with multiple fragmented systems [9].

Rising Demand for User-Friendly Healthcare Tech

With healthcare systems around the globe struggling with escalating costs, aging populations, and the growing burden of chronic disease, the need for accessible healthcare technology has never been higher. The following trends highlight the growing demand for health tech solutions that prioritize ease of use and accessibility. Patient-centered care is the most relevant to the healthcare domain and refers to an approach where patients remain engaged throughout treatment and decision-making. Powerful yet user-friendly technologies are crucial to supporting this change, allowing patients to access their health records, contact providers, and take control of their care. Telemedicine platforms are designed for ease of use, for example, enabling patients to seek timely treatment from the comfort of their own homes [10].

Mobile Health (mHealth) applications have gained popularity over recent years, from tracking fitness to managing chronic diseases. However, the success of these apps is a massive undertaking and boils down to their user experience and engagement components. Apps developed based on HCD principles, including intuitive interfaces, customized suggestions, and gamification features, are associated with increased user engagement and adherence [11].

Wearable health technologies, including trackers, smartwatches, and continuous glucose monitors, have grown in popularity as they offer real-time monitoring of health status. However, their effectiveness depends on a design that is easy to use. The implications of the use of difficult-to-set-up, difficult-to-interpret, and difficult-to-wear devices suggest that they are unlikely to be tolerated widely, reinforcing the need for HCD methods in their development [12].

With the expansion of digital health technologies, there is an increased awareness of the importance of addressing health disparities and ensuring equal access to healthcare. The key to achieving this goal is user-friendly technologies that can be accessed by different populations, including those with limited digital literacy or who may not have access to high-end devices. Design initiatives, such as building multilingual mobile health apps that can function offline, will also broaden their reach and impact [13].

Several standards, such as those from the FDA and ISO, have been established with a focus on usability in medical devices. These regulations are indicative of a larger shift in the industry towards focusing on user needs and user safety, which ultimately creates an increased demand for user-friendly health technologies. Adhering to these standards will not only lead to better user experiences but also increase the marketability of health tech solutions [14].

PRINCIPLES OF HUMAN-CENTERED DESIGN

Fig. (**1**) demonstrates the principles of HCD.

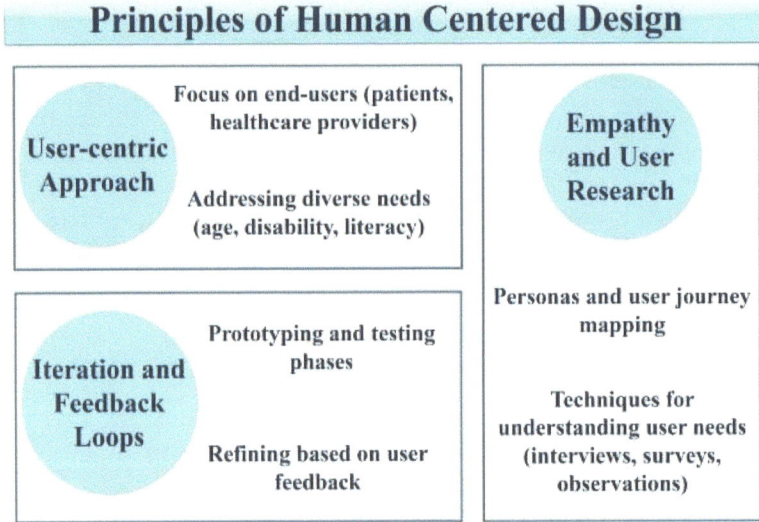

Principles of Human Centered Design

User-centric Approach

Focus on end-users (patients, healthcare providers)

Addressing diverse needs (age, disability, literacy)

Empathy and User Research

Iteration and Feedback Loops

Prototyping and testing phases

Refining based on user feedback

Personas and user journey mapping

Techniques for understanding user needs (interviews, surveys, observations)

Fig. (1). Principles of HCD.

User-Centric Approach

A user-centric approach is fundamental to HCD, ensuring that the needs, preferences, and behaviors of end-users guide every stage of the design process. In health tech, end-users cover a wide range of patients, healthcare providers, administrators, and caregivers, each with unique perspectives and requirements [15].

Focus on End-users

This method aims to create solutions that work well in the practical environments in which they are implemented. For example, a mobile health (mHealth) solution for chronic disease must not only deliver meaningful insights about the condition but also an interface that can accommodate patients across the spectrum of health literacy. For healthcare providers, solutions should streamline workflows and integrate easily with existing systems [16].

Addressing Diverse Needs

To be truly user-centric, health tech must cater to a wide spectrum of users, accounting for differences in age, physical abilities, cognitive capacities, and literacy levels. Designing for inclusivity ensures that no user group is overlooked.

For example, older adults may appreciate larger text sizes and simplified navigation in apps, while people with disabilities may rely on assistive technologies, such as screen readers or voice commands [17].

Empathy and User Research

Empathy is fundamental to HCD, as it involves deeply understanding the users' feelings, challenges, and experiences. When designers put themselves in the shoes of the user, they begin to develop solutions that align with their needs.

Techniques for Understanding User Needs

User research is a set of techniques used to gain insight. Surveys offer valuable insights into user attitudes, while in-depth interviews allow for more nuanced conversations about user experiences. In contrast, survey-based approaches gather quantitative data from larger populations, providing a more comprehensive view of user actions and preferences. Observations are also key; by watching users interact with existing systems or prototypes, designers can identify usability issues and unmet needs, which in turn reveal important opportunities [18].

Personas and User Journey Mapping

Creating detailed profiles of fictional users helps designers focus on specific user groups. Personas collect users' key traits, behaviors, and goals, helping to keep the design process user-centric. For instance, a persona for a telemedicine platform could include details about a middle-aged physician who values instant access to patient history and high-quality video. The visual approach makes it easier to understand the user journey in its entirety. They show pain points, areas for improvement, and the overall user experience as a whole [19].

Iteration and Feedback Loops

Iteration is a cornerstone of HCD, ensuring continuous improvement through repeated cycles of prototyping, testing, and refinement.

Prototyping and Testing Phases

Prototypes allow designers to experiment with concepts and receive user feedback at the earliest stages. For example, low-fidelity prototypes (*e.g.*, sketches or wireframes) can be useful for rapid concept testing, whereas high-fidelity prototypes are closer to the final product. Testing phases in healthcare may include simulated environments or controlled trials to assess usability and functionality [20].

Refining Based on User Feedback

Feedback loops involve collecting input from users after each testing phase and using it to refine the design. For example, a wearable health monitor could be tweaked for comfort or ease of use based on patient trial feedback. In addition to improving the product, this iterative refinement builds user trust by showing users that the company values their needs [21].

APPLICATION OF HCD IN HEALTH TECH INNOVATIONS

Fig. (**2**) demonstrates the applications of HCD.

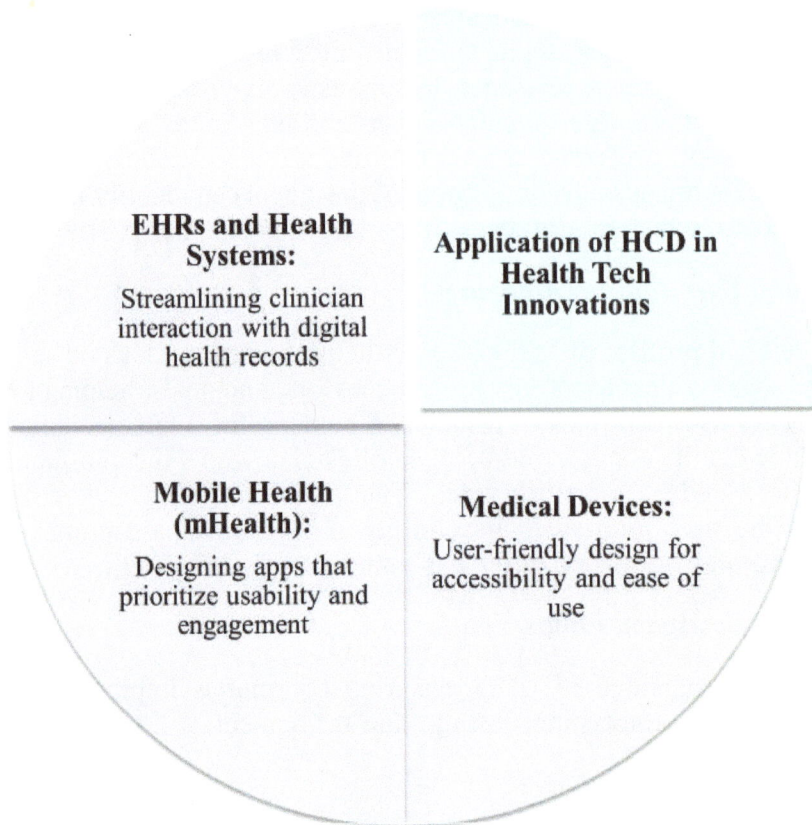

EHRs and Health Systems:

Streamlining clinician interaction with digital health records

Application of HCD in Health Tech Innovations

Mobile Health (mHealth):

Designing apps that prioritize usability and engagement

Medical Devices:

User-friendly design for accessibility and ease of use

Fig. (2). Applications of HCD.

Medical Devices

HCD has developed transformative designs that are easy to use, ensuring the devices can be adequately run by a wide variety of users, from patients with limited technical abilities to healthcare providers working under pressure. For instance, devices like smartwatches and fitness trackers are designed with very simple interfaces and real-time feedback systems that provide users instant access to their vitals whenever needed. Similarly, cutting-edge medical imaging equipment is equipped with intuitive dashboards, enabling technicians and doctors to analyze data and diagnose conditions more accurately and efficiently [22].

User-friendly Design for Accessibility and Ease of Use

Ergonomics is also a crucial part of the design of a user-friendly medical device, which means that the equipment or device must be physically comfortable, especially when worn for long durations or in high-stress environments. This involves designing lightweight, compact, and well-fitted devices, such as wearables, that do not hinder the user's daily activities. Additionally, when using the device, the interface should be obvious and simple, with little learning required. Similarly, when the device presents intricate health data, the controls must be easy to use, allowing users to access the insights they require easily [23].

In addition, the need for instant feedback allows users to clarify their clinical status and identify any possible problems they may have. These devices should provide specific feedback in various forms, like cues (*e.g.*, color-changing indicators), auditory signals (*e.g.*, beeps for irregular data), and vibration feedback (*e.g.*, vibrations) to alert users to detect important health changes or errors. Incorporating these elements can create a much more engaging experience for medical devices and ultimately lead to better patient outcomes [24].

Wearable Health Monitors

Devices such as fitness trackers, continuous glucose monitors (CGMs), or heart rate monitors need to be designed for simplicity, so they are easy to wear and use for all ages and technical abilities. For instance, a smartwatch showing a heart rate or activity levels should have a clean and easy-to-read screen, and it should reliably sync automatically with a smartphone app for streamlined data tracking [25].

Medical Imaging Interfaces

Medical imaging devices (such as CT scans, MRIs, and ultrasounds) play a vital role in diagnosing and monitoring medical conditions. HCD principles around these devices emphasize intuitive interfaces for radiologists, simplifying operational complexity and aiding image interpretation. Features may include touchscreens, customizable image settings, and real-time processing tools that provide clinicians with clearer images faster [26].

Mobile Health (mHealth) Applications

The advent of mobile health applications has revolutionized the delivery of healthcare services. HCD principles ensure that these apps will engage and suit users at various technological proficiency levels by focusing on usability and user engagement. For example, telemedicine platforms make virtual consultations easier with intuitive video conferencing tools and easy navigation. Mental health apps, for example, those that provide guided meditations or cognitive behavioral therapy exercises, rely on interactive tools and user-friendly content to keep users on track. HCD in mHealth applications helps overcome barriers to digital literacy and inclusivity, thereby improving user satisfaction and outcomes [27].

Designing Apps that Prioritize Usability and Engagement

Key design elements include intuitive navigation, ensuring that users can easily access essential features such as appointment scheduling, health tracking, and messaging with healthcare providers without confusion. Simple, easy-to-understand navigation minimizes barriers to consuming the app and allows users to engage with the app efficiently. The app can also focus on personalization, providing users with personalized health-related efforts based on the information collected through their wearable devices. This level of customization promotes engagement and relevance of the app to a user and their unique needs [28].

Finally, using interactive and engaging elements, such as gamification, progress tracking, and reminders, encourages users to return to the app regularly. Motivational messages or reminders (*e.g.*, "Great job! You have reached your 10,000 steps for today!"), create motivational rapport, support continued use, and motivate the user to work toward their health goals. This principle enables such applications, which are polished for continuous health management; thus, mHealth apps have become powerful tools for improving health quality [29].

Telemedicine Platforms

They include applications that provide patients with remote access to providers. The design of the application must revolve around video conferencing, messaging, and appointment scheduling, among other things. It should be easy to read, with large buttons for common actions (such as "Start Consultation" or "View Prescription"), and it should provide features like automatic calendar synchronization, prescription renewals, and digital notes from consultations. Teladoc has developed a user-friendly system that enables patients to schedule virtual visits with physicians, allowing people to access healthcare from the comfort of their own homes. It encompasses video calls, access to health records, and prescription management, all with an emphasis on user-friendly design [30].

Mental Health Apps

These apps focus on improving mental well-being, offering tools for stress relief, cognitive behavioral therapy (CBT), or mindfulness practices. Mental health apps should aim to create a calm, soothing aesthetic that helps lessen anxiety while providing easy updates and guided exercises. Headspace offers a stress-free interface for guided meditation and mental well-being. It incorporates soothing colors and uncomplicated navigation, allowing users to choose suitable meditation exercises according to their mood or stress levels [31].

Electronic Health Records (EHRs) and Health Systems

A major focus of integrating HCD into EHRs and systems of health more broadly lies in improving clinician interaction with digital interfaces. EHR platforms have built-in complexities that can contribute to clinician burnout and hinder efficiency. HCD principles make these systems easier to navigate and use by streamlining workflows, integrating predictive analytics, and structuring data in an intuitive way. Improving usability allows healthcare professionals to focus more on patient care rather than administrative work, which translates into better results [32].

Streamlining Clinician Interaction with Digital Health Records

Important design elements of user-friendly EHR systems include intuitive data entry and retrieval, enabling clinicians to input and retrieve patient information quickly and accurately. This means reducing duplicate data input, providing intelligent auto-completion, and using voice recognition or AI suggestions to help save time. Other key features include customizable dashboards, enabling clinicians to set up the interface according to their specific workflow. Customization allows clinicians to display the most relevant patient data, such as recent lab results or medication lists, prominently, ensuring that the information they need is easily accessible. Furthermore, error prevention and alerts are paramount to patient safety. EHRs should include validation checks on potential drug interactions, alerts for missed vaccinations, and an easy way to navigate sections of a patient's record to limit error potential [33].

Certain EHRs contain natural language processing (NLP), allowing providers to dictate patient notes, dramatically decreasing the time spent on data entry. Predictive text and automatic data filling are other features that simplify entering patient information. Electronic health records (EHRs) that are built with an intuitive interface and contextual prompts are more likely to be embraced and utilized by physicians. An example of an EHR provider that has implemented customizable dashboards is Epic Systems, which allows clinicians to prioritize tasks based on their specialty, thereby helping to eliminate clutter and focusing on the most important and relevant patient data. They also identify patient risks and recommend potential treatment options using predictive analytics as part of their system, facilitating better decision-making and improved patient care. Focusing on these design principles allows EHRs to work effectively for clinicians and produce better outcomes for patients [34].

Enhancing Usability for Efficient Patient Care

In busy healthcare environments, clinicians need to be able to interact efficiently with EHRs while maintaining high-quality patient care. HCD-oriented designs focus on usability, offering vital features such as structured patient charts, point-of-care lab results, and hospital-integration aspects (*e.g.*, pharmacy, radiology). All relevant patient data is available with just a few clicks, which reduces the cognitive load and time spent on administrative tasks for clinicians. Cerner is one of the most popular EHR systems, and it also focuses on user-centered design. It includes features such as customizable views for different clinical specialties, predictive alerts for patient care, and one-click access to patient histories. Adaptive systems allow for tailoring each system to the respective user's needs, and Cerner uses this approach to improve workflow and reduce errors that stem from data overload [35].

BENEFITS OF HCD IN HEALTH TECH

Table **1** illustrates how Human-Centered Design (HCD) can improve both patient outcomes and healthcare provider efficiency, while ensuring technology adoption in clinical settings.

Table 1. Summary of benefits of Human-Centered Design (HCD) in health tech.

Benefit	Description	Examples	References
Improved Patient Outcomes	• Minimizing mistakes *via* intuitive interfaces decreases confusion and enhances accuracy. • Helping patients to take control of their health by making tools more approachable and easier to understand.	• Medical devices with clear feedback signals (*e.g.*, wearable heart monitors with visual/auditory alerts). • mHealth apps that enable patients to track their symptoms and medication schedules.	[36, 37]
Enhanced Healthcare Provider Efficiency	• Streamlining workflows and automating repetitive tasks to decrease cognitive load for clinicians. • Supporting decision-making with consumer-friendly tools that deliver actionable insights at the point of care.	• EHRs with auto-population and voice recognition to speed up data entry. • Predictive analytics in EHRs to recommend patient treatment plans.	[38, 39]

(Table 1) cont.....

Benefit	Description	Examples	References
Increased Adoption of Technology	• Addressing technology adoption resistance by developing systems that are intuitive and easy to use. • Enabling seamless integration within clinical workflows to ensure technology works side by side with a person, not against them.	• Simple, intuitive interfaces for EHRs or mobile apps that require minimal training. • EHRs that integrate with pharmacy and radiology systems for quick access to patient data.	[40, 41]

INTEGRATING TECHNOLOGY WITH HCD

Integrating Technology with HCD is about combining the most progressive technological innovations with user-friendly approaches to building systems that are both powerful and efficient, but user-intuitive and approachable. This type of integration across systems is paramount in healthcare to drive better patient care, smarter clinician workflow, and the widespread adoption of new technologies.

Role of AI and Machine Learning in Understanding User Behavior

Artificial Intelligence (AI) and Machine Learning (ML) are transforming healthcare by offering new ways to understand and predict user behavior, ultimately improving the design and delivery of personalized healthcare services. These technologies allow health tech systems to examine large volumes of data, discover trends, and predict future outcomes based on user behaviors, preferences, and health status. AI and ML enable healthcare providers to deliver more tailored interventions, drive more engagement, and achieve better results. Machine learning can analyze this behavior and adapt the app's functions to increase engagement [42].

In wearables and IoT (Internet of Things) devices, AI and ML models can predict the user's health condition and adjust their personalized healthcare experience accordingly. For instance, a smartwatch that monitors a user's heart rate and activity level can feed data from heart rate sensors through an AI-powered algorithm that learns about a user's physical activity patterns. For example, suppose the AI recognizes that a person has been less active over time. In that case, it might send the user gentle reminders to increase activity or suggest exercises according to preferences determined by previous data. Moreover, when a wearable device detects unusual health signals (such as irregular heartbeats), AI-enabled systems can notify the user and their healthcare provider in real-time, allowing for timely interventions [43].

AI and ML also play an important role in the analysis of medical data to identify trends and predict potential future health events. For example, AI may analyse information on a patient's history and current behavior patterns to predict the possibility of a health issue, such as diabetes or cardiovascular disease, considering genetic predispositions, lifestyle, and past health conditions. These predictive insights can be incredibly valuable for personalized preventive care, where prompt attention can help mitigate the chances of the disease progressing further [44].

Using AI and ML can optimize the entire user experience through continuous evaluation of user behavior. As the system accumulates usage data, the algorithms behind it will become better at predicting, recommending, and personalizing the care experience for the user. This enables a highly personalized approach to healthcare that grows with time, supporting users with motivation and compliance in achieving their health goals [45].

IoT for Personalized Healthcare Experiences

The IoT is revolutionizing the healthcare industry, especially personalized healthcare. These data streams from IoT devices such as wearables, sensors, and connected medical devices can be used to analyze patient data and deliver highly personalized healthcare experiences. IoT technologies allow healthcare providers to collect real-time data on a patient's health and behavior, enabling personalized care plans and interventions that can be more effective, proactive, and adaptable as health conditions change.

IoT in healthcare allows organizations to perform continuous monitoring of patients, creating possibilities for personalized care that is time- and location-liberated. For example, a wearable device, such as a fitness tracker, can gather data on a person's physical activity, heart rate, sleep patterns, and other metrics. The data can be transmitted to a healthcare provider in real-time to monitor the patient and adjust their treatment plan accordingly. If the wearable device detects any frequent irregularities, such as a sudden increase in heart rate or decrease in activity, the system can alert the patient and doctors to take timely action [46].

IoT enables the creation of personalized health journeys by integrating data from multiple devices. For instance, IoT systems can integrate data from smart scales, glucose monitors, and blood pressure cuffs to provide a comprehensive picture of a patient's health. Through data analysis, AI-based systems can discover relationships and patterns between these inputs and provide personalized health advice. Individuals living with diabetes would be able to receive tailored recommendations on dietary changes, exercise routines, and medication adjustments based on real-time data pulled from their glucose monitor, activity tracker, and smart food scale [47].

The deployment of IoT devices in healthcare enables healthcare professionals to access real-time information, facilitating better decision-making and outcomes. For people with chronic conditions like heart disease or diabetes, continuous monitoring can reveal early signs that patients are deteriorating. As a specific example, a heart rate monitor can sense early-stage arrhythmias and trigger an intervention. The IoT provides valuable context to a patient's health status, allowing for more precise, evidence-based decisions and minimizing trial-and-error approaches to healthcare [48].

While streamlining care, the other benefit of IoT is the empowerment of patients. Patients can view personalized health data in real-time, track their progress, receive reminders based on the dataset, and set health goals. By being actively involved in making decisions about their care, patients become engaged partners in their treatment, which often leads to improved compliance with the treatment plan. For instance, a patient with asthma could utilize an IoT-enabled inhaler that tracks usage patterns and triggers, providing real-time feedback and recommendations on how to enhance inhaler technique and manage symptoms [49].

Leveraging Data Analytics for Continuous Improvement

Data analytics plays a crucial role in healthcare by transforming raw data into actionable insights, enabling continuous improvement in patient care and operational efficiency. Healthcare organizations can leverage data analytics to inform decision-making, improve care delivery, and drive better patient outcomes.

Identifying patterns and trends in patient data is the primary way data analytics supports continuous improvement in healthcare. Advanced algorithms and machine learning enable healthcare organizations to mine vast amounts of data from multiple sources, including patient records, connected devices, and mobile health (mHealth) apps. Analytical treatment of this data can provide information on preventive care, more accurate diagnoses, and effective targeted treatment plans for individual patients. For example, by reflecting on patient demographics, medical background, and real-time health statistics, data analytics can predict the probability of certain conditions or complications, leading to early interventions and a reduction in preventable health events [50].

Data analytics can not only improve individual patient care, but it can also increase the operational efficiency of healthcare systems as a whole. Healthcare administrators can study operational statistics, such as patient waitlists, staffing, and resource distribution, to detect areas where processes may be improved. The users can use predictive analytics to explain patient volumes and ensure timely schedules. This enhances the patient experience as well as decreases operational costs [51].

Another important element in utilizing data analytics is tracking and improving the quality of care. Through constant monitoring of patient outcomes, healthcare organizations can assess treatment efficacy, detect care gaps, and improve clinical treatments. For example, hospitals can monitor readmission rates based on particular conditions and analyze the causes of such readmissions. This information can help generate better care plans with reduced chances of patients returning to the hospital, improving patient care, and saving costs [52].

Data analytics also plays a crucial role in the continuous education and professional development of healthcare providers. Healthcare organizations can better train clinicians by analyzing their performance, identifying avenues for improvement, and providing targeted training. For instance, data can highlight trends in diagnostic accuracy, allowing for more targeted education (or mentorship) where needed. It is through the continuous collection and analysis of data that we take steps to create a culture of quality in healthcare. By harnessing the power of data analytics and artificial intelligence, healthcare providers can quickly gather insights into their operations and make informed decisions based on real-time information. This iterative process of continuous experimentation allows organizations to tailor their practices to real-world evidence, fostering a climate of blended innovation and the advancement of patient-centric care [53].

CHALLENGES AND BARRIERS

Fig. (**3**) illustrates the challenges associated with HCD.

Balancing Technological Innovation with Usability

One important aspect of health tech innovation is striking a balance between technological progress and usability. Although advanced health technologies such as AI-enabled diagnostic tools, wearable and remote devices, and machine learning algorithms hold great promise, they may often become too advanced for end users, patients, and healthcare providers. This complexity can hinder adoption, especially if the technology requires significant effort to operate or understand. For example, a highly sophisticated medical device may provide detailed health data. However, if it is too complicated to interpret or requires a steep learning curve, it will not be effective [54].

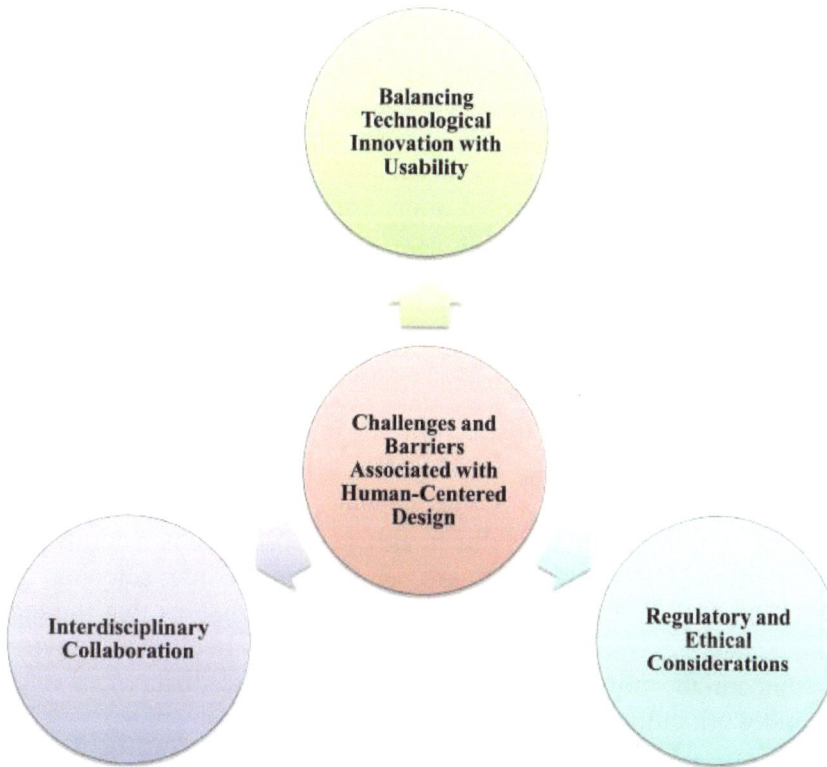

Fig. (3). Challenges associated with HCD.

The primary goal is to drive innovation; distinct innovations must address user needs, be innovative, yet not complicated or confusing. Consequently, developers need to embrace user-centered design principles, which focus on understanding end users' behaviors, preferences, and capabilities. The only way to square that circle is to integrate feedback from patients, clinicians, and other stakeholders into work on health tech tools, making them truly innovative and usable. This helps ensure that the health technology performs its role effectively, rather than creating too much strain on the user, by minimizing interfaces, increasing accessibility, and creating personalized features [55].

Regulatory and Ethical Considerations

Navigating regulatory and ethical considerations is another significant challenge in the development of health tech. Due to their potential impact on patient safety, privacy, and treatment outcomes, health-related technologies are subject to stringent regulation. Regulations like HIPAA (Health Insurance Portability and Accountability Act) in the U.S. govern how patient data must be protected, and

FDA (Food and Drug Administration) approval for medical devices can be a protracted and expensive process. It is therefore necessary for companies in this space to demonstrate that their products comply with the required regulatory standards and guidelines to gain access to the market and provide users with confidence that their technology is safe and reliable [56].

In addition to these regulatory hurdles, there are also ethical issues with the use of patient data. Since much health technology relies on personal health information to train AI, perform predictive analytics, and run devices, protecting this data from breaches is of utmost importance. All this comes with data encryption policies, consent forms, and transparent privacy policies. Balancing innovation with privacy protection is key to ensuring public trust and preventing the adoption of health tech from being stymied by fears over the misuse of data [57].

Interdisciplinary Collaboration

In many cases, building a successful health tech product is a multidisciplinary effort that involves design, healthcare, engineering, data science, and other disciplines. Collaboration with various disciplines guarantees that the technology will be advanced yet feasible and potent in actual healthcare environments. However, this collaboration can prove challengingdue to differences in expertise, priorities, and work cultures [58].

For instance, designers might prioritize usability and aesthetics, while healthcare professionals might prioritize clinical efficacy and safety. Engineers, by contrast, tend to focus more on technical feasibility and efficiency. Separate views can cause communication problems, which can delay development, and the product created may not satisfy the needs of all stakeholders. Bridging these gaps requires fostering open communication, mutual understanding, and respect for each discipline's contributions. Regular feedback loops, cross-functional teams, and co-design can help ensure that health tech innovations are both effective and usable [59].

CONCLUSION

Human-Centered Design (HCD) holds the potential to transform health tech innovations by placing the needs, behaviors, and experiences of users, patients, and healthcare providers at the core of the design process. This method helps solve the perennial problems of traditional health technology, such as lack of usability, low adoption rates, and misalignment with user needs. Through its focus on principles centered around humans, empathetic research processes, and iterative feedback loops, HCD encourages the development of technologies that are user-friendly, equitable, and meaningful. HCD has resurfaced as a framework across various health tech innovations. In the area of medical devices, it guarantees ease of use and accessibility, while in the areas of mobile health (mHealth) applications, it increases engagement and usability for diverse populations. HCD also enhances electronic health records (EHRs), which simplify clinician workflows and advance the quality of patient care. HCD, when paired with emerging technologies such as AI, IoT, and data analytics, greatly enhances opportunities for personalized as well as adaptive healthcare experiences. Despite its potential, implementing HCD in health tech comes with challenges, including balancing advanced technological innovation with simplicity, navigating complex regulatory frameworks, and fostering interdisciplinary collaboration among designers, engineers, and healthcare professionals. However, the benefits of HCD outweigh the challenges, with better patient outcomes, better provider efficiency, and increased adoption of health technology. As a vital framework for innovation, HCD moves beyond mere design methodology to become an increasingly integral component in ensuring healthcare systems deliver user-focused, efficient solutions. Its continuous development can not be understated for the field of health technology.

REFERENCES

[1]   Göttgens I, Oertelt-Prigione S. The application of human-centered design approaches in health research and innovation: a narrative review of current practices. JMIR Mhealth Uhealth 2021; 9(12): e28102.
[http://dx.doi.org/10.2196/28102] [PMID: 34874893]

[2]   Martinez L. Analyzing human-centered design approaches for involving end-users throughout the design process to create user-centric interactive systems. Hum Comput Interact Perspect 2023; 3(1): 14-28.

[3]   Melles M, Albayrak A, Goossens R. Innovating health care: key characteristics of human-centered design. Int J Qual Health Care 2021; 33 (Suppl. 1): 37-44.
[http://dx.doi.org/10.1093/intqhc/mzaa127] [PMID: 33068104]

[4]   Levander XA, VanDerSchaaf H, Barragán VG, et al. The role of human-centered design in healthcare innovation: a digital health equity case study. J Gen Intern Med 2024; 39(4): 690-5.
[http://dx.doi.org/10.1007/s11606-023-08500-0] [PMID: 37973709]

[5]   Akhtar MA, Kumar M, Nayyar A. The role of human-centered design in developing explainable AI. Towards Ethical and Socially Responsible Explainable AI: Challenges and Opportunities. Cham: Springer Nature Switzerland 2024; pp. 99-126.
[http://dx.doi.org/10.1007/978-3-031-66489-2_4]

[6]   Azim MA, Merry E, Gyalmo J, Alom Z. IoT in e-health, assisted living, and e-wellness. The Internet of Medical Things (IoMT) and Telemedicine Frameworks and Applications. IGI Global 2023; pp. 17-38.

[7]   Hyysalo S. Health technology development and use: from practice-bound imagination to evolving impacts. Routledge 2010.

[8]   Burrell DN, Ed. Innovations, Securities, and Case Studies Across Healthcare, Business, and Technology. IGI Global 2024.
[http://dx.doi.org/10.4018/979-8-3693-1906-2]

[9]   Iroju O, Soriyan A, Gambo I, Olaleke J. Interoperability in healthcare: benefits, challenges, and

resolutions. Int J Innov Appl Stud 2013; 3(1): 262-70.

[10] Penno E, Gauld R. Change, connectivity, and challenge: exploring the role of health technology in shaping health care for aging populations in Asia Pacific. Health Syst Reform 2017; 3(3): 224-35.
[http://dx.doi.org/10.1080/23288604.2017.1340927] [PMID: 31514665]

[11] Chib A, Lin SH. Theoretical advancements in mHealth: a systematic review of mobile apps. J Health Commun 2018; 23(10-11): 909-55.
[http://dx.doi.org/10.1080/10810730.2018.1544676] [PMID: 30449261]

[12] Jo A, Coronel BD, Coakes CE, Mainous AG III. Is there a benefit to patients using wearable devices such as Fitbit or health apps on mobiles? A systematic review. Am J Med 2019; 132(12): 1394-1400.e1.
[http://dx.doi.org/10.1016/j.amjmed.2019.06.018] [PMID: 31302077]

[13] Williams JS, Walker RJ, Egede LE. Achieving equity in an evolving healthcare system: opportunities and challenges. Am J Med Sci 2016; 351(1): 33-43.
[http://dx.doi.org/10.1016/j.amjms.2015.10.012] [PMID: 26802756]

[14] Singh J, Patel P. Methods for medical device design, regulatory compliance, and risk management. Journal of Engineering Research and Reports 2024; 26(7): 373-89.
[http://dx.doi.org/10.9734/jerr/2024/v26i71216]

[15] Pulicherla NV. Understanding human-centered design in the healthcare industry: a study of the application of HCD in healthcare. Master's thesis. Penn State – University Libraries 2023.

[16] An Q, Kelley MM, Hanners A, Yen PY. A Q, Kelley MM, Hanners A, Yen PY. Sustainable development for mobile health apps using the human-centered design process. JMIR Form Res 2023; 7: e45694.
[http://dx.doi.org/10.2196/45694] [PMID: 37624639]

[17] Ramos MO. Accessibility guidelines proposal for the interaction design of mobile applications: creating a more inclusive user experience. Master's thesis. Porto, University of Porto 2023.

[18] Hass C, Edmunds M. Understanding usability and human-centered design principles. Consumer Informatics and Digital Health. Solutions for Health and Health Care 2019; pp. 89-105.
[http://dx.doi.org/10.1007/978-3-319-96906-0_5]

[19] Harte R, Glynn L, Rodríguez-Molinero A, *et al.* A human-centered design methodology to enhance the usability, human factors, and user experience of connected health systems: a three-phase methodology. JMIR Human Factors 2017; 4(1): e8.
[http://dx.doi.org/10.2196/humanfactors.5443] [PMID: 28302594]

[20] Fischer M, Safaeinili N, Haverfield MC, Brown-Johnson CG, Zionts D, Zulman DM. Approach to human-centered, evidence-driven adaptive design (AHEAD) for health care interventions: a proposed framework. J Gen Intern Med 2021; 36(4): 1041-8.
[http://dx.doi.org/10.1007/s11606-020-06451-4] [PMID: 33537952]

[21] Or CK, Holden RJ, Valdez RS. Human factors engineering and user-centered design for mobile health technology: enhancing effectiveness, efficiency, and satisfaction. Human-Automation Interaction: Mobile Computing. Cham: Springer International Publishing 2022; pp. 97-118.

[22] Tahvanainen L, Tetri B, Ahonen O. Exploring and extending human-centered design to develop AI-enabled wellbeing technology in healthcare. Nordic Conference on Digital Health and Wireless Solutions. Cham: Springer Nature Switzerland 2024; pp. 288-306.
[http://dx.doi.org/10.1007/978-3-031-59091-7_19]

[23] Ahmad T. A critical analysis of ergonomics considerations in early medical device design planning. Cosmic J Biol 2023; 2(1): 235-43.

[24] Wiklund ME, Ed. Medical device and equipment design: usability engineering and ergonomics. CRC Press 1995.

[25] Takei K, Honda W, Harada S, Arie T, Akita S. Toward flexible and wearable human-interactive health-monitoring devices. Adv Healthc Mater 2015; 4(4): 487-500.
[http://dx.doi.org/10.1002/adhm.201400546] [PMID: 25425072]

[26] Hussain S, Mubeen I, Ullah N, *et al.* Modern diagnostic imaging technique applications and risk factors in the medical field: a review. BioMed Res Int 2022; 2022(1): 5164970.
[http://dx.doi.org/10.1155/2022/5164970] [PMID: 35707373]

[27] Schnall R, Rojas M, Bakken S, *et al.* A user-centered model for designing consumer mobile health (mHealth) applications (apps). J Biomed Inform 2016; 60: 243-51.
[http://dx.doi.org/10.1016/j.jbi.2016.02.002] [PMID: 26903153]

[28] Wei Y, Zheng P, Deng H, Wang X, Li X, Fu H. Design features for improving mobile health intervention user engagement: systematic review and thematic analysis. J Med Internet Res 2020; 22(12): e21687.
[http://dx.doi.org/10.2196/21687] [PMID: 33295292]

[29] Brunstein A, Brunstein J, Martin MK. Implementing behavior change: evaluation criteria and recommendations for mHealth applications based on the health action process approach and the quality of life technology framework in a systematic review. In: Adibi S, Ed. Mobile Health (mHealth): Multidisciplinary Verticals. Boca Raton: Taylor & Francis 2015; p. 133-56.

[30] Weinstein RS, Lopez AM, Joseph BA, *et al.* Telemedicine, telehealth, and mobile health applications that work: opportunities and barriers. Am J Med 2014; 127(3): 183-7.
[http://dx.doi.org/10.1016/j.amjmed.2013.09.032] [PMID: 24384059]

[31] Marzano L, Bardill A, Fields B, *et al.* The application of mHealth to mental health: opportunities and challenges. Lancet Psychiatry 2015; 2(10): 942-8.
[http://dx.doi.org/10.1016/S2215-0366(15)00268-0] [PMID: 26462228]

[32] Thayer JG, Ferro DF, Miller JM, *et al.* Human-centered development of an electronic health record-embedded, interactive information visualization in the emergency department using fast healthcare interoperability resources. J Am Med Inform Assoc 2021; 28(7): 1401-10.
[http://dx.doi.org/10.1093/jamia/ocab016] [PMID: 33682004]

[33] Kalsy M, Burant R, Ball S, Pohnert A, Dolansky MA. A human centered design approach to define and measure documentation quality using an EHR virtual simulation. PLoS One 2024; 19(8): e0308992.
[http://dx.doi.org/10.1371/journal.pone.0308992] [PMID: 39159187]

[34] Lee RY, Kross EK, Torrence J, *et al.* Assessment of natural language processing of electronic health records to measure goals-of-care discussions as a clinical trial outcome. JAMA Netw Open 2023; 6(3): e231204.
[http://dx.doi.org/10.1001/jamanetworkopen.2023.1204] [PMID: 36862411]

[35] Middleton B, Bloomrosen M, Dente MA, *et al.* Enhancing patient safety and quality of care by improving the usability of electronic health record systems: recommendations from AMIA. J Am Med Inform Assoc 2013; 20(e1): e2-8.
[http://dx.doi.org/10.1136/amiajnl-2012-001458] [PMID: 23355463]

[36] Liu P, Fels S, West N, Görges M. Human-computer interaction design for mobile devices based on a smart healthcare architecture. arXiv [Preprint] 2019.

[37] Beres LK, Simbeza S, Holmes CB, *et al.* Human-centered design lessons for implementation science: improving the implementation of a patient-centered care intervention. J Acquir Immune Defic Syndr 2019; 82(3) (Suppl. 3): S230-43.
[http://dx.doi.org/10.1097/QAI.0000000000002216] [PMID: 31764259]

[38] Mirabdolah A, Alaeifard M, Marandi A. User-centered design in HCI: enhancing usability and interaction in complex systems. Int J Adv Hum Comput Interact 2023; 1(1): 16-33.

[39] Salwei ME. Human-centered design of health information technology for workflow integration

[dissertation]. The University of Wisconsin-Madison, 2020.

[40]   Langote M, Saratkar S, Kumar P, *et al.* Human–computer interaction in healthcare: Comprehensive review. AIMS Bioeng 2024; 11(3): 343-90.
[http://dx.doi.org/10.3934/bioeng.2024018]

[41]   Lewis E. Looking ahead: the future of electronic health records. In: Patel D. Ed. Digital Health. Academic Press 2025; pp. 89-100.
[http://dx.doi.org/10.1016/B978-0-443-23901-4.00007-6]

[42]   Ahmed Z, Mohamed K, Zeeshan S, Dong X. Artificial intelligence with multi-functional machine learning platform development for better healthcare and precision medicine. Database (Oxford) 2020; 2020: baaa010.
[http://dx.doi.org/10.1093/database/baaa010] [PMID: 32185396]

[43]   Putra KT, Arrayyan AZ, Hayati N, *et al.* A review on the application of Internet of Medical Things in wearable personal health monitoring: a cloud-edge artificial intelligence approach. IEEE Access 2024; 12: 21437-52.
[http://dx.doi.org/10.1109/ACCESS.2024.3358827]

[44]   Panesar A. Machine learning and AI for healthcare. Coventry, UK: Apress 2019.
[http://dx.doi.org/10.1007/978-1-4842-3799-1]

[45]   Boppiniti ST. Exploring the synergy of AI, ML, and data analytics in enhancing customer experience and personalization. Int Mach Learn J Comput Eng 2022; 5(5)

[46]   Lan Hong T, Dave Y, Khant A, Verma L, Chauhan M, Parthasarathy S. The future of personalized medicine and Internet of Things reshaping healthcare treatment plans and patient experiences. J Intell Syst Internet Things 2025; 14(1)

[47]   Mamdiwar SD, R A, Shakruwala Z, Chadha U, Srinivasan K, Chang CY. Recent advances on IoT-assisted wearable sensor systems for healthcare monitoring. Biosensors (Basel) 2021; 11(10): 372.
[http://dx.doi.org/10.3390/bios11100372] [PMID: 34677328]

[48]   Zeadally S, Bello O. Harnessing the power of Internet of Things based connectivity to improve healthcare. Internet of Things 2021; 14: 100074.
[http://dx.doi.org/10.1016/j.iot.2019.100074]

[49]   Pramanik PK, Upadhyaya BK, Pal S, Pal T. Internet of Things, smart sensors, and pervasive systems: enabling connected and pervasive healthcare. In: Dey N, Ashour AS, Fong SJ, Eds. Healthcare Data Analytics and Management. Academic Press 2019; pp. 1-58.
[http://dx.doi.org/10.1016/B978-0-12-815368-0.00001-4]

[50]   Rehman A, Naz S, Razzak I. Leveraging big data analytics in healthcare enhancement: trends, challenges and opportunities. Multimedia Syst 2022; 28(4): 1339-71.
[http://dx.doi.org/10.1007/s00530-020-00736-8]

[51]   Kamble SS, Gunasekaran A, Goswami M, Manda J. A systematic perspective on the applications of big data analytics in healthcare management. Int J Healthc Manag 2019; 12(3): 226-40.
[http://dx.doi.org/10.1080/20479700.2018.1531606]

[52]   Wang Y, Kung L, Gupta S, Ozdemir S. Leveraging big data analytics to improve quality of care in healthcare organizations: a configurational perspective. Br J Manage 2019; 30(2): 362-88.
[http://dx.doi.org/10.1111/1467-8551.12332]

[53]   Willie MM. Strategies for enhancing training and development in healthcare management. SSRN 4567415.2023;
[http://dx.doi.org/10.2139/ssrn.4567415]

[54]   Goldberg L, Lide B, Lowry S, *et al.* Usability and accessibility in consumer health informatics current trends and future challenges. Am J Prev Med 2011; 40(5) (Suppl. 2): S187-97.
[http://dx.doi.org/10.1016/j.amepre.2011.01.009] [PMID: 21521594]

[55] Dakulagi V, Yeap KH, Nisar H, Dakulagi R, Basavaraj GN, Galindo MV. An overview of techniques and best practices to create intuitive and user-friendly human-machine interfaces. In: Subasi A, Qaisar SM, Nisar H, Eds. Artificial Intelligence and Multimodal Signal Processing in Human-Machine Interaction. Academic Press 2025; p. 63-77.
[http://dx.doi.org/10.1016/B978-0-443-29150-0.00002-0]

[56] Mennella C, Maniscalco U, De Pietro G, Esposito M. Ethical and regulatory challenges of AI technologies in healthcare: A narrative review. Heliyon 2024; 10(4): e26297.
[http://dx.doi.org/10.1016/j.heliyon.2024.e26297] [PMID: 38384518]

[57] Bala I, Pindoo I, Mijwil MM, Abotaleb M, Yundong W. Ensuring security and privacy in healthcare systems: a review exploring challenges, solutions, future trends, and the practical applications of artificial intelligence. Jor Med J 2024; 58(3)

[58] Fröhlich H, Balling R, Beerenwinkel N, *et al.* From hype to reality: data science enabling personalized medicine. BMC Med 2018; 16(1): 150.
[http://dx.doi.org/10.1186/s12916-018-1122-7] [PMID: 30145981]

[59] Ibikunle OE, Usuemerai PA, Adewale L, Abass VA, Nwankwo EI, Obianuju A. Fostering innovation through cross-functional teams in healthcare startups. Int J Eng Res 2024; 20(11): 392-410.

CHAPTER 10

Utilization of Machine Learning in Disease Anticipation and Prevention

Ashish Verma[1], Akhil Sharma[2], Shaikh Yahya[3], Shivkanya Fuloria[4] and **Shaweta Sharma[5,*]**

[1] *Department of Pharmacy, Mangalmay Pharmacy College, Greater Noida, Uttar Pradesh-201306, India*

[2] *R.J. College of Pharmacy, Raipur, Uttar Pradesh-202165, India*

[3] *Department of Pharmaceutical Chemistry, School of Pharmaceutical Education and Research, Jamia Hamdard, New Delhi-110062, India*

[4] *Department of Pharmaceutical Chemistry, Faculty of Pharmacy, AIMST University, Jalan Bedong—Semeling 08100 Bedong, Kedah, Malaysia*

[5] *Department of Pharmacy, School of Medical and Allied Sciences, Galgotias University, Greater Noida, Uttar Pradesh-201310, India*

Abstract: Predictive and preventative strategies for the disease have been transformed through ML (machine learning), which has created opportunities for earlier diagnosis and personalized care that were not previously available in healthcare. This chapter summarizes the role of ML in healthcare, emphasizing its importance in predicting diseases and preventing their onset. The key algorithms, including decision trees, neural networks, and support vector machines, and the fundamentals of ML (supervised, unsupervised, and reinforcement learning) are covered. It covers different data sources for ML applications, including genomic data, wearables, and public health data. Data preprocessing and feature engineering steps, such as cleaning, selection, and transformation, are also covered. The chapter delves into model training, evaluation metrics, and challenges such as handling imbalanced data, overfitting, and underfitting. It highlights personalized disease prediction models and risk factor assessments, which can show how individual health data can lead to more tailored predictions. The role of ML in preventive healthcare is also explored, with a focus on early intervention approaches and lifestyle change recommendations. It further explains the significant implementation of ML for disease prediction, including early detection of kidney diseases, infectious outbreaks, and mental health disorders. Finally, this chapter also discusses the challenges and limitations of the implementation of ML in healthcare.

Keywords: Data preprocessing, Disease prediction, Disease prevention, Early diagnosis, Health data, Healthcare, Machine learning, Personalized models.

* **Corresponding author Shaweta Sharma:** Department of Pharmacy, School of Medical and Allied Sciences, Galgotias University, Greater Noida, Uttar Pradesh-201310, India; E-mail: shawetasharma@galgotiasuniversity.edu.in

Shaweta Sharma, Akhil Sharma, Shivkanya Fuloria & Anurag Singh (Eds.)
All rights reserved-© 2025 Bentham Science Publishers

INTRODUCTION

Machine Learning (ML) has become a transformative technology in the realm of healthcare, leveraging its ability to analyze large and complex sets of data with remarkable speed and accuracy. This entails training algorithms to recognize patterns, forecast trends, and offer insights that were previously impossible to obtain through conventional methodologies. ML has dramatically improved healthcare delivery, ranging from automating diagnostic processes to tailoring treatment plans based on patient data. Applications of AI in healthcare include medical imaging, drug discovery, patient monitoring, and electronic health record management. Further, ML's synergy with wearables and mobile health applications has facilitated continuous monitoring of health, leading to proactive interventions. With the constantly rising global burden of diseases, ML is a promising, scalable, and cost-effective strategy to address healthcare challenges. ML represents the future of precision medicine and patient outcome improvement by enabling real-time clinical decision-making, and predictive analytics, and enhancing the ability of clinicians to tailor care responses [1].

Disease prediction and prevention are imperative for minimizing the global healthcare burden and improving the population's health. Predictive measures facilitate the early identification of individuals at risk, which can lead to timely intervention before the onset of severe symptoms. Preventive approaches can help prevent complications, decrease mortality rates, and reduce healthcare costs by avoiding the need for costly treatments for advanced diseases. This includes estimating the risk of cardiovascular disease or diabetes due to genetic, lifestyle, or environmental factors, which can help patients and clinicians implement lifestyle changes or initiate preventive medications. Moreover, prevention reduces the emotional and financial burden on patients and their families, ultimately leading to a healthier population. While chronic diseases, pandemics, and new diseases disrupt healthcare systems across the globe, prediction and prevention have become the greatest imperative to ensure care is sustainable and equitable. Shifting from reactive treatments to upstream healthcare interventions will help society move toward a holistic perspective of health [2].

ML helps clinicians with early diagnosis and prevention by revealing trends in patient information that would remain unnoticed using traditional tests. ML algorithms can examine parameters like genetics, lifestyle, and environmental factors to predict disease propensity for personalized risk estimation. These empower diagnostic precision and enable the early identification of chronic diseases, cancers, and infectious pathogens that allow timely interventions. From recommending lifestyle changes to monitoring adherence to treatment plans, ML-driven solutions enable preventive care approaches that can prevent long-term health complications and improve patient outcomes [3, 4].

FUNDAMENTALS OF MACHINE LEARNING

ML is a branch of artificial intelligence that enables computer systems to learn and improve from experience without being explicitly programmed, and its fundamentals are summarized in Fig. (1). This refers to the process of creating algorithms that break down massive amounts of data, recognize patterns, and make data-based predictions or choices. This is extensively used in recommendation systems and image recognition, as well as in healthcare for predicting and preventing diseases. ML models improve their performance over time as they learn from data, making it possible to detect anomalies, classify data, and perform regression. Its transformative potential lies in the ability to automate complex processes within various disciplines [5, 6].

Types of Machine Learning

Machine learning encompasses three primary types: supervised learning, unsupervised learning, and reinforcement learning. These approaches cater to diverse data patterns and applications, especially in disease prediction and prevention.

Supervised Learning

Supervised learning is the most widely used category of ML. In this category, models are trained on labeled datasets. Each input is paired with a corresponding output, enabling the model to learn the relationship between them. This is the most commonly opted method of training in healthcare for many tasks, such as disease diagnosis, prediction of patient outcomes, and personalized treatment planning. For example, in medical diagnosis, algorithms scrutinize past patient data to detect patterns signifying specific ailments, like diabetes or cancer. The labeled data offers a ground truth and allows the model to learn to make accurate predictions on new and unseen data. Popular techniques of this type include regression, decision trees, and support vector machines. The model's success relies heavily on the quality of the labeling. Challenges include obtaining high-quality labeled datasets and addressing potential biases. Nevertheless, supervised learning has played a crucial role in improving the accuracy and efficiency of diagnostic systems, which helps in early diagnosis and intervention [7 - 9].

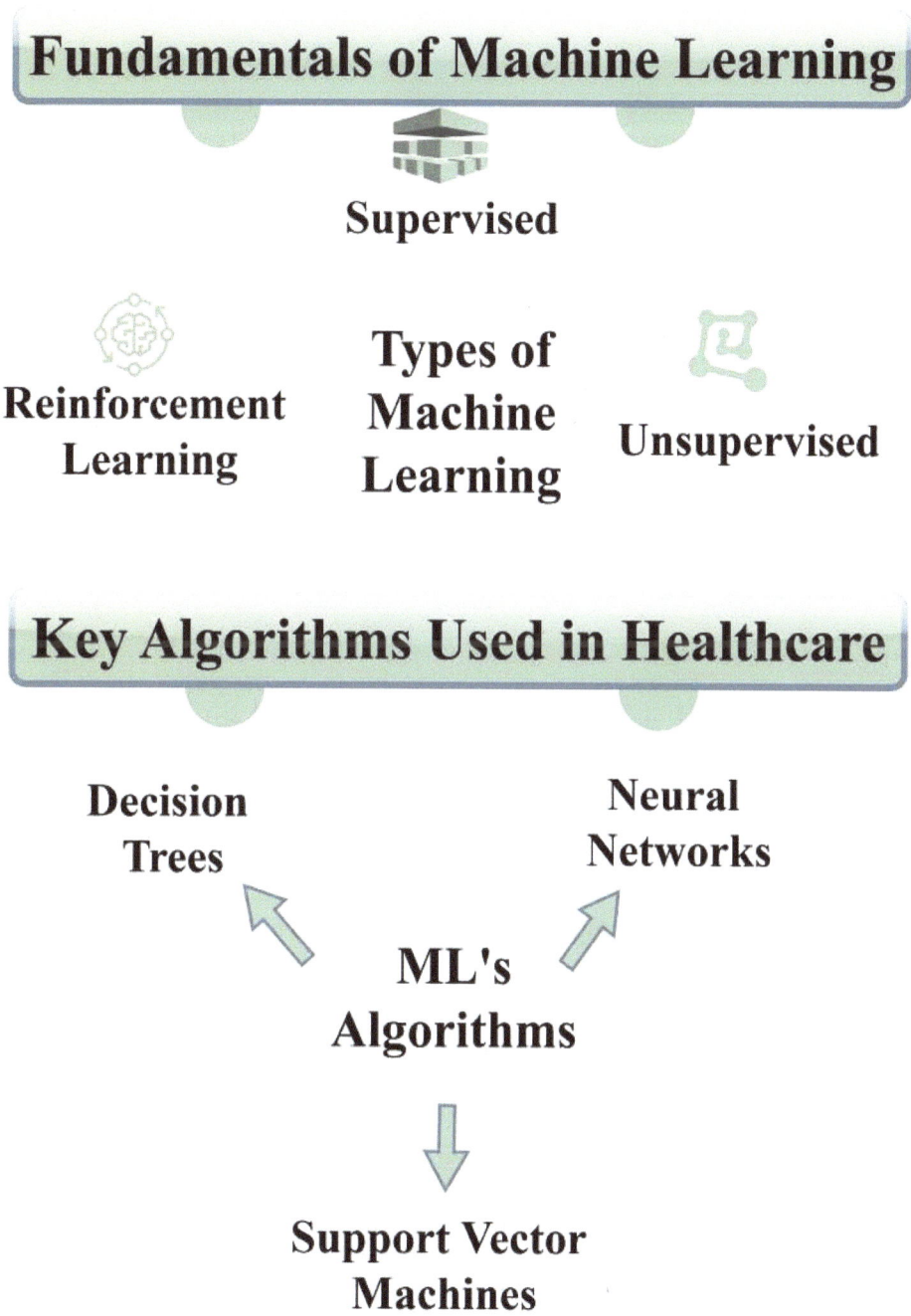

Fig. (1). Fundamentals of machine learning in healthcare.

Unsupervised Learning

Unsupervised learning deals with unlabeled data, finding hidden patterns and structures. It plays a key role in clustering, association, and dimensionality reduction tasks. Unsupervised learning is applied in healthcare to segment patients, identify at-risk groups, understand disease progression, *etc.* For instance, clustering techniques such as k-means or hierarchical clustering aggregate patients according to common attributes, facilitating personalized care plan development. Also, it could be used as any unsupervised approach to learning genomic data to identify new candidates of biomarkers or gene interactions. Techniques such as PCA (Principal Component Analysis) are used for dimensionality reduction to enable visualization and searchability for high-dimensional medical datasets. However, the absence of labeled data makes validation of results difficult. Despite this, unsupervised learning provides distinct insights that the supervised approaches would not, spurring developments in precision medicine and population health management [10].

Reinforcement Learning

Reinforcement learning (RL) is a type of feedback-based ML in which agents learn through interaction with their environments to maximize reward. Unlike supervised learning, RL does not rely on labeled data but instead uses a trial-and-error strategy. In healthcare, RL is increasingly being used to optimize treatment protocols, robotic surgery, and adaptive therapies. For instance, RL models could suggest the best drug dosage, trading efficacy with side effects based on how a patient responds. In medicine, it even works to train autonomous surgical robots to handle intricate surgeries with high accuracy. Approaches such as Q-learning and deep reinforcement learning underlie these applications. The dynamic and uncertain nature of healthcare environments makes RL particularly suitable. However, challenges include maintaining patient safety during real-world deployment and the computational demands of training RL models. Despite these, RL can revolutionize the delivery of healthcare, facilitating intelligent, adaptive decision-making systems [11].

Key Algorithms of Machine Learning Used in Healthcare

In healthcare, machine learning algorithms, including Decision Trees, Neural Networks, and Support Vector Machines (SVMs), enable efficient disease prediction, diagnosis, and treatment optimization. These algorithms process vast datasets, identify patterns, and predict outcomes, enhancing clinical decision-making and personalized care [12].

Decision Trees

Decision trees are one of the most readable ML algorithms utilized in healthcare for disease prediction and decision-making. A Decision Tree is a model that splits data branches based on the feature values, finally resulting in predictions going from the root to a leaf node. The advantage of decision trees is that they are easy to use and interpret, which is beneficial in healthcare applications where interpretability is important. For example, a decision tree can be used to classify a patient based on risk factors for diseases like diabetes or cardiovascular diseases. The tree uses data on characteristics of patients, including age, lifestyle, and medical history, to predict whether they are at risk of a condition. Because of its clear architecture, clinicians can interpret and validate decisions, therefore building trust in the algorithm. Moreover, Decision Trees are capable of handling both categorical and continuous data, adding to their versatility in various healthcare datasets. However, as more and more complex datasets are used, they tend to learn the training dataset too well, meaning they overfit and lose generalizability. Approaches to overcome this are by methods like pruning or ensemble methods like Random Forests, to make sure the model behaves more robustly and accurately [13, 14].

Neural Networks

Neural networks, which take inspiration from the structure of the human brain, are a class of very powerful machine learning algorithms used in various areas of healthcare, including disease detection, medical imaging, and patient outcome prediction. A neural network is a series of connected layers of nodes (neurons) that work with weighted connections. The network learns patterns in the data by adjusting these weights during training, enabling it to make predictions or classifications. Neural networks are especially effective in scenarios involving complex and high-dimensional data, such as medical imaging or genomic sequencing in health care. CNNs are commonly used in medical images to identify diseases, tumors, or fractures in images, and can detect the key features autonomously from an image without pre-extraction of features. Recurrent Neural Networks (RNNs), on the other hand, are designed to be applied to sequential data, which is typically suitable for patient vital signs or treatment outcomes over time. Neural networks are powerful models, yet their training requires a large number of labeled datasets and high computational resources. The other problem is overfitting, and techniques such as dropout and regularization solve that problem. The ability of Neural Networks to learn complex patterns and adapt to new data makes them invaluable for personalized medicine and precision healthcare [15, 16].

Support Vector Machines

Support Vector Machines (SVMs) are a powerful type of machine learning algorithm well-known for their performance in classification tasks, specifically in healthcare tasks such as disease diagnosis and prognosis prediction. SVM separates data into optimal hyperplanes with the maximum distance to obtain the highest accuracy. As an example in healthcare, SVMs can be found in applications related to classifying patient data into a set of categories (such as healthy or diseased), predicting whether a patient has a disease, or identifying disease subtypes. SVM has some benefits, including the fact that it works well in high-dimensional spaces, as in the case of complex healthcare-based datasets like genetic data or imaging data. SVMs can also handle non-linear separations by using kernel tricks, which transform data into higher-dimensional spaces to find a separating hyperplane. This flexibility allows SVMs to adapt to a wide range of healthcare problems. However, SVMs can be somewhat computationally expensive, particularly with larger datasets, and selecting the correct kernel and hyperparameters requires some tuning. Considering these obstacles, SVMs have been successfully adopted in cancer diagnosis, heart disease prediction, and other healthcare applications, and they have proven useful for making medical decisions [17 - 20].

DATA SOURCES FOR MACHINE LEARNING IN HEALTHCARE

Machine learning in healthcare relies on diverse data sources such as genomic data, wearables, IoT devices, public health data, and social determinants of health, each offering valuable insights for disease prediction and prevention.

Genomic Data

Genomic data is unique, and it conveys a depth of information for personalized healthcare, making it a critical source for machine learning for the prediction and prevention of diseases. With DNA sequencing technologies, researchers and clinicians can identify an individual's genetic makeup, which can give insights into gene mutations, variations, and predispositions to certain diseases. Machine learning models can use such data to recognize genetic predispositions relating to conditions such as cancer, cardiac problems, and neurological disorders. Machine learning algorithms can now process vast amounts of genomic data to identify intricate correlations between genetic mutations and health conditions, improving predictions of disease risk. Additionally, the genomic data can enhance precision medicine, where treatments and interventions are customized to an individual's genetic makeup, leading to improved efficacy and fewer adverse effects. However, the complexity of genomic data and their high dimensionality make genomic data difficult to interpret. Genetic data also raises privacy issues that need to be managed to avoid unethical practices. However, the combination of genomic data with other healthcare data sources such as EHRs and wearables holds great potential for accelerating predictive models in healthcare [21 - 23].

Wearables and IoT Devices

Real-time data generated by wearable sensors and IoT devices is being incorporated into the healthcare industry to predict certain diseases with the help of machine learning algorithms. Such devices also cover biosensors, smartwatches, and fitness trackers, which are parameter-measuring wearable devices. Wearables, through constant data collection, provide a rich and dynamic view of a person's health, supporting early detection of possible health problems. This data can be analyzed using machine learning models to predict the early onset of diseases such as diabetes, hypertension, or cardiovascular diseases [24, 25]. The summary of data sources for machine learning in healthcare using wearables and IoT devices is given in Table 1.

Table 1. Data sources for machine learning in healthcare using wearables and IoT devices.

S. No.	Data Source	Description	Example Devices
1	Physiological Indicators	Data related to vital signs and other physical parameters.	Smartwatches, fitness trackers (*e.g.*, Fitbit, Apple Watch) [26]
2	Physical Activity	Information about movement, activity levels, and exercise patterns.	Fitbit, Garmin, Apple Watch [27]
3	Dietary Habits & Medication	Data about food intake and medication schedules for personalized healthcare.	Apps for nutrition tracking (*e.g.*, MyFitnessPal), medication reminder devices [28]
4	Electrocardiogram (ECG)	Electrical activity of the heart is used for detecting arrhythmias and heart conditions.	KardiaMobile, Apple Watch ECG, Omron HeartGuide [29]
5	Electroencephalogram (EEG)	Brainwave patterns are useful for monitoring neurological conditions such as epilepsy.	Muse Headband, Emotiv EPOC, NeuroSky MindWave [30]
6	Blood Glucose	Real-time monitoring of blood sugar levels, particularly for diabetic patients.	Abbott Freestyle Libre, Dexcom G6 [31]
7	Sweat	Data related to sweat composition (*e.g.*, hydration levels, lactate, electrolytes).	E-skin patches, Sweat sensors, Hexoskin Smart Shirt [32]

Public Health Data

Machine learning using public health data, *e.g.*, epidemiological data, is widely used for disease prediction and prevention. Using epidemiological studies gives insight into the distribution and determinants of health conditions across populations while also identifying risk factors, including environmental exposure, lifestyle choices, and genetic predisposition. Machine learning algorithms can analyze public health data to discover patterns and trends regarding the spread of infectious diseases, the impact of public health interventions, or the emergence of new health threats. For example, during an outbreak, machine learning models can utilize public health data to forecast how the disease will spread, compare the effectiveness of different containment measures, and identify populations that are at higher risk. Epidemiological data have the potential to inform long-term health outcomes by characterizing the natural history of disease and tracking outcomes over time across demographic groups. A key challenge with using public health data in machine learning is that there is a heterogeneity of data sources, ranging from quality, granularity, and geographic coverage. Despite the challenges, the merging of public health data with other healthcare sources has great potential for predicting disease and improving prevention efforts [33, 34].

Social Determinants of Health

Social determinants of health (SDOH) refer to conditions in which people are born, live, work, and age, and play a significant role in determining health outcomes. These include socioeconomic status, employment, education, social support, and health care access and quality. Similarly, SDOH data integrated into a machine learning model can help predict disease development likelihood and allow for the identification of populations at risk. For instance, those with lower socioeconomic statuses often have less access to healthcare and subsequently receive diagnoses more often than those in higher socioeconomic brackets. This is because machine learning can add information about income, education, and employment to predictive models, and identify people who might benefit from targeted intervention to upstream factors. Additionally, SDOH data can enable the development of actionable, proactive, and personalized care plans that incorporate the broader context of an individual's life to improve preventative and treatment plans. However, this integration is not without its challenges, and the use of SDOH data within machine learning algorithms can be limited by data accuracy, coverage from a variety of data sources, and confidentiality considerations. Nevertheless, understanding and addressing the social factors that affect health is essential for creating more equitable healthcare solutions [35, 36].

DATA PREPROCESSING AND FEATURE ENGINEERING

Data preprocessing is a crucial step in the machine-learning pipeline for disease prediction and prevention. It involves data cleaning, feature selection, extraction, and normalization to enhance model accuracy and reliability.

Data Cleaning (Missing Values, Outliers)

Data cleaning is an essential phase of machine learning for disease prediction and prevention. Predictive models in healthcare are often developed from datasets that have missing values, errors, or outliers, which can negatively impact the model's performance. Data can be missing for many reasons, including but not limited to incomplete patient records, failed sensors, *etc*. There are various approaches to address missing values, like imputation methods (*e.g.*, using mean, median, or mode), more sophisticated approaches like K-nearest neighbors (KNN) imputation, or regression imputation. The approach is specific to the type and distribution of the data. The importance of detecting and dealing with outliers cannot be overstated, as they can distort the results. For example, outliers in medical datasets may represent rare diseases or data entry errors. Techniques such as Z-scores, IQR (Interquartile Range), or visual methods like box plots can be used to detect and remove or treat outliers. Additionally, ensuring consistency in data types and ranges is vital for creating a uniform dataset for model training. Cleaning the data ensures that the dataset is of higher quality and reduces the level of noise, allowing models to learn patterns relevant to predicting and preventing disease. Appropriate treatment of missing values and outliers is directly related to the predictive accuracy and generalization capabilities of machine learning algorithms in the healthcare domain [37, 38].

Feature Selection and Extraction

In the domain of machine learning for disease risk prediction and prevention, proper feature selection and extraction are vital, since they can influence the accuracy and explainability of the models. It is used to reduce dimensionality and decrease overfitting by selecting the best features available in the chosen dataset. Some of the popular techniques are filter methods, wrapper methods, and embedded methods. They are evaluated and filtered based on statistical tests that capture relevance (*e.g.*, association or mutual information with the target variable), which enables the elimination of irrelevant and redundant features. In contrast, wrapper methods select a subset of features based on the performance of the model, instead of using evaluation on the model, to compute a feature set iteratively. Embedded methods select features as part of the model training process; for example, Lasso regression can shrink the coefficients of irrelevant features to zero. Feature extraction is just the task of converting the original set of features to a new representation that is more informative. Dimensionality reduction techniques such as principal component analysis (PCA) or independent component analysis (ICA) construct new features through linear combinations of existing features to maximize either variance or independence between components. Therefore, both the focus on key patterns and the reduction of computation time lead to higher accuracy in the model as well as increased interpretability; this is another real impact in a field like healthcare, where the explainability of a model is important for trust and adoption in healthcare areas [39, 40].

Data Normalization and Transformation

Training data needs to be appropriately scaled, so data normalization and transformation are important preprocessing steps. There are often features in healthcare datasets having different magnitudes and units, such as the age (years), blood pressure (mmHg), or blood glucose (mg/dL) levels of the patient, which can dominate the learning process and end up generating biased models. Normalization is the process of rescaling data to a range of 0 to 1 or standardizing data by removing the mean and scaling it to unit variance. When using algorithms where the distance between data points is important, such as K-nearest neighbors (KNN) and support vector machines (SVM), these algorithms are sensitive to the scale of the features. Some common methods include normalizing the data with log or Box-Cox transformation, which can help stabilize variance and make the data closer to a normal distribution. Transforming variables is important for this purpose in the case of highly skewed data, which can also improve the performance of models that are based on the normality assumption. For example, a log transformation can convert exponential growth patterns (*e.g.*, the spread of a disease) into a linear form, making it easier for models to detect trends. Normalization and transformation of data not only ensure that homogeneous scale features are used to train models but also lead to faster convergence, better prediction performance, and quicker learning. These steps are crucial since the predictions of these models are likely to be optimal only if they account for the interplay of multiple features in complex healthcare datasets [41, 42].

MODEL TRAINING AND EVALUATION

Machine learning relies heavily on model training and evaluation to ensure robust and accurate prediction of disease, which is depicted in Fig. (**2**). Training refers to providing historical data (training dataset) for a model to learn the patterns and relations inferred from it, and evaluation tests the learned model on unseen data (testing dataset) to see how well the model generalizes. It usually consists of dividing the dataset into training and test datasets and may contain cross-validation to guarantee that the performance of the model is not sensitive to a single division. Metrics for evaluation include accuracy, precision, recall, F1-score, AUC (Area Under the Curve), *etc*. The aim is to reduce error, increase generalizability, and avoid overfitting or underfitting [43, 44].

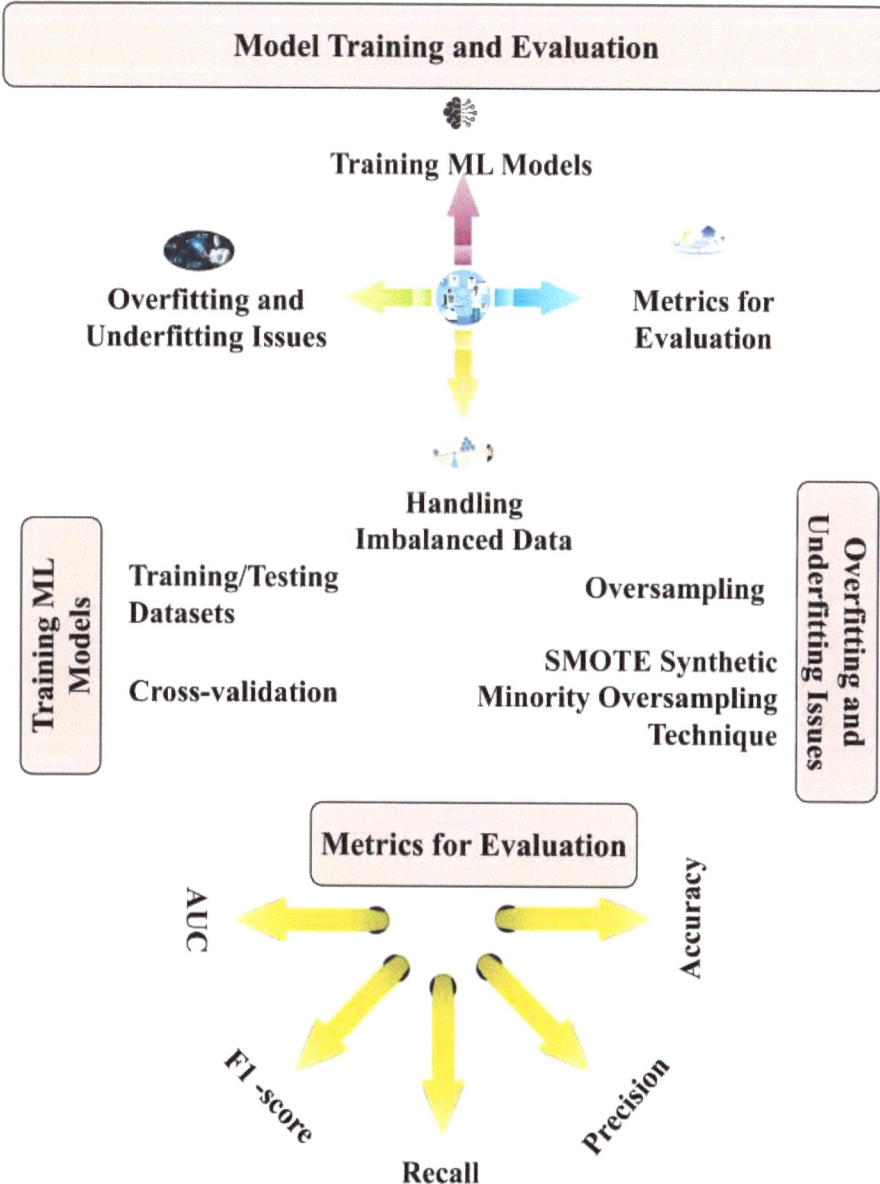

Fig. (2). Model training and evaluation in machine learning for accuracy in disease prediction.

Training ML Models (Training/Testing Datasets, Cross-Validation)

Training machine learning models for disease prediction involves several steps. Initially, the available data is split into training and testing datasets. In the training dataset, the model is provided with input features and their associated target label, on which it builds the model. The model, once trained, is evaluated on how well it can predict data it has not yet seen by running predictions on the testing dataset, which is critical to verifying that the model can generalize to new situations. A popular method to improve model reliability is cross-validation, where the training dataset is split into several subsets, and the model is trained and validated on different splits iteratively. This minimizes the risk of bias that a single train-test split can introduce, helping to ensure that the model has been evaluated from various perspectives. A common example is k-fold cross-validation, where the dataset is divided into k-folds and the model is trained k-1 times, each time using a different fold for validation. This is done recursively until all k-folds have been used as the validation set. It gives a better estimate of model performance by reducing the variance of evaluation results. This mix of training and testing sets allows for examining the symptoms of overfitting to determine whether the model is memorizing general patterns. The model's success is also heavily dependent on pre-processing, feature selection, and data cleaning [45, 46].

Metrics for Evaluation (Accuracy, Precision, Recall, F1-Score, AUC)

Disease prediction models can be evaluated using metrics, which are important for evaluating this model's prediction performance. Accuracy is the easiest and most intuitive metric to calculate, as it simply represents the ratio of correct predictions to the total number of predictions made. For imbalanced datasets, the accuracy may not reflect the actual effectiveness of the model. Precision (which calculates the ratio of true positive predictions to all positive predictions made) captures the quality of positive predictions, where you want to decrease false positives. Recall, or sensitivity, is the proportion of true positive predictions against all actual positives, and ensures the model captures most positive instances. F1-score is a single measure that combines precision and recall into a single value, balancing the two. That becomes especially important when the classes are imbalanced, as it balances precision with recall. The Area Under the Curve (AUC) of the Receiver Operating Characteristic (ROC) curve is a good metric that describes how well your model can distinguish between positive and negative classes at varying thresholds. AUC values range from 0 to 1, where a value closer to 1 indicates better performance. All of these metrics are usually used together to provide the complete picture of model performance. For example, a disease prediction model with very high accuracy but low precision and recall is not an ideal model, as it would fail to classify several sick patients and/or falsely classify healthy patients as sick. Thus, a combination of metrics, including F1-score and AUC, gives you a clearer picture of the model's strengths and weaknesses [47, 48].

Handling Imbalanced Data (SMOTE, Oversampling)

Class imbalance causes many problems that reduce good predictions and thus can lead to adverse effects by predicting disease where there is none, or vice versa. Models trained on imbalanced datasets typically exhibit bias toward predicting the majority class. This problem is resolved using a variety of techniques. The most widely used approach is oversampling, which artificially creates new synthetic data points for the minority class to balance the class distribution. The Synthetic Minority Oversampling Technique (SMOTE) is a widely used technique to make synthetic examples by interpolating between neighboring minority class examples. Instead of copying the existing datasets, SMOTE generates more realistic data points to expand the decision boundaries of the minority class. Another approach is undersampling, where the excess data points from the majority class are reduced to bring it to an equal scale. However, this can lead to a loss of information from the majority class. A different option is to use ensemble methods, such as Random Forests or boosting algorithms, which can handle class imbalance by giving more importance to the minority class. When the preservation of the real data is critical, cost-sensitive learning and focal loss can be applied, which imposes a higher penalty for misclassification of the minority class. These techniques help alleviate class imbalance problems, thus enhancing the model's sensitivity and overall prediction accuracy, resulting in more accurate predictions of diseases, especially in rare diseases or parts of diseases that occur infrequently [49, 50].

Overfitting and Underfitting Issues

In machine learning, two common problems that can hamper disease prediction effectiveness are overfitting and underfitting. This happens when the model memorizes the noise and patterns from the training data rather than learning generalizable relationships. This results in a model that achieves a perfect score on the training set but does not fare well when predicting the same model on the test set. Regular (*e.g.*, L1/L2 regularization) and simpler models (fewer parameters) are used to mitigate the overfitting problem. It is also a good way to detect overfitting because no single part of the data is overly tuned to the model (cross-validation). In contrast, underfitting happens when the model is not complex enough to adequately learn the properties hidden in the data. This leads to weak results on both the training and test sets. To overcome underfitting, the model complexity can be increased, more sophisticated algorithms can be used, or more features that may help enhance predictive power can be added. Finding the right balance between overfitting and underfitting is essential, as either side could severely compromise the practicality of disease prediction models. Both problems can be prevented with hyperparameter tuning, early stopping whilst training, and adjusting the algorithm to fit the type of data. A model that finds the middle ground can produce reliable disease predictions in different situations [51, 52].

PERSONALIZED DISEASE PREDICTION MODELS

Personalized disease prediction models use individual-specific health data to provide more accurate risk assessments. By analyzing a person's unique biological, lifestyle, and environmental factors, these models tailor predictions to anticipate potential health conditions, enabling targeted prevention strategies.

Tailored Predictions Based on Individual Health Data

Disease prediction models are typically personalized on data regarding medical history, genetics, lifestyle choices, and environmental exposures, which can help provide a more accurate prediction of future health risks. Unlike traditional models, which generalize risk for a population, these are person-centered. ML algorithms, particularly supervised learning methods (random forests, support vector machines, *etc.*), are trained on large datasets with varying health parameters. This allows them to recognize sophisticated patterns and connections among variables, enhancing their predictions based on the particularized context of an individual [53].

For instance, in the problem of predicting the risk of diabetes, ML models can include input features like blood sugar levels, family history, exercise, diet, and age. By analyzing these variables, models can find early signs of disease long before traditional diagnostic methods would. As such, aspects of these models are valuable in healthcare, enabling early intervention, tailored treatment plans, and optimized healthcare resource allocation; they would indeed find their place in healthcare for better outcomes and patient adherence. These models can also get better over time (*i.e.*, the models can learn more from the processing of individual-level data, leading to higher predictive performance). Even more, it can help the patients by providing them with insights that are relevant to their unique situation [54].

Risk Factor Assessment (Age, Genetics, Lifestyle)

Various machine learning algorithms use factors like age, genetics, and lifestyle to predict health risks to a patient, which accounts for a huge component of disease prediction. By integrating these variables with extensive datasets, ML models generate a complete risk profile that predicts future health conditions. Age is a critical factor, with certain diseases being more prevalent in older populations. Genetic predisposition also plays a significant role, as individuals with a family history of conditions like cancer or heart disease are at higher risk. ML can use genetic analysis to detect mutations or hereditary patterns associated with these diseases, which can improve the predictive power [55].

The other primary inputs in personalized prediction models are lifestyle factors like diet, physical activity, smoking, and alcohol consumption. For example, an individual who leads a sedentary lifestyle and has poor dietary habits may be more prone than someone who engages in a lifestyle of physical activity and proper dietary practices to conditions like hypertension or diabetes. ML models can help merge the data available for the patient from different sources, such as wearable devices, health trackers, and more, to gather live lifestyle data, providing more accurate benchmarks. By ongoing surveillance of such factors, tailored models can update risk estimations and recommendations for personalized management, leading to such methods for more precise preventive healthcare and enhancing these long-term health outcomes [56].

ML in Predicting Heart Disease Risk

Machine learning models are increasingly used to predict the risk of heart disease, offering valuable insights for early diagnosis and prevention. Utilizing a combination of risk factors, including age, blood pressure, cholesterol levels, smoking habits, and family history, ML algorithms can identify those patients who are at greater risk. As an example, a supervised learning model can work on a dataset containing health records of people, and that dataset also has a label that tells whether the person developed heart disease or not. Then, the algorithm identifies patterns from the training data and applies them to new patients to predict the risk of heart disease [57].

In addition, ML can discover hidden associations among risk factors, for example, the interplay of elevated cholesterol and smoking, which may not be obvious by traditional statistical approaches. Advanced models, including neural networks and ensemble learning, can integrate diverse data sources like genetic information, medical imaging, and patient-reported outcomes, refining the prediction further. This tailored strategy allows for early intervention, whether it be through lifestyle changes, medication, or increased surveillance, all of which can drastically mitigate the chances of developing heart disease. As ML models progress, they may transform preventive cardiology, yielding more accurate, personalized health advice [58].

MACHINE LEARNING IN PREVENTIVE HEALTHCARE

Machine learning (ML) is revolutionizing preventive healthcare by enabling predictive models that analyze vast amounts of patient data to identify risk factors, predict potential diseases, and optimize interventions.

Predicting Risk Factors before Disease Onset

By examining different datasets such as genetic information, environmental influences, and lifestyle choices, machine learning can detect early indications of possible health hazards. For example, ML algorithms can analyze data from biometric sensors and wearable devices to determine the risk of failure from chronic diseases like diabetes, cardiovascular diseases, and specific cancers. ML models can flag early signs of deterioration, even before symptoms develop, by recognizing patterns and trends in patient history, like blood pressure or glucose level changes. Genetic data can also be used by machine learning algorithms to predict the risk of genetic disorders, allowing for preventive measures. Such complex predictive models help identify risks, but they are also personalized because they mix individual data, thus making predictions clear and actionable. Healthcare providers may intervene early, taking preventive measures to prevent disease progression by predicting disease onset before clinical detection. The ability to predict outcomes and risks is a game-changer, leading to better patient outcomes and lower healthcare expenses; it is far more cost-effective to prevent disease than to treat it. By recognizing who is most in danger in advance, ML expands resources provided to those who are most in need of targeted help, which can help reverse or slow disease progression [59, 60].

Early Intervention Strategies

Early intervention is one of the pillars of preventive healthcare, and machine learning plays a significant role in finding the right time to intervene. Machine learning algorithms are trained on historical data to recognize risk profiles that predict adverse health events like heart attacks, strokes, or exacerbations of chronic conditions. Identifying potential patients in this way allows for early interventions to be undertaken, including personalized medication adjustments, lifestyle changes to address risk factors, or increased screening to monitor the progression of these risk factors. ML enables providers to intervene before a disease has advanced too far or to an irreversible degree by identifying these patterns of deterioration early on in the progression of a disease. Screening becomes even more important, as these public health measures can considerably reduce the occurrence of worse health conditions or prevent them completely, achieving better results for patients. In addition, ML can help determine the best timing and approach for interventions tailored to a patient's unique healthcare condition, genetic make-up, and environmental factors. For instance, if a patient shows a strong ML profile for hypertension, that could lead to early interventions like more regular blood pressure checks or dietary or exercise modifications. Data-driven, personalized approaches like these can constitute early intervention strategies capable of preventing diseases from escalating, which can complement both individual health and the efficiency of healthcare systems. Early intervention also contributes to the overall healthcare economy by decreasing the need for future costly treatments [61, 62].

Lifestyle Modification Recommendations

Lifestyle modification is a powerful tool in disease prevention, and machine learning can provide personalized recommendations tailored to an individual's specific needs. ML model assesses a patient's demographic data, medical history and health status to recommend an ideal change in diet, exercise and other behaviors that can help improve overall health outcomes. For instance, it could be simple for an ML algorithm to learn that someone with a family history of heart problems, coupled with a lazy lifestyle, would do better with a low-saturated-fat diet and a cardiovascular-based exercise plan. Machine learning can do the same for conditions that have already appeared, like encouraging a diabetic patient with insulin resistance to change their diet or suggesting which types of exercises and routines to follow to avoid triggering an arthritis flare. Moreover, mobile health apps or wearables powered by ML can monitor progress and provide immediate feedback, rendering lifestyle modifications easier. Moreover, this degree of customization and adaptability guarantees that the interventions are feasible and sustainable, promoting compliance in the long run. Additionally, as these systems combine data from multiple sources, including sleep patterns, stress levels, and environmental factors, they help offer a more comprehensive approach to lifestyle management *via* machine learning. ML-based personalized suggestions enable individuals to adopt preventative measures in managing their health by preventing the onset of chronic disorders or reducing the intensity of existing disorders [63, 64].

APPLICATIONS AND CHALLENGES OF MACHINE LEARNING IN DISEASE PREDICTION

ML has revolutionized healthcare by providing predictive models that aid in early diagnosis, monitoring disease progression, and suggesting preventive measures. Its applications span diverse domains, including early detection, infectious disease outbreak prediction, and mental health predictions, making it a vital tool for disease management and prevention.

Early Detection of Diseases (Kidney Diseases, Pneumonia, Waterborne Diseases)

Machine learning plays a critical role in early disease detection by analyzing patient data and identifying patterns that humans might overlook. For kidney diseases, ML models are capable of predicting kidney failure based on routine biomarker tests and a range of other clinical data. If detected early, kidney disease can respond well to treatment, including dialysis and other forms of medication management. In pneumonia, machine learning models can process the information from chest X-rays or CT scans and help doctors diagnose the disease faster and with better accuracy than traditional methods. Algorithms learn from large datasets of imaging and clinical data, enabling them to recognize subtle signs of pneumonia that may be missed by the human eye, thus improving diagnostic accuracy and minimizing errors.

For waterborne diseases, machine learning aids in predicting outbreaks by analyzing environmental conditions, including water quality, temperatures, and rainfall patterns. Models like these can trace the propagation of pathogens such as cholera and other waterborne diseases, giving health authorities time to take preventive measures before an epidemic strikes. In addition, machine learning allows for continuous surveillance to identify and direct resources toward at-risk populations, particularly in regions with limited healthcare infrastructure [65, 66].

Predicting Infectious Disease Outbreaks (Flu, COVID-19)

ML is used to predict potential infectious disease outbreaks in advance, to avoid loss of life or property. For instance, with the flu, ML models are trained on historical data such as flu seasonality, vaccination rates, and demographic information to predict outbreaks. Seamlessly integrating real-time data like temperature variations and viral mutations, these models can predict outbreaks on a regional scale so that health organizations can allocate resources more effectively and deploy vaccines [67].

Machine learning showed its potential for global health crisis management, as evidenced by the COVID-19 pandemic. For example, ML models were used early in the pandemic to forecast how quickly the virus spread based on information from case reports, patterns of movement, and even the genetic sequences of the virus. These models also helped predict strain on the health care system, guiding decisions about how to allocate critical resources such as the I.C.U. beds and ventilators. Besides predicting how the virus would spread, ML models also identified hotspots of high risk, enabling the implementation of travel restrictions and social distancing. Furthermore, ML techniques also accelerated the rapid development of vaccines and therapeutic drugs with the identification of promising compounds and optimization of clinical trial designs. Using vaccination rates, viral mutations, and socio-behavioral patterns, ML models are capable of predicting future waves of infectious diseases and the best public health strategy to implement in these cases [68].

Mental Health Predictions (Depression, Anxiety)

Machine learning is also being used to predict and diagnose mental health conditions such as depression and anxiety. For example, ML models that analyze behavioral data (including social media posts, smartphone usage patterns, and speech patterns) can detect early signs of mental health issues before formal diagnosis occurs. Algorithms can analyze how often particular keywords appear in social media content or the tone of voice in recorded conversations, identifying potential indicators of depression or anxiety. These models can also detect shifts in a person's day-to-day rhythms, sleep behaviors, and levels of physical activity, linking those behavioral changes to mental health disorders. This early identification and treatment can lead to a better prognosis overall for every patient and a decrease in the impact of unaddressed mental health concerns long term. For example, ML tools used in clinical practice can analyze the patients' surveys, medical histories, and transcripts of their therapy sessions to predict the onset or recurrence of mental health conditions. Such forecasts enable healthcare professionals to assess personalized treatment plans and tailor therapies according to the patient's changing conditions. Additionally, analytics based on machine learning algorithms can anticipate the best course of treatment for an individual patient by examining treatment outcomes from large datasets, allowing clinicians to determine the most effective approach. By leveraging data from various sources (*e.g.*, patient history, genetics, and neuroimaging), ML can contribute to more accurate diagnosis and treatment, allowing patients to receive the most effective therapy as early as possible [69, 70].

CHALLENGES AND LIMITATIONS

The challenges and limitations of machine learning (ML) for disease prediction and prevention are summarized in Table **2**.

Table 2. Challenges and limitations of machine learning (ML) for disease prediction and prevention.

S. No.	Challenge/ Limitation	Description
1	Data Quality	Data that is of poor quality, incomplete, or noisy can result in poor predictions. The quality of the input data plays a critical role in the accuracy of the ML models [71].

(Table 2) cont.....

S. No.	Challenge/ Limitation	Description
2	Data Bias	Bias in training data can lead to unfair or inaccurate predictions, especially when certain demographics are underrepresented or misrepresented in datasets [72].
3	Interpretability and Transparency	Deep learning and similar advanced ML models are usually perceived as black boxes that deliver predictions without transparency or explanation and understanding of the model behavior [73].
4	Computational Resources	Training advanced ML needs a lot of computational power and resources, which may not be affordable for some healthcare institutions [74].
5	Complexity in Model Deployment	Deploying and maintaining machine learning models in clinical environments can be difficult, as they require continuous updates, validation, and monitoring [75].
6	Data Privacy and Security	Health data is sensitive, and using it for training ML models can lead to privacy and security issues. The protection of patient confidentiality is essential [76].
7	Integration with Existing Systems	Integrating ML models into current healthcare workflows and systems may be complex and costly, and may require significant infrastructure changes [77].

CONCLUSION

In the ever-evolving landscape of healthcare, machine learning has come forth as a game-changer, especially concerning disease prediction and prevention. Machine learning algorithms can assist in developing predictive models by harnessing large volumes of data from various sources, including wearables, lab results, and genomic information, to deliver early and accurate diagnoses, allowing timely interventions. The capability to personalize disease prediction according to patients' risk factors, including age, susceptible genes, and lifestyle, has turned personalized medicine from a dream into reality. In addition, predictive models can enable the prevention of disease onset, transforming healthcare delivery from reactive to proactive care. While the potential for these innovations is encouraging, various issues remain, including concerns over data privacy, the high demand for clean and diverse data, and the transparency of algorithms. Scaling ML in healthcare would require solving issues surrounding model overfitting, imbalanced data, and fairness, among other challenges, to give clinicians and patients the best possible care with the generalization of its models. Nonetheless, the increasing use of machine learning in disease prediction and prevention strategies offers a future where healthcare is more efficient, accessible, and personalized. Ensuring the appropriate use of ML remains a challenge in developing patient-centered health care, and this should be addressed as research continues.

REFERENCES

[1]   Callahan A, Shah NH. Machine learning in healthcare. Key Advances in Clinical Informatics. Academic Press 2017; pp. 279-91.
[http://dx.doi.org/10.1016/B978-0-12-809523-2.00019-4]

[2]   Atkinson JG, Atkinson eg. Machine learning and health care: potential benefits and issues. J Ambul Care Manage 2023; 46(2): 114-20.
[http://dx.doi.org/10.1097/JAC.0000000000000453] [PMID: 36649491]

[3]   Huttunen J. Benefits of machine learning in operational management systems in the social and healthcare sectors. Master's thesis. LUT University; 2024.

[4]   Ngiam KY, Khor IW. Big data and machine learning algorithms for health-care delivery. Lancet Oncol 2019; 20(5): e262-73.
[http://dx.doi.org/10.1016/S1470-2045(19)30149-4] [PMID: 31044724]

[5]   Trappenberg TP. Fundamentals of Machine Learning Oxford Academic 2019.
[http://dx.doi.org/10.1093/oso/9780198828044.001.0001]

[6]   Du KL, Swamy MN. Fundamentals of Machine Learning. Neural Networks and Statistical Learning 2014; pp. 15-65.

[7]   Ayodele TO. Types of machine learning algorithms. In: Zhang Y, Ed. New advances in machine learning. London: IntechOpen; 2010. pp. 3-32.

[8]   Nasteski V. An overview of the supervised machine learning methods. Horizons B 2017; 4: 56.
[http://dx.doi.org/10.20544/HORIZONS.B.04.1.17.P05]

[9]   Muhammad I, Yan Z. Supervised machine learning approaches: a survey. ICTACT J Soft Comput 2015; 5(3)
[http://dx.doi.org/10.21917/ijsc.2015.0133]

[10] Naeem S, Ali A, Anam S, Ahmed MM. An unsupervised machine learning algorithm: a comprehensive review. Int J Comput Digit Syst 2023.
[http://dx.doi.org/10.12785/ijcds/130172]

[11] Fayaz SA, Jahangeer Sidiq S, Zaman M, Butt MA. Machine learning: an introduction to reinforcement learning. In: Agrawal P, Gupta C, Sharma A, Madaan V, Joshi N, Eds. Machine learning and data science: fundamentals and applications. 1st ed. Wiley 2022 p. 1–22.
[http://dx.doi.org/10.1002/9781119776499.ch1]

[12] Ferdous M, Debnath J, Chakraborty NR. Machine learning algorithms in healthcare: a literature survey. 11th International Conference on Computing, Communication and Networking Technologies (ICCCNT) 2020; 1-6.
[http://dx.doi.org/10.1109/ICCCNT49239.2020.9225642]

[13] Abdulqader HA, Abdulazeez AM. A review of the decision tree algorithm in healthcare applications. J Comp Sci 2024; 13(3)
[http://dx.doi.org/10.33022/ijcs.v13i3.4026]

[14] Zhang M, Chen Y, Susilo W. Decision tree evaluation on sensitive datasets for secure e-healthcare systems. IEEE Trans Depend Secure Comput 2023; 20(5): 3988-4001.
[http://dx.doi.org/10.1109/TDSC.2022.3219849]

[15] Saleem TJ, Chishti MA. Exploring the applications of machine learning in healthcare. Int J Sensors Wirel Commun Control 2020; 10(4): 458-72.
[http://dx.doi.org/10.2174/2210327910666191220103417]

[16] Javaid M, Haleem A, Pratap Singh R, Suman R, Rab S. Significance of machine learning in healthcare: Features, pillars and applications. Int J of Intell Net 2022; 3: 58-73.
[http://dx.doi.org/10.1016/j.ijin.2022.05.002]

[17] Salcedo-Sanz S, Rojo-Álvarez JL, Martínez-Ramón M, Camps-Valls G. Support vector machines in engineering: an overview. Wiley Interdiscip Rev Data Min Knowl Discov 2014; 4(3): 234-67.
[http://dx.doi.org/10.1002/widm.1125]

[18] Cristianini N, Scholkopf B. Support vector machines and kernel methods: the new generation of learning machines. AI Mag 2002; 23(3): 31.

[19] Dua S, Acharya UR, Dua P, Eds. Machine Learning in Healthcare Informatics. Berlin: Springer 2014.
[http://dx.doi.org/10.1007/978-3-642-40017-9]

[20] Poongodi T, Sumathi D, Suresh P, Balusamy B. Deep learning techniques for electronic health record (EHR) analysis. In: Bhoi A, Mallick, P, Liu, CM, Balas, V. Eds. Bio-inspired Neurocomputing. Studies in Computational Intelligence. Singapore, Springer 2021; pp. 73-103.
[http://dx.doi.org/10.1007/978-981-15-5495-7_5]

[21] Wong J, Murray Horwitz M, Zhou L, Toh S. Using machine learning to identify health outcomes from electronic health record data. Curr Epidemiol Rep 2018; 5(4): 331-42.
[http://dx.doi.org/10.1007/s40471-018-0165-9] [PMID: 30555773]

[22] Chafai N, Bonizzi L, Botti S, Badaoui B. Emerging applications of machine learning in genomic medicine and healthcare. Crit Rev Clin Lab Sci 2024; 61(2): 140-63.
[http://dx.doi.org/10.1080/10408363.2023.2259466] [PMID: 37815417]

[23] Sunil Krishnan G, Joshi A, Kaushik V. Bioinformatics in personalized medicine. In: Advances in Bioinformatics. Singapore: Springer 2021; pp. 303-315.
[http://dx.doi.org/10.1007/978-981-33-6191-1_15]

[24] Sabry F, Eltaras T, Labda W, Alzoubi K, Malluhi Q. Machine learning for healthcare wearable devices: the big picture. J Healthc Eng 2022; 2022(1): 1-25.
[http://dx.doi.org/10.1155/2022/4653923] [PMID: 35480146]

[25] Poongodi T, Krishnamurthi R, Indrakumari R, Suresh P, Balusamy B. Wearable devices and IoT. In: Balas VE, Solanki VK, Kumar R, Ahad MAR, Eds. A handbook of internet of things in biomedical and cyber physical system. 1st ed. Academic Press; 2020. p. 245-73.

[26] Masoumian Hosseini M, Masoumian Hosseini ST, Qayumi K, Hosseinzadeh S, Sajadi Tabar SS. Smartwatches in healthcare medicine: assistance and monitoring; a scoping review. BMC Med Inform Decis Mak 2023; 23(1): 248.
[http://dx.doi.org/10.1186/s12911-023-02350-w] [PMID: 37924029]

[27] Bort-Roig J, Gilson ND, Puig-Ribera A, Contreras RS, Trost SG. Measuring and influencing physical activity with smartphone technology: a systematic review. Sports Med 2014; 44(5): 671-86.
[http://dx.doi.org/10.1007/s40279-014-0142-5] [PMID: 24497157]

[28] Samad S, Ahmed F, Naher S, *et al.* Smartphone apps for tracking food consumption and recommendations: Evaluating artificial intelligence-based functionalities, features and quality of current apps. Intelligent Systems with Applications 2022; 15: 200103.
[http://dx.doi.org/10.1016/j.iswa.2022.200103]

[29] Dahiya ES, Kalra AM, Lowe A, Anand G. Wearable technology for monitoring electrocardiograms (ECGs) in adults: a scoping review. Sensors (Basel) 2024; 24(4): 1318.
[http://dx.doi.org/10.3390/s24041318] [PMID: 38400474]

[30] Sugden RJ, Pham-Kim-Nghiem-Phu VLL, Campbell I, Leon A, Diamandis P. Remote collection of electrophysiological data with brain wearables: opportunities and challenges. Bioelectron Med 2023; 9(1): 12.
[http://dx.doi.org/10.1186/s42234-023-00114-5] [PMID: 37340487]

[31] Blum A. Freestyle Libre glucose monitoring system. Clin Diabetes 2018; 36(2): 203-4.
[http://dx.doi.org/10.2337/cd17-0130] [PMID: 29686463]

[32] Gao F, Liu C, Zhang L, *et al.* Wearable and flexible electrochemical sensors for sweat analysis: a

review. Microsyst Nanoeng 2023; 9(1): 1-21.
[http://dx.doi.org/10.1038/s41378-022-00443-6] [PMID: 36597511]

[33]   Khoury MJ, Iademarco MF, Riley WT. Precision public health for the era of precision medicine. Am J Prev Med 2016; 50(3): 398-401.
[http://dx.doi.org/10.1016/j.amepre.2015.08.031] [PMID: 26547538]

[34]   Kamel Boulos MN, Zhang P. Digital twins: from personalised medicine to precision public health. J Pers Med 2021; 11(8): 745.
[http://dx.doi.org/10.3390/jpm11080745] [PMID: 34442389]

[35]   Braveman P, Egerter S, Williams DR. The social determinants of health: coming of age. Annu Rev Public Health 2011; 32(1): 381-98.
[http://dx.doi.org/10.1146/annurev-publhealth-031210-101218] [PMID: 21091195]

[36]   Marmot M, Allen J, Bell R, Bloomer E, Goldblatt P. WHO European review of social determinants of health and the health divide. Lancet 2012; 380(9846): 1011-29.
[http://dx.doi.org/10.1016/S0140-6736(12)61228-8] [PMID: 22964159]

[37]   Dong G, Liu H, Eds. Feature Engineering for Machine Learning and Data Analytics. CRC Press 2018.

[38]   Kang M, Tian J. Eds. Machine learning: data pre-processing. Prognostics and Health Management of Electronics. Fundamentals, Machine Learning, and the Internet of Things 2018; pp. 111-30.
[http://dx.doi.org/10.1002/9781119515326.ch5]

[39]   Khalid S, Khalil T, Nasreen S. A survey of feature selection and feature extraction techniques in machine learning. 2014 Science and Information Conference. IEEE 2014; pp. 372-8.
[http://dx.doi.org/10.1109/SAI.2014.6918213]

[40]   Zebari R, Abdulazeez A, Zeebaree D, Zebari D, Saeed J. A comprehensive review of dimensionality reduction techniques for feature selection and feature extraction. J App Sci Tech Tren 2020; 1(1): 56-70.
[http://dx.doi.org/10.38094/jastt1224]

[41]   Singh D, Singh B. Investigating the impact of data normalization on classification performance. Appl Soft Comput 2020; 97: 105524.
[http://dx.doi.org/10.1016/j.asoc.2019.105524]

[42]   Ha TN, Lubo-Robles D, Marfurt KJ, Wallet BC. An in-depth analysis of logarithmic data transformation and per-class normalization in machine learning: Application to unsupervised classification of a turbidite system in the Canterbury Basin, New Zealand, and supervised classification of salt in the Eugene Island minibasin, Gulf of Mexico. Interpretation (Tulsa) 2021; 9(3): T685-710.
[http://dx.doi.org/10.1190/INT-2021-0008.1]

[43]   Uddin S, Khan A, Hossain ME, Moni MA. Comparing different supervised machine learning algorithms for disease prediction. BMC Med Inform Decis Mak 2019; 19(1): 281.
[http://dx.doi.org/10.1186/s12911-019-1004-8] [PMID: 31864346]

[44]   Barboza F, Kimura H, Altman E. Machine learning models and bankruptcy prediction. Expert Syst Appl 2017; 83: 405-17.
[http://dx.doi.org/10.1016/j.eswa.2017.04.006]

[45]   Lee SB, Gui X, Manquen M, Hamilton ER. Use of training, validation, and test sets for developing automated classifiers in quantitative ethnography. First International Conference, ICQE 2019 Madison, WI, USA. October 20–22, 2019; 117-27.
[http://dx.doi.org/10.1007/978-3-030-33232-7_10]

[46]   Martens HA, Dardenne P. Validation and verification of regression in small data sets. Chemom Intell Lab Syst 1998; 44(1-2): 99-121.
[http://dx.doi.org/10.1016/S0169-7439(98)00167-1]

[47]   Juba B, Le HS. Precision-recall versus accuracy and the role of large data sets. Proc Conf AAAI Artif

Intell 2019; 33(1): 4039-48.
[http://dx.doi.org/10.1609/aaai.v33i01.33014039]

[48]   Alvarez SA. An exact analytical relation among recall, precision, and classification accuracy in information retrieval. Boston College, Boston 2002; 1-22.

[49]   Matharaarachchi S, Domaratzki M, Muthukumarana S. Enhancing SMOTE for imbalanced data with abnormal minority instances. Machine Learning with Applications 2024; 18: 100597.
[http://dx.doi.org/10.1016/j.mlwa.2024.100597]

[50]   Pradipta GA, Wardoyo R, Musdholifah A, Sanjaya IN, Ismail M. SMOTE for handling imbalanced data problem: A review. Sixth International Conference on Informatics and Computing (ICIC) 2021; 1-8.
[http://dx.doi.org/10.1109/ICIC54025.2021.9632912]

[51]   Reilly J. Overfitting and underfitting in machine learning. Great Learning 2024.

[52]   Montesinos López OA, Montesinos López A, Crossa J. Overfitting, model tuning, and evaluation of prediction performance. In: Multivariate Statistical Machine Learning Methods for Genomic Prediction. Cham: Springer International Publishing 2022; pp. 109-39.
[http://dx.doi.org/10.1007/978-3-030-89010-0_4]

[53]   Damaševičius R, Jagatheesaperumal SK, Kandala RNVPS, Hussain S, Alizadehsani R, Gorriz JM. Deep learning for personalized health monitoring and prediction: A review. Comput Intell 2024; 40(3): e12682.
[http://dx.doi.org/10.1111/coin.12682]

[54]   van der Leeuw J, Ridker PM, van der Graaf Y, Visseren FLJ. Personalized cardiovascular disease prevention by applying individualized prediction of treatment effects. Eur Heart J 2014; 35(13): 837-43.
[http://dx.doi.org/10.1093/eurheartj/ehu004] [PMID: 24513790]

[55]   Weitzel JN, Blazer KR, MacDonald DJ, Culver JO, Offit K. Genetics, genomics, and cancer risk assessment. CA Cancer J Clin 2011; 61(5): 327-59.
[http://dx.doi.org/10.3322/caac.20128] [PMID: 21858794]

[56]   Jeon J, Du M, Schoen RE, *et al.* Determining the risk of colorectal cancer and the starting age of screening based on lifestyle, environmental, and genetic factors. Gastroenterology 2018; 154(8): 2152-2164.e19.
[http://dx.doi.org/10.1053/j.gastro.2018.02.021] [PMID: 29458155]

[57]   Bertsimas D, Orfanoudaki A, Weiner RB. Personalized treatment for coronary artery disease patients: a machine learning approach. Health Care Manage Sci 2020; 23(4): 482-506.
[http://dx.doi.org/10.1007/s10729-020-09522-4] [PMID: 33040231]

[58]   Dogan A, Li Y, Peter Odo C, Sonawane K, Lin Y, Liu C. A utility-based machine learning-driven personalized lifestyle recommendation for cardiovascular disease prevention. J Biomed Inform 2023; 141: 104342.
[http://dx.doi.org/10.1016/j.jbi.2023.104342] [PMID: 36963450]

[59]   Xu D, Xu Z. Machine learning applications in preventive healthcare: A systematic literature review on predictive analytics of disease comorbidity from multiple perspectives. Artif Intell Med 2024; 156: 102950.
[http://dx.doi.org/10.1016/j.artmed.2024.102950] [PMID: 39163727]

[60]   Yadav V. Machine learning and the economics of preventive healthcare: studying cost-benefit analysis of machine learning-driven preventive healthcare measures. N Am J Eng Res 2022; 3(1)

[61]   Ibrahim MS, Saber S. Machine learning and predictive analytics: Advancing disease prevention in healthcare. J Contemp Healthc Anal 2023; 7(1): 53-71.

[62]   Licea D. Early intervention through AI: redefining the future of preventive healthcare. Bachelor's thesis. Lima (PE): UTEC Universidad de Ingeniería y Tecnología 2024.

[63]   Chiang PH, Wong M, Dey S. Using wearables and machine learning to enable personalized lifestyle recommendations to improve blood pressure. IEEE J Transl Eng Health Med 2021; 9: 1-13.
[http://dx.doi.org/10.1109/JTEHM.2021.3098173] [PMID: 34765324]

[64]   Vodovotz Y, Barnard N, Hu FB, *et al.* Prioritized research for the prevention, treatment, and reversal of chronic disease: recommendations from the lifestyle medicine research summit. Front Med (Lausanne) 2020; 7: 585744.
[http://dx.doi.org/10.3389/fmed.2020.585744] [PMID: 33415115]

[65]   Jeyakumar V, Sundaram P, Ramapathiran N. Artificial intelligence-based predictive tools for life-threatening diseases. In: Kanagachidambaresan G.R, Bhatia D, Kumar, D, Mishra, A. Eds. System Design for Epidemics Using Machine Learning and Deep Learning. Cham: Springer International Publishing 2023; pp. 123-52.
[http://dx.doi.org/10.1007/978-3-031-19752-9_8]

[66]   Khew CY, Akbar R, Assaad NM. Progress and challenges for the application of machine learning for neglected tropical diseases. arXiv preprint arXiv:221201027 2022.

[67]   Heidari A, Jafari Navimipour N, Unal M, Toumaj S. Machine learning applications for COVID-19 outbreak management. Neural Comput Appl 2022; 34(18): 15313-48.
[http://dx.doi.org/10.1007/s00521-022-07424-w] [PMID: 35702664]

[68]   Lalmuanawma S, Hussain J, Chhakchhuak L. Applications of machine learning and artificial intelligence for Covid-19 (SARS-CoV-2) pandemic: A review. Chaos Solitons Fractals 2020; 139: 110059.
[http://dx.doi.org/10.1016/j.chaos.2020.110059] [PMID: 32834612]

[69]   Balraj CS, Nagaraj P. Prediction of mental health issues and challenges using hybrid machine and deep learning techniques. In: Giri D, Vaidya J, Ponnusamy S, Lin Z, Joshi KP, Yegnanarayanan V, Eds. Proceedings of the Tenth International Conference on Mathematics and Computing (ICMC 2024). Singapore: Springer 2024; pp. 15-27.
[http://dx.doi.org/10.1007/978-981-97-2069-9_2]

[70]   Shatte ABR, Hutchinson DM, Teague SJ. Machine learning in mental health: a scoping review of methods and applications. Psychol Med 2019; 49(9): 1426-48.
[http://dx.doi.org/10.1017/S0033291719000151] [PMID: 30744717]

[71]   Amann J. Machine learning in stroke medicine: opportunities and challenges for risk prediction and prevention. In: Jotterand F, Ienca M, Eds. Artificial Intelligence in Brain and Mental Health. Philosophical, Ethical & Policy Issues 2022; pp. 57-71.

[72]   Cai YQ, Gong DX, Tang LY, *et al.* Pitfalls in developing machine learning models for predicting cardiovascular diseases: challenges and solutions. J Med Internet Res 2024; 26: e47645.
[http://dx.doi.org/10.2196/47645] [PMID: 38869157]

[73]   Rahmani AM, Yousefpoor E, Yousefpoor MS, *et al.* Machine learning (ML) in medicine: review, applications, and challenges. Mathematics 2021; 9(22): 2970.
[http://dx.doi.org/10.3390/math9222970]

[74]   Gogoi P, Valan JA. Machine learning approaches for predicting and diagnosing chronic kidney disease: current trends, challenges, solutions, and future directions. Int Urol Nephrol 2024; 57(4): 1245-68.
[http://dx.doi.org/10.1007/s11255-024-04281-5] [PMID: 39560857]

[75]   Xie S, Yu Z, Lv Z. Multi-disease prediction based on deep learning: a survey. Comput Model Eng Sci 2021; 128(2): 489-522.
[http://dx.doi.org/10.32604/cmes.2021.016728]

[76]   Naser MA, Majeed AA, Alsabah M, Al-Shaikhli TR, Kaky KM. A review of machine learning's role in cardiovascular disease prediction: recent advances and future challenges. Algorithms 2024; 17(2): 78.

[http://dx.doi.org/10.3390/a17020078]

[77]   Alfred R, Obit JH. The roles of machine learning methods in limiting the spread of deadly diseases: A systematic review. Heliyon 2021; 7(6): e07371.
[http://dx.doi.org/10.1016/j.heliyon.2021.e07371] [PMID: 34179541]

CHAPTER 11

Virtual Reality and Augmented Reality in Medical Training and Therapy

Sunita[1], Akhil Sharma[1], Akanksha Sharma[1], Ashish Verma[2] and **Shaweta Sharma[3,*]**

[1] *R.J. College of Pharmacy, Raipur, Uttar Pradesh-202165, India*

[2] *Department of Pharmacy, Mangalmay Pharmacy College, Greater Noida, Uttar Pradesh-201306, India*

[3] *Department of Pharmacy, School of Medical and Allied Sciences, Galgotias University, Greater Noida, Uttar Pradesh-201310, India*

Abstract: The virtual reality (VR) and augmented reality (AR) revolutionize medical training and therapy. VR immerses users in a completely simulated environment, whereas AR enhances real-world experiences by layering digital information. VR and AR provide groundbreaking advancements over traditional methods in medical training, such as virtual dissections, streaming of datasets visualizing anatomy, and even surgical simulations. These training methods boost skills development, crisis management skills, and tailor-made learning, which can further improve both student and professional proficiency. VR is changing the field of pain management in therapeutic settings, supporting rehabilitation for physical recovery and providing treatment strategies for mental health conditions such as anxiety, PTSD, and phobias. VR-based cognitive rehabilitation programs are enhancing the outcome of brain injury and disorder. Despite these advancements, challenges remain, such as expensive equipment, integration with healthcare systems, and acceptance among medical professionals and patients. In the future, continuing developments of immersive technology, increased accessibility, and remote applications will expand the role of VR and AR in the treatment of healthcare. This chapter focuses on the technological background, current applications, and future directions of VR and AR in medicine, as well as their possibilities of transforming the landscape of medicine as the foundation of future medical education, patient care, and therapy.

Keywords: Augmented reality, Healthcare innovation, Immersive technology, Medical simulation, Medical therapy, Medical training, Virtual reality.

---

* **Corresponding author Shaweta Sharma:** Department of Pharmacy, School of Medical and Allied Sciences, Galgotias University, Greater Noida, Uttar Pradesh-201310, India; E-mail: shawetasharma@galgotiasuniversity.edu.in

Shaweta Sharma, Akhil Sharma, Shivkanya Fuloria & Anurag Singh (Eds.)
All rights reserved-© 2025 Bentham Science Publishers

INTRODUCTION

Virtual Reality (VR) is a computer-generated virtual environment that can either replicate or be similar to the real world. It allows the user to interact with three-dimensional (3D) settings by utilizing devices such as controllers, headsets, and gloves. VR replaces the real world with a simulated one, offering an isolated yet interactive experience. Unlike VR, AR enhances the existing surroundings rather than replacing them, providing a blended view of virtual and physical elements. From hardware to software, the combination of VR and AR is a great way to give experiences beyond other interface systems, thus becoming a great tool in many industries. In healthcare, these technologies are reshaping how training, treatment, and patient engagement are conducted, providing innovative solutions to complex challenges [1, 2].

The applications of VR and AR are becoming popular and are being used as disruptive technologies in the healthcare field because they can help improve training, diagnosis, and therapy. VR provides realistic simulations of clinical scenarios for medical training, enabling students and practicing medical professionals to practice surgical operations without the risk. AR complements this by providing real-time guidance during live surgeries, overlaying critical information like anatomy information or imaging scans onto the surgical field. They enhance the patient education experience as patients find it easier to visualize the condition as well as the treatment. In therapy, VR is used for exposure therapy in mental health treatments, which gives patients the opportunity to face their fears or PTSD (Post-traumatic stress disorder) in a controlled environment. AR enhances physical rehab by visualizing exercises and providing better feedback for more efficient workouts. Moreover, the use of these in pain management and telemedicine highlights their usefulness for a variety of healthcare needs. AR and VR must also be integral to modern healthcare innovation because their ability to merge virtual and physical realities streamlines processes that promote accessibility and personalized care [3 - 5].

TECHNOLOGICAL COMPONENTS OF VR AND AR

Medical training and therapy use VR and AR based on their capability to simulate and augment scenarios in the real world. VR provides completely digital environments, and AR interactively blends our digital information with the physical world. To provide their function in healthcare, both technologies depend on efficient hardware and software. Whether it be realistic simulations for training purposes or real-time guidance during procedures, the dynamic interaction between VR and AR promises precision, accessibility, and efficiency. Using cutting-edge computing, sensing, and visualization technologies, these innovations are poised to revolutionize medicine [6].

Virtual Reality (VR)

Virtual reality generates non-exploratory digital environments, replicating real-world scenarios or cultivating new ones for training, education, and therapy. The immersive nature of VR allows medical professionals to practice complex procedures or simulated patient interactions without any real-world repercussions. This increases the amount of time on task, results in fewer mistakes, and builds self-efficacy. VR has become a key feature of new healthcare technology as it can tailor a person-specific environment to individuals, providing realistic experiences to users to adjust to different situations [7].

Hardware

VR is dependent on its hardware, such as VR headsets, motion sensors, and haptic feedback devices, which make it effective. Headsets like the Oculus Quest, HTC Vive, and PlayStation VR provide you with immersive visuals and sound to interact with 3D environments. Motion sensors monitor real-life physical movements and transfer them to the virtual space in real-time. Haptic devices like gloves and suits, which provide tactile sensations to users, enable them to feel the virtual world. In the health sector, these technologies act as virtual human beings to perform effective simulations of surgeries, helping in training for upcoming trainees. A critical feature of such devices is haptic feedback, which simulates the texture and stiffness of human tissue and is essential to practicing the fundamentals of performance. The progress in hardware is making it lighter, cheaper, and more accessible, and it has led to the general adoption of VR in the medical field [8, 9].

Software

VR software is important for developing these dynamic simulations specific to the medical field and is important for practicing and practical learning. Platforms like Osso VR and ImmersiveTouch provide a realistic 3D visualisation of surgical procedures featuring 3D anatomical models and procedural training modules. These applications replicate real-world situations like conducting surgeries, diagnosing diseases, and managing emergencies. AI and machine learning in VR software can measure a user's performance and offer personalized feedback for improvement. For example, pain VR is an application that provides parallel environments for pain relief and cognitive therapy in a therapeutic environment. VR software is also more useful in health care because it has certain EHR interactivity and training analytics built into it for seamless interoperability [10].

Augmented Reality (AR)

Through AR, the real world becomes a platform for digital content, including images, instructions, or 3D models. The main benefit it offers is that it can deliver information without removing the user from the environment. From guided surgeries to patient education, AR applications in healthcare provide context-specific interactive insights that allow for improved outcomes [11].

Hardware

AR hardware refers to equipment such as AR glasses (*e.g.*, Microsoft HoloLens, Magic Leap), smartphones, and tablets. With the application of AR glasses, surgeons can be directed to digital overlays that can provide critical patient data or anatomical guides in a hands-free manner. With powerful cameras and sensors built in, smartphones and tablets become portable AR platforms for patient education and diagnostic assistance. These devices require accurate tracking technologies to register digital data to the real world consistently and accurately. In healthcare, AR hardware is designed to be lightweight and ergonomic, enabling prolonged use in clinical settings. Continued improvements in display resolution, battery life, and connectivity are making AR devices more efficient and reliable for medical applications [12].

Software

AR Software can enable seamless integration of digital content with a physical setting in real-time to improve the accuracy of decision-making and procedural tasks. Applications such as AccuVein and Medivis use AR to project vein maps or anatomical guides onto patients, helping with surgeries or injections. AR software uses AI to evaluate data and offer specific interpretations, such as marking areas of interest in medical imaging. Healthcare professionals can customize the interface to fit a range of clinical scenarios. As machine vision and data processing keep getting better, AR software is quickly becoming a must-have for enhancing human expertise within the healthcare sector [13, 14].

Difference Between VR and AR

Virtual Reality (VR) and Augmented Reality (AR) are both immersive technologies, but they differ in their approach and application, as shown in Table 1.

VR/AR IN MEDICAL TRAINING

VR and AR are currently changing medical training by offering the opportunity for hands-on experiences without the dangers that come with traditional methods.

VR and AR can be used in medical education to simulate complex medical procedures, allowing students to practice and refine their skills in a controlled environment. This is done through the combination of interactive models and instant feedback on their performance during exercises, in this case, including anatomy, surgeries, and diagnostics, and an overview of students is necessary for better skill enhancement. They are also a great assessment and evaluation tool that the instructor uses to test competency, monitor progress, pinpoint where improvement is needed, and provide improved, individualized medical training, as depicted in Fig. (1) [20].

Table 1. Key differences between virtual reality and augmented reality.

Aspect	Virtual Reality (VR)	Augmented Reality (AR)	References
User Interaction	Users' engagement with an entire virtual environment.	Users interact with both virtual and real environments.	[15]
Immersion	Complete immersion in a 3D virtual environment.	Partial immersion is where digital elements overlay the real world.	[16]
Environment	Has no physical surroundings and is completely virtual.	Real-world surroundings are enhanced with digital content.	[17]
Level of Reality	Complete disconnection from reality.	Augments real-world experience with virtual objects.	[18]
Primary Focus	Creating a new, self-contained reality.	Increasing or altering the real world with digital information.	[19]

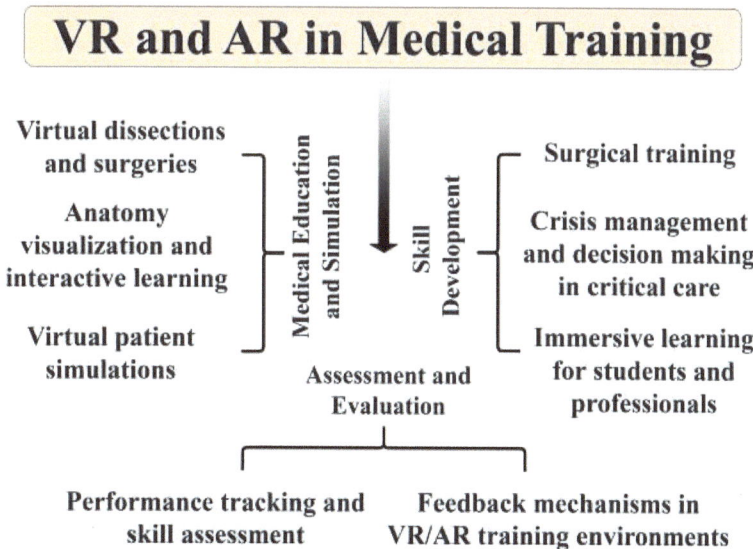

Fig. (1). Use of VR and AR in medical training.

Medical Education and Simulation

VR and Augmented Reality (AR) have made medical education come to life through realistic simulations and interactive learning experiences. Such technologies close the gap between academic theory and practical experience, providing students with opportunities to practice and develop critical decision-making and procedural skills.

Virtual Dissections and Surgeries

Medical students can use virtual reality platforms to conduct dissections or surgical procedures in an immersive, yet controlled setting. These simulations mimic anatomy perfectly in real life, letting learners peel back layers of anatomy. The virtual dissections have no ethical implications and can be practiced as many times as desired, which is not possible with traditional cadaver-based dissections. Finally, augmented reality takes these experiences a step further by displaying digital information over physical models, giving those learning the opportunity to experience mixed-reality learning. VR surgical simulations replicate the operating room for surgeons, who practice procedures, develop dexterity, and perfect decisions. Simulation-based training frequently includes haptic feedback, replicating the tactile sensations associated with real surgical procedures, providing enhanced motor skill practice, and a higher level of confidence. With the advancement in technology, virtual dissections and surgeries are becoming valuable assets in medical science education; they reduce cadaver dependence while ensuring quality training [21].

Anatomy Visualization and Interactive Learning

VR and AR also provide an interactive three-dimensional representation of the human body, which gives a unique ability to understand human anatomy better. With the possibility to examine complex anatomical systems from all angles, zoom in on elaborate structures, and comprehend spatial relationships at a deep level, medical students can learn it. Classroom-based AR applications projecting realistic anatomical models can provide collaborative and interactive learning. Such methods of anatomy education, where one method is more dynamic and engaging, help in understanding and retention of knowledge, which cannot be achieved so well by traditional methods. Users can also simulate physiological processes, such as blood circulation and neural transmission, within the same application in a more interactive manner, which can make textbook content a lot more appealing. This interactive mindset suits a variety of learning methods, making it possible for anatomy education to be even more accessible and engaging. VR and AR are changing how medics learn and apply anatomical concepts by closing the gap between theory and practice [22].

Virtual Patient Simulations

Virtual patient simulations (VPS) use VR to put medical students and professionals in a simulated, realistic environment where they can practice diagnosing and treating virtual patients. These simulations replicate different clinical scenarios, allowing trainees to practice theoretical applications in realistic but safe environments. VPS scenarios include patient histories, vital signs, and responses to treatments, forcing the participant to think fast and make decisions. This can improve diagnostic accuracy, ability to communicate, and teamwork across disciplines. While VPS helps to visualize actual structures in 3D space, AR helps to augment these structures with patient information like imaging results or lab reports in the practitioner's field of view to support decision-making. VPS not only aids in training but also helps to evaluate clinical competencies and provide learners with objective feedback. By offering a safe yet realistic environment to practice and refine skills, virtual patient simulations are paving the way for the future of standards in medical education and training [23].

Skill Development

VR and AR offer unique environments that allow users to learn and practice skills where they are completely safe and free to test out their skills in environments tailored to their exact needs. From mastering intricate surgical procedures to developing critical thinking skills under pressure, these technologies cater to diverse learning needs. This provides the best opportunity for practice in a safe and controlled environment, limitless environments to practice and advance their skills through VR and AR before gaining real-life experience out in the marketplace. From excelling in complex surgical procedures to honing decision-making abilities in time-pressured scenarios, the technologies serve an array of learning functions. They are even more useful for instant feedback and progress tracking in many areas, securing a continuous feedback loop of learning [24].

Surgical Training

VR and AR have revolutionized surgical training due to realistic simulations that mimic the intricacies of real operating rooms. Virtual devices replicate actual equipment, allowing trainees to perform complex processes. These platforms provide a safe space for learners to play, whereby they can make mistakes and repeat the process repeatedly until they gain proficiency in relative safety without putting any patients at risk. VR and AR are transforming the surgical training sector, given how these technologies replicate the dynamics of a physical operating room. This creates virtual devices that reproduce real devices and enable trainees to execute intricate processes using them. These platforms afford learners a protected environment to practice by letting them be wrong and repeating the process over and over until they have mastered a skill safely and without risking any patients [25].

Crisis Management and Decision-making in Critical Care

VR and AR training facilitate healthcare professionals in developing crisis management and instantaneous decision-making skills during critical care. The technologies offer teachers high-pressure environments, like cardiac arrests or mass casualty incidents, where learners must make difficult decisions within seconds. The VR simulations re-enact such scenarios, filled with realistic patient responses, environmental challenges, and time constraints, where learners only have to practice prioritizing, resource allocation, and team coordination. AR can greatly assist real-time decision-making by projecting vital signs, diagnosis information, and other relevant data into the practitioner's view. These tools, designed for emergency protocols, allow teams to naturally practice and hone their responses to the high pressure of real-time crisis conditions. Moreover, being exposed to simulated crises over and over generates resilience and self-confidence that minimizes the chances of mistakes during real events [26, 27].

Immersive Learning for Students and Professionals

VR and AR provide a platform for an interactive and immersive learning-enabled environment for medical students and professionals. These technologies allow for the execution of clinical skills and interaction with patients by facilitating learners in immersive, virtual experiences. An example has even more unique and beneficial options, offering students the opportunity to conduct diagnostic assessments, practice bedside manner, or explore human anatomy in three-dimensional form, all of which greatly benefit understanding and compassion. Looking to the future, AR applications may complement traditional learning by providing overlaid visual input during dissections or clinical simulations that reinforce theoretical knowledge. With unparalleled attention, the learning experience provided by VR ensures quality engagement, whereas the flexible characteristics of these platforms allow for training that may very easily be tailored to the individual. In addition, gamification features such as points and challenges encourage the user to attain greater levels of proficiency. VR and AR are ushering in a new age of competency-based medical training that combines education with technology [28, 29].

Assessment and Evaluation

VR and AR provide a new approach to assessing and evaluating medical training. These technologies provide a realistic clinical environment for educators to evaluate a trainee's performance under controlled but realistic dynamics. In

VR/AR training, evaluations can not only be objective and accurate but also track clinical decision-making, procedural performance, and patient interaction. They can also assess elements like time taken to respond, correctness, and number of steps taken to complete a process, and curate detailed analytics to inform the next steps for learners. This marks an objective evaluation that makes it more bias-free, consistent, and reproducible [30].

Performance Tracking and Skill Assessment in VR/AR Training

Real-time performance tracking and assessment is one of the most important uses of VR and AR in medical training. Such systems are built with motion sensors, haptic feedback, and eye-tracking technology, allowing continuous monitoring of the trainee's actions. Similarly, for VR, motion sensors can identify whether a trainee performs the procedure optimally, including all aspects from incision accuracy to instrument handling. AR enhances the trainee's view with real-time data, assisting with skill learning and clinical practice performance tracking. This real-time data collection supports holistic feedback, including objective measures of time management, technique execution, and decision-making.

VR and AR technologies provide the opportunity to design contexts and closely copy all types of clinical situations, from simple to complicated cases, so the trainees can observe all necessary conditions and emergencies. Performance tracking not only assesses technical skills but also cognitive functions, such as accurate diagnosis and clinical reasoning. This type of evaluation also helps in the process of identifying gaps over time so that trainers can customize the training experience according to the needs of the individual. Ultimately, VR and AR provide an invaluable tool for assessing medical skills in a highly realistic, controlled, and measurable way, enhancing both learner confidence and competency [31].

Feedback Mechanisms in VR/AR Training Environments

Feedback is an essential aspect of the VR and AR training environment that makes the learning process possible. They offer on-demand contextual training feedback, and trainees can see the corrections to their errors instantly. For instance, in a surgical VR simulator, if a trainee makes a mistake, the system can give corrective feedback on handling, suggesting that the trainee change the positioning of the hand or make a more accurate incision. Likewise, feedback in AR settings can involve visual overlays illuminating regions in need of adaptation, for instance, wrong anatomy or improper tool use. In the training session, raw data can be used to create detailed feedback reports, offering quantitative and qualitative evaluations. Both trainees and instructors can access these reports to discuss strengths, weaknesses, and further development opportunities. They can also get tailored responses based on their performance, thus focusing on what they need to practice and improve on [32, 33].

VR/AR IN MEDICAL THERAPY

Medical therapy is another area where VR and AR have high importance, as elaborated in Fig. (**2**). For pain management, VR and AR serve to distract the patient and take their minds off the pain, helping to reduce its perception. They can also guide rehabilitation exercises and improve motor skills. Moreover, VR and AR help in mental health therapy and cognitive rehabilitation by presenting therapeutic situations to manage mental health problems such as stress, anxiety, and cognitive disorders [34].

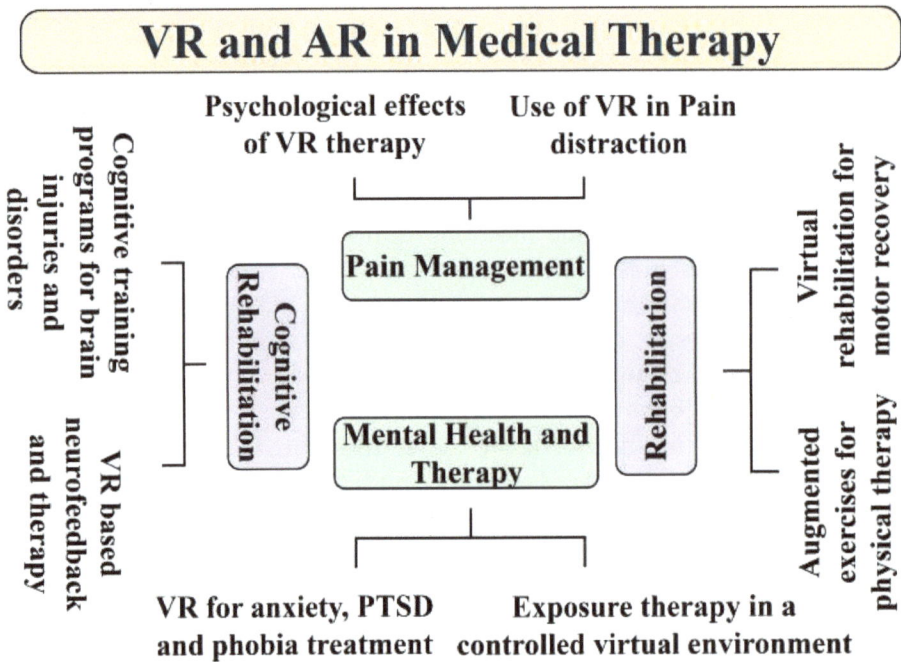

Fig. (2). Use of VR and AR in medical therapy.

Pain Management

VR and AR have emerged as innovative tools in pain management. Patients suffering from acute and chronic pain, such as burn victims or those affected by fibromyalgia, can greatly benefit from VR and AR. They offer a different sensory experience that reduces the awareness of the pain, thus providing substantial comfort without the use of medication. It can be used alongside conventional pain management methods as a non-invasive adjunct, increasing treatment efficacy [35, 36].

Use of VR in Pain Distraction

VR, originally a research tool for understanding the sensory and emotional pathways to pain, has been recognized over the years, especially in clinical contexts (eg, for burn patients and chronic conditions) as an effective method for distraction from pain. Burn victims, who often feel severe burning pain as wounds are treated, can use VR to distract themselves from the pain associated with the trauma. VR environments, such as a calming beach scene or a game that requires active engagement, can immerse the patient in an alternate reality, thereby decreasing the brain's processing of pain signals. The VR environment helps to reduce anxiety, enhance relaxation, and provide a sense of control, which can be empowering for the patient [37].

Similarly, for those patients who suffer from chronic pain, it can provide a non-pharmacological alternative that can decrease the use of opioids and other pain medications that can cause unwanted side effects and substance abuse. Not only do guided experiences take patients through coping strategies that build those skills over time for pain management in day-to-day life, but VR also immerses them in different environments. Additionally, high percentages of patients who engage in therapy with VR experience apparent reductions in the intensity and emotional distress associated with pain. In many cases, VR has also demonstrated prolonged relief in many patients, with continued pain decreasing well after the end of the VR session [38].

Psychological Effects of VR Therapy

VR therapy has a strong psychological component as it completely changes both the way patients experience physical pain and the way they identify mentally with the experience. VR experiences can be an effective form of distraction, so immersing patients in VR experiences can relieve them from anxiety and stress, which is a common emotional response to pain. Studies show that when patients are immersed in such distracting virtual environments, the centers of the brain that process pain become less active, yielding reduced emotional and physical pain experience. This advantage is especially helpful with those who suffer from chronic pain since the mental aspect can amplify the pain. Additionally, patients can escape from the real world, burdened with pain, and experience the feeling of control, participation, and social engagement in a safe environment through VR. This quick psychological separation proves crucial in stopping the pain and stress feedback loop [38].

The patients feel a great sense of self-efficacy, and taking part in therapeutic activities in the virtual world can also boost their mood and overall mental health level, which VR therapy can represent better. In studies of individuals experiencing chronic pain conditions, VR treatment has led to emotional benefits as well, with decreases in learning, depression and anxiety being reported. VR not only focuses on the physical aspects of pain but also strengthens their minds and spirits, instilling hope and greater long-term confidence in treatment capabilities among patients [39].

Rehabilitation

VR and AR have changed the old method of rehabilitation therapy with a new approach for motor disabled patients. These technologies can completely immerse the patient in simulated environments, thus engaging them and improving recovery processes. Combining VR and AR with physical therapy exercises provides patients with gamified therapy that increases motivation, decreases pain perception, and accelerates rehabilitation. Because VR and AR provide real-time feedback, they can identify when a user is making progress and when a change in their therapeutic exercise is needed to cater to individual needs, maximizing rehabilitation potential. The field is still emerging, but it holds great potential to enrich the quality of clinical care [40].

Virtual Rehabilitation for Motor Recovery

Virtual rehabilitation has become a cornerstone in motor recovery therapies among patients with stroke, spinal cord injuries, and other diseases. Through VR simulations, they can perform active, interactive activities that target motor function recovery. These exercises more often include actual actions, like stretching, walking, or grabbing things. In this virtual environment, patients can do movements that they otherwise might not be able to do in the real world, which reduces the psychological barriers to recovery. It enables therapists to customize the individual patient, as they can manipulate the difficulty of the tasks. It offers a safe environment for the patient to rehearse certain movements without the tangible threat of injury ensuing from practice. In addition, the VR is highly immersive, which motivates the patient to participate in and enjoy the rehabilitation process itself, helping to solve one of the most important challenges in conventional physical rehabilitation [41].

Also, VR therapies have been proven to improve motor function, coordination, and balance, which are essential for recovery among stroke patients. Individuals with spinal cord injury also have an advantage, as VR can also maintain strength in muscles, and joints, and prevent complications of immobility. VR promotes neuroplasticity too, where the brain forms new connections in response to rehabilitation, a crucial factor in stroke and spinal cord injury recovery [42].

Augmented Exercises for Physical Therapy

Augmented reality is used in physical therapy, providing immediate and responsive feedback to the patient and creating an interactive rehabilitation process. AR enables patients to have a visual representation of exercises, where they can observe themselves executing movements in sync with contextual visual clues that teach them how to perform tasks correctly. This immediate feedback is critical for ensuring accurate movement patterns, which are essential for preventing further injury and promoting recovery.

For example, in physical therapy for joint replacement or rehabilitation following a sports injury, AR can overlay markers on the patient's body, guiding them through exercises to improve joint alignment, flexibility, and strength. It can also track the progress of the rehabilitation process, adjusting the difficulty and complexity of the exercises based on performance. AR has been particularly beneficial in post-operative rehabilitation, where patients can follow structured routines in real-time, while being guided by virtual elements that show them the correct form and technique [43].

AR is one of the applications that keep the patient engaged and motivated in the rehabilitation process. AR gamification makes it fun for patients to be involved in their therapy rather than consider it a boring task. Furthermore, AR provides convenience to the therapists in terms of tracking a patient remotely, which you cannot physically do in face-to-face sessions. The virtual exercises combined with AR feedback have made AR a powerful tool in contemporary physical therapy, allowing for enhanced results for patients with a variety of conditions [44].

Mental Health and Therapy

VR and AR technologies are rapidly changing the landscape for mental health and therapeutic interventions, offering high-value content and controlled virtual spaces for patients to process their challenges. Virtual reality has the potential to provide compelling, multisensory environments that mimic real-life experiences, where patients can meet challenges and rehearse skills to cope with them in a safe, controllable environment. In contrast, AR overlays digital components on top of the physical world, thereby making it possible to engage with virtual elements without being detached from actual reality. Each technology has shown breakthrough potential for many mental health disorders (anxiety, depression, and PTSD) by providing innovative means of patient engagement and therapeutic delivery [45, 46].

VR for Anxiety, PTSD, and Phobia Treatment

VR has had a big impact on treating anxiety disorders, PTSD, and phobias, where patients are immersed in a controlled therapeutic environment that focuses on confronting their fears in a safe environment. When first treating anxiety, VR provides simulated scenarios that people with an addiction can slowly face their triggers, such as public speaking or social interactions, without any real-life implications. VR exposure therapy for PTSD recreates scenarios associated with trauma, allowing patients to cope with memories and feelings in a safe environment where therapists are present. Eventually, this slow exposure lessens the emotional reactivity from painful memories and reframes patients' reactions [47].

VR gives patients the opportunity to face their specific phobias in a virtual world- be it heights, spiders, or small spaces. Therapists control the amount of exposure to this and keep the patients at an optimal level of stress. Research has demonstrated that VR therapy decreases phobia severity through gradual desensitization of phobic triggers in a safe and controllable environment. By facing their fears in a virtual space, patients gain confidence and experience resilience that carries over into their everyday lives and prepares them for future encounters with these anxieties. Moreover, because VR is immersive, it can encourage more patient engagement and satisfaction with the treatment. Additionally, the immersive nature of the technology can help patients stick with the therapy process, which can be difficult with other modes of treatment. The interactive elements of VR allow for the management of psychological conditions to take a more interactive and less invasive approach, expanding the role and scale of the use of VR in the management of a range of mental health conditions [48].

Exposure Therapy in a Controlled Virtual Environment

When it comes to treating anxiety, PTSD, and phobias, exposure therapy remains a central paradigm of treatment, and recently, there has been much appeal to providing exposure in VR as it allows for a high level of administration control with less concern about the safety of potential stressors. Usually, exposure therapy requires facing your fear step by step, which is relatively unmanageable in reality. VR overcomes these limitations by creating an immersive and safe environment, enabling gradual exposure for the patients in a way that is impossible to replicate in physical reality.

During VR-based exposure therapy, individuals are navigated through virtual environments that resemble their particular phobias, for example, confined spaces, dark places, or traumatic experiences, while supervised by a qualified therapist. The patient can step into a virtual world in which the level of intensity of the exposure can be controlled, from less threatening to progressively more challenging as the client becomes desensitized to their triggers in a safe environment. This enables therapists to allow the patient to progress with the therapy at their own pace, so they are neither overwhelmed nor still moving forward, overcoming their fear [49].

Perhaps the most significant advantage of virtual exposure therapy is its flexibility. It means patients can sit in the comfort of their own homes to have their therapy sessions, eliminating the need for traveling or encountering real-world stimuli that can be triggering and impede learning. Not only does it allow patients to face their fears over and over again in a safe environment, but it has also been shown to hasten the desensitization process more than standard methods would. In person, it is easy to feel embarrassed or ashamed, but VR eliminates this, generating more openness for the patients to be involved in the process. Virtual reality exposure therapy is an exciting, highly efficacious treatment modality for mental health disorders. By combining the power of technology with psychological principles, VR can provide meaningful therapeutic experiences that are both practical and impactful in helping individuals confront and manage their fears [50].

Cognitive Rehabilitation

Cognitive rehabilitation encompasses the use of therapeutic interventions to improve mental abilities, including memory, attention, and executive functions, which may be impaired owing to chronic neurological conditions. VR and AR provide novel platforms for cognitive rehabilitation by exposing the patient to interactive environments that simulate real-world situations. That means the technology offers both a safe environment for patients to rehearse cognitive challenges while also tracking progress and providing real-time feedback. For patients suffering from brain injury, dementia, or neurodegenerative diseases, VR and AR can provide tailored therapeutic experiences that are attractive and motivating for patients and can stimulate cognitive function improvement [51].

Cognitive Training Programs for Brain Injuries and Disorders

Cognitive training programs using VR and AR have emerged as valuable solutions in the rehabilitation of brain-impaired individuals, including those with Alzheimer's disease, traumatic brain injury (TBI), and stroke. The programs involve cognitive exercises, delivered through these immersive simulations, which work to rebuild the neural pathways in the brain that are frail and need some restructuring; memory improves, and mental sharpness is regained. In the case of those suffering from Alzheimer's, VR environments can simulate regular day-to-day activities, making them reassert their memories and problem-solving skills. They can simulate real-world scenarios, including cooking, shopping, or moving through public areas, where patients can rehearse in a safe environment. It presents repeated adaptive challenges that can be calibrated to individual progress to make it possible to make tasks successively more challenging as cognitive capacity increases [52].

VR-based training can be useful to activate specific brain regions related to spatial memory, executive functions, and motor control so that it represents a more holistic rehabilitation approach. VR environments can be crafted to reflect everyday obstacles associated with regaining motor skills, cognitive functions, and attention spans for patients with traumatic brain injury and stroke. These cognitive training programs are frequently integrative with biofeedback, providing the individual with an immediate response to their performance. Such positive reinforcement serves to enhance cognitive links and increase brain capacity overall. Therefore, VR and AR-based cognitive training programs are effective, enjoyable, and possibly game-changing technology for rehabilitation [53].

VR-Based Neurofeedback and Therapy

Combining virtual reality with neurofeedback therapy, VR-based neurofeedback therapy allows patients to modulate their brain activity as they experience immersive environments, creating a new way to treat neurological and psychological disorders. Neurofeedback is a technique that depends on instant brainwave feedback, most often based on EEG sensor signals, to help patients learn to control their brain activity. Patients use a VR-based neurofeedback system while wearing EEG caps or sensors that measure their brain waves during the play of interactive VR. These systems offer visual or auditory feedback in real-time based on the patient's brain activity, rewarding changes in the brainwave patterns in the desired direction, and prompting self-regulation. Patients can literally see and change their brains, which has proven effective for treating ADHD, anxiety, depression, and PTSD [54].

Moreover, the immersive nature of VR offers a distinctive space to recreate stress-inducing situations or relaxing surroundings and allows patients to apply emotional regulation skills immediately. A powerful feature of VR-based neurofeedback is that it makes it possible to create highly individualized interventions, meaning therapists can adjust the difficulty and type of stimuli depending on patient specifics. Not only does this tailor the neurofeedback therapy treatment to the individual, but the immersive nature of VR therapy can also help to keep patients engaged and interested in their own recovery. Patients gain the ability to change neural circuit activation, resulting in cognitive and emotional regulation improvements maintained over time. Such an innovative method particularly helps patients who may struggle to stick to traditional means due to boredom or complexity [55].

CHALLENGES IN IMPLEMENTATION

There are also a lot of challenges to the implementation of VR and AR in medical training and therapy, are represented in Fig. (**3**). Technological hurdles include high-end hardware, high costs, and continuous software updates. A few medical institutions may also not even have the proper infrastructure to enable such technologies. Another significant challenge is acceptance and adaptation, as healthcare professionals and patients may be hesitant to adopt new technologies due to unfamiliarity or skepticism about their efficacy. These challenges can be overcome through thorough training, providing user-friendly interfaces, and showing the potential benefits of VR and AR in medical education or therapy approaches [56].

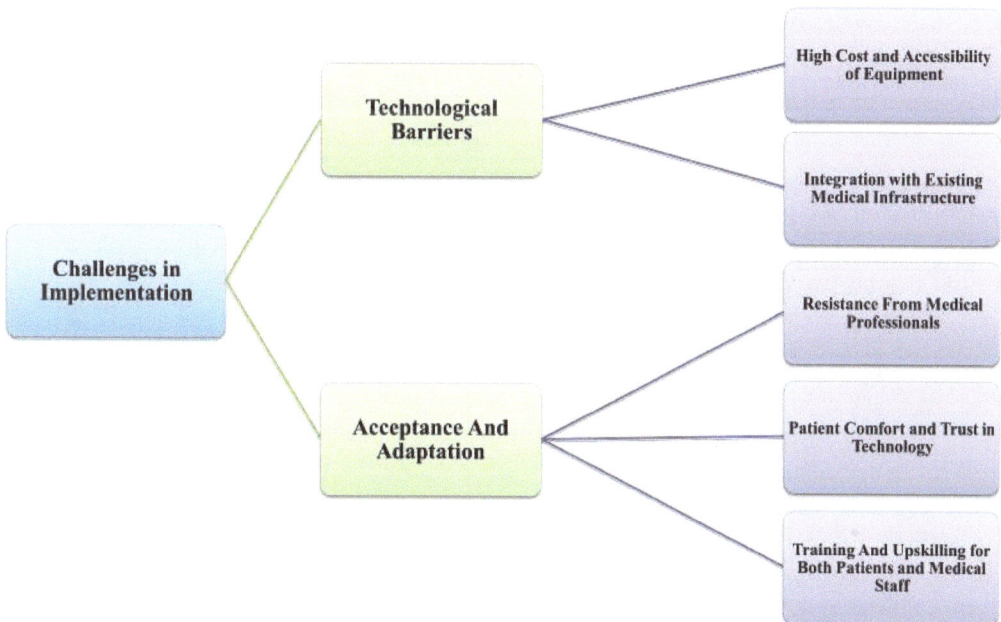

Fig. (3). Challenges associated with implementing virtual reality (VR) and augmented reality (AR).

Technological Barriers

The use of VR and AR in medical training and therapy faces multiple technological issues. They comprise the difficulty of providing realistic and effective simulations, seamless functionality, and the ability to maintain stability and reliability during prolonged use. Additionally, the hardware requirements for these technologies, which require powerful processing units and high-definition displays, also make it difficult to scale them up [57].

High Cost and Accessibility of Equipment

One of the primary barriers to the widespread adoption of VR and AR in medical training and therapy is the high cost of the necessary equipment. The sophisticated hardware, such as headsets, motion tracers, and haptic feedback devices, is usually expensive. Thus, posing a barrier to hospitals, medical schools, and clinics with small budgets. Also, ongoing maintenance and upgrading of these systems contribute to the cost. Though costs are expected to drop over time as the technology matures and becomes more ubiquitous, this initial financial barrier is significant. Access to these technologies is also limited, as almost every VR/AR technology is usually exclusively accessible to larger medical institutions or those within the most technologically advanced areas, disadvantaging smaller or less-funded institutions. For these reasons, making VR and AR more affordable and accessible will be crucial in enhancing the reach and efficacy of these technologies in the medical field [58, 59].

Integration with Existing Medical Infrastructure

Another major challenge is integrating VR and AR technologies into existing medical infrastructure. Existing systems for medical imaging, patient records, and training, which are already widely used by hospitals and clinics, may not be compatible with the new VR/AR system. This integration often requires substantial investments in upgrading existing IT systems, as well as the development of new workflows to incorporate VR/AR solutions into daily operations. Moreover, it is important to have trained personnel who can help doctors and healthcare professionals use these technologies without changing their routine processes. The complexity of aligning VR/AR technologies with existing tools like Electronic Health Records (EHR) and diagnostic systems, while maintaining patient safety and care continuity, requires a well-coordinated effort and a significant commitment of resources. Successful integration will rely on public protocols and open-source platforms to enable seamless interaction across the old system and the new [60].

Acceptance and Adaptation

The acceptance and adaptation of VR and AR in medical training and therapy face significant challenges. Healthcare professionals might be resistant to adopting new technologies, as they may be unfamiliar with them and skeptical about their effectiveness or potential risks. Additionally, the costs associated with implementing VR and AR systems, alongside the need for ongoing maintenance and upgrades, can deter institutions from adopting these innovations. Overcoming these hurdles requires a shift in mindset, starting with understanding the long-term benefits such as improved patient outcomes, enhanced training simulations, and cost savings. Positive early results, coupled with tailored training programs, can help in building trust and acceptance.

Resistance from Medical Professionals

The most frequent barrier to the use of VR and AR technologies in a healthcare environment is resistance from medical professionals. Virtual simulations are a relatively new area of research in the field of education and health care, so many practitioners may have doubts about their effectiveness and reliability compared to other methods. Additionally, some professionals may feel overwhelmed by the technological complexity of VR and AR, fearing that it may disrupt established workflows or require significant time and effort to master. Solving this resistance is showing how these technologies can improve clinical outcomes, with a literature review evidencing their potential and possible effectiveness to improve diagnosis, treatment planning, or patient care. In addition, encouraging collaboration between technology developers and medical practitioners can help ensure VR and AR systems are easy to use and well-established in healthcare routines. Over time, ongoing training, education, and experience with these innovations will allow medical professionals to become more receptive to using them as beneficial components in both training and therapeutic settings [61].

Patient Comfort and Trust in Technology

These advances can only be introduced in medical therapy if the patient is comfortable with and trusts the VR and AR technology. A lot of patients might be tentative about using virtual platforms, and this could be due to not being accustomed to the technology or feeling that the technology can be invasive. Trust in virtual environments can also be hindered by doubts about their accuracy, safety, and privacy. Resolving these issues needs to be handled by thoughtfully designing VR and AR applications, considering user experience, and making clear how these technologies function and what benefits they provide. Showing patients that these technologies are safe, effective, and useful for treating their own disease may help alleviate these fears. Furthermore, simulation of the device, soliciting feedback, and engaging the patient in the design process can allow the patient to feel a sense of control and understanding. Trust by patients is built upon their perception that the care will be transparent and focused on their well-being, knowing that caregivers will use the best tools available to optimize their health [62].

Training and Upskilling for Both Patients and Medical Staff

Effective incorporation of VR and AR in healthcare would require extensive training and upskilling of both the patients and the medical staff. It is crucial for healthcare professionals to learn the ways in which they will use these technologies to ensure they are seamlessly integrated into clinical practice. It mandates training on the usage of VR and AR tools, comprehension of the software that comes along, and the usage of innovative techniques related to virtual diagnosis and other treatment procedures. Accommodating technological advances and their medical applicability will also need to be a core element of ongoing professional development. Patients also benefit from tailored training sessions designed to meet their specific needs and comfort level, which helps decrease patient anxiety and increase engagement with the technology. This can include becoming comfortable with VR headsets, instruction for traveling through virtual spaces, and assistance in using these tools for rehabilitation or treatment. Providing instant and actionable training for everyone involved will also increase the general effectiveness of virtual and augmented reality applications in healthcare, as both medical institution staff and patients will be more assured in operating technology and ensuring the best outcome [63].

FUTURE PROSPECTS

VR and AR stand for use in medical training and therapy, with even more potential in the future, with the evolution of immersive technologies, expanding availability, and rising use in telemedicine and remote implementations.

The revolution of VR and AR in the field of medical science can be foreseen as technology advances, bringing learning and treatment within its purview. Similarly, in medical training, VR simulations allow students and healthcare professionals to practice complex procedures in a controlled, safe setting. As graphics, haptic feedback, and real-time interaction improve, VR should continue to provide increasingly accurate simulations to allow users to perform more complex surgeries, diagnostic tests, and clinical skills exercises without physical models or cadavers. Learning experiences and competency in certain medical fields can be fortified by these advancements without extensive real-time training, thus decreasing possible mistakes in real-life scenarios [64].

The expanding accessibility and affordability of VR and AR in healthcare is one of the most important trends shaping the future of VR and AR design in general. Over the next few years, the cost of VR and AR devices is expected to decrease as technology becomes more mainstream, making these tools more accessible to a larger pool of medical institutions, practitioners, and patients. Science and technology have a long history of democratizing the availability of these tools for underserved and rural minorities who have limited or no access to quality medical care, training, or targeted types of therapy. Specifically, AR shows great potential in helping patients during physical therapy, cognitive impairment, or mental health treatment. For example, AR can project visual guides and interactive components onto the real-world environment that can assist a patient with exercises or exercises in behavioral therapy to promote healing or improvement [65].

The expansion of VR and AR technologies into telemedicine and remote healthcare applications is poised to play a pivotal role in the future of healthcare. These technologies will facilitate access to remote consultation, diagnosis, and therapy *via* immersive experiences, connecting patients and health professionals in areas where in-person care is rare. Practitioners can also have virtual consultations with patients living in remote areas, simulating real-life interactions, thanks to VR and AR technology. The continuous evolution of telehealth platforms integrates immersive technology, which will drive new growth of real-time remote treatment, enhancing patient outcomes at lower costs and logistical complexity. VR and AR promise to change the way health care is delivered to patients by improving both medical education and clinical applications and providing alternative approaches to health care delivery shortly [66].

CONCLUSION

Virtual Reality (VR) and Augmented Reality (AR) are revolutionizing medical training and therapy by providing innovative and immersive solutions that surpass traditional approaches. The unique immersive nature of VR and its ability to mimic high-fidelity surgical simulations create a safe, repetitive, and highly immersive training environment. At the same time, AR has the potential to augment operational workflow and improve clinical efficiency by displaying contextual data and information in real-time decision-making. One of the most important benefits that these technologies provide is education in the field of medicine, as they can simulate dissections, surgeries, and simulations that will broaden knowledge and allow for accurate practice and improvement of skills. Moreover, virtual reality and augmented reality are enriching patient care in therapeutic environments, with the widespread implementation of VR in pain management, rehabilitation, and mental health treatments. Some applications serve as target platforms for motor rehabilitation for stroke, exposure therapy for anxiety and PTSD, as well as cognitive rehabilitation for neurological disorders.

However, the use of VR and AR in healthcare does not go without challenges, including the expensive costs of technology, integration with existing medical infrastructure, and concerns regarding patient comfort and professional adoption.

However, hardware and software improvements, as well as access to technology, are eliminating these barriers over time. VR and AR may provide opportunities for expanded accessibility, remote applications, and telemedicine integration. As the technology matures and becomes more affordable, it is poised to become a cornerstone of medical training, therapy, and patient care, offering more personalized, effective, and immersive healthcare experiences.

REFERENCES

[1]   Mustafa IS, Nahmatwlla LL, Ahmed WA, Balaji B. Virtual reality roles in the society using web technology and distributed systems. J Biomech Sci Eng 2023 Apr 17; 74-94.

[2]   Dargan S, Bansal S, Kumar M, Mittal A, Kumar K. Augmented reality: A comprehensive review. Arch Comput Methods Eng 2023; 30(2): 1057-80.
[http://dx.doi.org/10.1007/s11831-022-09831-7]

[3]   Hiran KK, Doshi R, Patel M, Eds. Modern technology in healthcare and medical education: blockchain, IoT, AR, and VR: blockchain, IoT, AR, and VR. IGI Global 2024.

[4]   Javaid M, Haleem A. Virtual reality applications toward medical field. Clin Epidemiol Glob Health 2020; 8(2): 600-5.
[http://dx.doi.org/10.1016/j.cegh.2019.12.010]

[5]   Akpan EE. Healthcare applications of augmented reality. Creating immersive learning experiences through virtual reality (VR) 2024 Sep 16; 201.

[6]   Ivanova AV VR. VR & AR technologies: opportunities and application obstacles. Strategic Decis Risk Manag 2018 Oct; 9(3): 88-107.

[7]   Ruthenbeck GS, Reynolds KJ. Virtual reality for medical training: the state-of-the-art. J Simul 2015; 9(1): 16-26.
[http://dx.doi.org/10.1057/jos.2014.14]

[8]   Anthes C, García-Hernández RJ, Wiedemann M, Kranzlmüller D. State of the art of virtual reality technology. 2016 IEEE Aerospace Conference 2016; 1-19.
[http://dx.doi.org/10.1109/AERO.2016.7500674]

[9]   Helou S, Khalil N, Daou M, El Helou E. Virtual reality for healthcare: A scoping review of commercially available applications for head-mounted displays. Digit Health 2023; 9: 20552076231178619.
[http://dx.doi.org/10.1177/20552076231178619] [PMID: 37312952]

[10]   Gupta A, Scott K, Dukewich M. Innovative technology using virtual reality in the treatment of pain: does it reduce pain *via* distraction, or is there more to it? Pain Med 2018; 19(1): 151-9.
[http://dx.doi.org/10.1093/pm/pnx109] [PMID: 29025113]

[11]   Arena F, Collotta M, Pau G, Termine F. An overview of augmented reality. Computers 2022; 11(2): 28.
[http://dx.doi.org/10.3390/computers11020028]

[12]   Kress BC. Digital optical elements and technologies (EDO19): applications to AR/VR/MR. Digital Optical Technologies. SPIE 2019; 11062: pp. 343-55.

[13]   Prieto Gomà M. Improvement and development of SurgicAR: an intraoperative Augmented Reality application for Hospital del Mar. Bachelor's thesis. Barcelona: Universitat Pompeu Fabra 2020.

[14]   Pugliesi RA. The Synergy of Artificial Intelligence and Augmented Reality for Real-time Decision-Making in Emergency Radiology. Int J Intell Autom Comp 2018; 1(1): 21-32.

[15]   Tang A, Biocca F, Lim L. Comparing differences in presence during social interaction in augmented reality versus virtual reality environments: An exploratory study. Proceedings of PRESENCE 2004;

204-8.

[16]   Verhulst I, Woods A, Whittaker L, Bennett J, Dalton P. Do VR and AR versions of an immersive cultural experience engender different user experiences? Comput Human Behav 2021; 125: 106951.
[http://dx.doi.org/10.1016/j.chb.2021.106951]

[17]   Krichenbauer M, Yamamoto G, Taketom T, Sandor C, Kato H. Augmented reality versus virtual reality for 3d object manipulation. IEEE Trans Vis Comput Graph 2018; 24(2): 1038-48.
[http://dx.doi.org/10.1109/TVCG.2017.2658570] [PMID: 28129181]

[18]   Caudell TP. Introduction to augmented and virtual reality. Telemanipulator and Telepresence Technologies 1995; 2351: 272-81.

[19]   Doerner R, Broll W, Jung B, Grimm P, Göbel M, Kruse R. Introduction to virtual and augmented reality. In: Doerner R, Broll W, Grimm P, Jung B. eds. Virtual and Augmented Reality (VR/AR) Foundations and Methods of Extended Realities (XR). Cham: Springer International Publishing 2022; pp. 1-37.
[http://dx.doi.org/10.1007/978-3-030-79062-2_1]

[20]   Hsieh MC, Lee JJ. Preliminary study of VR and AR applications in medical and healthcare education. J Nurs Health Stud 2018; 3(1): 1.
[http://dx.doi.org/10.21767/2574-2825.100030]

[21]   B Douglas D, A Wilke C, Gibson D, F Petricoin E, Liotta L. Virtual reality and augmented reality: Advances in surgery. Biol Eng Med 2017; 3(1): 1-8.
[http://dx.doi.org/10.15761/BEM.1000131]

[22]   Moro C, Štromberga Z, Raikos A, Stirling A. The effectiveness of virtual and augmented reality in health sciences and medical anatomy. Anat Sci Educ 2017; 10(6): 549-59.
[http://dx.doi.org/10.1002/ase.1696] [PMID: 28419750]

[23]   Zielke MA, Zakhidov D, Hardee G, *et al.* Developing virtual patients with VR/AR for a natural user interface in medical teaching. 2017 IEEE 5th International Conference on Serious Games and Applications for Health (SeGAH) 2017 Apr 2; 1-8.

[24]   Zhou Y, Hou J, Liu Q, *et al.* VR/AR Technology in Human Anatomy Teaching and Operation Training. J Healthc Eng 2021; 2021(1): 1-13.
[http://dx.doi.org/10.1155/2021/9998427] [PMID: 34211684]

[25]   Lahanas V, Georgiou E, Loukas C. Surgical simulation training systems: box trainers, virtual reality and augmented reality simulators. Int J Adv Robot Autom 2016; 1(2): 1-9.

[26]   Jallah JK, Kanyal D, Lalwani L, Flahn STL, Dweh TJ. Navigating tomorrow's healthcare: Exploring the future of healthcare navigation with VR, AR, and emerging technologies: A comprehensive review. Multidis Rev 2024; 8(5): 2025140.
[http://dx.doi.org/10.31893/multirev.2025140]

[27]   Chakal K. A virtual reality training application for administering basic life support in stressful scenarios. Master's thesis. Oulu (Finland): University of Oulu 2024.

[28]   Ryan GV, Callaghan S, Rafferty A, Higgins MF, Mangina E, McAuliffe F. Learning outcomes of immersive technologies in health care student education: systematic review of the literature. J Med Internet Res 2022; 24(2): e30082.
[http://dx.doi.org/10.2196/30082] [PMID: 35103607]

[29]   Khan MNR, Austal,, Lippert K. Immersive technologies in healthcare education. In: Nguyen NG, Reddy CK, Anisha PR, Eds. Intelligent systems and machine learning for industry advancements, challenges, and practices. Boca Raton (FL): CRC Press 2022; p. 115-38.

[30]   Barsom EZ, Graafland M, Schijven MP. Systematic review on the effectiveness of augmented reality applications in medical training. Surg Endosc 2016; 30(10): 4174-83.
[http://dx.doi.org/10.1007/s00464-016-4800-6] [PMID: 26905573]

[31]   Yazdi M. Augmented reality (AR) and virtual reality (VR) in maintenance training. Advances in Computational Mathematics for Industrial System Reliability and Maintainability 2024 Feb 25; 169-83.

[32]   Lampropoulos G, Fernández-Arias P, del Bosque A, Vergara D. Augmented Reality in Health Education: Transforming Nursing, Healthcare, and Medical Education and Training. Nur Rep. 2025 Aug 8;15(8):289.

[33]   Shafarenko MS, Catapano J, Hofer SOP, Murphy BD. The role of augmented reality in the next phase of surgical education. Plast Reconstr Surg Glob Open 2022; 10(11): e4656.
[PMID: 36348749]

[34]   Vashishth TK, Sharma V, Sharma KK, Kumar B, Chaudhary S, Panwar R. Virtual reality (VR) and augmented reality (AR) transforming medical applications. In: Khang A, Ed. AI and IoT-Based Technologies for Precision Medicine. IGI Global 2023; pp. 324-48.

[35]   Freitas DMO, Spadoni VS. Is virtual reality useful for pain management in patients who undergo medical procedures? Einstein (Sao Paulo) 2019; 17(2): eMD4837.
[http://dx.doi.org/10.31744/einstein_journal/2019MD4837] [PMID: 31116237]

[36]   Matthie NS, Giordano NA, Jenerette CM, *et al.* Use and efficacy of virtual, augmented, or mixed reality technology for chronic pain: a systematic review. Pain Manag (Lond) 2022; 12(7): 859-78.
[http://dx.doi.org/10.2217/pmt-2022-0030] [PMID: 36098065]

[37]   Moreau S, Thérond A, Cerda IH, *et al.* Virtual reality in acute and chronic pain medicine: an updated review. Curr Pain Headache Rep 2024; 28(9): 893-928.
[http://dx.doi.org/10.1007/s11916-024-01246-2] [PMID: 38587725]

[38]   Riva G, Baños RM, Botella C, Mantovani F, Gaggioli A. Transforming experience: the potential of augmented reality and virtual reality for enhancing personal and clinical change. Front Psychiatry 2016; 7: 164.
[http://dx.doi.org/10.3389/fpsyt.2016.00164] [PMID: 27746747]

[39]   Bell IH, Pot-Kolder R, Rizzo A, *et al.* Advances in the use of virtual reality to treat mental health conditions. Nature Reviews Psychology 2024; 3(8): 552-67.
[http://dx.doi.org/10.1038/s44159-024-00334-9]

[40]   Alamri A, Cha J, El Saddik A. AR-REHAB: An augmented reality framework for poststroke-patient rehabilitation. IEEE Trans Instrum Meas 2010; 59(10): 2554-63.
[http://dx.doi.org/10.1109/TIM.2010.2057750]

[41]   Ng YS, Chew E, Samuel GS, Tan YL, Kong KH. Advances in rehabilitation medicine. Singapore Med J 2013; 54(10): 538-51.
[http://dx.doi.org/10.11622/smedj.2013197] [PMID: 24154577]

[42]   Huang D, Mao Y, Chen P, Li L. Virtual reality training improves balance function. Neural Regen Res 2014; 9(17): 1628-34.
[http://dx.doi.org/10.4103/1673-5374.141795] [PMID: 25368651]

[43]   Da Gama AEF, Chaves TM, Figueiredo LS, *et al.* MirrARbilitation: A clinically-related gesture recognition interactive tool for an AR rehabilitation system. Comput Methods Programs Biomed 2016; 135: 105-14.
[http://dx.doi.org/10.1016/j.cmpb.2016.07.014] [PMID: 27586484]

[44]   Elizabeth A. Gamification for activation, motivation, and engagement. Phd dissertation. Salford (UK): University of Salford 2019.

[45]   Barak A, Grohol JM. Current and future trends in internet-supported mental health interventions. J Technol Hum Serv 2011; 29(3): 155-96.
[http://dx.doi.org/10.1080/15228835.2011.616939]

[46]   Singh G, Sandhu JK. Virtual and augmented reality technology for the treatment of mental health

disorders: an overview. 13th International Conference on Computing, Communication and Networking Technologies (ICCCNT) 2022; 1-5.

[47] Maples-Keller JL, Yasinski C, Manjin N, Rothbaum BO. Virtual reality-enhanced extinction of phobias and post-traumatic stress. Neurotherapeutics 2017; 14(3): 554-63.
[http://dx.doi.org/10.1007/s13311-017-0534-y] [PMID: 28512692]

[48] Freitas JRS, Velosa VHS, Abreu LTN, *et al.* Virtual reality exposure treatment in phobias: a systematic review. Psychiatr Q 2021; 92(4): 1685-710.
[http://dx.doi.org/10.1007/s11126-021-09935-6] [PMID: 34173160]

[49] Wechsler TF, Kümpers F, Mühlberger A. Inferiority or even superiority of virtual reality exposure therapy in phobias?—A systematic review and quantitative meta-analysis on randomized controlled trials specifically comparing the efficacy of virtual reality exposure to gold standard *in vivo* exposure in agoraphobia, specific phobia, and social phobia. Front Psychol 2019; 10: 1758.
[http://dx.doi.org/10.3389/fpsyg.2019.01758] [PMID: 31551840]

[50] Rizzo A, Reger G, Gahm G, Difede J, Rothbaum B. Virtual reality exposure therapy for combat-related PTSD. In: LeDoux J, Keane T, Shiromani P, eds. Post-traumatic stress disorder. Totowa (NJ): Humana Press 2009; p. 375–99.
[http://dx.doi.org/10.1007/978-1-60327-329-9_18]

[51] Velagaleti SB. A Study on Feasibility and Acceptability of an AI-Powered VR/AR Cognitive Rehabilitation Platform for Patients with Alzheimer's Disease and Dementia. International Conference on Data Science, Machine Learning and Applications 2023; 1079-83.Singapore. 2023; pp.

[52] De Luca R, Portaro S, Le Cause M, *et al.* Cognitive rehabilitation using immersive virtual reality at young age: A case report on traumatic brain injury. Appl Neuropsychol Child 2020; 9(3): 282-7.
[http://dx.doi.org/10.1080/21622965.2019.1576525] [PMID: 30838889]

[53] Riva G, Mancuso V, Cavedoni S, Stramba-Badiale C. Virtual reality in neurorehabilitation: a review of its effects on multiple cognitive domains. Expert Rev Med Devices 2020; 17(10): 1035-61.
[http://dx.doi.org/10.1080/17434440.2020.1825939] [PMID: 32962433]

[54] Cai H, Wang Z, Zhang Y, Chen Y, Hu B. A virtual-reality-based neurofeedback game framework for depression rehabilitation using a pervasive three-electrode EEG collector. Proceedings of the 12th Chinese Conference on Computer Supported Cooperative Work and Social Computing 2017; 173-6.
[http://dx.doi.org/10.1145/3127404.3127433]

[55] Prasad AA. Unveiling neurophysiological signatures of interaction in immersive worlds: A multimodal study. Master's thesis. Charlotte (NC): University of North Carolina at Charlotte 2024.

[56] Musamih A, Yaqoob I, Salah K, *et al.* Metaverse in healthcare: Applications, challenges, and future directions. IEEE Consum Electron Mag 2023; 12(4): 33-46.
[http://dx.doi.org/10.1109/MCE.2022.3223522]

[57] Ullah H, Manickam S, Obaidat M, Laghari SUA, Uddin M. Exploring the potential of metaverse technology in healthcare: Applications, challenges, and future directions. IEEE Access 2023; 11: 69686-707.
[http://dx.doi.org/10.1109/ACCESS.2023.3286696]

[58] Glegg SMN, Levac DE. Barriers, facilitators, and interventions to support virtual reality implementation in rehabilitation: a scoping review. PM R 2018; 10(11): 1237-51.
[http://dx.doi.org/10.1016/j.pmrj.2018.07.004] [PMID: 30503231]

[59] Chengoden R, Victor N, Huynh-The T, *et al.* Metaverse for healthcare: a survey on potential applications, challenges, and future directions. IEEE Access 2023; 11: 12765-95.
[http://dx.doi.org/10.1109/ACCESS.2023.3241628]

[60] Gupta I, Dangi S, Sharma S. Augmented reality-based human-machine interfaces in healthcare environment: benefits, challenges, and future trends. 2022 International Conference on Wireless Communications, Signal Processing, and Networking (WiSPNET) 2022; 251-7.

[http://dx.doi.org/10.1109/WiSPNET54241.2022.9767119]

[61]   Giblin TB, Sinkowitz-Cochran RL, Harris PL, *et al.* Clinicians' perceptions of the problem of antimicrobial resistance in health care facilities. Arch Intern Med 2004; 164(15): 1662-8.
[http://dx.doi.org/10.1001/archinte.164.15.1662] [PMID: 15302636]

[62]   Willaert WIM, Aggarwal R, Van Herzeele I, Cheshire NJ, Vermassen FE. Recent advancements in medical simulation: patient-specific virtual reality simulation. World J Surg 2012; 36(7): 1703-12.
[http://dx.doi.org/10.1007/s00268-012-1489-0] [PMID: 22532308]

[63]   Gasteiger N, van der Veer SN, Wilson P, Dowding D. How, for whom, and in which contexts or conditions augmented and virtual reality training works in upskilling health care workers: realist synthesis. JMIR Serious Games 2022; 10(1): e31644.
[http://dx.doi.org/10.2196/31644] [PMID: 35156931]

[64]   Jha G, Sharma LS, Gupta S. Future of augmented reality in healthcare department. In: Singh PK, Wierzchoń ST, Tanwar S, Ganzha M, Rodrigues JJPC, Eds. Proceedings of second international conference on computing, communications, and cyber-security. Lecture notes in networks and systems. Singapore: Springer 2021.
[http://dx.doi.org/10.1007/978-981-16-0733-2_47]

[65]   Narayanan S, Ramesh NN, Tyagi AK, Anbarasi LJ, Raj BE. Current Trends, Challenges, and Future Prospects for Augmented Reality and Virtual Reality. In: Tyagi A, Ed. Multimedia and sensory input for augmented, mixed, and virtual reality. Hershey (PA): IGI Global Scientific Publishing 2021. p. 275-81.
[http://dx.doi.org/10.4018/978-1-7998-4703-8.ch015]

[66]   Riva G, Gamberini L. Virtual reality in telemedicine. Telemed J E Health 2000; 6(3): 327-40.
[http://dx.doi.org/10.1089/153056200750040183] [PMID: 11110636]

CHAPTER 12

Digital Therapeutics: Prescribing Software for Health

Yatindra Kumar[1], Akhil Sharma[2], Sunita[2], Shilpa Thukral[3] and Sagar Pamu[4],*

[1] *Department of Pharmacy, GSVM Medical College, Kanpur, Uttar Pradesh-208002, India*

[2] *R.J. College of Pharmacy, Raipur, Uttar Pradesh-202165, India*

[3] *Dnyan Ganga College of Pharmacy, Thane, Maharashtra-400615, India*

[4] *Pharmacy Practice Department, Institute of Pharmacy, Nirma University, Ahmedabad, Gujarat-380001, India*

Abstract: Digital Therapeutics (DTx) is a new way of providing health care, and delivering evidence-based therapeutic interventions to patients using high-quality software programs to prevent, manage, or treat a medical disorder or disease. Distinct from traditional therapies and the rise of mobile health apps, DTx addresses the need for targeted treatment of diseases and behavioral health conditions, filling therapy gaps that are not addressed by current treatment options. This chapter explores the core principles of DTx, including human-centered design to promote accessibility and usability, integration with electronic health records (EHR), and the incorporation of AI and machine learning for personalized, data-driven interventions. Different kinds of DTx are mentioned, such as disease-specific therapeutics for chronic conditions like diabetes and cardiovascular diseases, behavioral health interventions including cognitive behavioral therapy (CBT) apps, and tools for chronic disease management. Next-gen technologies, such as virtual reality (VR), augmented reality (AR), wearables, and blockchain, play a crucial role in enhancing DTx by providing real-time patient feedback, immersive therapies, and security. This chapter also discusses how DTx could integrate into healthcare, its clinical adoption, the need to train healthcare providers, and plans to engage with patients. Challenges to DTx integration, including resistance to technology and interoperability issues, are examined alongside strategies to overcome these obstacles.

Keywords: AI and machine learning, Behavioral health, Chronic disease management, Digital therapeutics, Health systems integration, Healthcare technology.

* **Corresponding author Sagar Pamu:** Pharmacy Practice Department, Institute of Pharmacy, Nirma University, Ahmedabad, Gujarat-380001, India; E-mail: dr.sagar@live.com

Shaweta Sharma, Akhil Sharma, Shivkanya Fuloria & Anurag Singh (Eds.)
All rights reserved-© 2025 Bentham Science Publishers

INTRODUCTION

Digital Therapeutics (DTx) is a part of the fast-growing field of digital health, where software-based interventions are implemented to help with evidence-based therapeutic interventions. These are technology-based tools that are used to prevent, manage, or treat medical problems in patients. In contrast to traditional methods, DTx provides a scalable and accessible way to facilitate healthcare, filling current treatment deficiencies. As a consequence of these advances in digital health, DTx has come into prominence for its advantage of enhanced clinical outcomes, better patient engagement, and reduced healthcare costs [1].

By employing a targeted, evidence-based approach with clinical validation, digital therapeutics differentiate themselves from traditional therapy and mHealth (mobile health) apps. Conventional therapies, whether in the form of medications or in-person therapies, depend on physical intervention, whereas DTx utilizes software as a means of treatment. In contrast to general wellness or fitness apps, the design of DTx solutions typically emphasizes scientific rigor, regulatory compliance, and clinical testing to demonstrate therapeutic value. DTx provides therapeutic interventions with measurable clinical outcomes, whereas mHealth apps have been primarily used to monitor and improve health habits. Furthermore, DTx is often integrated within healthcare systems, with physician involvement, and supports chronic disease management based on data-informed decisions [2].

Addressing Gaps in Current Treatments

DTx overcomes many of the accessibility, affordability, and scalability limitations of current treatment options. In more traditional healthcare settings, patients living in more remote areas are frequently unable to obtain treatment, and the costs of care for the long term may be prohibitive. However, DTx circumvents these barriers through scalable, remote interventions delivered *via* smartphones, tablets, or computers. Moreover, DTx bridges the gap in chronic disease management through continuous monitoring, personalized feedback, and enhanced adherence to treatment regimens. DTx brings new solutions that improve patient engagement and outcomes for diseases that classical therapies can not treat, like mental health disorders, substance use, or rehabilitation. DTx combines the ability to draw data-driven inferences to enable clinicians to make better decisions and hence significantly improves the quality of care [3].

Role in Healthcare Technology

Digital therapeutics are designed to work with the existing healthcare ecosystems, such as Electronic Health Records (EHRs), telehealth platforms, and even wearable devices to promote eHealth. DTx provides the healthcare provider with remote, data-driven tools to monitor a patient's progress, optimize treatment decisions, and deliver the highest quality of personalized care possible. From a treatment perspective, DTx provides an accessible and interactive platform to give patients the tools to take charge of their health, which, in turn, improves adherence and long-term outcomes. DTx also plays a role in preventative care, with such solutions able to reduce risks and manage early symptoms through non-invasive means, before they develop into a known disease [4].

TECHNOLOGY AND DESIGN PRINCIPLES FOR DIGITAL THERAPEUTICS

Human-centered design (HCD) is not the same as software utility; DTx optimizes usability, retention, and efficacy by focusing on patient needs and behaviors contrary to many existing models of treatment; the goal of DTx is to improve treatment adherence. When integrated with health systems, it allows the seamless flow of data, interoperability, and clinician involvement and helps deliver personalized care to improve outcomes [5].

AI (Artificial Intelligence) and ML (Machine Learning) are also essential to DTx because they analyze huge datasets, predict responses from patients, and adjust interventions dynamically. They improve accuracy, automate decisions, and streamline therapeutic delivery. By harnessing user-centric design, system integration, and AI-driven insights, DTx can provide scalable, evidence-based interventions that help improve patient health whilst minimizing healthcare system burden [6]. The technology and design principles for digital therapeutics are shown in Fig. (**1**).

Human-Centered Design in DTx

In HCD, the end-user is kept at the center of the design and development process, including research, prototyping, testing, and refinement. In DTx, this method includes working closely with patients, providers, and other stakeholders to recognize pain points and co-design solutions that boost user engagement and treatment adherence. HCD not only drives empathically-informed insights but also employs iterative feedback loops to ensure DTx applications reflect actual use cases and clinical needs. The importance of user trust, satisfaction, and commitment to long-term adoption is pivotal to the desired therapeutic outcomes in DTx, and effective HCD gives rise to the same. It also focuses on design simplicity and intuitiveness, allowing users to easily integrate the DTx solutions into their everyday lives. Ultimately, HCD ensures that digital interventions are not just likely to work technically but also are practical, user-friendly, and deeply attuned to the human experience of healthcare [7].

Technology and Design Principles for DTx

Human Centered Design in DTx

Integration with Health Systems

Ensuring usability, accessibility and inclusivity

EHR compatibility

AI and Machine Learning in DTx

Personalization and predictive analytics

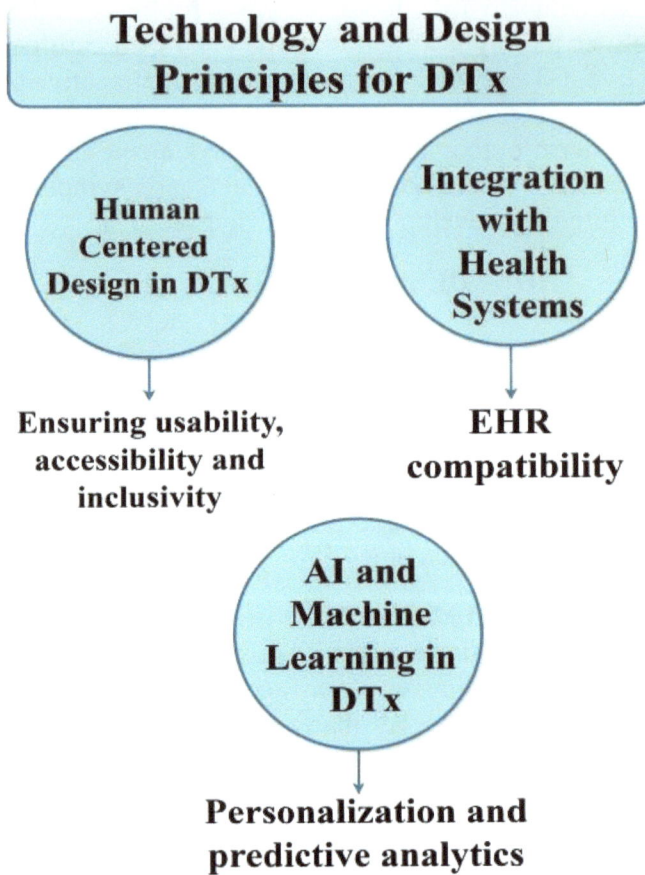

Fig. (1). Technology and design principles for digital therapeutics.

Ensuring Usability, Accessibility, and Inclusivity

However, usability, accessibility, and inclusivity are key pillars of success for DTx. Usability reduces the cognitive load on patients and clinicians by ensuring that DTx solutions are intuitive, efficient, and easy to use. High usability depends on clear navigation, simplified interfaces, and personalized user experiences. Focusing on usability and continuous improvement through testing helps developers identify and remove barriers to adoption, allowing for effortless interactions with the technology [8].

Efficiency is concerned with how well DTx solutions meet the functional needs of users with different capabilities and those with disabilities or with limited digital literacy. Facilities like screen readers, increasing or decreasing text size, voice commands, and multilingual support will help all users to use the software properly. Then, once again, accessibility needs to break any technological impediments through compatibility with varied devices, operating systems, and levels of internet connectivity [9].

While usability and accessibility are critical components of DTx solutions, inclusivity reaches beyond those concepts, making sure that DTx solutions are equitable with respect to different socioeconomic, cultural, and demographic backgrounds. This engages underrepresented populations as part of the design process to prevent bias and promote fairness. Therapeutic access for underprivileged individuals can be made possible by the utilization of inclusive design, which supports equality between all ages, genders, ethnicities, and even economic status. Focusing on usability, accessibility, and inclusivity in an integrated manner can enable DTx solutions to provide accessible, effective, and user-friendly care for a larger segment of the population, thereby enhancing health outcomes and quality of life [10].

Integration with Health Systems

Integration within the current health systems is fundamental for DTx to reach its full potential. Integration allows DTx solutions to become naturally integrated into the patient care continuum and make clinical workflows more efficient rather than hindering them. A crucial element for this integration is allowing DTx platforms to communicate with other services, healthcare providers, and larger health systems to provide holistic care. When integrated well, they enable greater access to timely patient information, increase decision-making capabilities, and offer customized treatment plans. Furthermore, DTx solutions will need to adhere to different regulations and interoperability frameworks to be secure, reliable, and scalable directly into the healthcare infrastructures. Through integration, DTx platforms connect innovative technology with traditional healthcare, allowing healthcare providers to track treatment adherence, clinical outcomes, and timely interventions. This holistic approach ensures that digital therapeutics are not isolated solutions but fully embedded tools that contribute to improving patient outcomes, lowering the cost of healthcare, and maximizing care delivery [11, 12].

EHR (Electronic Health Records) Compatibility

The successful deployment and adoption of DTx requires paying special attention to EHR compatibility. EHR systems serve as centralized repositories of patient data, and compatibility with EHRs enables DTx platforms to be incorporated into existing healthcare workflows. With the ease of EHR compatibility, DTx is available outside of the EHR workflow. Still, outputs such as patient progress, treatment adherence, and clinical outcomes can be made available to healthcare providers in real-time. Moreover, because it allows for seamless data exchange between programs, it eliminates duplicate data entry, reduces administrative overhead, and decreases the chances of erroneous data [13].

Integration with EHRs enables continuity of care as insights can be shared among multidisciplinary teams who can then pivot treatment plans as needed. As an example, data from a DTx app that helps patients with chronic diseases, like diabetes or hypertension, may be uploaded to the patient's EHR automatically so that providers on the care team have access to the most current information. Furthermore, DTx solutions can be integrated with patients' EHRs, which increases patient engagement by providing access to their treatment progress and engaging patients to participate in their care [14].

Interoperability standards such as HL7 FHIR (Fast Healthcare Interoperability Resources) and compliance with privacy regulations are essential to ensuring seamless EHR integration. By aligning with these standards, DTx platforms can securely exchange data with EHR systems, fostering trust and adoption among healthcare providers and patients. Overall, EHR compatibility streamlines clinical workflows, enhances care coordination, and ensures that digital therapeutics contribute effectively to evidence-based, patient-centered care [15].

AI and Machine Learning in DTx

With the help of AI and ML technologies, DTx solutions can process large quantities of data, learn from interactions with users, and provide specific, evidence-based interventions. DTx applications with AI capabilities track user behavior, monitor physiological signals, and recognize signals that might give an early indication of a change in a patient's condition. Using previous patient outcomes and feedback, machine learning algorithms keep improving the accuracy and effectiveness of the treatment. The iterative process of learning enhances the personalisation of recommendations, optimizing patient engagement and adherence to therapy. Moreover, AI allows DTx to provide real-time monitoring and predictive capabilities, enabling healthcare professionals to detect early signs of health problems and provide early intervention. DTx applications utilize AI and ML to manage chronic diseases, mental health disorders, and lifestyle-related conditions that are highly scalable, accessible, and cost-effective, ultimately mitigating the burden on healthcare systems [16, 17].

Personalization and Predictive Analytics

A cornerstone of effective DTx is personalization, which can be achieved with the help of AI-driven predictive analytics. AI analyzes user-related data like medical history, lifestyle habits, genetic predispositions, and real-time health numbers to produce customized treatment plans that address the specific needs of each person. For instance, a DTx solution for diabetes management can analyze concentrations of glucose, levels of physical activity, and food consumption in order to provide tips on insulin dosing, dietary changes, and exercise programs, tailored specifically to the patient [18]. ML models keep learning from new data points and hence refining the treatment strategy over time, and consequently delivering better results. AI predictive analytics takes personalisation to the next level, predicting likely health issues before they arise. For example, in cases such as asthma or depression, AI algorithms may be able to predict an imminent asthma exacerbation or depressive episode based on patterns observed in user behavior and biometric data, and prompt appropriate behavioral changes [19].

DTx combines personalization with predictive analytics to deliver timely, relevant, and actionable insights to keep patients engaged. Interventions are more likely to be effective when patients feel aligned with their unique circumstances and therefore are more likely to adhere to the treatments. In addition, predictive capabilities enable healthcare providers to allocate resources more effectively to those high-risk patients who need to be addressed first or the most. As DTx evolves, the combination of AI-driven personalization and predictive analytics will continue to revolutionize care delivery to be more precise, proactive, and patient-centered [20].

TYPES OF DIGITAL THERAPEUTICS

Digital therapeutics can be classified into mainly 3 types: disease-specific therapeutics, which target diseases such as diabetes and cardiovascular diseases; behavioral health interventions such as cognition behavioral therapy (CBT) mobile apps for mental health and addiction; and chronic disease management that involves remote monitoring and patient adherence tools that support both ongoing care and outcomes are illustrated in Fig. (2) [21].

Disease-Specific Therapeutics

DTx designed for a specific disease helps to supplement or replace traditional medical treatments by making it easy for patients to access cost-effective, scalable options for effective management of their conditions. These therapies also provide customized interventions with real-time tracking, reminders, education, and behavior-changing features, allowing patients to participate in their health management, leading to better outcomes and high-quality healthcare at low costs [22].

Types of Digital Therapeutics

Cardiovascular Diseases

Diabetes Management

1. Disease Specific Therapeutics

Cognitive Behavioral Therapy (CBT) Apps

2. Behavioral Health Interventions

Addiction Treatment

Remote Monitoring Software

3. Chronic Disease Management

Patient Adherence Tools

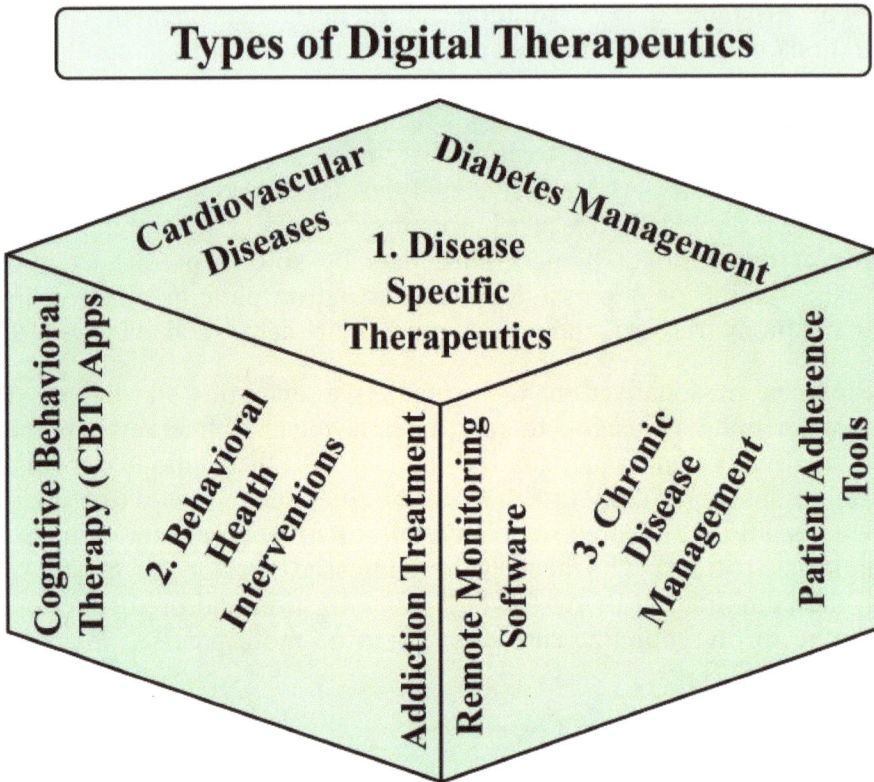

Fig. (2). Types of digital therapeutics.

Diabetes Management

Diabetes, specifically type 2 diabetes, is a worldwide health challenge that needs monitoring and management of blood glucose levels, adherence to lifestyle modifications, and medication compliance. Mobile apps, wearables, and telehealth platforms that monitor glucose levels, dietary intake, physical activity, medication adherence, and other related variables are among the digital therapeutics for diabetes management. These tools typically leverage algorithms to provide tailored suggestions, reminders for medication intake, and educational materials to assist the user in informed decision-making behaviours regarding the health condition. For example, apps can track food intake, estimate insulin dosage, and offer real-time feedback to optimize glucose control [23].

Such digital interventions have proven helpful for greater patient involvement by adhering to treatment plans and making the necessary lifestyle adjustments, such as daily exercises and balanced meals. The work of monitoring also makes it feasible for patients to be alerted to potential health issues before they occur, so that steps can be taken to avert them. There are also applications for ML and AI to avoid low or high glucose levels. Additionally, few DTx platforms offer virtual coaching or peer support to help users remain motivated and adhere to long-term diabetes management [24, 25].

Cardiovascular Diseases

Cardiovascular diseases (CVDs) are responsible for the most deaths worldwide, and millions of people suffer from hypertension, coronary artery disease, or heart failure. Digital therapeutics for CVD prevent risk factors management, lifestyle changes, and medication adherence. These therapies usually involve heart rate, blood pressure, activity detection, physical activity encouragement, and diet suggestions. Real-time data is collected through wearable devices, smartphone apps, and telemedicine platforms to track progress so that patients and healthcare providers can make necessary treatment plan adjustments [26].

Digital tools can be used in dealing with cardiovascular disease, allowing patients to track vital signs such as blood pressure, cholesterol levels, and weight. For example, certain applications are capable of synchronizing with smart devices to automatically monitor heart rate and activity, deliver exercise program feedback, and recommend lifestyle modifications that can reduce the risk of heart attack or stroke. Moreover, few DTx solutions for cardiovascular health may provide virtual coaching and facilitate desirable behavior changes such as smoking cessation, physical activity, and dietary modification, which have an important role in cardiovascular risk reduction. By leveraging ML capabilities on the collected data, AI can predict future cardiovascular events and help doctors intervene on time to provide better preventive care. The combination of personalized care and real-time data enables patients to take an active role in their treatment to enhance long-term cardiovascular health outcomes. Table **1** summarizes the different types of disease-specific digital therapeutics [27, 28].

Behavioral Health Interventions

Digital therapeutics featuring behavioral health interventions use technology to strengthen mental health through online-based treatment of anxiety, depression, stress, and more. These are interventions that can help the person cope with their symptoms outside traditional therapy settings. Behavioral health interventions can offer real-time monitoring, motivation, and behavior change *via* interactive methods, including mobile apps, online platforms, and wearables. These are especially beneficial for individuals who may be limited from in-person care because of cost, stigma, or location. In turn, this can help drive patient engagement and improve long-term outcomes, making digital behavioral interventions a powerful tool for the future [34].

Table 1. Different types of disease-specific digital therapeutics.

Digital Therapeutic	Therapeutic Area	Description	References
Propeller Health	Chronic Respiratory Diseases	Digital inhaler technology that aids asthma and COPD patients by tracking medication usage and symptoms.	[29]
Pear Therapeutics (reSET)	Mental Health and Behavioral Health	A digital therapy that enables patients to reduce cravings for a substance use disorder.	[30]
Noom	Obesity and Weight Loss	A weight loss program combining behavioral science and mobile technology to help users with obesity or weight management.	[31]
Oshi Health	Irritable Bowel Syndrome (IBS)	An evidence-based IBS dietary management guidance, behavioral therapy, and a digital therapeutic tracking.	[32]
Sleepio	Sleep Disorders	A cognitive behavioral therapy program that helps patients with insomnia manage and improve their sleep quality.	[33]

Cognitive Behavioral Therapy (CBT) Apps

Cognitive Behavioral Therapy (CBT) is a popular method where patients learn to identify and dispute negative thought habits, resulting in changes in behaviors and control over emotions. CBT apps are digital platforms that can provide CBT-based interventions through more interactive means. Such modules usually consist of cognitive restructuring, mindfulness, mood tracking, and goal setting. This is both more flexible and more accessible than traditional therapy, as it allows users to access evidence-based CBT techniques at any time. CBT apps have generated a lot of interest in the treatment of anxiety, depression, and stress. Studies have shown that these apps are effective; for instance, various studies indicate that several apps substantially decrease symptoms of a mental health disorder. CBT apps often contain features such as reminders and tracking progression, which can also reinforce positive behavioral change. A key benefit of these applications is that they provide a private and self-paced intervention, enabling individuals to undergo therapy in the comfort of their own homes without the pressure of attending in-person appointments. Additionally, many of the CBT apps are meant to work in a complementary fashion with traditional in-person therapy for a more holistic treatment approach. As digital health solutions are growing, CBT apps will likely play an increasingly integral role in promoting mental well-being [35, 36].

Addiction Treatment

Similarly, DTx is also being used in the key addiction treatment, providing a new way and access to help those with substance use disorders and behavioral addictions. These apps and platforms sometimes use a combination of behavioral therapies, individualized coaching, and support networks to help people manage cravings, avoid relapse, and achieve long-term recovery. Such digital interventions also often contain principles of effective approaches to intervention, such as CBT, motivational interviewing, and contingency management, that are frequently used in successful addiction treatment programs. Using these methods, users are trained to reframe negative thought patterns, come up with less harmful coping strategies, and are rewarded for gradually changing their behavior for the better. Most apps that support addiction treatment feature a real-time progress tracker to monitor substance use, mood, and triggers, so users can identify patterns and take active steps to avoid relapsing. Additionally, many of these apps have support groups and community forums that offer social support, hence decreasing social isolation and enhancing accountability. There are several apps that provide virtual coaching or counseling to help people access professional assistance from home. This is abusing because digital addiction treatment tools provide easy access and anonymity that promise a solution for individuals who may not feel comfortable pursuing traditional treatment options due to stigma, cost, or lack of transportation. These platforms are emerging as the cornerstones of integrated addiction care models as treatment shifts into the digital age [37, 38].

Chronic Disease Management

DTx for chronic disease management uses software solutions to assist patients with long-term chronic conditions like diabetes, hypertension, and cardiovascular diseases. Such personalized interventions are usually based on real-time data and are designed to promote self-management and prevent disease progression. Patients can use digital tools to record important health metrics, get personalized recommendations, and interact with healthcare providers. These tools aim to provide patient outcomes and quality of life improvements while minimizing hospitalizations and dependence on medication by becoming an integral part of the patient's daily care. There is evidence of the effectiveness of digital therapeutics for chronic disease management, with greater reductions in complications and hospitalizations (*e.g.*, diabetes) seen in several studies [39, 40].

Remote Monitoring Software

Remote monitoring software is essential in digital therapeutics, primarily for chronic illness management. From sensors and wearables to connected devices, healthcare providers can monitor the health data of patients continuously, often in real-time. This software can also gather various data, such as blood glucose, heart rate, sleep, and physical activity. As these parameters can be monitored remotely, healthcare professionals can get notified about the early signs of deterioration and take timely action to adjust the plans of treatment as required. This improves patient outcomes through more personalized care and higher patient engagement in their health management. The benefit of remote monitoring is that it reduces the need for frequent in-person visits, reduces healthcare costs, and improves accessibility to care. It also encourages a two-way interaction between patients and caregivers, which aids adherence and prompts treatments. Such systems can empower patients with chronic disease to take control of their condition, help them learn those skills that foster long-term health, and minimize chronic disease burden [40, 41].

Patient Adherence Tools

DTx includes patient adherence tools that ensure patients are more consistent and adherent to their treatment regimens. They provide reminders, alerts, and tracking features so that patients can maintain adherence to prescribed treatments such as medications or lifestyle changes. Others connect to wearables to track live health data, providing patients with insights into their improvement and feedback with results. Using behavioral science principles, these tools prompt adherence by gamifying good behaviors and overcoming common barriers to adherence (*i.e.*, forgetting, lack of motivation, confusion with instructions). They can also include educational content to educate the patient about their disease and the importance of adherence. Consequently, patient adherence tools help improve treatment efficiency, lower hospital readmission rates, and save money in the healthcare sector. They also integrate with telemedicine platforms to facilitate patient-provider communication, which enables a more comprehensive strategy for managing chronic conditions [42].

ROLE OF EMERGING TECHNOLOGIES IN ENHANCING DIGITAL THERAPEUTICS

The evolution of emerging technologies, such as AI, VR, IoT, and Blockchain, is transforming DTx with the ability to provide personalized, data-driven, and real-time therapeutic interventions, as shown in Fig. (**3**). Such technologies enhance patient engagement, treatment outcomes, and overall healthcare delivery. AI & ML enhance decision-making and personalize therapies, and VR/AR provide engaging, interactive experiences to treat mental health and rehabilitation. The combination of IoT & wearables improves monitoring & feedback, whereas Blockchain makes data both useful and secure, which in turn increases trust in digital health solutions [43].

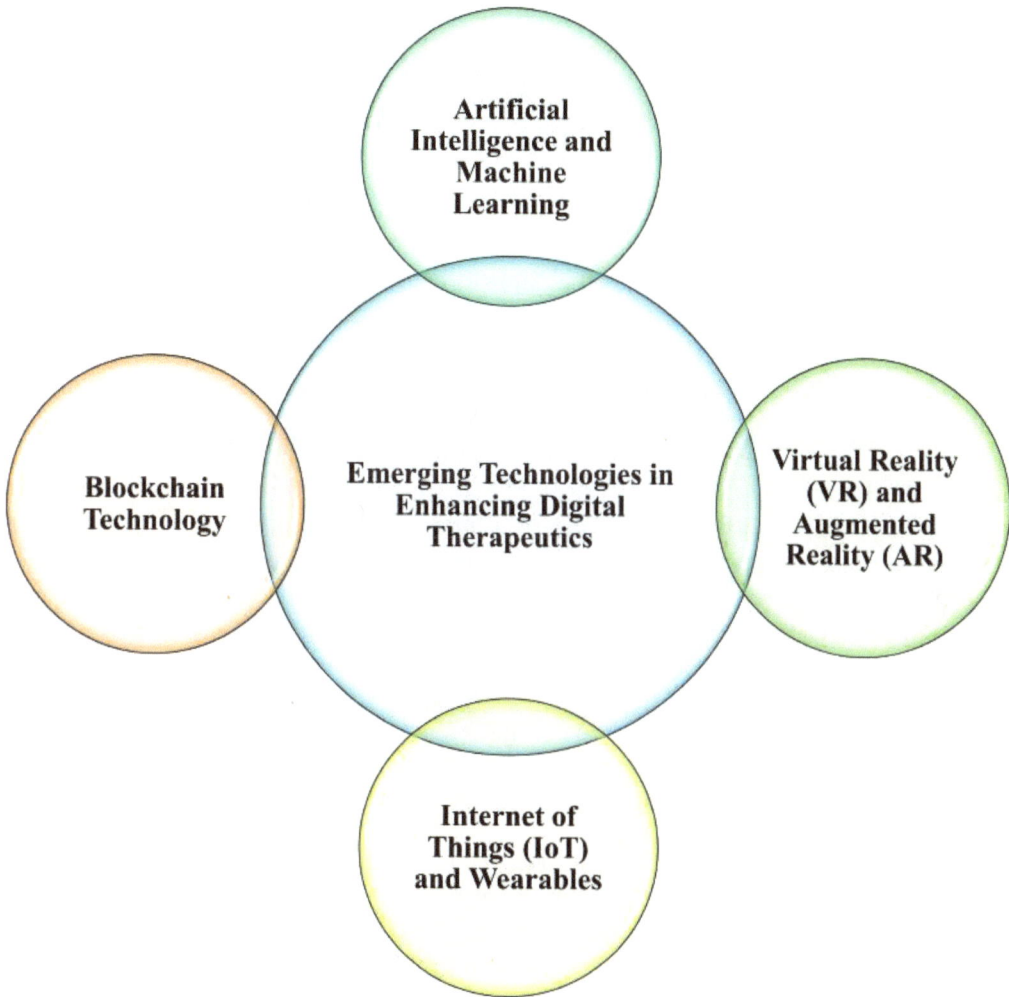

Fig. (3). Role of emerging technology in enhancing DTx.

Artificial Intelligence and Machine Learning

DTx has a key role in AI and ML since it provides personalized treatment plans and clinical outcomes. Using huge datasets of patient data, AI/ML can identify patterns, make predictions of how a disease may progress, and even develop personalized therapies. With the help of AI algorithms, patients can be monitored in real-time so treatments can be modified and tailored for every individual patient. In chronic disease management, for instance, AI models can monitor the vitals of the patients continuously and modify the therapeutic regimen in real-time to enhance the treatment effect. These technologies also help identify patients at risk of complications to trigger timely interventions. Moreover, the ability of AI-based systems to adapt also means that therapies can be designed to adapt as a patient changes over time, potentially allowing for better health outcomes over the long term at a lower healthcare cost [44].

Real-time Patient Monitoring and Adaptive Therapies

The ability to monitor patients in real-time, powered by AI and ML, is an absolute breakthrough aspect of DTx. Continuous monitoring of health status enables dynamic adjustment of therapies to changing health data. For example, in chronic disease, diabetes, real-time data from a continuous glucose monitor is transmitted to the AI systems, which then adjust insulin dosages automatically. Moreover, ML can be used to make predictions about disease progression and can potentially enable intervention at an early stage when the presence of critical symptoms is identifiable. This continuous data flow enables adaptive therapies that can develop with the changing patient throughout treatment, thereby leading to more responsive, individualized treatment plans. Moreover, timely monitoring facilitates better intervention methods, leading to a reduction in hospital readmission, an increase in patient engagement, and improved compliance with treatment protocols. Digital health solutions can deliver the increasing precision and effectiveness required to improve patient outcomes while simultaneously optimizing the burden of designated resources on healthcare systems by integrating AI and real-time data into the therapeutic process [45, 46].

Virtual Reality (VR) and Augmented Reality (AR)

Virtual reality (VR) and augmented reality (AR) are changing the landscape of DTx by embedding therapy within immersive environments. VR is a fully immersive experience commonly used in the treatment of pain, mental health, and rehabilitation. In contrast, AR supplements the real world with digital information, which can be used to improve physical therapy and rehabilitation by providing real-time guidance and feedback. Combined, these technologies allow for personalized and interactive therapies that increase patient adherence and therapeutic effectiveness [47].

Immersive Therapies for Mental Health and Rehabilitation

Within the domain of DTx, immersive therapies using VR and AR have also demonstrated their effectiveness in the treatment and rehabilitation of mental disorders. VR-based exposure therapy offers patients an alternative to traditional exposure therapy by helping to desensitize them to their triggers *via* a more controlled, gradual, and likely even safer experience. Additionally, VR has also been used for pain control as a method for distracting people from chronic pain and providing them with a sense of control and relaxation in the process. AR, meanwhile, enhances rehabilitation exercises by overlaying instructional cues onto the patient's surroundings, promoting greater engagement in physical therapy. That improves the accuracy of their movements, motivates the patients, and enhances their recovery. Both VR and AR take experiences that might be boring and difficult and create an interactive therapy environment, improving patient compliance, decreasing the perceived challenge of treatments, and providing a sense of achievement, ultimately leading to better mental health outcomes and accelerated physical rehabilitation [48].

Internet of Things (IoT) and Wearables

The Internet of Things (IoT) and wearables allow us to continuously monitor patients with real-time feedback. Smartwatches, fitness trackers, and medical sensors are all types of Wearable devices that collect large volumes of data about a patient's vital signs, activity levels, and sleep quality. With the help of IoT, these devices connect to a central system with which the healthcare provider can monitor the patient's health from a remote location and respond to any deviation in condition on the spot. IoT and wearables encourage continuous monitoring, thus gaining valuable information about the patient's health status on a daily basis, which will lead to timely intervention and a personalized treatment plan [49].

Data-driven Insights and Continuous Patient Feedback

IoT devices and wearables play an essential role in developing DTx, which provides continuous patient feedback and generates data-driven insights. They automatically collect live data on multiple health parameters, like heart rate, blood pressure, oxygen saturation, and physical activity, and transmit them to health care providers or cloud platforms. The steady flow of data also provides a better understanding of health trends, enabling the identification of early warning signs of health problems. For example, a wearable glucose monitor for diabetic patients, which allows for immediate analysis of blood glucose levels, could be used to adjust insulin doses or effect lifestyle changes. Furthermore, constant monitoring ensures that therapies can be adapted promptly based on the feedback received, optimizing treatment outcomes. Now, patients are able to monitor their upfront journey while tracking their decision-making about their health. Consequently, a data-driven approach allows for a more personalized mode of treatment, thereby enhancing treatment compliance or even improving health outcomes. Hence, IoT and wearables enable patients to improve care delivery and practice proactive health or well management, making digital therapeutic solutions more efficient and effective [50].

Blockchain Technology

Blockchain technology is transforming DTx by increasing the privacy, security, and transparency of health data. Blockchain, with its decentralized and immutable ledger where data cannot be tampered with, provides a powerful solution in a healthcare ecosystem where data integrity is at the core. This is especially important for sensitive health information exchanged between patients, providers, and third parties. Thus, Blockchain ensures that patient data and transactions are secure and that authorization is possible for people who need it. It can also simplify administrative tasks, like processing claims and reconciling payments, by providing a transparent, auditable history of interactions [51].

Ensuring Security and Transparency in DTx

An important technology that contributes to DTx security and transparency is blockchain. Blockchain is decentralized, which means that patients' information is saved all over the network, which makes it highly safe from any hacking or corruption. This allows details of medical information like treatment plans and personal health records to be kept secure yet accessible to authorized healthcare providers only. Also, the immutability of blockchain ensures that once any data is stored, it is immutable and cannot be changed or deleted, creating an auditable trail for all data interactions. Blockchain is decentralized, which means that patients' information is saved all over the network, which makes it highly safe from any hacking or corruption. This allows details of medical information like treatment plans and personal health records to be kept secure yet accessible to authorized healthcare providers only. Also, the immutability of blockchain ensures that once any data is stored, it is immutable and cannot be changed or deleted, creating an auditable trail for all data interactions. Ultimately, blockchain technology improves the integrity and credibility of DTx, promoting its widespread adoption in modern healthcare [52].

INTEGRATION INTO HEALTHCARE SYSTEMS

The integration of DTx into the healthcare system could represent a paradigm shift in the delivery of care and impact patient outcomes. More healthcare providers have begun to integrate DTx into their practices alongside traditional therapies. Integration success relies on compatibility with EHRs, clear regulatory parameters, and adequate support for clinicians. The wider adoption of DTx is contingent on the effectiveness in the management of chronic diseases and the successful delivery of more tailored, accessible, and patient-centered care. DTx integrated into healthcare systems can improve the management of diabetes, depression, cardiovascular diseases, and many others [53].

Adoption in Clinical Practice

Clinicians are slowly incorporating DTx in clinical practice, which is changing the delivery of health care. Providers use DTx as adjuncts to traditional therapies to treat chronic disease, mental health, and lifestyle diseases by incorporating them into their treatment protocols. They are used not only as monotherapy but also combined with other therapeutic modalities, providing comprehensive patient care. Adoption is aided by increasing evidence supporting DTx efficacy, alongside growing familiarity with digital solutions in healthcare. This growth of various medical innovations is paired with medical practices and hospital digital infrastructure growth, as seen within telemedicine and remote patient monitoring trends. Moving to DTx demands the evolution of both care delivery models and patient data coalescing into a powerful new driver of decision-making, enabling increased precision of treatment and clinician outcomes [54].

How Healthcare Providers Incorporate DTx into Their Practices?

Healthcare providers are becoming aware of the importance of incorporating DTx into their workflow, especially in the management of chronic conditions, as a means of enhancing patient engagement and as a tool for remote care. They commonly recommend DTx in combination with conventional therapeutics, where they serve as adjunctive therapies to improve overall patient benefit. For instance, a doctor can prescribe a DTx for chronic pain, depression, or diabetes and prescribe it in parallel to medication or physical therapy. DTx requires changes to clinical workflows to include seamless integration with existing technology, where healthcare providers review patient data *via* digital means and provide real-time feedback with remote monitoring. Healthcare providers may also work with DTx companies to ensure that these digital therapeutics remain aligned with evidence-based guidelines and regulatory standards. In some instances, DTx platforms are utilized strictly for the provision of patient education, facilitated through behavior change, self-management, and symptom monitoring. As healthcare providers gain confidence in the effectiveness and convenience of DTx solutions, their role in clinical practice becomes more integral, expanding beyond the traditional face-to-face consultation model to encompass digital tools that help patients manage their health remotely [55].

Training Clinicians for DTx Prescriptions

A successful integration of these healthcare innovations relies on training clinicians to prescribe and implement DTx in their practice. Healthcare providers need to be educated about the clinical effectiveness of different DTx solutions and where they fit as complementary or additive to existing therapies. There has been a gradual shift in medical education and healthcare professional development programs to include modules on digital health, with increasing emphasis on the use of DTx for specific conditions, including chronic, mental health, and lifestyle diseases. Physicians and clinicians are trained in evaluating and choosing appropriate DTx based on patient needs, health conditions, and treatment goals. They also learn how to prescribe DTx and how to adjust treatment when patients report outcomes *via* digital tools. It also includes teaching clinicians to interpret data produced by DTx platforms so that they can use that information to manage patients more effectively. In addition, providers will need training on the DTx regulatory and reimbursement environment so that they can ensure compliance with and take advantage of such policies. Incorporating DTx into clinical practice requires a shift in the way healthcare providers interact with patients and technology, and comprehensive training programs are essential for ensuring that clinicians are adequately prepared to use these tools in their care practices [56].

Patient-centric Approaches

Patient-centric approaches to DTx highlight the importance of aligning technology with patient needs and preferences to improve engagement, outcomes, and satisfaction. DTx solutions should be made accessible, user-friendly, and appropriately grounded in the immediate health challenges of patients. With an emphasis on the individual, patient-centric DTx promotes adherence to treatment regimens, effectively allowing patients to take control of their conditions. This not only empowers patients but also supports long-term compliance with digital interventions. Integrating patients into the development and ongoing refinement of DTx tools ensures that these solutions are aligned with their needs and engenders a sense of ownership that can facilitate optimal health outcomes [57].

Patients are the primary end users of DTx applications. Therefore, they need to be able to easily observe and track their health, input data, and receive feedback in a non-frustrating manner. Accessibility provisions, like smartphone compatibility, voice commands, or simple dashboards, allow patients of all ages and experience with technology to utilize digital therapeutics, interacting directly with the platform. Furthermore, the integration of interactive features, notifications, and game-like elements can help make the process less tedious for patients. Features such as chatbots or customer service hotlines, alongside clear instructions, can ensure that patients are supported throughout their DTx journey. By taking these design elements into account, digital therapeutics could serve as an easy, integrated part of a patient's treatment plan for chronic disease and health more broadly [58].

Challenges to Integration

Although the interest in DTx has grown, there are still barriers that need to be overcome to facilitate the integration of novel DTx into healthcare systems. A few major challenges that exist in this realm are regulatory clarity surrounding DTx, educating patients about their use, and having platforms be widely accessible and seamlessly implemented alongside standard treatment practices at healthcare centres. Such barriers can hamper widespread implementation, as many key stakeholders may be reluctant to adopt digital solutions without sufficient clinical evidence. Finally, there are important challenges regarding data privacy, reimbursement models, and training clinicians on how to use these solutions successfully and safely. Addressing these challenges is essential to unlocking the full potential of DTx in healthcare [59].

Resistance to DTx technology in healthcare is a complex issue, and approaches to overcome it consist of dealing with doubts about its effectiveness, complexity, integration with existing systems, *etc*. Clinicians and patients alike may be slow to adopt DTx for fear that they won't understand the technology or have skepticism about its efficacy compared to traditional forms of treatment. Demonstrating evidence of DTx efficacy and safety through appropriate studies is vital to gaining traction in overcoming this resistance. Training and professional development can educate healthcare providers on the benefits and proper use of DTx solutions, thus giving their clients peace of mind that these tools now have a greater chance of successfully entering their practices. Incorporating positive examples of trend case studies and patient testimonials can boost acceptance. Part of overcoming resistance is connecting with the patients as well and explaining to them how DTx allows patients to take control of their health. Reducing the perceived barriers through intuitive DTx solutions, ease of use, and support from the clinical world. Once it treats usability, reliability, and effectiveness, DTx will eventually find its way into acceptance and then trust, like the rest of the healthcare ecosystem [60, 61].

Interoperability is a significant challenge when integrating DTx into healthcare systems. DTx solutions must be interoperable with present electronic health records (EHRs), health information systems, and clinical workflows to ensure seamless integration. The technical infrastructure that supports healthcare IT systems is often not robust enough to facilitate DTx platforms, resulting in problems with data exchange, patient tracking, and treatment coordination. It can be difficult for clinicians to monitor patient progress over time and adjust treatment plans without that interoperability. To address this, DTx providers need to collaborate with the healthcare system to ensure their platforms are compatible with electronic health record (EHR) systems and other health IT tools. This could mean that data formats need to be standardized, protocols commonly used, and application programming interfaces (APIs) used to help facilitate communication between systems. Additionally, healthcare organizations may have to invest in IT infrastructure to support these technologies. By addressing interoperability issues, digital therapeutics can be more effectively adopted, enabling comprehensive, coordinated care and improved patient outcomes [62, 63].

CONCLUSION

Digital Therapeutics (DTx) is a paradigm shift in health care that provides precision, evidence-based interventions that can be personalized and scaled. Unlike conventional therapies and mobile health apps, DTx is specifically designed to treat medical conditions through software, addressing unmet needs in current treatment paradigms. DTx fills care voids and improves outcomes by treating disease-specific characteristics alongside behavioral health interventions and chronic disease management. DTx solutions are based on human-centered design principles, which make them highly accessible, inclusive, and user-friendly. The integration with existing health systems, such as Electronic Health Records, ensures seamless information exchange between patients and healthcare providers, while the embedded AI and machine learning allow for real-time, adaptive treatments tailored to the unique needs of each patient. New technologies, including VR, AR, and the IoT, can provide immersive, data-rich solutions and real-time feedback from patients to make DTx even more powerful. Blockchain technology adds an additional layer of security, ensuring patient data privacy and promoting trust in digital healthcare solutions. To enable the successful implementation of DTx in clinical practice, healthcare practitioners need to be trained to prescribe these therapies, and patient-centered practices need to be adopted to maximize engagement and adherence. However, they will need to overcome the challenges of resistance to technology and interoperability with existing systems for more widespread adoption. Ultimately, Digital Therapeutics represents a significant advancement in healthcare, giving patients personalized, effective, and accessible treatments that enhance overall health outcomes. With the continuous evolution of technology to leverage, the scope of DTx to change the future of healthcare is endless.

REFERENCES

[1]   Rijcken C. Digital therapeutic mangroves. In: Rijcken C, Ed. Pharmaceutical care in digital revolution: insights towards circular innovation. Amsterdam: Academic Press 2019; p. 169-79.
        [http://dx.doi.org/10.1016/B978-0-12-817638-2.00015-8]

[2]   Sverdlov O, van Dam J, Hannesdottir K, Thornton-Wells T. Digital therapeutics: an integral component of digital innovation in drug development. Clin Pharmacol Ther 2018; 104(1): 72-80.
        [http://dx.doi.org/10.1002/cpt.1036] [PMID: 29377057]

[3]   Cho CH, Lee HJ, Kim YK. The new emerging treatment choice for major depressive disorders: digital

therapeutics. Adv Exp Med Biol 2024; 1456: 307-31.

[4]   Khan PA. Telemedicine and digital health: the future for pharmaceutical companies & healthcare. Pristyn Research Solutions 2024 May 16;

[5]   Hong JS, Wasden C, Han DH. Introduction of digital therapeutics. Comput Methods Programs Biomed 2021; 209: 106319.
[http://dx.doi.org/10.1016/j.cmpb.2021.106319] [PMID: 34364181]

[6]   Lee AG. AI-and XR-powered digital therapeutics (DTx) innovations. Digital Frontiers- Healthcare, Education, and Society in the Metaverse Era. IntechOpen 2024.

[7]   Bolpagni M, Pardini S, Gabrielli S. Human centered design of AI-powered Digital Therapeutics for stress prevention: Perspectives from multi-stakeholders' workshops about the SHIVA solution. Internet Interv 2024; 38: 100775.
[http://dx.doi.org/10.1016/j.invent.2024.100775] [PMID: 39314669]

[8]   Vaccaro G. Assessing the role of Extended Reality in Healthcare Industry: a systematic inquiry to process optimization MSc thesis. Milan (IT): Politecnico di Milano 2024.

[9]   Kim M, Patrick K, Nebeker C, *et al.* The Digital Therapeutics Real-World Evidence Framework: An Approach for Guiding Evidence-Based Digital Therapeutics Design, Development, Testing, and Monitoring. J Med Internet Res 2024; 26: e49208.
[http://dx.doi.org/10.2196/49208] [PMID: 38441954]

[10]   Viglione AC, Hekler E. The Digital Therapeutics Real World Evidence Framework: An approach for guiding evidence-based DTx design, development, testing, and monitoring 2.

[11]   Fürstenau D, Gersch M, Schreiter S. Digital therapeutics (DTx). Bus Inf Syst Eng 2023; 65(3): 349-60.
[http://dx.doi.org/10.1007/s12599-023-00804-z]

[12]   Prodan A, Deimel L, Ahlqvist J, *et al.* Success factors for scaling up the adoption of digital therapeutics towards the realization of P5 medicine. Front Med (Lausanne) 2022; 9: 854665.
[http://dx.doi.org/10.3389/fmed.2022.854665] [PMID: 35492346]

[13]   Carrera A, Zoccarato F, Mazzeo M, *et al.* What drives patients' acceptance of Digital Therapeutics? Establishing a new framework to measure the interplay between rational and institutional factors. BMC Health Serv Res 2023; 23: 145.

[14]   Singh B, Hazra P, Roy S, *et al.* Exploring the Need and Benefits of Digital Therapeutics (DTx) for the Management of Heart Failure in India. Cureus 2023; 15(11): e49628.
[http://dx.doi.org/10.7759/cureus.49628] [PMID: 38161874]

[15]   Aziz SUA, Askari M, Shah SN. Standards for digital health. In: Klonoff DC, Kerr D, Mulvaney SA, Eds. Diabetes digital health 2020; p. 231-42.
[http://dx.doi.org/10.1016/B978-0-12-817485-2.00017-1]

[16]   Carrera A, Manetti S, Lettieri E. Rewiring care delivery through Digital Therapeutics (DTx): a machine learning-enhanced assessment and development (M-LEAD) framework. BMC Health Serv Res 2024; 24(1): 237.
[http://dx.doi.org/10.1186/s12913-024-10702-z] [PMID: 38395905]

[17]   Palanica A, Docktor MJ, Lieberman M, Fossat Y. The need for artificial intelligence in digital therapeutics. Digit Biomark 2020; 4(1): 21-5.
[http://dx.doi.org/10.1159/000506861] [PMID: 32399513]

[18]   Foktas Ž. AI-based digital therapeutics in diabetes management. Master's thesis. Lisbon (Portugal): Universidade Católica Portuguesa; 2024.
[http://dx.doi.org/10.1007/s12325-023-02743-3]

[19]   Molfino NA, Turcatel G, Riskin D. Machine learning approaches to predict asthma exacerbations: a narrative review. Advances in therapy 2024; 41(2): 534-2.

[20]   Vasdev N, Gupta T, Pawar B, Bain A, Tekade RK. Navigating the future of health care with AI-driven

digital therapeutics. Drug Discov Today 2024; 29(9): 104110.
[http://dx.doi.org/10.1016/j.drudis.2024.104110] [PMID: 39034025]

[21] Recchia G, Maria Capuano D, Mistri N, Verna R. Digital Therapeutics-What they are, what they will be. Acta Sci Med Sci 2020; 4(3): 1-9.
[http://dx.doi.org/10.31080/ASMS.2020.04.0575]

[22] Stewart WK. Digital therapeutics: a new era of technology for treatment. In: Patel D, Ed. Digital health: telemedicine and beyond. Amsterdam: Academic Press; 2025. p. 205-25.
[http://dx.doi.org/10.1016/B978-0-443-23901-4.00014-3]

[23] Ramakrishnan P, Yan K, Balijepalli C, Druyts E. Changing face of healthcare: digital therapeutics in the management of diabetes. Curr Med Res Opin 2021; 37(12): 2089-91.
[http://dx.doi.org/10.1080/03007995.2021.1976737] [PMID: 34511002]

[24] Nordyke RJ, Appelbaum K, Berman MA. Estimating the impact of novel digital therapeutics in type 2 diabetes and hypertension: health economic analysis. J Med Internet Res 2019; 21(10): e15814.
[http://dx.doi.org/10.2196/15814] [PMID: 31599740]

[25] Hu P, Hu L, Wang F, Mei J. Editorial: Computing and artificial intelligence in digital therapeutics. Front Med (Lausanne) 2024; 10: 1330686.
[http://dx.doi.org/10.3389/fmed.2023.1330686] [PMID: 38249985]

[26] Willis M, Darwiche G, Carlsson M, Nilsson A, Wohlin J, Lindgren P. Real-world long-term effects on blood pressure and other cardiovascular risk factors for patients in digital therapeutics. Blood Press Monit 2023; 28(2): 86-95.
[http://dx.doi.org/10.1097/MBP.0000000000000633] [PMID: 36729897]

[27] Moshawrab M, Adda M, Bouzouane A, Ibrahim H, Raad A. Smart wearables for the detection of cardiovascular diseases: a systematic literature review. Sensors (Basel) 2023; 23(2): 828.
[http://dx.doi.org/10.3390/s23020828] [PMID: 36679626]

[28] Chen C, Liu A, Zhang Z, Chen J, Huang H. Digital therapeutics in hypertension: How to make sustainable lifestyle changes. J Clin Hypertens (Greenwich) 2024; 26(10): 1125-32.
[http://dx.doi.org/10.1111/jch.14894] [PMID: 39248244]

[29] Sykes DL, See YY, Chow ECY, *et al.* Digitally monitored inhaled therapy: a 'smart' way to manage severe asthma? J Asthma 2024; 61(9): 970-5.
[http://dx.doi.org/10.1080/02770903.2024.2316726] [PMID: 38323583]

[30] Velez FF, Ruetsch C, Maricich Y. Evidence of long-term real-world reduction in healthcare resource utilization following treatment of opioid use disorder with reSET-O, a novel prescription digital therapeutic. Expert Rev Pharmacoecon Outcomes Res 2021; 21(4): 519-20.
[http://dx.doi.org/10.1080/14737167.2021.1939687] [PMID: 34148473]

[31] Mitchell ES, Fabry A, Ho AS, *et al.* The Impact of a Digital Weight Loss Intervention on Health Care Resource Utilization and Costs Compared Between Users and Nonusers With Overweight and Obesity: Retrospective Analysis Study. JMIR Mhealth Uhealth 2023; 11(1): e47473.
[http://dx.doi.org/10.2196/47473] [PMID: 37616049]

[32] Hamilton MJ. The use of mobile applications in the management of patients with inflammatory bowel disease. Gastroenterol Hepatol (N Y) 2018; 14(9): 529-31.
[PMID: 30364254]

[33] Hames P, Miller CB. Digital therapeutics for sleep and mental health. In: Sverdlov O, van Dam J, Eds. Digital therapeutics. 1st ed. Amsterdam: Chapman and Hall/CRC 2022 p. 261-80.
[http://dx.doi.org/10.1201/9781003017288-12]

[34] Ebert DD, Harrer M, Apolinário-Hagen J, Baumeister H. Digital interventions for mental disorders: key features, efficacy, and potential for artificial intelligence applications. In: Kim YK, Ed. Frontiers in psychiatry: artificial intelligence, precision medicine, and other paradigm shifts. Singapore: Springer; 2019. p. 583-627.

[http://dx.doi.org/10.1007/978-981-32-9721-0_29]

[35]   Stawarz K, Preist C, Tallon D, Wiles N, Coyle D. User experience of cognitive behavioral therapy apps for depression: an analysis of app functionality and user reviews. J Med Internet Res 2018; 20(6): e10120.
         [http://dx.doi.org/10.2196/10120] [PMID: 29875087]

[36]   Wright JH, Mishkind M, Eells TD, Chan SR. Computer-assisted cognitive-behavioral therapy and mobile apps for depression and anxiety. Curr Psychiatry Rep 2019; 21(7): 62.
         [http://dx.doi.org/10.1007/s11920-019-1031-2] [PMID: 31250242]

[37]   Hao W, Wang X, Li D, Wang G. Overview of the expert consensus on the digital therapeutics in addictive-related disorders. Gen Psychiatr 2024; 37(3): e101392.
         [http://dx.doi.org/10.1136/gpsych-2023-101392]

[38]   Jacobson NC, Kowatsch T, Marsch LA, Eds. Digital therapeutics for mental health and addiction: The state of the science and vision for the future. 1st ed. London: Academic Press 2022.

[39]   Chengyu Z, Xueyan H, Ying F. Research on disease management of chronic disease patients based on digital therapeutics: A scoping review. Digit Health 2024; 10: 20552076241297064.
         [http://dx.doi.org/10.1177/20552076241297064] [PMID: 39525556]

[40]   Marier-Tétrault E, Bebawi E, Béchard S, *et al.* Remote Patient Monitoring and Digital Therapeutics Enhancing the Continuum of Care in Heart Failure: Nonrandomized Pilot Study. JMIR Form Res 2024; 8: e53444.
         [http://dx.doi.org/10.2196/53444] [PMID: 39504548]

[41]   Piccini JP, Mittal S, Snell J, Prillinger JB, Dalal N, Varma N. Impact of remote monitoring on clinical events and associated health care utilization: A nationwide assessment. Heart Rhythm 2016; 13(12): 2279-86.
         [http://dx.doi.org/10.1016/j.hrthm.2016.08.024] [PMID: 27544748]

[42]   Schwartz DG, Spitzer S, Khalemsky M, *et al.* Apps don't work for patients who don't use them: Towards frameworks for digital therapeutics adherence. Health Policy Technol 2024; 13(2): 100848.
         [http://dx.doi.org/10.1016/j.hlpt.2024.100848]

[43]   Pooja P, Chikhale MM, Dhir S. Uncovering the strategic potential of blockchain technology adoption: a systematic literature review. Strategic Change. 2025 Mar; 34(2): 151-80.

[44]   Hu P, Hu L, Wang F, Mei J. Editorial: Computing and artificial intelligence in digital therapeutics. Front Med (Lausanne). 2024 Jan 5; 10: 1330686.

[45]   Rath KC, Khang A, Rath SK, Satapathy N, Satapathy SK, Kar S. Artificial intelligence (AI)-enabled technology in medicine-advancing holistic healthcare monitoring and control systems. In: Khang A, Abdullayev V, Hrybiuk O, Shukla AK Eds. Computer Vision and AI-Integrated IoT Technologies in the Medical Ecosystem. CRC Press 2024; pp. 87-108.
         [http://dx.doi.org/10.1201/9781003429609-6]

[46]   Awad A, Trenfield SJ, Pollard TD, *et al.* Connected healthcare: Improving patient care using digital health technologies. Adv Drug Deliv Rev 2021; 178: 113958.
         [http://dx.doi.org/10.1016/j.addr.2021.113958] [PMID: 34478781]

[47]   Ciubean AD, Popa T, Ciortea VM, *et al.* Digital therapeutics in musculoskeletal pain management: a narrative review of gamification, virtual reality and augmented reality approaches. Balneo PRM Res J 2024 Aug 23; 15(2)

[48]   Singha R, Singha S. Mental health treatment: exploring the potential of augmented reality and virtual reality. Applications of Virtual and Augmented Reality for Health and Wellbeing 2024; pp. 91-110.

[49]   Mamdiwar SD, R A, Shakruwala Z, Chadha U, Srinivasan K, Chang CY. Recent advances on IoT-assisted wearable sensor systems for healthcare monitoring. Biosensors (Basel) 2021; 11(10): 372.
         [http://dx.doi.org/10.3390/bios11100372] [PMID: 34677328]

[50] Lee U, Jung G, Ma EY, *et al.* Toward data-driven digital therapeutics analytics: literature review and research directions. IEEE CAA J Autom Sin 2023 Jan 6; 10(1): 42-66.

[51] Srivastava S, Singh SV, Singh RB, Shukla HK. Digital transformation of healthcare: a blockchain study. Int J Innov Sci Eng Technol 2021 May; 8(5): 414-25.

[52] Raj R, Raja SP. Revolutionizing healthcare: blockchain's transformative applications for data security, privacy, and interoperability. 2024 IEEE 9th International Conference for Convergence in Technology (I2CT) 2024 Apr 5; 1-9.

[53] Bélisle-Pipon JC, David PM. Digital therapies (DTx) as new tools within physicians' therapeutic arsenal: Key observations to support their effective and responsible development and use. Pharmaceut Med 2023; 37(2): 121-7.
[http://dx.doi.org/10.1007/s40290-022-00459-3] [PMID: 36653600]

[54] Dang A, Arora D, Rane P. Role of digital therapeutics and the changing future of healthcare. J Family Med Prim Care 2020; 9(5): 2207-13.
[http://dx.doi.org/10.4103/jfmpc.jfmpc_105_20] [PMID: 32754475]

[55] Coder M. Building the digital therapeutic industry: regulation, evaluation, and implementation. In: Jacobso NC, ed. Digital therapeutics for mental health and addiction [Internet]. Cambridge (MA): Elsevier 2023. p. 165-77.

[56] Shafai G, Aungst TD. Prescription digital therapeutics: A new frontier for pharmacists and the future of treatment. J Am Pharm Assoc 2023; 63(4): 1030-4.
[http://dx.doi.org/10.1016/j.japh.2023.03.012] [PMID: 37019379]

[57] Stegemann L, Gubser R, Gersch M, *et al.* Future-oriented and patient-centric? A qualitative analysis of digital therapeutics and their interoperability. The 31st European Conference on Information Systems (ECIS 2023). Association for Information Systems. 2023.

[58] Aminabee S. The future of healthcare and patient-centric care: Digital innovations, trends, and predictions. Emerging Technologies for Health Literacy and Medical Practice. IGI Global Scientific Publishing 2024; pp. 240-62.
[http://dx.doi.org/10.4018/979-8-3693-1214-8.ch012]

[59] Butt JS. Navigating the grey area: Legal frameworks for digital health monitoring & use of ai for elderly patients in the nordics. Int J Technol Emerg Sci 2024; 4: 1-8.

[60] Kapur R. Digital platforms and transformation of healthcare organizations: integrating digital platforms with advanced IT systems and work transformation. 1st ed. New York: Productivity Press; 2023.

[61] Armeni P, Polat I, De Rossi LM, Diaferia L, Meregalli S, Gatti A. Exploring the potential of digital therapeutics: An assessment of progress and promise. Digit Health 2024; 10: 20552076241277441.
[http://dx.doi.org/10.1177/20552076241277441] [PMID: 39291152]

[62] Stegemann L, Gubser R, Gersch M, *et al.* Future-oriented and patient-centric? A qualitative analysis of digital therapeutics and their interoperability. Proceedings of the 31st European Conference on Information Systems (ECIS); Kristiansand, Norway. AIS 2023.

[63] Abernethy A, Adams L, Barrett M, *et al.* The promise of digital health: then, now, and the future. NAM Perspect 2022 Jun 27; 2022: 10-31478.
[http://dx.doi.org/10.31478/202206e]

CHAPTER 13

Cybersecurity in the Age of Connected Healthcare

Chanchla Devi Haldkar[1], Shaweta Sharma[2], Sunita[3], Akanksha Sharma[3] and **Akhil Sharma[3,*]**

[1] *Shri Rawatpura Sarkar Institute of Pharmacy, Jabalpur, Madhya Pradesh-482001, India*

[2] *Department of Pharmacy, School of Medical and Allied Sciences, Galgotias University, Greater Noida, Uttar Pradesh-201310, India*

[3] *R.J. College of Pharmacy, Raipur, Uttar Pradesh-202165, India*

Abstract: In the digital age, interconnected technologies are essential for healthcare systems, ranging from the Internet of Medical Things (IoMT) to telemedicine. This chapter discusses the importance of cybersecurity in protecting patient data and ensuring the continuity of services in the healthcare sector. The gradual transition of the healthcare sector to more advanced technologies such as cloud computing, artificial intelligence (AI), and mHealth (mobile health) apps creates several new security challenges, such as data breaches, ransomware, and vulnerabilities in medical devices. The chapter discusses the challenges of securing these systems, taking into account risks from interconnected devices, remote monitoring, and data sharing between different constituents in a healthcare ecosystem. Best practices for mitigating cybersecurity threats, including encryption, authentication, and risk management strategies, are discussed. Additionally, new technologies such as AI and blockchain provide new ways to increase security. The chapter also highlights the importance of training healthcare providers, developing robust cybersecurity policies, and complying with regulatory frameworks to protect against evolving cyber threats. As healthcare technology continues to advance, it is essential to adopt comprehensive cybersecurity measures to ensure patient safety and data privacy.

Keywords: Cybersecurity, Data breaches, Encryption, Healthcare policies, Healthcare technology, IoMT, Medical devices, Ransomware, Risk management.

INTRODUCTION

Cybersecurity in healthcare refers to the strategies, technologies, and practices designed to protect sensitive health data and systems from unauthorized access, cyberattacks, and breaches. With the increasing reliance on digital technologies in the healthcare sector, safeguarding patient information and ensuring the availabi-

---

* **Corresponding author Akhil Sharma:** R. J. College of Pharmacy, Raipur, Uttar Pradesh-202165, India; E-mail: xs2akhil@gmail.com

Shaweta Sharma, Akhil Sharma, Shivkanya Fuloria & Anurag Singh (Eds.)
All rights reserved-© 2025 Bentham Science Publishers

lity of critical systems have become paramount. Cyberattacks in healthcare can result in dire consequences, including compromised patient safety, financial losses, and erosion of trust in healthcare providers. Unlike other industries, healthcare faces unique challenges due to the high value of medical data on the black market, the complexity of interconnected systems, and the need for uninterrupted operations. Effective cybersecurity measures in healthcare not only protect sensitive information but also enable compliance with regulations such as HIPAA and GDPR, ensuring ethical and legal data handling [1, 2].

Overview of Healthcare Systems in the Digital Era

The introduction of digital technologies is reshaping the landscape of modern healthcare systems to become an ecosystem of interconnected devices, platforms, and stakeholders. Wearable health monitors and smart diagnostic tools, for example, closed-loop systems that adapt to lifestyle or behavioral inputs in real-time, could provide personalized care through the Internet of Things (IoT). Cloud computing has completely transformed how data is stored and shared, while telemedicine platforms have increased the accessibility of healthcare services. This improves efficiency, provides high-level patient outcomes, and allows data-driven decisions. At the same time, they can expose them to cybersecurity risks through more entry points, and securing heterogeneous systems can be difficult. Such a transition to digital healthcare highlights the urgent requirement of cybersecurity to secure the availability, confidentiality, and durability of these systems [3, 4].

Evolution of Healthcare Technology

Healthcare technology has evolved with massive innovations that redefine care delivery. Smart devices introduced by IoT, which range from implantable defibrillators to home monitoring systems, allow for more proactive health management. Telemedicine has changed the way patients and providers engage with one another, especially in the context of a crisis such as the COVID-19 pandemic. AI has also transformed diagnostics, where machine learning algorithms have diagnosed diseases based on patterns in medical imaging and genomic data for some time now. Blockchain is growing in popularity to secure medical records and ensure data integrity. Together, these developments enable a super-connected healthcare ecosystem to revolutionize efficiencies, accessibility, and personalization. However, dependence on technology only increases the threat of cyberattacks, which makes it necessary to keep innovating in the cybersecurity field to protect it [5, 6].

HEALTHCARE TECHNOLOGY LANDSCAPE

The connected healthcare space is witnessing robust growth, led by innovations in the space such as the Internet of Medical Things (IoMT), cloud computing, mHealth apps, and telemedicine, as shown in Fig. (**1**) . By integrating machine learning, artificial intelligence, and big data, predictive analytics and personalized care are on the verge of becoming a reality. However, the interoperability issue limits data sharing across the healthcare ecosystem, which requires a rigorous framework of interconnected features to guarantee that there is seamless data exchange while still keeping the data secure and compliant in this interconnected environment [7, 8].

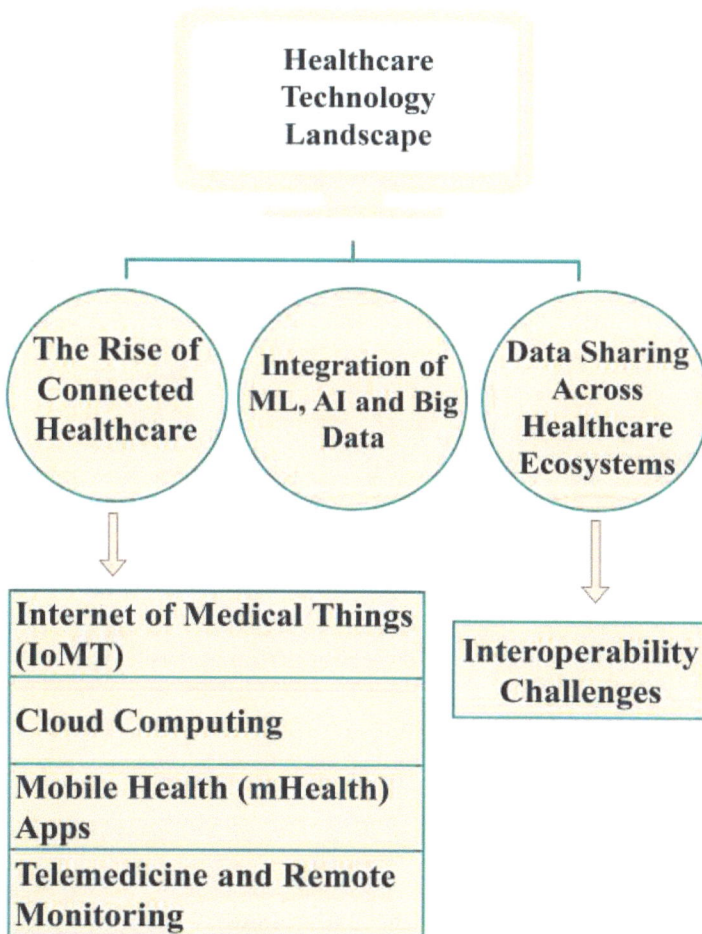

Fig. (1). Various technologies used in healthcare systems.

The Rise of Connected Healthcare

Connected healthcare integrates digital technologies to provide continuous care to patients. Advanced technologies such as IoMT, mobile apps, telemedicine, and cloud computing help improve provider-patient interaction. It allows for real-time health monitoring, immediate diagnostics, and customized medicines. However, increased connectivity comes with higher vulnerability to cyber threats. Protecting healthcare networks, devices, and patient data is critical to realizing the full potential of connected healthcare without compromising security or privacy [9, 10].

Internet of Medical Things (IoMT)

The Internet of Medical Things (IoMT) refers to the collection of devices and sensors to monitor and analyse the health data of patients connected and transmitted over the Internet. These devices include smart wearables such as fitness trackers, smart insulin pumps, and patient monitoring devices. By notifying providers when health anomalies arise, IoMT empowers proactive care before issues become critical. However, this connectivity increases exposure to cyber threats like unauthorized access, data breaches, and malware attacks. To ensure the safety of IoMT devices, it is essential to have encrypted communication, secure device authentication, and regular software updates. The safety of such IoMT-enabled healthcare systems comes only by adopting comprehensive security strategies [11, 12].

Cloud Computing

Cloud computing technology has transformed the world of healthcare and helps store, access, and share huge amounts of data securely. Cloud services are becoming appealing to healthcare organizations due to their cost-efficient and scalable nature. However, challenges such as data breaches and unauthorized access demand stringent cybersecurity measures. Multi-factor authentication, encryption, and robust access controls are critical. Engaging with a trusted cloud provider means engaging with best cloud practices and unleashing the potential of cloud technology in healthcare without hindering security [13, 14].

Mobile Health (mHealth) Apps

Mobile health (mHealth) applications such as fitness tracking, medication reminders, and virtual consultations give patients the tools to manage their health. Such applications boost involvement and accessibility, particularly in unserved parts. Even though the applications have an edge over the rest, mHealth apps collect sensitive personal and medical data, and thereby, the apps can also be susceptible to cyberattacks. Developers need to use secure coding techniques, and data encryption, and follow the law on data protection. This means that the app updates should be frequent, and the privacy policy should be transparent. User education about proper app use is another way to mitigate risks, helping to create a secure foundation for mobile healthcare solutions [15].

Telemedicine and Remote Monitoring

Telemedicine and remote monitoring have transformed patient care by allowing consultations and diagnostics to take place from a distance. Telehealth will enable patients to consult with specialists without geographic barriers, minimize hospital visits, and enhance chronic disease management. Remote monitoring tools measure vital signs to keep healthcare providers updated in real-time. However, such technologies come with an increase in cybersecurity risks, including the possibility of eavesdropping, device tampering, and data breaches. Deploying end-to-end encryption, together with secure networks and device authentication protocols, protects all sensitive information. Enhanced measures and protocols for cybersecurity ensures the utilization of telemedicine and remote monitoring in the connected healthcare age [16].

Integration of Machine Learning, AI, and Big Data in Healthcare

Machine Learning (ML), along with Artificial Intelligence (AI) and Big Data, has transformed the landscape of healthcare. These technologies utilize large, complex datasets to discover trends, make predictions, and improve decision-making in response to the complex challenges of contemporary health care. Big Data is the cornerstone, aggregating diverse information, such as medical imaging, genomics, wearable devices, and even social determinants of health. AI and ML algorithms harness this power to convert the structured and unstructured data from these sources into actionable insights [17].

Natural language processing (NLP) and computer vision-supported solutions can further boost the diagnostic accuracy by evaluating medical images either by detecting abnormalities or by extracting information from unstructured documents such as text. ML models within the field of radiology can automatically raise awareness of the earliest signs of a disease, such as cancer or neurological disorders, thereby minimizing people's diagnostic mistakes and optimizing results. AI-based systems also aid in predictive analytics and predictions about disease progression and patient readmissions, enabling healthcare providers to take early action and personalize care.

The intersection of ML and Big Data is especially visible in fields like genomics and precision medicine. ML algorithms can study large-scale databases of genetic resources to find mutations related to diseases and investigate how a person will respond to a therapy and another will not. Such an experience allows for building individualized but useful treatment modalities that would significantly increase effectiveness and minimize side effects [18].

Data Sharing Across Healthcare Ecosystems

Data sharing is essential in health care delivery to provide patient-centered, efficient, and high-quality care. Healthcare systems have become digitized, allowing for effortless and inexpensive data sharing between hospitals, clinics, laboratories, pharmacists, and even the patients themselves. Health information exchanges (HIEs) and cloud-based platforms have popularized technologies that simplify the combination of medical histories, diagnostic reports, and treatment plans. The seamlessly connected ecosystem helps healthcare providers make real-time, balanced decisions, which finally leads to more positive health results. In addition, data sharing aids in research, which can lead to new therapeutic options and the development of personalized medicine. Differences often hamper the exchange of data in data formats, standards, and technological capabilities. Moreover, protecting delicate patient records remains essential in preventing and mitigating access breaches. Despite these hurdles, initiatives such as the adoption of Fast Healthcare Interoperability Resources (FHIR) and incentivized government policies aim to bridge the gaps in data sharing. With the collaboration of all stakeholders and the focus on secure and standardized practices, the modern healthcare industry can realize the full potential of interconnected platforms for data [19, 20].

Interoperability Challenges

Interoperability, or the ability of different healthcare systems to exchange and use information, is a key component of modern healthcare. However, making interoperability a reality is still difficult because of technical, organizational, and regulatory obstacles. A fundamental technical hurdle is the variation in data formats and coding systems across healthcare organizations.

Organizational challenges, like resistance to adopting new technologies and inadequate training among healthcare professionals, make this even worse. Healthcare institutions often operate in silos, focusing on internal processes rather than engaging externally, which results in barriers to data flow. Institutions with limited resources face even higher costs and hurdles because of the need for strong cybersecurity measures to avoid violations of sensitive data. It will take a team effort from technology providers, policymakers, and healthcare organizations to address these issues. Through universal standards, system interoperability, and security policies that support access and ease of use over heavy-handed technical features, these barriers can be attacked in a way that will further enable the delivery of data-driven care across the healthcare ecosystem [21, 22].

TYPES OF CYBERSECURITY THREATS IN HEALTHCARE

The healthcare sector experiences a variety of cybersecurity threats, ranging from data breaches and ransomware attacks to phishing and malware infiltrations, which are elaborated in Fig. (**2**) . Many of these threats aimed at sensitive systems and personal health information (PHI) lead to financial loss, disruption of care, and endangerment of patient safety. Denial-of-service (DoS) attacks targeting vulnerable medical devices and networked systems can also render healthcare facilities inoperable. Such challenges require strong, multi-layered defenses for resilience and continuity of healthcare services [23].

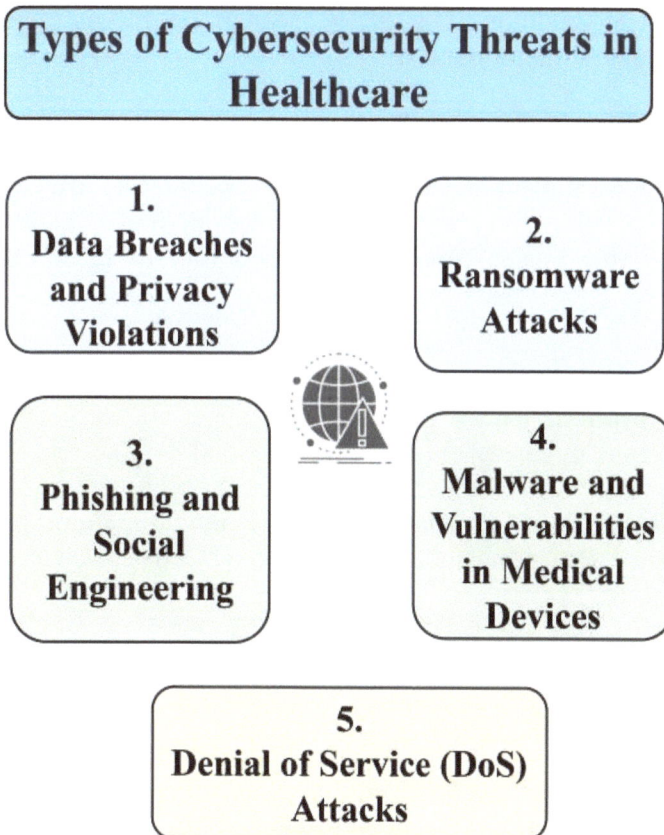

Types of Cybersecurity Threats in Healthcare

1. **Data Breaches and Privacy Violations**

2. **Ransomware Attacks**

3. **Phishing and Social Engineering**

4. **Malware and Vulnerabilities in Medical Devices**

5. **Denial of Service (DoS) Attacks**

Fig. (2). Different types of cybersecurity threats in healthcare.

Data Breaches and Privacy Violations

Data breaches are when unauthorized individuals access patient records and render them vulnerable, thus breaching their privacy. Cybercriminals take advantage of vulnerable systems to steal and/or expose PHI. These breaches can be attributed to hacking, insider threat personnel, or human error. This fallout consists of lost confidence, legal consequences, and identity fraud. Protecting PHI demands encrypted communication, stringent access controls, and regular employee training, creating a culture of cybersecurity awareness across healthcare institutions.

Personal health information (PHI) is a prime target for cybercriminals due to its value on the black market and its critical role in patient care. PHI includes medical records, billing, and insurance information that can be exploited to commit identity theft or fraud. Data breaches remain a challenge for healthcare organizations due to vulnerabilities like old software, weak encryption standards, and the need for many interconnected systems [24].

Attackers use tactics like phishing emails, credential theft, or exploiting unsecured networks to infiltrate systems. For example, ransomware attacks encrypt PHI, holding it hostage for ransom payments, while breaches may expose sensitive data publicly or sell it illegally. Patients face potential harm, including financial exploitation or compromised care due to altered records [25].

Ransomware Attacks

Ransomware attacks encrypt healthcare data, disrupting access and demanding a ransom for decryption. These events cause complete suspension of patient services, disruptions in care provision, and financial destruction. Cybercriminals take advantage of system vulnerabilities, which often take place in critical infrastructure areas. A robust data backup regime, endpoint protection, and employee vigilance against phishing attempts are effective measures to reduce the risks of ransomware [26].

Phishing and Social Engineering

Never-ending phishing and social engineering attacks are the most frequent hazards that healthcare organizations face. In phishing, hackers pose as a real organization (like a health insurer, hospital, or government agency, for example) to trick consumers into giving up sensitive data. They are typically sent through emails where fake messages urge the recipients to click on harmful links or attachments that can invade systems [27].

Social engineering, on the other hand, is the act of manipulating individuals in a way that allows the hacker to extract secret details from the unsuspecting person or otherwise do something that threatens the security of the individual. In healthcare, this might be people pretending to be colleagues, technicians, or support staff so that they can access secure systems or perform some other type of malicious act. The success of these attacks relies heavily on human error or ignorance of security protocols. Social engineering attacks leverage psychological triggers (like fear, urgency, or authority) to convince you to give up your information or take action without considering the risk.

Cybercriminals use it as an entry point to write letters in systems that are missing login credentials to access patients ' records, or some other confidential data, by giving it to healthcare workers. This means that healthcare providers have no choice but to provide employees with thorough cybersecurity training, stressing the need to check emails and communications, spot suspicious behavior, and adhere to good practices [28].

Malware and Vulnerabilities in Medical Devices

The rise of medical devices, attached to hospital networks and used in patient treatment, poses an enormous cyber attacks. Infusion pumps, pacemakers, and diagnostic tools are just a few examples of medical devices that are at risk for malware attacks since many operate on decades-old operating systems without sufficient security, according to the report. Medical devices can be infected with malware in several ways, such as an infected USB drive, an email attachment, or a compromised software update. Exploitable weaknesses in these types of configurations are serious since they may allow attackers to gain access to or manipulate critical systems, with the result of endangerment to those in care or a violation of privacy [29].

A major issue is that many medical devices were designed with functionality as the primary focus and security as an afterthought. The nature of these devices, with weak authentication mechanisms, open ports, and unpatched software, makes them lucrative targets for cybercriminals. Some manufacturers may not issue security patches promptly, leaving healthcare organizations vulnerable. Moreover, with the essentiality of these devices, healthcare cannot have enough cybersecurity. A broad security approach is required for healthcare organizations, including regular vulnerability assessments, strong access controls, and monitoring of connected devices for unusual activity. Collaboration between manufacturers and healthcare providers is also essential to ensure that medical devices meet the required cybersecurity posture to protect patient safety [30].

Denial of Service (DoS) Attacks

Denial of Service (DoS) attacks pose an ever-increasing threat to healthcare organizations as they can disrupt essential healthcare operations and subsequently patient care. In the case of a DoS attack, cybercriminals flood the network, servers, or services of a healthcare provider, making them unusable, and forcing the system to shut down and no longer be able to serve legitimate users. As a result, this can take down hospital systems, leaving healthcare workers unable to view patient records, book procedures, or render care within critical timelines [31].

In healthcare, for instance, a DoS attack can postpone medical treatments, hamper emergency response systems, and disturb communication between healthcare professionals, which can result in life-threatening situations for patients. The emergence of distributed denial of service (DDoS) attacks, in which the same attack traffic originates from many different systems, has made the problem so much worse. Since a DDoS attack is effective mainly because it uses many infected devices to overwhelm a healthcare network, it is particularly hard to prevent. Even worse, DoS attacks in healthcare can be directed toward mission-critical infrastructure like medical imaging tools and the telemedicine platforms they rely on to carry out their daily operations [32].

As a result, DoS attacks are sometimes used as a smokescreen for other malicious activities, such as a data breach or installation of ransomware, making remediation difficult. To avoid the risk of DoS attacks in healthcare, organizations must invest in active security such as load balancing, traffic filtering, and other firewalls capable of detecting unusual activities and attempts to block them. Finally, healthcare providers need to have an incident response plan to aid a quick recovery and lessen the impact on patient care. Further preparation can be helped by regular resilience tests and working in close partnership with cybersecurity specialists [33].

CYBERSECURITY CHALLENGES IN CONNECTED HEALTHCARE

The cybersecurity concerns of connected healthcare systems are immense due to the large amounts of sensitive patient data stored by these organizations. As more devices, networks, and applications get connected, there is a rise in the potential for cyberattacks, system failures, unauthorized access, and data breaches. The complexity of interconnected systems and the changing nature of cyber threats make it nearly impossible to achieve good security as different sectors of healthcare embrace new technologies and patient care solutions, as shown in Table **1** [34].

Table 1. Description of challenges associated with connected healthcare.

S. No.	Category	Challenge	Description
1	**Complexity of Healthcare Systems**	Multiple Stakeholders	Hospitals, insurance providers, pharmacies, and patients with diverse access points and data requirements
		Legacy Systems and Their Security Gaps	Older systems often lack modern security protocols, making them susceptible to cyberattacks [35].
2	**Security of IoT and Wearable Devices**	Vulnerabilities in Medical Devices	Potential for hacking or data breaches in connected medical equipment and wearables [36].

BEST PRACTICES AND SOLUTIONS FOR CYBERSECURITY IN HEALTHCARE

Cybersecurity in healthcare is critical for protecting patient data, ensuring privacy, and maintaining trust, as depicted in Fig. (**3**) .

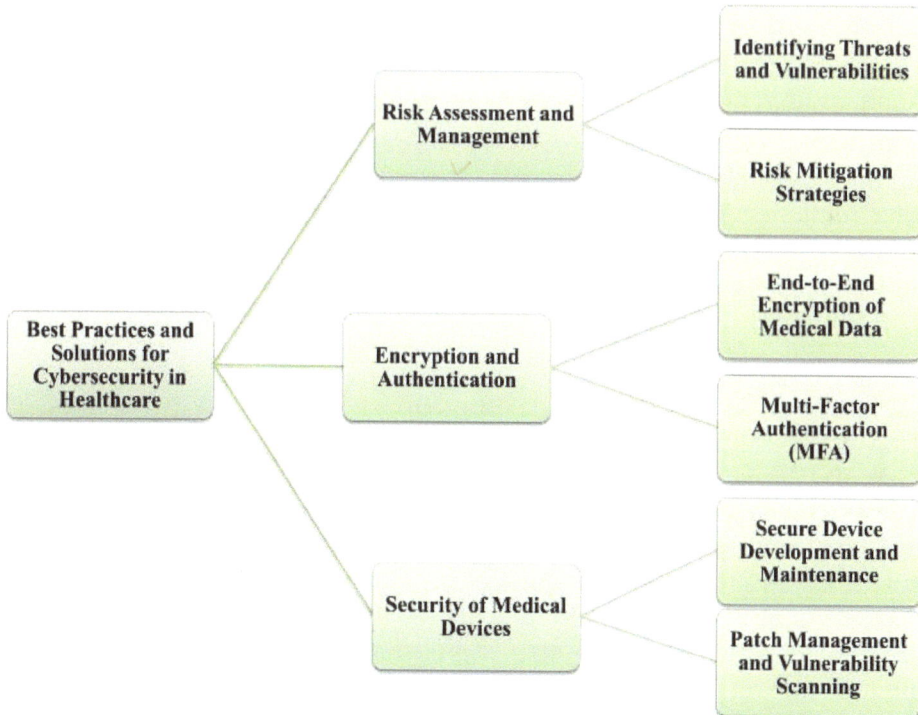

Fig. (3). Solution for cybersecurity in healthcare.

Risk Assessment and Management

Risk assessment and management are crucial to help identify potential weaknesses and reduce their impact. This includes analyzing the threats, creating risk assessments, and making mitigation plans to protect healthcare data from various cyber threats. A good risk management plan effectively directs resources to those areas that have the potential to result in the highest possible impact, leading to greater security [37].

Identifying Threats and Vulnerabilities

Threats and vulnerabilities are an integral part of any healthcare cybersecurity. Cybercriminals, insider threats, or even system weaknesses are all examples of potential origins of threats. Healthcare organizations need to identify relevant risks like malware, ransomware, data breaches, and phishing that can expose patient data or disrupt healthcare functions. Vulnerabilities can include outdated software, poor coding practices, and untrained personnel who handle sensitive data. In order to decrease risk, it is imperative to frequently conduct vulnerability scans, keep software up-to-date, and train employees on software security practices. The threat-intelligence systems that measure external and internal factors can participate in the proactive detection of emerging threats. The assessment must be comprehensive, including potential entry points like network connections, open medical devices, and legacy databases. Moreover, human error is a contributing factor to many vulnerabilities, including insecure passwords and mishandling of sensitive data. The staff training is given utmost importance here and later implemented by technical means such as firewalls, intrusion detection systems, and encryption to reduce the number of weak points and to protect the system from cyber threats and breaches [38].

Risk Mitigation Strategies

In healthcare, the emphasis of risk mitigation is on cyber threats, focusing on reducing the consequences as well as the chance of specific threats. One of the most popular strategies is the application of a layered security approach, with multiple levels of defenses to guard the information. Firewalls, intrusion detection systems, and encryption technologies prevent unauthorized access. Moreover, implementing strong password policies, multi-factor authentication, and role-based access control (RBAC) allows sensitive information to be accessed only by authorized personnel. They are also amongst the most significant practices for reducing the impact of a ransomware attack, as appropriate data backups can help the healthcare provider recover their data in the event of a breach. One of the most critical aspects of risk remediation is patch management, which ensures that software and systems are updated as soon as new patches are released [39].

Vulnerability scanning tools help to discover vulnerabilities within systems and applications so they can be fixed before a malicious attacker does. Healthcare organizations should also have a robust organization-wide incident response plan that includes detection, investigation, and remediation of security incidents. Regular staff training on cybersecurity threats and what needs to be done will help cultivate a culture of awareness around security. Third-party vendors also need to collaborate to ensure shared risk management since certain medical devices and software used by healthcare providers can contain vulnerabilities. In addition, implementing a zero-trust security model, in which zero access is granted without verification of both users and devices, can go a long way in minimizing the possibility of internal threats [40].

Encryption and Authentication

Encryption and authentication are essential to secure sensitive healthcare data. While using encryption secures patient information from being stored and transmitted, authentication systems help to verify the identity of users and devices that access medical systems. These practices offer protection against unauthorized access and data breaches [41].

End-to-End Encryption of Medical Data

The E2EE also protects medical data when it is sent over the network and only decrypts the data once it gets to the desired destination. This encryption ensures that even if the data is intercepted (which generally falls under the category of authorized penetration), a stranger cannot read it, nor alter any of its contents. For example, in the case of medical records or lab results being transmitted over the internet to a healthcare provider, E2EE protects data between the healthcare provider and patient, regardless of the level of security in the network. E2EE can also safeguard data when medical devices, like a wearable health tracker or diagnostic tool, transmit information to centralized systems or healthcare [42].

This prevents hackers from accessing personal health information during transmission. Moreover, when E2EE is combined with secure storage protocols, the overall security level of medical data attained is even stronger. Healthcare organizations should ensure that keys are stored securely and can only be accessed by authorized personnel. Audits and an update of encryption protocols must continuously occur to sustain the security and structure of the data. The lack of E2EE makes sensitive medical data susceptible to interception, and breaches of confidentiality can easily take place [43].

Multi-Factor Authentication (MFA)

Multi-factor authentication (MFA) is a security measure that requires users to enter more than one type of verification to gain access to sensitive medical systems or data. MFA enhances access by combining two or more authentication factors (what the user knows (password), what the user has (their smartphone or hardware token), and something the user is (biometric), which the user has to provide to reduce the likelihood of a successful access attempt to zero. MFA is critical in the healthcare sector, as it prevents unauthorized access to medical records that contain a treasure trove of sensitive information that cybercriminals can use for identity theft, fraud, or ransom. Both hospitals and clinics in the healthcare sector are implementing MFA more frequently to protect personal health information. MFA is known to reduce the risks related to password-based attacks like phishing and brute-force attacks. Metrics Keep Passwordless: The combination of biometrics, such as a fingerprint or facial recognition, provides a more secure option than traditional password authentication. Nevertheless, healthcare organizations need to balance security and usability so that they do not impede the work of healthcare professionals, who require rapid, efficient access to patient information [44, 45].

Security of Medical Devices

Protecting against cyberattacks on medical devices is challenging yet crucial to ensure patient care is not disrupted and sensitive data is not compromised. Security by design, periodic patching, and monitoring ensure the devices cannot be compromised and that remote access control is not taken over [46].

Secure Device Development and Maintenance

Securing devices is one of the most crucial aspects of healthcare cybersecurity as it plays a major role in device development and maintenance. Ensuring the security of medical devices is just as important as the connectivity and integration of medical devices with any or all of the healthcare systems. During the planning phase of development, manufacturers can build security by using strong encryption, secure communication protocols, and strong authentication to prevent cyberattacks. Developers should incorporate built-in security capabilities that facilitate software updates and patches to fix recent vulnerabilities. Also, manufacturers ought to offer healthcare organizations thorough guidance on the secure deployment and maintenance of devices [47].

Maintaining the security of medical devices throughout their lifecycle is also crucial. This encompasses regular risk assessments, vulnerability scanning, and penetration testing to detect and remediate possible threats. Healthcare providers should establish partnerships with medical device manufacturers to ensure that devices are updated with the latest security patches. In addition, the network segmentation would keep medical devices separate from other important system sectors. Therefore, best practice would recommend that the healthcare organization adopt such a strategy to reduce the number of critical systems that the attacker can breach. It also lists practices such as secure device decommissioning to reduce the risk of unauthorized access to sensitive patient information [48].

Patch Management and Vulnerability Scanning

Managing patches and scanning devices for vulnerabilities is critical to securing the medical devices themselves. Patch management involves the quick application of software updates, also known as patches, from the manufacturer, which will include updates to address security vulnerabilities. Medical devices without patching will always be vulnerable to cyberattacks using well-known exploits. Healthcare organizations need to ensure a robust patch management plan, defined not just by the timeliness of patches but also by what goes into identifying, testing, and applying them. This process must involve cooperation with device manufacturers to ensure that patches do not disrupt the operation of the device. This is where vulnerability scanning comes in, and the same goes for medical devices with potential exploits to discover [49].

Automated vulnerability scanning tools can help identify legacy software, unaddressed security weaknesses, and misconfigurations that could expose devices to attack. Constant scanning and security testing ensure that vulnerabilities are discovered as early as possible before attackers can exploit them. With medical devices becoming even more connected, vulnerability scanning should be a key part of any cybersecurity strategy for healthcare organizations. In addition, a risk-based approach to the vulnerability management process is necessary to identify and prioritize which vulnerabilities are absorbing time and resources that can better be spent to protect patient safety and data from harm [50].

EMERGING TECHNOLOGIES IN CYBERSECURITY

While AI boosts the ability to identify and respond to threats, blockchain can provide secure storage of personal data and patient privacy. While quantum computing is still under development, it has the potential to transform encryption methods, providing stronger and speedier adaptive mechanisms for defense. These technologies provide a competitive advantage in an ever more complicated cybersecurity world [51].

AI for Threat Detection and Response

AI has been a strong technology to be used for cybersecurity, especially threat detection and response. Traditional security methods often struggle to keep up with the volume and complexity of modern cyber threats. AI, however, relies on analyzing massive amounts of data and detecting anomalies that a human analyst may miss, with tons of data coming in at the same time. AI systems can use algorithms and machine learning models to discover anomalies, identify patterns in malicious behavior, and even anticipate potential cyberattacks before they occur. Upon detecting a threat, AI can trigger automatic responses like quarantining affected machines or cutting off access, usually without human input. The ongoing learning mechanisms of AI also help with adapting to new threats, which means organizations have to do everything possible to shore up their cybersecurity stance. Especially in high-stakes industries such as healthcare, finance, and government, it is necessary to apply this to mitigate risks [52, 53].

Machine Learning Models for Predicting Cyber Threats

ML models are the most common in predicting and preventing cyber threats. These models study past data and recognize patterns, then predict possible future cyberattacks before they occur. Recognizing patterns in data can identify subtle anomalies indicating malicious activity, such as a login at an unusual time or abnormal network traffic. These models learn and develop with time and thus become more accurate in identifying the latest threats. Among the most obvious benefits of ML in cybersecurity is the ability to discover zero-day vulnerabilities (new exploits that conventional security tools may not have detected). Because it is predictive in nature, machine learning can help organizations to mitigate risks by enabling proactive defenses, such as fixing vulnerabilities or changing network access policies before a cyber-attack occurs. ML models are scalable to increasing data volumes, allowing organizations to keep pace with the dynamic nature of cyber threats. As these technologies develop, they will form an integral part of a proactive cybersecurity strategy [54, 55].

Blockchain for Secure Patient Data Sharing

Blockchain can provide a secure and efficient framework to allow patient data to be viewed by many healthcare service providers. Interoperability, privacy concerns, and the risks of unauthorized access are issues of data sharing that tend to have a relatively low concern level using traditional approaches. This means that hospitals, doctors, and any other health facility can easily and securely exchange information thanks to the decentralized and permanent ledger of Blockchain technology. For example, when a patient shares their medical records, this transaction is publicly and transparently stored on a blockchain, ensuring authenticity. This means that only authorized parties have access to the patient's data, and access is granted *via* safe, blockchain-based authentication mechanisms [56, 57].

Smart Contracts for Healthcare Transactions

Blockchain technology enables a new form of healthcare smart contracts, which can effectively provide automation and trust for healthcare transactions. A smart contract is a self-executing contract with the terms of the agreement between buyer and seller directly written into lines of code. They do not require an intermediary because they automatically perform actions when certain conditions are fulfilled. Smart contracts can automate insurance claims and payment processing, as well as to help manage consent tracking in healthcare. For example, a smart contract can automatically verify the details of a claim to ensure it matches the patient's insurance policy after a healthcare provider submits a claim and processes payment if all criteria are met. This automation reduces administrative overhead, minimizes human error, and enhances the speed of transactions. Furthermore, smart contracts are secured, transparent, and immutable by virtue of being written on a blockchain, which means that everyone involved may trust the transaction and its execution. That is why smart contracts can be more useful in reducing fraud and making healthcare more efficient [58, 59].

THE ROLE OF HEALTHCARE PROVIDERS AND POLICY MAKERS

Healthcare providers and policymakers play a crucial role in ensuring the protection of patient data and healthcare infrastructure. They support organizations in developing risk mitigation strategies, formulate and implement robust cybersecurity policies and procedures, train employees, and collaborate with cybersecurity specialists, thereby reducing risks, improving data and application security, and increasing overall trust in the healthcare system [60].

Training and Awareness Programs for Healthcare Workers

Training and awareness programs are mandatory for healthcare workers to get insight into cybersecurity risks and best practices. Such programs must emphasize the development of a proactive culture of security awareness and encourage employees to identify potential threats as well as respond with suitable actions to protect patient data and other organizational assets [61].

Role of Staff in Maintaining Cybersecurity Hygiene

Staff members are integral to maintaining cybersecurity hygiene in healthcare environments. Employees minimize the likelihood of cyberattacks by following the right security protocols. Such as password management guidelines, avoiding outdated software and systems, and being careful with sensitive information. Healthcare professionals should be cautious while retrieving patient records, as only authorized personnel should access sensitive information. They also need to refrain from using unsecured devices or networks to access the organization's systems. Regular training sessions should continue to stress the significance of cybersecurity hygiene and ensure the staff is easy with the resources and skills to safeguard these healthcare systems from threats. When staff are secure in their culture, they are more likely to follow the stages of cybersecurity and report any potential threats. Encouraging the staff to stay up to date on new threats like phishing and ransomware also helps bring about an extra line of defense for the organization, protecting patient data and the integrity of the system [62].

Healthcare Leadership and Cybersecurity Policies

Healthcare leadership is essential in shaping and implementing cybersecurity policies that protect sensitive patient information and healthcare infrastructure. By prioritizing cybersecurity at the organizational level, leaders ensure the allocation of necessary resources, establish clear security guidelines, and foster a culture of compliance and vigilance [63].

Developing Cybersecurity Frameworks

A cybersecurity framework in healthcare is essential for mitigating risks and protecting patient data. This framework should consist of policies, procedures, and technical security safeguards that cover a wide range of potential threats and vulnerabilities. Such should encompass risk assessments, incident response plans, access controls, and continual monitoring. It must also be in conjunction with national and international standards, which dictate industries that need to adhere to specific guidelines. Important components of a strong cybersecurity framework include encrypted confidential information, secure channels of communication, and regular software updates to plug security holes. In addition, the healthcare organizations should follow a multi-layered security approach, such as strong firewalls, and intrusion detection and prevention systems to restrict unauthorized access, providing and promoting regular employee training to keep up with cybersecurity best practices and new threats. The framework is set up in a way that requires collaboration between different departments, like IT, compliance, and more clinical staff, to make sure it meets the unique cybersecurity challenges in the industry. The importance of this audit and frequent framework updates guarantees that it is relevant and protects vital healthcare data [64, 65].

Collaborations with Cybersecurity Experts

Collaborating with cybersecurity experts is vital for healthcare organizations to stay ahead of emerging threats. They can identify the vulnerabilities, review the existing practices, and recommend best practices to improve the security policies specific to healthcare systems. By collaborating with cybersecurity experts, fortresses can obtain access to state-of-the-art tools, threat intelligence, and incident response techniques. They can also help design tailored training software that strengthens cybersecurity awareness among employees while ensuring that all employees are abreast with the best practices. Additionally, professionals can guide healthcare organizations in the adoption of advanced technologies, like AI-driven threat detection and immediate monitoring systems, to help detect and thwart threats before they manifest. Cybersecurity specialists can give not only information on threats but also point to trends in their profession, which will allow healthcare providers to adapt. Engaging experts enables healthcare organizations to fortify their cybersecurity defenses and ensures that care providers are protected against cyberattacks targeting sensitive patient data or critical infrastructure [66, 67].

Government Regulations and Industry Standards

Government regulations and industry standards are essential to ensure that healthcare organizations maintain strong cybersecurity practices. These regulations help establish consistent security protocols, safeguard patient data, and promote compliance with best practices across the sector, strengthening the overall cybersecurity posture in healthcare [68].

Strengthening Legal and Regulatory Frameworks

Strengthening legal and regulatory frameworks in healthcare is crucial for addressing the rising threat of cyberattacks and ensuring the protection of patient data. Governments and regulatory organizations need to provide a concrete set of standards regarding cybersecurity, which health organizations should be compliant with, similar to HIPAA in the U.S. This regulation appropriately orders the healthcare institutes to practice the best security practices, practice regular risk assessments, and report the breaches immediately. It should also respond to emergent threats, whether it be ransomware or advanced persistent threats, with clearly defined penalties for non-compliance. Regulations can promote the use of cybersecurity technologies, such as encryption and multi-factor authentication, that healthcare organizations should be using to better defend themselves. Instead, governments and industry should work together to develop national cybersecurity frameworks that are in line with global standards to help ensure that health organizations are aware of enemy attacks. This will help build public trust regarding the ability of sectors to protect sensitive information [69, 70].

Global Cybersecurity Standards in Healthcare

These global cybersecurity standards in healthcare represent a harmonized strategy to ensure patient data and healthcare systems are cyberattack-proof. For instance, standards like ISO/IEC 27001 and the NIST Cybersecurity Framework provide guidelines for healthcare organizations to implement sound security practices and protect the confidentiality, integrity, and availability of health data. Compliance with global standards benefits organizations in minimizing the risk of cyber threats, including data breaches and ransomware attacks, through best practices in data protection and incident response. There are more than a few standards that highlight the implementation of measures like continuous monitoring, risk management, staff training, *etc*, to keep cybersecurity resilience intact. These standards should be proactively adapted for emerging threats and technologies through global dialogue between healthcare providers, policymakers, and cybersecurity experts. The adoption of international standards in cybersecurity helps healthcare organizations show their commitment to ensuring the protection of patients and patient data, hence maintaining the trust of the customers and stakeholders of the organization. Although they do help facilitate cross-border collaboration, global standards also enhance the security and efficiency of the healthcare systems by providing a common framework between the systems [71, 72].

CONCLUSION

Connected healthcare cybersecurity is an important part of protecting patient data, maintaining healthcare services, and growing trust in digital health solutions. The trend toward connected healthcare through IoT, cloud computing, and AI also brings an escalation in the risk of data breaches, ransomware, and the security of medical devices. These challenges need to be met with a strong combination that involves risk management, encryption, and multi-factor authentication. Innovative technologies like artificial intelligence and blockchain are viable options, as they help detect threats better while ensuring the security of patient's data. Nevertheless, the multi-stakeholder, antiquated infrastructure environment of healthcare systems presents significant challenges. A multi-stakeholder approach is vital as providers, policymakers, and cybersecurity experts must design robust frameworks and policies that protect the data and systems upon which the industry relies. Continuous education of health workers and compliance with the world's cybersecurity regulations can decrease the risk. As healthcare continues to evolve in the digital age, a proactive and coordinated approach to cybersecurity is imperative to protect both patients and the healthcare ecosystem from cyber threats.

REFERENCES

[1]   Weber K, Kleine N. Cybersecurity in health care. International Library of Ethics, Law and Technology 2020; 21: 139-56.
[http://dx.doi.org/10.1007/978-3-030-29053-5_7]

[2]   Alanazi AT. Clinicians' perspectives on healthcare cybersecurity and cyber threats. Cureus 2023; 15(10): e47026.
[http://dx.doi.org/10.7759/cureus.47026] [PMID: 37965389]

[3]   Belliger A, Krieger DJ. The digital transformation of healthcare. In: North K, Maier R, Haas O, Eds. Knowledge management in digital change: new findings and practical cases 2018; 311-26.
[http://dx.doi.org/10.1007/978-3-319-73546-7_19]

[4]   Kraus S, Schiavone F, Pluzhnikova A, Invernizzi AC. Digital transformation in healthcare: Analyzing the current state-of-research. J Bus Res 2021; 123: 557-67.
[http://dx.doi.org/10.1016/j.jbusres.2020.10.030]

[5]   Yelton SJ, Schoener B. The evolution of healthcare technology management in leading healthcare delivery organizations. Biomed Instrum Technol 2020; 54(2): 119-24.
[http://dx.doi.org/10.2345/0899-8205-54.2.119] [PMID: 32186916]

[6]   Kaur M, Thakur S, Hussain U. Evolution in the health care sector with emerging technologies. Tenth International Conference on Wireless and Optical Communications Networks (WOCN) 2013; 1-4.
[http://dx.doi.org/10.1109/WOCN.2013.6616213]

[7]   Tabish SA, Nabil S. Future of healthcare delivery: Strategies that will reshape the healthcare industry landscape. Int J Sci Res 2015; 4(2): 727-58.

[8]   Mantaleon D. The evolving landscape of healthcare: challenges, innovations, and a vision for the future. Health Sci J 2023; 17(8): 1-3.

[9]   Bohr A, Memarzadeh K. The rise of artificial intelligence in healthcare applications. In: Artificial Intelligence in healthcare. Academic Press 2020; pp. 25-60.
[http://dx.doi.org/10.1016/B978-0-12-818438-7.00002-2]

[10]   Nayak S, Blumenfeld NR, Laksanasopin T, Sia SK. Point-of-care diagnostics: recent developments in a connected age. Anal Chem 2017; 89(1): 102-23.
[http://dx.doi.org/10.1021/acs.analchem.6b04630] [PMID: 27958710]

[11]   Vishnu S, Ramson SJ, Jegan R. 5th International Conference on Devices, Circuits and Systems (ICDCS) 2020; 101-4.

[12]   Ashfaq Z, Rafay A, Mumtaz R, *et al.* A review of enabling technologies for Internet of Medical Things (IoMT) Ecosystem. Ain Shams Eng J 2022; 13(4): 101660.
[http://dx.doi.org/10.1016/j.asej.2021.101660]

[13]   Qian L, Luo Z, Du Y, Guo L. Cloud computing: an overview. In: Jaatun MG, Zhao G, Rong C, Eds. Cloud computing: first international conference, CloudCom 2009; 2009 Dec 1-4; Beijing, China. Berlin, Heidelberg: Springer; 2009. p. 626–31.

[14]   Sunyaev A, Sunyaev A. Cloud computing. Internet computing: principles of distributed systems and emerging internet-based technologies 2020; 195-236.

[15]   Schnall R, Rojas M, Bakken S, *et al.* A user-centered model for designing consumer mobile health (mHealth) applications (apps). J Biomed Inform 2016; 60: 243-51.

[http://dx.doi.org/10.1016/j.jbi.2016.02.002] [PMID: 26903153]

[16]   Field MJ, Grigsby J. Telemedicine and remote patient monitoring. JAMA 2002; 288(4): 423-5.
        [http://dx.doi.org/10.1001/jama.288.4.423] [PMID: 12132953]

[17]   Ngiam KY, Khor IW. Big data and machine learning algorithms for health-care delivery. Lancet
        Oncol 2019; 20(5): e262-73.
        [http://dx.doi.org/10.1016/S1470-2045(19)30149-4] [PMID: 31044724]

[18]   Beam AL, Kohane IS. Big data and machine learning in health care. JAMA 2018; 319(13): 1317-8.
        [http://dx.doi.org/10.1001/jama.2017.18391] [PMID: 29532063]

[19]   Lovestone S. The European medical information framework: A novel ecosystem for sharing healthcare
        data across Europe. Learn Health Syst 2020; 4(2): e10214.
        [http://dx.doi.org/10.1002/lrh2.10214] [PMID: 32313838]

[20]   Islam S, Grigoriadis C, Papastergiou S. Information sharing for creating awareness for securing the
        healthcare ecosystem. 2023, the 19th International Conference on the Design of Reliable
        Communication Networks (DRCN) 2023 Apr 17; 1-5.
        [http://dx.doi.org/10.1109/DRCN57075.2023.10108266]

[21]   Iroju O, Soriyan A, Gambo I, Olaleke J. Interoperability in healthcare: benefits, challenges and
        resolutions. Int J Innov Appl Stud 2013; 3(1): 262-70.

[22]   Albouq SS, Sen AAA, Almashf N, Yamin M, Alshanqiti A, Bahbouh NM. A survey of
        interoperability challenges and solutions for dealing with them in an IoT environment. IEEE Access
        2022; 10: 36416-28.
        [http://dx.doi.org/10.1109/ACCESS.2022.3162219]

[23]   Chua JA. PMP C. Cybersecurity in the healthcare industry. J Med Pract Manage 2021; 36: 229-31.

[24]   Javaid M, Haleem A, Singh RP, Suman R. Towards insighting cybersecurity for healthcare domains:
        A comprehensive review of recent practices and trends. Cyber Security and Applications 2023; 1:
        100016.
        [http://dx.doi.org/10.1016/j.csa.2023.100016]

[25]   Manworren N, Letwat J, Daily O. Why you should care about the Target data breach. Bus Horiz 2016;
        59(3): 257-66.
        [http://dx.doi.org/10.1016/j.bushor.2016.01.002]

[26]   Minnaar A, Herbig FJ. Cyberattacks and the cybercrime threat of ransomware to hospitals and
        healthcare services during the COVID-19 pandemic. Acta Criminologica: African Journal of
        Criminology & Victimology 2021; 34(3): 155-85.

[27]   Gupta S, Singhal A, Kapoor A. A literature survey on social engineering attacks: phishing attack.
        International conference on computing, communication and automation (ICCCA) 2016 Apr 29; 537-
        40.

[28]   Al-Otaibi AF, Alsuwat ES. A study on social engineering attacks: Phishing attack. International
        Journal of Recent Advances in Multidisciplinary Research 2020; 7(11): 6374-80.

[29]   Williams PA, Woodward AJ. Cybersecurity vulnerabilities in medical devices: a complex environment
        and multifaceted problem. 2015; 305-16.
        [http://dx.doi.org/10.2147/MDER.S50048]

[30]   Bracciale L, Loreti P, Bianchi G. Cybersecurity vulnerability analysis of medical devices purchased by
        national health services. Sci Rep 2023; 13(1): 19509.
        [http://dx.doi.org/10.1038/s41598-023-45927-1] [PMID: 37945583]

[31]   Ray S, Mishra KN, Dutta S. Detection and prevention of DDoS attacks on M-healthcare sensitive data:
        a novel approach. International Journal of Information Technology 2022; 14(3): 1333-41.
        [http://dx.doi.org/10.1007/s41870-022-00869-1]

[32]   Ashu MR. DDoS attacks impact on data transfer in IOT-MANET-based E-Healthcare for tackling

COVID-19. In: Khanna A, Gupta D, Pólkowski Z, Bhattacharyya S, Castillo O, Eds. Data Analytics and Management: Proceedings of ICDAM 2021; 301-9.

[33] Kotkova B. Cybersecurity in the healthcare sector- current threats. International Multidisciplinary Scientific GeoConference: SGEM 2022; 22(2.1): 11-8.

[34] Sendelj R, Ognjanovic I. Cybersecurity challenges in healthcare. Achievements, milestones and challenges in biomedical and health informatics. IOS Press 2022; pp. 190-202.
[http://dx.doi.org/10.3233/SHTI220951]

[35] Pool J, Akhlaghpour S, Fatehi F, Burton-Jones A. A systematic analysis of failures in protecting personal health data: A scoping review. Int J Inf Manage 2024; 74: 102719.
[http://dx.doi.org/10.1016/j.ijinfomgt.2023.102719]

[36] Affia AO, Finch H, Jung W, Samori IA, Potter L, Palmer XL. IoT health devices: exploring security risks in the connected landscape. IoT 2023; 4(2): 150-82.
[http://dx.doi.org/10.3390/iot4020009]

[37] Giuca O, Popescu TM, Popescu AM, Prostean G, Popescu DE. A survey of cybersecurity risk management frameworks. Proceedings of the 8th International Workshop Soft Computing Applications (SOFA 2018) Vol. I2021; : 240-72.
[http://dx.doi.org/10.1007/978-3-030-51992-6_20]

[38] He Y, Aliyu A, Evans M, Luo C. Health care cybersecurity challenges and solutions under the climate of COVID-19: Scoping review. J Med Internet Res 2021; 23(4): e21747.
[http://dx.doi.org/10.2196/21747] [PMID: 33764885]

[39] Iso I. Risk management–Principles and guidelines. Geneva, Switzerland: International Organization for Standardization 2009.

[40] Pennock MJ, Haimes YY. Principles and guidelines for project risk management. Syst Eng 2002; 5(2): 89-108.
[http://dx.doi.org/10.1002/sys.10009]

[41] Pradeep Kumar K, Prathap BR, Thiruthuvanathan MM, Murthy H, Jha Pillai V. Secure approach to sharing digitized medical data in a cloud environment. Data Science and Management 2024; 7(2): 108-18.
[http://dx.doi.org/10.1016/j.dsm.2023.12.001]

[42] Hale B, Komlo C. On end-to-end encryption. Cryptology ePrint Archive 2022.

[43] Bai W, Pearson M, Kelley PG, Mazurek ML. Improving non-experts' understanding of end-to-end encryption: an exploratory study. IEEE European Symposium on Security and Privacy Workshops (EuroS&PW) 2020 Sep 7; 210-9.

[44] Ibrokhimov S, Hui KL, Al-Absi AA, Sain M. Multi-factor authentication in cyber-physical systems: a state-of-the-art survey. the 21st International Conference on Advanced Communication Technology (ICACT) 2019 Feb 17; 279-84.
[http://dx.doi.org/10.23919/ICACT.2019.8701960]

[45] Henricks A, Kettani H. On data protection using multi-factor authentication. Proceedings of the 2019 International Conference on Information Systems and System Management 2019; 1-4.

[46] Rindfleisch TC. Privacy, information technology, and health care. Commun ACM 1997; 40(8): 92-100.
[http://dx.doi.org/10.1145/257874.257896]

[47] Meingast M, Roosta T, Sastry S. Security and privacy issues with health care information technology. International Conference of the IEEE Engineering in Medicine and Biology Society 2006 Aug 30; 5453-8.
[http://dx.doi.org/10.1109/IEMBS.2006.260060]

[48] Layode O, Naiho HN, Adeleke GS, Udeh EO, Labake TT. The role of cybersecurity in facilitating

sustainable healthcare solutions: Overcoming challenges to protect sensitive data. Int Med Sci Res J 2024; 4(6): 668-93.
[http://dx.doi.org/10.51594/imsrj.v4i6.1228]

[49]   Colarik AM. A secure patch management authority. PhD dissertation. Auckland (New Zealand): University of Auckland 2003.

[50]   Dissanayake N, Jayatilaka A, Zahedi M, Babar MA. Software security patch management - A systematic literature review of challenges, approaches, tools and practices. Inf Softw Technol 2022; 144: 106771.
[http://dx.doi.org/10.1016/j.infsof.2021.106771]

[51]   Lewallen J. Emerging technologies and problem definition uncertainty: The case of cybersecurity. Regul Gov 2021; 15(4): 1035-52.
[http://dx.doi.org/10.1111/rego.12341]

[52]   Katiyar N, Tripathi MS, Kumar MP, Verma MS, Sahu AK, Saxena S AI. Educational Administration: Theory and Practice 2024; 30(4): 6273-82.

[53]   Shutenko V. AI in Cybersecurity: Exploring the Top 6 Use Cases. TechMagic 2023.

[54]   Samia N, Saha S, Haque A. Predicting and mitigating cyber threats through data mining and machine learning. Comput Commun 2024; 228: 107949.
[http://dx.doi.org/10.1016/j.comcom.2024.107949]

[55]   Sarker IH. Machine learning for intelligent data analysis and automation in cybersecurity: current and future prospects. Annals of Data Science 2023; 10(6): 1473-98.
[http://dx.doi.org/10.1007/s40745-022-00444-2]

[56]   Kunal S, Gandhi P, Rathod D, Amin R, Sharma S. Securing patient data in the healthcare industry: A blockchain-driven protocol with advanced encryption. J Educ Health Promot 2024; 13(1): 94.
[http://dx.doi.org/10.4103/jehp.jehp_984_23] [PMID: 38726083]

[57]   Ali O, Jaradat A, Kulakli A, Abuhalimeh A. A comparative study: Blockchain technology utilization benefits, challenges, and functionalities. IEEE Access 2021; 9: 12730-49.
[http://dx.doi.org/10.1109/ACCESS.2021.3050241]

[58]   Khatoon A. A blockchain-based smart contract system for healthcare management. Electronics (Basel) 2020; 9(1): 94.
[http://dx.doi.org/10.3390/electronics9010094]

[59]   Sharma A, Sarishma , Tomar R, Chilamkurti N, Kim B-G. Blockchain Based Smart Contracts for Internet of Medical Things in e-Healthcare. Electronics (Basel) 2020; 9(10): 1609.
[http://dx.doi.org/10.3390/electronics9101609]

[60]   Harries J, Cooper D, Myer L, Bracken H, Zweigenthal V, Orner P. Policy maker and health care provider perspectives on reproductive decision-making amongst HIV-infected individuals in South Africa. BMC Public Health 2007; 7(1): 282.
[http://dx.doi.org/10.1186/1471-2458-7-282] [PMID: 17919335]

[61]   Mackert M, Ball J, Lopez N. Health literacy awareness training for healthcare workers: Improving knowledge and intentions to use clear communication techniques. Patient Educ Couns 2011; 85(3): e225-8.
[http://dx.doi.org/10.1016/j.pec.2011.02.022] [PMID: 21474264]

[62]   Clarke M, Martin K. Managing cybersecurity risk in healthcare settings. Healthcare Management Forum 2024; 37(1): 17-20.
[http://dx.doi.org/10.1177/08404704231195804]

[63]   Burrell DN, Aridi AS, McLester Q, *et al.* Exploring systems thinking leadership approaches to the healthcare cybersecurity environment. Int J of Ext Auto Conn Health 2021; 3(2): 20-32. [IJEACH].
[http://dx.doi.org/10.4018/IJEACH.2021070103]

[64] Oyeniyi LD, Ugochukwu CE, Mhlongo NZ. Developing cybersecurity frameworks for financial institutions: A comprehensive review and best practices. Comp Sci IT Res J 2024; 5(4): 903-25.
[http://dx.doi.org/10.51594/csitrj.v5i4.1049]

[65] Jacobs PC, von Solms SH, Grobler MM. Towards a framework for the development of business cybersecurity capabilities. Business & Management Review 2016; 7(4): 51.

[66] Tully J, Selzer J, Phillips JP, O'Connor P, Dameff C. Healthcare challenges in the era of cybersecurity. Health Secur 2020; 18(3): 228-31.
[http://dx.doi.org/10.1089/hs.2019.0123] [PMID: 32559153]

[67] Adebukola AA, Navya AN, Jordan FJ, Jenifer NJ, Begley RD. Cybersecurity as a threat to health care. Journal of Technology and Systems 2022; 4(1): 32-64.
[http://dx.doi.org/10.47941/jts.1149]

[68] Tompkin RB. Interactions between government and industry food safety activities. Food Control 2001; 12(4): 203-7.
[http://dx.doi.org/10.1016/S0956-7135(00)00038-4]

[69] Elendu C, Omeludike EK, Oloyede PO, Obidigbo BT, Omeludike JC. Legal implications for clinicians in cybersecurity incidents: A review. Medicine (Baltimore) 2024; 103(39): e39887.
[http://dx.doi.org/10.1097/MD.0000000000039887] [PMID: 39331908]

[70] Rahim MJ, Rahim MI, Afroz A, Akinola O. Cybersecurity threats in healthcare IT: challenges, risks, and mitigation strategies. J Artif Intell Gen Sci 2024 Dec; 6(1): 438-62.

[71] Luidold C, Jungbauer C. Cybersecurity policy framework requirements for the establishment of highly interoperable and interconnected health data spaces. Front Med (Lausanne) 2024; 11: 1379852.
[http://dx.doi.org/10.3389/fmed.2024.1379852] [PMID: 38784226]

[72] Kandasamy K, Srinivas S, Achuthan K, Rangan VP. Digital healthcare-cyberattacks in asian organizations: an analysis of vulnerabilities, risks, NIST perspectives, and recommendations. IEEE Access 2022; 10: 12345-64.
[http://dx.doi.org/10.1109/ACCESS.2022.3145372]

CHAPTER 14

Remote Patient Monitoring and Home Healthcare Solutions

SK Abdul Rahaman[1,*], Afroz Khan[1], MD Kaif[1], Naga Rani Kagithala[1], Arfa Shams[1] and **Niranjan Kaushik[1]**

[1] *Department of Pharmacy, School of Medical and Allied Sciences, Galgotias University, Greater Noida, Uttar Pradesh-201310, India*

Abstract: Remote Patient Monitoring (RPM) enables patient observation outside traditional medical settings, such as at home or remote locations, enhancing care access and reducing healthcare costs. By using digital technologies, RPM collects health data like vital signs, blood pressure, and sleep quality from patients in one particular location and securely transmits it to healthcare providers elsewhere for analysis and recommendations. This method promotes real-time monitoring using mobile medical devices, helping prevent unnecessary hospitalizations, improve recovery, and ensure patient safety. RPM gathers biometric data such as heart rate and blood oxygen level, analyzes it, and shares insights with caregivers remotely. These programs can perform bedside-like observations, reducing optional readmissions and in-person visits. The approach revolutionizes healthcare by shifting from reactive to proactive care, improving patient outcomes, engagement, and satisfaction while lowering costs. Future advancements in RPM, powered by wearable technology and artificial intelligence, aim to personalize care, enhance early disease detection, and support secure data exchange. As these innovations grow, ensuring patient data privacy and security will remain critical, alongside developing integrated home healthcare ecosystems. RPM and home healthcare solutions are transforming healthcare delivery, prioritizing accessible, effective, and patient-centered care.

Keywords: AI, Biosensor, Case studies, Challenge, Chronic disease management, Cloud computing, Healthcare, Integration of RPM, IoT, Mhealth, Real-time remote monitoring, Remote patient monitoring, Wearable.

INTRODUCTION

Remote Patient Monitoring stands as a novel approach to enhance well-being and optimize patient management and care [1]. Patient disease-related and physiological data are communicated digitally over the telephone, Internet, or

* **Corresponding author SK Abdul Rahaman:** Department of Pharmacy, School of Medical and Allied Sciences, Galgotias University, Greater Noida, Uttar Pradesh-201310, India; E-mail: rahamandr123@gmail.com

Shaweta Sharma, Akhil Sharma, Shivkanya Fuloria & Anurag Singh (Eds.)
All rights reserved-© 2025 Bentham Science Publishers

videoconferencing from the patient's residence to a healthcare facility, facilitating clinical input. It facilitates the early identification of illness decompensation, hence permitting timely treatments and decreasing mortality and hospitalization rates, while also enhancing patient education and self-management. Technology has experienced several alterations, facilitating the extensive adoption of telemedicine [2]. Currently, equipment includes intelligent sensors, wearable or handheld gadgets, Internet-connected smartphones, and implanted monitoring devices that are readily accessible. The substantial volume of articles on telemonitoring in the last decade indicates the growing significance of technology in healthcare, notwithstanding the increasing interest in telemonitoring treatments and evidence.

Remote Patient Monitoring

Remote Patient Monitoring (RPM) is a technology-based system that captures a variety of health-related data directly from the point of care, such as vital signs, blood pressure, oxygen levels, body temperature, and brain activity, among other metrics [3]. Following collection, the data is distributed to healthcare professionals working in medical institutions such as hospitals, clinics, critical care units, and nursing homes. Remote Patient Monitoring (RPM) uses a variety of monitoring technologies, such as wearables, sensors, and mobile applications, to gather and transmit patients' health data to healthcare practitioners.

The purpose of remote patient monitoring systems is to collect various physiological data from patients. Electrocardiograms (ECGs), electroencephalograms (EEGs), heartbeats and respiration rate, blood oxygen levels (also known as pulse oximetry), nervous system signals, blood pressure, body/skin temperature, and blood glucose levels are the most commonly collected data. In addition to these, patient weight, activity level, and sleep information are occasionally gathered. Numerous studies have been conducted for applications in sleep monitoring and wound care [4].

The COVID-19 pandemic disrupted normal healthcare practices, necessitating the employment of inventive ways to ensure treatment continuity. RPM has become an essential tool, allowing healthcare practitioners to oversee patients' health state and deliver personalised treatment without requiring patients to leave their residences [5].

Data processing and acquisition systems, hospital end terminals, and communication networks are the fundamental components of a remote monitoring system. The various sensors or devices with embedded sensors that have wireless data transmission capabilities make up the data acquisition system. As technology advances, sensors may be more than just medical ones; they may also be cameras or smartphones. This is due to current studies that examine contactless techniques, in which the surgical instruments do not come into contact with the patient's body [6].

Telemonitoring collects real-time data from patients so that medical professionals can assess their health state remotely, regardless of the technology used. The observed advantages and disadvantages of telemonitoring must be assessed in order to keep improving this technique, which is becoming more and more pertinent to patient care. Thus, the purpose of this systematic review was to determine how medical professionals felt about and dealt with RPM.

The Role of Home Healthcare in Modern Medicine

Given that it protects people's health, health care might be regarded as vital to our existence. Hospitals and private clinics have had fewer beds for the past 20 years. At the same time, as the population ages, more people are experiencing chronic degenerative diseases, which result in both handicaps and functional limitations. In actuality, the financial circumstances surrounding the care of elderly have led them to focus on Home Health Care (HHC) outside of hospital facilities. In order to feel more comfortable, patients receiving palliative care or therapies for various chronic diseases prefer care that removes them from their family context as little as possible.

Importance and Benefits of Remote Patient Monitoring

A healthcare provider initially evaluates and determines a patient's condition suitable for remote patient monitoring and initiates a program to deliver the service [7]. Upon concluding that a patient will gain from remote monitoring, the physician secures the patient's permission and prescribes a suitable gadget such as a blood pressure monitor or glucose meter, which is electronically linked *via* a selected network. The gathered data is subsequently communicated electronically to the clinician, who analyses it and offers guidance to the patient based on the findings. Providers are required to undertake additional measures, including ascertaining coverage, establishing patient intake procedures, and training personnel to administer the RPM services. Patients may necessitate support in using the technology, and their user-friendliness is contingent upon the design and intricacy of the equipment supplied. Collaborating with an RPM vendor like Patient One can assist healthcare providers in establishing effective patient programs. The use of RPM has shown several advantages in healthcare provision and home care, which are elaborated and shown in Fig. (**1**) .

Improved Patient Outcomes

RPM enables healthcare professionals to monitor patients' health in real-time, facilitating the early detection of potential health issues and timely intervention. This, therefore, results in improved patient outcomes, reduced hospital readmissions, and diminished healthcare costs.

Increased Patient Comfort and Convenience

RPM enables patients to get medical care in the comfort of their homes, hence diminishing the need for recurrent hospitalizations. This alleviates patients' stress and suffering, enhances their quality of life, and enables them to live autonomously.

Personalized Care

RPM allows healthcare professionals to collect and evaluate patients' health data, facilitating the provision of tailored treatment regimens that meet specific patient needs and enabling adjustments as necessary to optimise outcomes. Public health and individualized healthcare are connected and made easier by digital health. In the modern world, personalized healthcare has become a vital strategy for enhancing patient satisfaction and health outcomes. It has been demonstrated that the application of artificial intelligence (AI) in personalized healthcare holds great promise for disease prediction, early identification, tailored treatment, medication creation, and remote patient monitoring.

Enhanced Patient Safety

Since patient safety directly affects the standard of care and individual results, it is a core concern in the healthcare industry. The introduction of wireless monitoring equipment has completely changed how medical professionals monitor and treat patients' ailments, improving efficiency and safety. These systems eliminate the risk of infections or discomfort associated with traditional wired systems by enabling continuous, real-time monitoring of a patient's vital signs, including temperature, oxygen levels, blood pressure, and heart rate, without the need for physical connections.

Efficient Healthcare Delivery

In addition to having an impact on people's lives, subpar treatment is a waste of time and money. It is both a question of aiming for longer and better lives and a matter of economic need to make quality a key component of universal health coverage. Countries of all economic levels can afford to improve the quality of their health systems. In actuality, the expense of low quality is prohibitive, particularly for the most impoverished nations. In addition to adding to the worldwide burden of disease and unmet medical requirements, poor quality of care has a significant financial impact on communities and health systems worldwide. Correcting avoidable treatment problems and patient harm accounts for about 15% of hospital spending in high-income nations.

Increased Patient Engagement

Because wireless monitoring technologies allow for real-time data collection, continuous monitoring, and remote health tracking, they have drastically changed patient engagement in the healthcare industry. By offering real-time feedback, tailored alarms, and smooth connections with medical professionals, these technologies enable people to participate in their own health management actively [8].

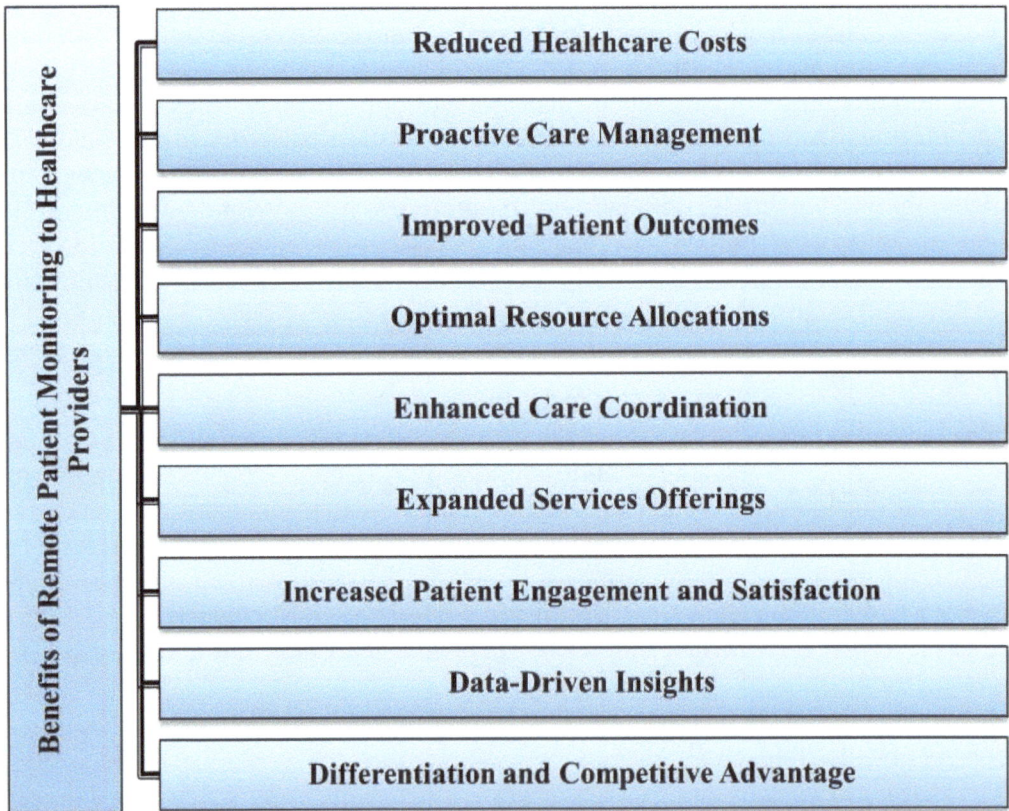

Benefits of Remote Patient Monitoring to Healthcare Providers

- Reduced Healthcare Costs
- Proactive Care Management
- Improved Patient Outcomes
- Optimal Resource Allocations
- Enhanced Care Coordination
- Expanded Services Offerings
- Increased Patient Engagement and Satisfaction
- Data-Driven Insights
- Differentiation and Competitive Advantage

Fig. (1). Benefits of remote patient monitoring in healthcare.

TECHNOLOGIES ENABLING REMOTE PATIENT MONITORING

Wearable Devices

From physiological conditions like heart disease, high blood pressure, and muscular problems to neurocognitive conditions like Parkinson's disease, Alzheimer's disease, and other mental illnesses, wearable technology has found many uses in the medical field. For this aim, a variety of wearables are utilized, such as skin-based wearables, which include textile-based wearables, biofluidic-based wearables, and tattoo-based wearables [9]. Wearable technology has recently demonstrated promising advancements as a medication delivery system, increasing its applicability to individualized healthcare. Before being marketed as a completely customized healthcare system, these wearables must overcome several fundamental issues [10].

Types of Wearable Technology in Healthcare

Fitness Trackers

The general public can now easily use fitness trackers in their daily lives thanks to technological advancements. This kind of device provides information regarding our exercise and physical activity. Steps, distance traveled, and heart rate can all be tracked with the majority of fitness trackers [11, 12]. This alliance promotes a proactive approach to personal health and fitness.

Smartwatches

It has evolved from basic timekeeping to sophisticated health-monitoring technology. They are outfitted with sensors like heart rate monitors, accelerometers, and gyroscopes, which provide real-time data on cardiovascular health, identify irregularities, and assist with medication compliance. Hydration reminders and medication alerts are essential components for overseeing daily health obligations and promoting healthier lifestyles [13].

Enhancing Healthcare Outcomes

The goal of healthcare is to alleviate patients of as much of the agony they encounter on a daily basis as is medically feasible. As a result, patients can fully exercise and move around freely in a totally private environment. In the past, cable sensors that were directly connected to hospital computers made up the majority of patient monitoring systems. One of the main disadvantages of these devices was that they significantly restricted the patient's mobility. In addition to being expensive and unwieldy, the equipment used was limited in its ability to monitor multiple patients simultaneously [14, 15].

When healthcare facilities began providing home-based care, they expanded those services, and this technology, like earlier patient monitoring methods, was not very user-friendly. As technology has advanced over time, researchers have been able to develop strategies for both wirelessly connected patient monitoring and remote patient monitoring. An increasing number of researchers and organizations are using remote patient monitoring systems to improve patient care, and the market for these systems is growing at a rapid rate. This is helping the health industry make great advancements towards improvement, which is a positive development [16].

Biosensors in Patient Health Monitoring

Advancements and Innovations

Advances in Biosensor Technology

In recent years, the use of aptamers or nucleotides, affibodies, peptide arrays, and molecule-imprinted polymers provides tools to develop innovative biosensors over classical methods. Integrated approaches provided a better perspective for developing specific and sensitive biosensors with high regenerative potential. Various biosensors, ranging from nanomaterials, and polymers to microbes, have wider potential applications. Recent advances in biological techniques and instrumentation involving fluorescence tags to nanomaterials have increased the sensitivity limit of biosensors.

Miniaturization and Wearable Biosensors

The majority of biomarker testing is still carried out in centralized, specialized labs today, with large, cumbersome equipment, automated analyzers, and more time and money spent on analysis. It is highly predicted that these traditional laboratory-oriented assays will be replaced by smaller, quicker, and less expensive microdevices that use a cloud server to send diagnostic data straight to the patient's smartphone. In order to properly understand the measured biomarkers of numerous bioanalytes, including DNA, RNA, urine, and blood, several problems and limitations need to be addressed before the development and use of multiple biosensors. However, innovative biosensor-based approaches may enable reliable biomarker testing in a decentralized setting [17].

Integration of Artificial Intelligence

A complex integration of multimodal systems, the use of AI in healthcare systems requires fundamental breakthroughs in areas including privacy, large-scale machine learning, optimization, and model performance. Data with security and analytics with insights are two essential ideas that must be addressed in order to successfully integrate AI into healthcare. Effective integration requires total transparency and confidence with regard to data and security. Likewise, data analytics and insight play a critical role. Because of recent developments in computer science and informatics, among other things, artificial intelligence is quickly becoming a significant part of modern healthcare. Medical professionals are being helped in clinical settings and ongoing research by AI-powered algorithms and tools. At the moment, the most widely used AI applications in medical settings are image analysis and clinical decision assistance. Clinical decision support systems offer clinicians quick access to current information and research pertinent to the patient's condition, addressing treatment, medicine, and other patient needs [18].

Multi-Parameter Biosensors

Modern biosensors are progressing towards multi-parameter capabilities, enabling simultaneous evaluation of several health metrics. This integrated approach offers a comprehensive view of patient well-being, enabling customised treatment strategies. Multi-parameter biosensors enhance diagnostic accuracy by integrating data from several physiological signals, enabling tailored treatments.

Applications in Patient Monitoring

The AD8232 electrocardiogram (ECG) biosensor and the MAX30102 biosensor for heart rate and pulse oximetry exemplify significant advancements in biosensor technology. These new technologies underscore the role of biosensors in real-time patient monitoring [19].

ECG Biosensors

ECG biosensors, in particular the AD8232, are employed in the continuous observation of the heart's electrical activities. They use properly positioned electrodes to transform electrical impulses generated during heartbeats into graphical ECGs [20]. These devices are crucial for identifying cardiac issues because of their many benefits, which include versatile electrode combinations, high signal resolution, and compact designs that ensure mobility and efficacy. With the help of ECG biosensors, real-time abnormal event detection is possible, which in turn helps in decreasing the risk of negative cardiac events.

Heart Rate and Pulse Oximetry Biosensors

For contactless measurement of heart rate as well as blood oxygen, biosensors such as MAX30102 are important. Blood flow changes are detected by a PPG sensor, which utilizes changes in light absorption. Features that aid in reliable performance in difficult environments include high temperature accuracy, advanced LED technology, and low power consumption. These biosensors provide necessary information for stress reactions, the cardiovascular system, and the general physical fitness of the patients, thus facilitating complete patient management [21].

MOBILE HEALTH APPLICATION

The development of m-Health services and applications has gained significant attention from the research community owing to its profound impact on the field. M-Health has mostly been used for monitoring, risk assessment, disease detection, and basic treatment. Healthcare delivery system. These advancements have greatly improved areas such as cardiology, diabetes, obesity, smoking cessation, elderly care, as well as the treatment of chronic diseases, as depicted in Fig. (**2**) [22]. It has become prevalent in poorer nations, where healthcare services are frequently unattainable. The fast proliferation of mobile healthcare applications signifies the increasing interest and diversification within this domain. In the United States, more than 40,000 healthcare applications exist, classified by therapeutic domains including prevention, diagnostics, education, and chronic illness management. Instruments such as the IMS Health Appscore assess these applications according to their functionality, user evaluations, and capacity to decrease healthcare expenses.

Internet of Things (IOT) in Healthcare

The Internet of Things (IoT) is a prevalent subject of research. Progress in electronics, the use of IPv6, and the deployment of wireless networks have contributed to the expansion of IoT technology. With the ongoing advancement of IoT devices and technology. The Internet of Things (IoT) has proliferated extensively and is utilised across many settings, including residential areas, healthcare facilities, aerospace, and numerous modes of transportation. The integration of control systems with the Internet of Things is a primary topic for academics. A variety of methods have been suggested to regulate IoT devices. IoT security is of paramount significance and has emerged as the primary focus of study in the IoT domain [23].

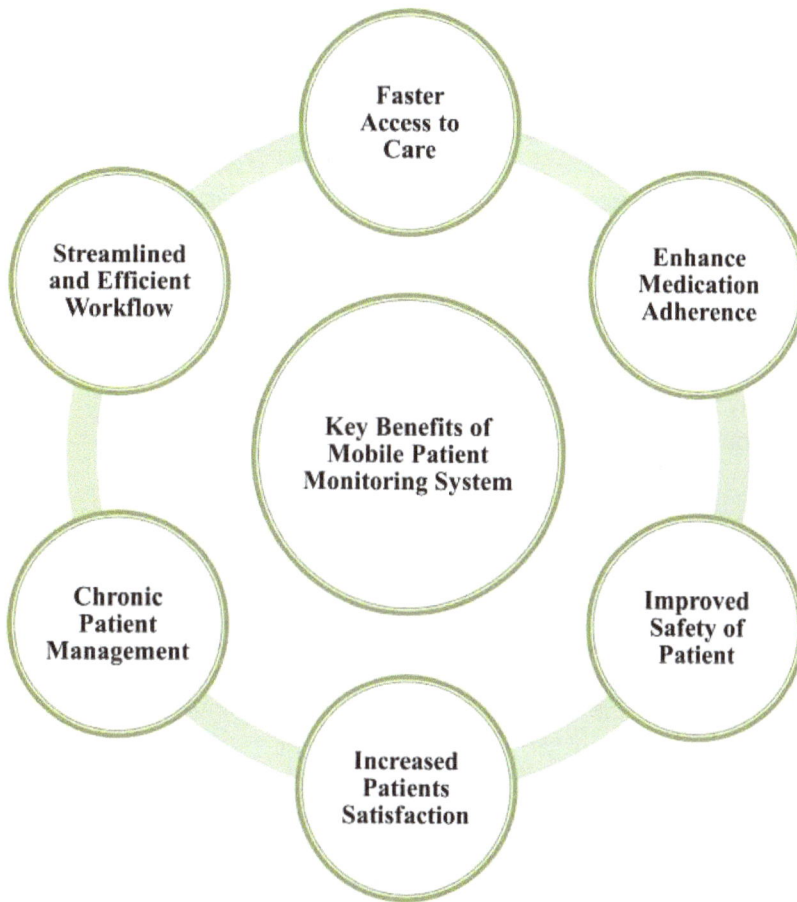

Fig. (2). Mobile health application.

The increasing interest in body-worn sensors has lately established them as potent instruments for healthcare applications, with several devices being commercially accessible for diverse uses, including personal health monitoring, activity tracking, and fitness enhancement. Researchers have suggested novel clinical uses of these technologies for remote health monitoring systems, which encompass long-term status recording and physician access to patient's physiological information. Most proposed frameworks for remote health monitoring feature a three-tier architecture: the first tier comprises a body sensor network that includes wearable sensors for data acquisition, such as blood pressure, heart status, and body temperature; the second tier encompasses communication and networking services that collect data from the sensors and forward it. The third layer comprises the processing and analysis nodes.

Cloud Computing and Data Storage Solutions

Cloud computing is a parallel and distributed system made up of a pool of networked, virtualised computers that are dynamically provided and presented to customers as a single resource under Service Level Agreements (SLAs). This paradigm enables users to execute apps and store data remotely, taking advantage of on-demand services without the need to manage local hardware or software [24]. Unlike traditional data storage, which depends on dedicated servers, cloud storage uses several third-party servers, with the real locations of data concealed for security reasons. This transition from local infrastructure to cloud services has changed IT by allowing consumers to pay based on consumption, directing resources towards utilisation rather than upkeep. Cloud computing is the process of relocating services, computations, or data off-site to centralised facilities, either internally or externally, for cost and operational efficiency.

Cloud computing may be deployed in four ways: private, public, community, and hybrid clouds. A private cloud is owned and controlled by a single organisation, whether on or off-premises, and provides a secure environment with internal administration. Large cloud service providers (CSPs) administer public clouds by owning data centres, which are frequently scattered across numerous locations and provide services that reduce the cost of in-house equipment. Community clouds are shared by organisations that have similar aims and can be administered by the community or a third party. Hybrid clouds incorporate features of private, public, and community clouds, allowing for different organisational needs while sharing infrastructure [25].

Storage is an important feature of cloud computing. Data is kept on several third-party servers rather than on typical dedicated servers. Although customers interact with virtual servers and believe data is kept in permanent places, the actual storage might fluctuate and is dynamically controlled by the cloud provider. Users experience a consistent storage interface, comparable to accessing a local disc, even if the data may change physical locations over time. The dynamic nature of cloud storage optimises resources and improves accessibility [26].

APPLICATIONS OF RPM IN HEALTHCARE

Remote Patient Monitoring (RPM) revolutionizes healthcare by allowing real-time tracking of patient health through wearable sensors, mobile apps, and connected devices. It enhances patient care, decreases hospital visits, and improves disease management across various conditions, as illustrated in Fig. (**3**) .

Chronic Disease Management

Remote patient monitoring (RPM) for chronic disease management has emerged as an effective alternative for those with chronic diseases [27]. Research indicates that the use of RPM reduces emergency department visits, avoids hospital readmissions, and shortens hospital stays. This article delineates five primary advantages of remote patient monitoring in the optimal management of patients with chronic illnesses, including diabetes, heart failure, and hypertension.

Promotes Early Identification of Chronic Disease

The majority of individuals consult their physician only when their condition deteriorates or when their subsequent visit is due. What if an issue arises between appointments? If the patient is unaware of what to monitor, difficulties may arise [28]. Remote patient monitoring for chronic illness management enhances treatment between appointments. Regular monitoring of patients' vital signs provides physicians with daily insights into their illnesses. A physician is promptly notified if medical intervention is required. The RPM gadget transmits real-time data to the remote patient monitoring platform for instant clinician access. Clinicians will get automated alerts for prompt intervention when a patient's reading exceeds or falls below the established threshold. Remote patient monitoring facilitates the prompt detection of chronic illness signs. The earlier symptoms or problems are recognized, the sooner patients can receive therapy and mitigate disease development.

RPM Prompts Adjustments to Treatment Plans

Remote patient monitoring utilising at-home health equipment enhances chronic care management by facilitating prompt modifications to treatment strategies. Clinicians can monitor their patients' status at any time using the RPM portal. Consequently, they may observe patient responses to drugs and modify prescriptions accordingly [29]. In the absence of remote patient monitoring for chronic illness management, numerous patients endure prolonged periods with suboptimal or ineffective treatment plans. RPM assists patients in identifying an effective treatment regimen while mitigating the advancement of chronic diseases.

Increased Patient Engagement

Implementing healthy lifestyle behaviours in daily life may be arduous. Digital health and remote patient monitoring include extending healthcare outside traditional settings and integrating it into the patient's everyday routine and lifestyle. RPM assists people in effectively managing their health with a sense of support. Patients are inherently motivated to adopt healthier lifestyle choices and comply with their management plans, since they are aware that their care professionals consistently monitor their health data. Patients are integral to remote patient monitoring in the management of chronic diseases [30]. They are obligated to measure their vital signs a minimum of 16 times each month. This offers physicians vital knowledge, and patients also participate more effectively in their health management when they comprehend their situation. Regular measurements enable patients to identify the usual range for their bodies. They may monitor whether their health is enhancing or deteriorating over time and assess the impact of lifestyle modifications on their readings. The more the patient's comprehension of their disease and involvement, the higher the likelihood of adopting healthy behaviours, monitoring for problems, and communicating with their physician.

Lower Healthcare Costs

Patients are less likely to need complex operations, visit emergency rooms, and be admitted to hospitals when chronic illness is managed using remote patient monitoring. As a consequence, healthcare expenses are reduced. RPM is very cost-effective for treating heart conditions like heart failure, hypertension, and chronic obstructive pulmonary disease, according to research [31].

Remote patient monitoring can help manage several chronic illnesses, including stroke, heart disease, diabetes, and chronic heart failure. For chronic obstructive pulmonary disease and kidney disease, vital signs need to be checked according to the patient's condition. For instance, a remote blood pressure monitor will be helpful for people who are at risk for renal disease or stroke. Those who have diabetes also need to monitor their blood glucose levels.

Post-Surgical Recovery and Rehabilitation

Rehabilitation and post-operative care are essential parts of the patient journey in the medical field. These two services alone place a significant burden on the US healthcare system, since 15 million patients require post-surgical care each year, of whom 8.6 million need rehabilitation [32]. Thanks to remote patient monitoring (RPM), medical practitioners may now follow their patients' progress without having to deal with the dangers, costs, and inconveniences of in-person visits. Better treatment and better results have been provided by this technology, which has changed the playing field. Utilising RPM in Rehabilitation and Post-Surgical Care Environments. There are several uses for remote monitoring technologies in post-operative care and rehabilitation environments. Typical uses include:

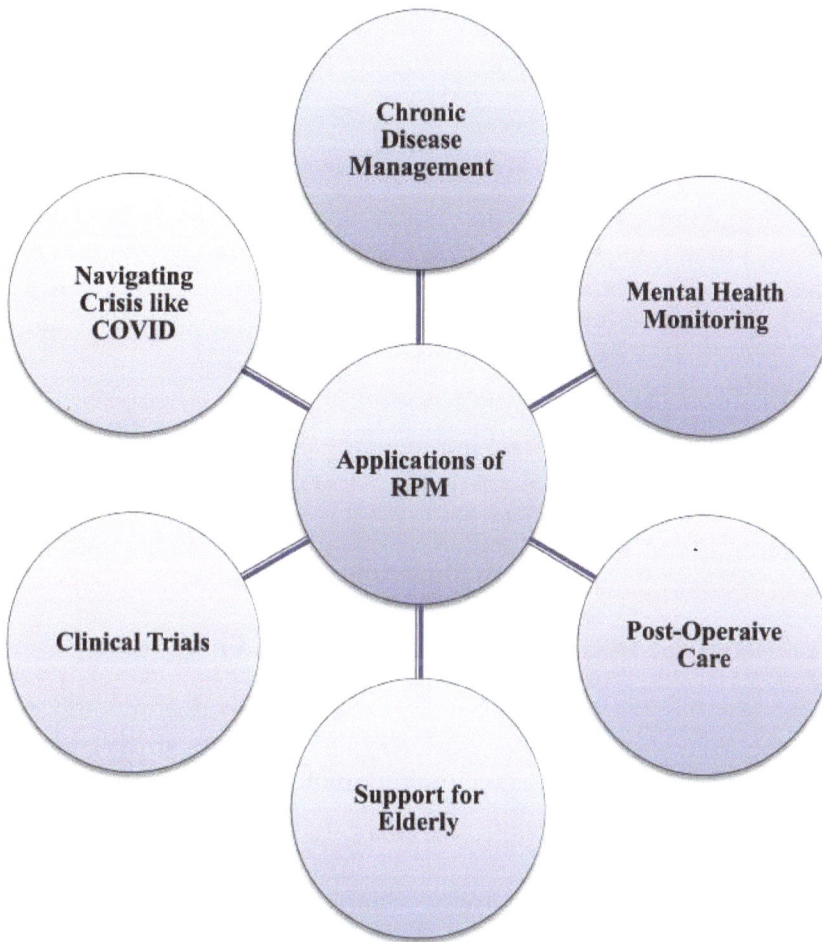

Fig. (3). Applications of RPM in healthcare.

Vital Signs Monitoring

One of the most popular uses of remote monitoring technologies in rehabilitation and post-operative care is vital sign tracking. Clinicians can remotely monitor vital signs such as heart rates, oxygen saturation, and blood pressure using wearable sensors and other smart devices [33]. This enables them to see any significant changes in signs and take appropriate action before issues emerge.

Medication Adherence Tracking

In post-surgical treatment and rehabilitation, medication non-adherence is a major challenge. According to medical literature, over half of patients do not take their prescribed medications as directed. Individuals recovering from an illness or injury may require many medications and strict adherence to precise dosage standards. Health monitoring devices alert patients about the timing and manner of medicine ingestion, allowing clinicians to watch adherence to treatment regimens [34].

Activity Levels Observing

Patients who are recovering from illness or injury may require a progressive increase in their regular physical activity. Remote patient monitoring technologies, such as activity sensors, allow post-surgical patients to register and record their physical activity levels and monitor their progress over time.

Wound Healing Overseeing

Wearable sensors or other tracking devices are used by patients who have undergone surgery or who have wounds that need ongoing care to monitor the healing process. Healthcare professionals keep an eye on indicators like vital signs to determine if a wound is healing adequately and take appropriate action [35].

Benefits of RPM for Post-surgical Care and Rehabilitation

There are several benefits of using remote monitoring technologies in rehabilitative and post-operative care settings. In these situations, the primary advantages of implementing this technology include [36].

Improved Patient Outcomes

Improved patient outcomes are a major benefit of remote monitoring technologies. Regularly keeping an eye on their patients' health and well-being allows doctors to promptly identify any changes in their condition and take action before problems develop. Better results, fewer readmissions to the hospital, and quicker recovery durations result from this.

Increased Patient Engagement

RPM technology makes patients more involved in their treatment. Because they are more likely to adhere to treatment programs and actively participate in their recovery, people who are very engaged in their therapy typically experience better outcomes. Patients may keep an eye on their health and well-being with remote patient monitoring, which gives them a sense of control over their circumstances and keeps them motivated while they rehabilitate.

Reduced Healthcare Costs

According to the American Medical Association, healthcare spending in 2022 is expected to reach US$5 trillion. RPM reduces ER visits and hospital readmissions by identifying potential problems early [37]. Additionally, by shortening hospital stays, remote monitoring technology adds value and generates further cost savings.

Revolutionizing Post-surgical Care and Rehabilitation

Technology for remote monitoring has the potential to revolutionize rehabilitation and post-operative care while lowering medical costs [38]. When RPM technology is implemented correctly and the right steps are taken to make full use of it, providers benefit. Working with an experienced and reputable remote patient monitoring service may help the organization get rid of poor results and give patients better treatment while also expediting the procedures in the clinic.

Elderly Care and Fall Prevention

Remote monitoring for older people is increasingly essential in healthcare due to the rapid increase in the ageing population [39]. As approximately 20% of the U.S. population is projected to exceed 65 years of age by 2050, the demand for efficient, scalable solutions is pressing. Remote monitoring technologies, frequently integrated with artificial intelligence and machine learning, are essential in facilitating ageing in place, enhancing quality of life, and meeting the specific requirements of older folks and their carer.

Elderly Remote Monitoring and Aging in Place

Ageing in place, the capacity for seniors to reside autonomously in their own homes, is the chosen option for over 90% of older persons. It correlates with increased life satisfaction, superior quality of life, and heightened well-being. Nonetheless, facilitating this autonomy needs strong support networks, especially as ageing frequently introduces health issues that require ongoing care.

Remote monitoring for older people is addressing this issue by offering solutions that enable carers to oversee vital signs, administer prescription regimens, and observe everyday activities from a distance [40]. Wearable sensors, smart home connections, and AI-driven applications are employed to gather real-time data, which is subsequently analysed to detect possible health hazards or patterns. These technologies alleviate the responsibilities of carers while promoting active ageing and decreasing the necessity for institutional care.

Understanding Innovations in Elderly Remote Monitoring

Remote monitoring for older people is an effective response to the issues presented by an ageing demographic [41]. These solutions enable older people to stay in their homes while providing the caregivers all the help needed to provide care, thus solving pressing problems and developing sustainable care models. The elderly remote monitoring gives healthcare providers, caregivers, and families a tool to offer better care for older people while ensuring their independence.

Mental Health and Behavioral Monitoring

Remote patient monitoring has the potential to increase accessibility, foster targeted treatment, and increase results in a particular area of mental health [42]. This paper examines the impact of remote patient monitoring on mental health services, its role in the improvement of patients in the mental health area, expansion of access to care, and provision of customized treatment using new technologies.

Understanding Remote Patient Monitoring for Mental Health

The Method of using Tech to gather and send patient information remotely is known as remote patient monitoring for mental health. This enables checkup practitioners to value and proctor associates in nursing individuals' moral health through square goal settings. This approach is specifically decisive for people with long-term illnesses, including diabetes, cancer, and heart disease. The World Health Organization emphasizes the importance of regular health checkups and early detection to report potential mental health issues and ensure timely intervention.. People who suffer from depression are also more likely to develop certain medical conditions. This is applicable to people of all ages. In addition, 45 percent of Americans who have a clinically serious mental illness do not seek or receive treatment. The main reasons include a preference for independence, doubts about the effectiveness of the help, and ambiguity about what kind of help to seek [43]. People could also fear change, the unknown, and scrutiny, or they might worry that others will find out about their situation. One of the main advantages of remote patient monitoring for mental health is its ability to remove geographic restrictions and make mental health treatment services accessible in the comfort of one's own home. People who live in remote areas or have limited mobility can now receive continuous monitoring and support, removing barriers to mental health treatment.

Remote Patient Monitoring for Mental Health: Early Detection and Intervention

The use of remote patient monitoring enables the prompt detection of potential mental health concerns [44]. By monitoring many indicators, including sleep patterns, activity levels, and mood fluctuations, healthcare workers can detect early signals of anxiety before they escalate. Timely intervention is essential in mental health treatment, and remote monitoring offers a pre-emptive strategy to tackle problems before they escalate. The subsequent sections delineate equipment suitable for the remote surveillance of patients' mental health to identify potential issues.

Remote Patient Monitoring Scale

Significant alterations in dietary patterns frequently signify mental health concerns. A remote patient monitoring scale is an essential device for monitoring substantial weight fluctuations. Depression, as delineated in the Diagnostic and Statistical Manual of Mental Disorders, is frequently correlated with fluctuations in weight. Providers, notified by the remote patient monitoring scale, can swiftly modify treatment procedures to avert worsening.

Remote Patient Monitoring Blood Pressure Monitor

Stress, grief, and worry can influence heart rate, resulting in palpitations or elevated rates. A remote patient monitoring device for blood pressure enables authorized healthcare professionals to observe these physiological variations [45]. Utilizing the gathered data, physicians can customize treatment regimens to avert the intensification of anxiety or depressive episodes.

Remote Patient Monitoring Sleep Devices

Sleep disturbances, such as insomnia, may signify underlying mental health issues [46]. Remote patient monitoring sleep devices are crucial for alerting doctors to insomnia, changes in sleep patterns, or manic behaviours. Timely identification of these signs allows healthcare professionals to adjust treatment approaches and address the root causes of sleep-related mental health disorders.

Remote Patient Monitoring Thermometer

A psychogenic fever is an elevation in body temperature induced by stress. It is occasionally termed stress-induced hyperthermia. It is occasionally termed stress-induced hyperthermia. It illustrates the kinship between emotions and natural welfare. These fevers are identified when body temperature exceeds 98.6 degrees Fahrenheit during episodes of acute or chronic stress. Associate in Nursing Rev thermometer is an important tool used by healthcare professionals to evaluate variations in trunk temperature. A fluctuation may indicate an imminent mental health crisis necessitating prompt treatment to alleviate the consequences.

RPM for Mental Health Treatment Plans

Remote patient watching enables healthcare practitioners to formulate tailored treatment strategies that are informed by specific patient information [47]. This customized scheme ensures that therapies are focused and modified to each patient's clear requirements, enhancing the effectiveness of mental health care interventions. Traditional in-person meetings for mental health treatment can be challenging due to several factors, including stigma, scheduling disagreements, and transportation problems. Telehealth and remote monitoring help ease these challenges by offering a convenient and accessible option. Patients can remotely transmit their information to healthcare providers, reducing the need for frequent in-person consultations and improving the accessibility and flexibility of mental health therapy.

INTEGRATION OF RPM IN HOME HEALTHCARE

Remote Patient Monitoring, by its abbreviation RPM, is changing the nature of home healthcare for the better by ensuring that correlated devices are tracking and monitoring the health of the patients. This interface allows doctors to access real-time data about a patient's vital signs, medication intake, and symptoms, hence eradicating the delays associated with notification of potential health problems. With the use of RPM, patients can receive fast treatment, and there is a reduction in patients being readmitted to the hospital. Patients also practice self-care management, which improves their overall well-being. It offers low-cost options for the management of chronic diseases and post-surgical recovery care, giving a more holistic philosophy that integrates the clinic and home care [48]. Integrating Remote Patient Monitoring (RPM) and Telehealth (as shown in Fig. **4**)) enables continuous patient data collection through wearable devices while allowing remote consultations *via* Telehealth platforms.

Workflow and Communication Between Patients and Providers

Remote patient monitoring (RPM), according to evidence, boosts effectiveness in multiple aspects of home care, particularly the interaction between patients and providers [49]. Creatively, RPM systems may be considered as software programs provided with digital instruments for constant control of such health parameters as heart rate, blood pressure, glucose levels, or even oxygen saturation. These parameters are relayed in real-time to healthcare practitioners, enabling them to oversee patients without necessitating frequent in-person consultations.

An RPM integration improves workflow by making the collection and input of the data less dependent on human efforts. Automated alerts and notifications ensure that medical professionals are up to date with important health events and can act rapidly. On the other side, patients are able to report their symptoms, upload relevant information, and get responses using secure mobile apps or web portals. This two-way communication fosters collaboration, addresses inefficiencies, and enhances the patient's role in the entire treatment process. Clearly defined communication channels are important for the effective incorporation of RPM into home care services. Standard operating procedures for data sharing, communication about specific actions to all parties in case of crises, and frequent tele-consultations allow for universal coordination, in addition to improving the quality of healthcare. These principles also reduce the burden of caregivers by enhancing time allocation [50].

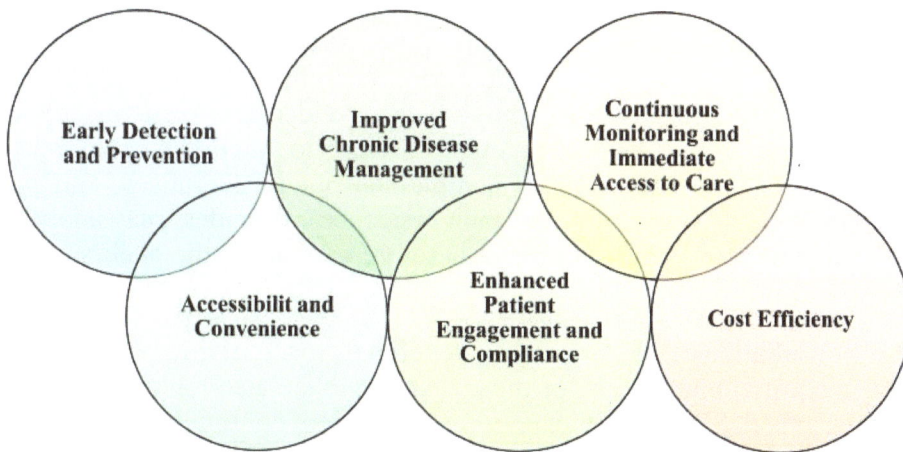

Fig. (4). Integrating RPM and tele-health.

Real-Time Data Sharing and Analysis

RPM encompasses the ability to share real-time information, making it possible to maintain oversight and make decisions at home across a healthcare setting [51]. Devices worn by patients and sensors are able to record information about the patient and send such data to the cloud for interpretation with algorithms. This study provides meaningful materials that assist healthcare practitioners in spotting aberrations, in anticipating dangers to a person's health, and customizing treatment. Real-time data exchange guarantees that clinicians are always aware of their patients' health state. For example, an RPM system monitoring a diabetic patient can notify the clinician if glucose levels fall outside the usual range, allowing for prompt adjustments to treatment regimens. Patients gain from obtaining immediate feedback and advice, allowing them to manage their health proactively.

The combination of artificial intelligence (AI) with machine learning (ML) expands the possibilities of real-time data processing [52]. AI-driven analytics can detect minor patterns and connections that manual review may miss, allowing for early diagnosis and personalised care strategies. Data privacy and security are crucial in this setting, necessitating adherence to regulations such as HIPAA (Health Insurance Portability and Accountability Act) and GDPR (General Data Protection Regulation).

Remote Consultations and Virtual Care

Remote consultations and virtual care have revolutionised home healthcare by making medical expertise accessible from any place [53]. RPM systems improve these services by providing healthcare practitioners with up-to-date patient information before consultations, therefore enabling informed and efficient decision-making. Virtual care systems integrate video conferencing, encrypted texting, and electronic health records (EHRs) to facilitate comprehensive consultations. Patients can express complaints, obtain diagnoses, and procure medications from the convenience of their residences. Providers may analyse real-time data trends during consultations, therefore enhancing the accuracy of their evaluations.

Remote consultations are especially beneficial for individuals with chronic diseases, mobility impairments, or those residing in isolated regions. They reduce the need for travel, lower healthcare costs, and ensure continuity of service. RPM systems facilitate post-consultation oversight, ensuring patient adherence to treatment regimens and promoting effective recovery. A number of challenges, such as a lack of digital literacy, network issues, and regulatory compliance, must be solved in order to fully utilise the possibilities of remote online consultations [54]. These problems can be solved by training patients and providers, building the necessary infrastructure, and setting appropriate regulations to ensure fair conditions for the provision of virtual care.

CHALLENGES AND BARRIERS

The application of RPM while a patient is undergoing home care brings about some hurdles owing to several issues. Some of the problems that RPM poses to patients under home care include:

Technical Challenges

The deployment of Remote Patient Monitoring Systems (RPMS) requires the integration of several technological devices, which include wearables, home construction monitoring devices, and mobile health apps. Failing to ensure the integration of any devices into the system could render the entire project a failure [55].

Data Management Challenges

At times, potential RPM generates a high volume of clinical data, which will require storage, analysis, and management after sufficient health surveillance activities. All forms of sensitive data generated must be safe and fall under a medical record system in a format that integrates all data to avoid fragmentation [56].

Patient Education and Support

To ensure proper use of RPM devices, each patient must receive thorough education on their operation, with continuous guidance provided throughout their usage. This brings in more requirements of resources and manpower for educating and supporting users [57].

Reimbursement and Cost

Using RPM devices may demand an elaborate expenditure, and receiving payment for RPM services may be a hassle for healthcare practitioners. Furthermore, providers could face a difficult situation if insurers refuse to reimburse for clinical devices [58].

Regulatory and Legal Challenges

Several legal requirements on the security of data and patient privacy must be complied with when handling RPM. In order to protect the patient's privacy and avoid lawsuits, healthcare professionals are required to follow some rules and laws. Nevertheless, by managing these difficulties, the RPM's advantages can be taken by the healthcare providers to deliver quality services to clients from a distance [59].

FUTURE TRENDS

The RPM, or Remote Patient Monitoring, is something that can sustain potential growth and innovation in the future. Advanced technologies such as the IoT, AI, and 5G allow the creation of new RPM devices and solutions to be developed and deployed. These technologies facilitate remote health monitoring by trained professionals in the field and extend personalized care solutions to patients. Smart home devices are capable of monitoring the surrounding space and could alert for safety measures such as fall detection for patients [60].

Shifting the focus back to RPM, it is now becoming complex yet simpler to use and understand. For example, systems using AI for RPM coping mechanisms and learning can look at the general data and patients of a particular region to form conclusions about them in order to flag any potential health risks to them. Such technology can then alert the essentials involved, offering a chance to curtail the problem and its repercussions. The shift towards value-based care is another important trend that will determine the future of RPM and home care. In value-based care, high-quality care can be provided by the healthcare providers while also lowering the costs, which moves the burden away from the patient. RPM supports patients in tracking and sharing their key health indicators, aligning with our goals at Patient-One [61].

CASE STUDIES

Successful Implementation of RPM Programs

A number of healthcare organisations have successfully deployed Remote Patient Monitoring (RPM) initiatives in an effort to save costs and enhance patient care. By using RPM devices to monitor vital signs on a daily basis, a large hospital network decreased readmission rates for patients with heart failure [62]. RPM technologies have also been shown to significantly increase patient involvement and treatment plan adherence in chronic illness management programs [63]. These case studies demonstrate how RPM has the potential to revolutionise healthcare delivery, especially in marginalised and rural regions.

Lessons Learned from Real-World Deployments

Practical applications of RPM programs yield substantial insights into scalability and sustainability. Widespread issues encompass data security management, ensuring interoperability with Electronic Health Records (EHRs), and instructing both patients and physicians for appropriate technology utilisation [64]. Effective programs emphasise the need for intuitive interfaces, robust support systems, and clear information about the benefits of RPM. These insights provide direction for healthcare professionals aiming to initiate or improve RPM initiatives, ensuring ongoing success and patient satisfaction.

CONCLUSION

Remote Patient Monitoring (RPM) with home healthcare is transforming the healthcare sector, providing continuous, real-time care outside conventional clinical environments. RPM utilises sophisticated technology to enhance patient outcomes and save expenses, corresponding with the need for individualised, proactive treatment. Remote Patient Monitoring (RPM) utilises wearable devices, biosensors, and mobile health applications to link patients with healthcare practitioners, facilitating the remote acquisition and analysis of health data. This enables prompt treatments, assists in chronic illness management, aids in post-surgical rehabilitation, and simplifies the monitoring of physical and mental health. Augmented by technologies such as IoT, cloud computing, and mHealth applications, RPM facilitates uninterrupted communication and data analysis. Its applications encompass diabetes and hypertension control, fall detection, and mental health care, enhancing accessibility and quality of life. Nonetheless, obstacles such as data privacy, legal concerns, and user-friendliness require attention. Innovations like artificial intelligence and predictive analytics are poised to enhance RPM, underscoring its increasing significance in revolutionizing healthcare into a more efficient, patient-centric approach.

REFERENCES

[1]   Wootton R. Twenty years of telemedicine in chronic disease management – an evidence synthesis. J Telemed Telecare 2012; 18(4): 211-20.
[http://dx.doi.org/10.1258/jtt.2012.120219] [PMID: 22674020]

[2]   Shane-McWhorter L, McAdam-Marx C, Lenert L, *et al.* Pharmacist-provided diabetes management and education *via* a telemonitoring program. J Am Pharm Assoc (Wash DC) 2015; 55(5): 516-26.
[http://dx.doi.org/10.1331/JAPhA.2015.14285] [PMID: 26359961]

[3]   Bhambri P, Khang A. Managing and Monitoring Patient's Healthcare Using AI and IoT Technologies InDriving Smart Medical Diagnosis Through AI-Powered Technologies and Applications. IGI Global 2024; pp. 1-23.

[4]   Ong MK, Romano PS, Edgington S, *et al.* Effectiveness of remote patient monitoring after discharge of hospitalized patients with heart failure: the better effectiveness after transition–heart failure (BEAT-HF) randomized clinical trial. JAMA Intern Med 2016; 176(3): 310-8.
[http://dx.doi.org/10.1001/jamainternmed.2015.7712] [PMID: 26857383]

[5]   Mahmmod BM, Naser MA, Al-Sudani AHS, *et al.* Patient Monitoring System Based on Internet of Things: A Review and Related Challenges With Open Research Issues. IEEE Access 2024; 12: 132444-79.
[http://dx.doi.org/10.1109/ACCESS.2024.3455900]

[6]   Muller AE, Ormstad SS, Jardim P, Johansen TB, Berg R. Managing chronic illnesses with remote patient monitoring in primary health care. Systematic review. Oslo (Norway): Norwegian Institute of Public Health; 2020.

[7]   Blount M, Batra VM, Capella AN, *et al.* Remote health-care monitoring using Personal Care Connect. IBM Syst J 2007; 46(1): 95-113.
[http://dx.doi.org/10.1147/sj.461.0095]

[8]   Su CR, Hajiyev J, Fu CJ, Kao KC, Chang CH, Chang CT. A novel framework for a remote patient

monitoring (RPM) system with abnormality detection. Health Policy Technol 2019; 8(2): 157-70.
[http://dx.doi.org/10.1016/j.hlpt.2019.05.008]

[9]   Gao S, Tang G, Hua D, *et al.* Stimuli-responsive bio-based polymeric systems and their applications. J
        Mater Chem B Mater Biol Med 2019; 7(5): 709-29.
        [http://dx.doi.org/10.1039/C8TB02491J] [PMID: 32254845]

[10]   Adeghe EP, Okolo CA, Ojeyinka OT. A review of wearable technology in healthcare: Monitoring
        patient health and enhancing outcomes. OARJ of Multidisciplinary Studies 2024; 7(01): 142-8.

[11]   Chan M, Estève D, Fourniols JY, Escriba C, Campo E. Smart wearable systems: Current status and
        future challenges. Artif Intell Med 2012; 56(3): 137-56.
        [http://dx.doi.org/10.1016/j.artmed.2012.09.003] [PMID: 23122689]

[12]   Okeme AB, Akeju O, Enyejo LA, Ibrahim A. Exploring the Impact of Wearable Health Devices on
        Chronic Disease Management. Intl J of Adv Res Pub Rev 2025; 2(2): 43-69.

[13]   Lee JG, Lee B, Choe EK. Decorative, evocative, and uncanny: reactions on ambient-to-disruptive
        health notifications via plant-mimicking shape-changing interfaces. Proceedings of the 2023 CHI
        Conference on Human Factors in Computing Systems 2023; 1-16.

[14]   Dias D, Paulo Silva Cunha J. Wearable health devices—vital sign monitoring, systems and
        technologies. Sensors (Basel) 2018; 18(8): 2414.
        [http://dx.doi.org/10.3390/s18082414] [PMID: 30044415]

[15]   Vijayan V, Connolly JP, Condell J, McKelvey N, Gardiner P. Review of wearable devices and data
        collection considerations for connected health. Sensors (Basel) 2021; 21(16): 5589.
        [http://dx.doi.org/10.3390/s21165589] [PMID: 34451032]

[16]   Aggarwal P, Mathan N, Karthikeyan MP, Kalia P, Guntaj J, Das M. Wearable Sensors and Systems
        for Personalized Healthcare Monitoring. 2025 International Conference on Networks and Cryptology
        (NETCRYPT) 2025 May 29 (pp. 978-982).

[17]   Vigneshvar S, Sudhakumari CC, Senthilkumaran B, Prakash H. Recent advances in biosensor
        technology for potential applications–an overview. Front Bioeng Biotechnol 2016; 4: 11.
        [http://dx.doi.org/10.3389/fbioe.2016.00011] [PMID: 26909346]

[18]   Kirsch J, Siltanen C, Zhou Q, Revzin A, Simonian A. Biosensor technology: recent advances in threat
        agent detection and medicine. Chem Soc Rev 2013; 42(22): 8733-68.
        [http://dx.doi.org/10.1039/c3cs60141b] [PMID: 23852443]

[19]   Bhatia D, Paul S, Acharjee T, Ramachairy SS. Biosensors and their widespread impact on human
        health. Sens Int 2024; 5: 100257.
        [http://dx.doi.org/10.1016/j.sintl.2023.100257]

[20]   Luo K, Li J, Wu J. A dynamic compression scheme for energy-efficient real-time wireless
        electrocardiogram biosensors. IEEE Trans Instrum Meas 2014; 63(9): 2160-9.
        [http://dx.doi.org/10.1109/TIM.2014.2308063]

[21]   Rossi P. Rate-responsive pacing: biosensor reliability and physiological sensitivity. Pacing Clin
        Electrophysiol 1987; 10(3): 454-66.
        [http://dx.doi.org/10.1111/j.1540-8159.1987.tb04507.x] [PMID: 2439993]

[22]   Istepanian R, Laxminarayan S, Pattichis CS, Eds. M-health: Emerging mobile health systems. Springer
        Science & Business Media 2007.

[23]   Lu Y, Xu LD. Internet of Things (IoT) cybersecurity research: A review of current research topics.
        IEEE Internet Things J 2019; 6(2): 2103-15.
        [http://dx.doi.org/10.1109/JIOT.2018.2869847]

[24]   Deshpande PS, Sharma SC, Peddoju SK. Security and Data Storage Aspect in Cloud Computing 2019.
        [http://dx.doi.org/10.1007/978-981-13-6089-3]

[25]   Pal S, Le DN, Pattnaik PK, Eds. Cloud Computing Solutions: Architecture, Data Storage,

Implementation, and Security. John Wiley & Sons 2022.
[http://dx.doi.org/10.1002/9781119682318]

[26] Zhao L, Sakr S, Liu A, Bouguettaya A. Cloud data management 2014.
[http://dx.doi.org/10.1007/978-3-319-04765-2]

[27] Wagner EH. The role of patient care teams in chronic disease management. BMJ 2000; 320(7234):
569-72.
[http://dx.doi.org/10.1136/bmj.320.7234.569] [PMID: 10688568]

[28] Fernandes RA, Zanesco A. Early physical activity promotes lower prevalence of chronic diseases in
adulthood. Hypertens Res 2010; 33(9): 926-31.
[http://dx.doi.org/10.1038/hr.2010.106] [PMID: 20574424]

[29] Lang R, Harbison Tostanoski A, Travers J, Todd J. The only study investigating the rapid prompting
method has serious methodological flaws but data suggest the most likely outcome is prompt
dependency. Evid Based Commun Assess Interv 2014; 8(1): 40-8.
[http://dx.doi.org/10.1080/17489539.2014.955260]

[30] Su D, Michaud TL, Estabrooks P, *et al.* Diabetes management through remote patient monitoring: the
importance of patient activation and engagement with the technology. Telemed J E Health 2019;
25(10): 952-9.
[http://dx.doi.org/10.1089/tmj.2018.0205] [PMID: 30372366]

[31] Olsen L, Saunders RS, Yong PL, Eds. The healthcare imperative: lowering costs and improving
outcomes: workshop series summary 2010.

[32] Donati D, Aroni S, Tedeschi R, *et al.* Exploring the impact of rehabilitation on post-surgical recovery
in elbow fracture patients: a cohort study. Musculoskelet Surg 2024; 109(1): 33-9.
[http://dx.doi.org/10.1007/s12306-024-00848-8] [PMID: 39026047]

[33] Kyriacos U, Jelsma J, Jordan S. Monitoring vital signs using early warning scoring systems: a review
of the literature. J Nurs Manag 2011; 19(3): 311-30.
[http://dx.doi.org/10.1111/j.1365-2834.2011.01246.x] [PMID: 21507102]

[34] Ahmed I, Ahmad NS, Ali S, *et al.* Medication adherence apps: review and content analysis. JMIR
Mhealth Uhealth 2018; 6(3): e62.
[http://dx.doi.org/10.2196/mhealth.6432] [PMID: 29549075]

[35] Charkviani M, Simonetto DA, Ahrens DJ, *et al.* Conceptualization of Remote Patient Monitoring
Program for Patients with Complex Medical Illness on Hospital Dismissal. Mayo Clinic Proceedings:
Digital Health 2023; 1(4): 586-95.
[http://dx.doi.org/10.1016/j.mcpdig.2023.09.005] [PMID: 40206304]

[36] Serrano LP, Maita KC, Avila FR, *et al.* Benefits and challenges of remote patient monitoring as
perceived by health care practitioners: a systematic review. Perm J 2023; 27(4): 100-11.
[http://dx.doi.org/10.7812/TPP/23.022] [PMID: 37735970]

[37] Birkett SL. Remote Patient Monitoring as a Means to Reduce 30-Day Readmissions in Skilled
Patients: An Integrative Review. PhD dissertation. Lynchburg (VA): Liberty University; 2022.

[38] Benzon HM, Rathmell JP, Wu CL, *et al.* Eds. Practical Management of Pain. 6th ed. Philadelphia:
Elsevier; 2022.

[39] Majumder S, Aghayi E, Noferesti M, *et al.* Smart homes for elderly healthcare—Recent advances and
research challenges. Sensors (Basel) 2017; 17(11): 2496.
[http://dx.doi.org/10.3390/s17112496] [PMID: 29088123]

[40] Perryman EM. A Qualitative Description of In-Home Remote Monitoring Acceptance Among Older
Adults, Informal Caregivers and Home and Community-Based Service Providers (Doctoral
dissertation, The University of Oklahoma Health Sciences Center), 2024.

[41] Ahmad I, Asghar Z, Kumar T. Li G, Manzoor A, Mikhaylov K. Emerging technologies for next

generation remote health care and assisted living. IEEE Access 2022; 10: 56094-132.
[http://dx.doi.org/10.1109/ACCESS.2022.3177278]

[42] Tsvetanov F, Integrating AI. Technologies into Remote Monitoring Patient Systems. Engineering Proceedings 2024; 70(1): 54.

[43] Tao X, Shaik TB, Higgins N, Gururajan R, Zhou X. Remote patient monitoring using radio frequency identification (RFID) technology and machine learning for early detection of suicidal behaviour in mental health facilities. Sensors (Basel) 2021; 21(3): 776.
[http://dx.doi.org/10.3390/s21030776] [PMID: 33498893]

[44] Tsvetanov F, Integrating AI. Technologies into Remote Monitoring Patient Systems. Engineering Proceedings 2024; 70(1): 54.

[45] Noah B, Keller MS, Mosadeghi S, *et al.* Impact of remote patient monitoring on clinical outcomes: an updated meta-analysis of randomized controlled trials. NPJ Digit Med 2018; 1(1): 20172.
[http://dx.doi.org/10.1038/s41746-017-0002-4] [PMID: 31304346]

[46] Freeman D, Sheaves B, Waite F, Harvey AG, Harrison PJ. Sleep disturbance and psychiatric disorders. Lancet Psychiatry 2020; 7(7): 628-37.
[http://dx.doi.org/10.1016/S2215-0366(20)30136-X] [PMID: 32563308]

[47] Prasad SS, Devi RM, Keerthika P, Suresh P, Macedo AR. From remote monitoring to personalized care. In: Kumar Rana A, Sharma V, Rana A, Alam M, Lata Tripathi S, Eds. Convergence of blockchain and internet of things in healthcare. 1st ed. Boca Raton (FL): CRC Press; 2024. p 26.
[http://dx.doi.org/10.1201/9781003466949-17]

[48] De Leon A, Pajardo JC. Using mobile health applications in postoperative care: patients' and healthcare providers' experiences. Bachelor's thesis. Helsinki: Metropolia University of Applied Sciences; 2024.

[49] L S P, Khurdi S, G PT, Mary S P. Impact of Remote Patient Monitoring Systems on Nursing Time, Healthcare Providers, and Patient Satisfaction in General Wards. Cureus 2024; 16(6): e61646.
[http://dx.doi.org/10.7759/cureus.61646] [PMID: 38966455]

[50] Joglekar GS, Giridhar A, Reklaitis G. A workflow modeling system for capturing data provenance. Comput Chem Eng 2014; 67: 148-58.
[http://dx.doi.org/10.1016/j.compchemeng.2014.04.006]

[51] Uddin R, Koo I. Real-Time Remote Patient Monitoring: A Review of Biosensors Integrated with Multi-Hop IoT Systems *via* Cloud Connectivity. Appl Sci (Basel) 2024; 14(5): 1876.
[http://dx.doi.org/10.3390/app14051876]

[52] Paramesha M, Rane N, Rane J. Big data analytics, artificial intelligence, machine learning, internet of things, and blockchain for enhanced business intelligence. SSRN 2024; 1(2): 110-33.
[http://dx.doi.org/10.2139/ssrn.4855856]

[53] Haleem A, Javaid M, Singh RP, Suman R. Telemedicine for healthcare: capabilities, features, barriers, and applications. Sensors Int 2021; 2: 100117.

[54] Omboni S, Padwal RS, Alessa T, *et al.* The worldwide impact of telemedicine during COVID-19: current evidence and recommendations for the future. Connected Health 2022; 1: 7.

[55] Shaik T, Tao X, Higgins N, *et al.* Remote patient monitoring using artificial intelligence: Current state, applications, and challenges. Wiley Interdiscip Rev Data Min Knowl Discov 2023; 13(2): e1485.
[http://dx.doi.org/10.1002/widm.1485]

[56] El-Rashidy N, El-Sappagh S, Islam SMR, M El-Bakry H, Abdelrazek S. Mobile health in remote patient monitoring for chronic diseases: Principles, trends, and challenges. Diagnostics (Basel) 2021; 11(4): 607.
[http://dx.doi.org/10.3390/diagnostics11040607] [PMID: 33805471]

[57] Abdolkhani R, Gray K, Borda A, DeSouza R. Recommendations for the quality management of

patient-generated health data in remote patient monitoring: mixed methods study. JMIR Mhealth Uhealth 2023; 11(1): e35917.
[http://dx.doi.org/10.2196/35917] [PMID: 36826986]

[58]   Wallace EL, Rosner MH, Alscher MD, *et al.* Remote patient management for home dialysis patients. Kidney Int Rep 2017; 2(6): 1009-17.
[http://dx.doi.org/10.1016/j.ekir.2017.07.010] [PMID: 29634048]

[59]   Condry MW, Quan XI. Remote patient monitoring technologies and markets. IEEE Eng Manage Rev 2023; 51(3): 59-64.
[http://dx.doi.org/10.1109/EMR.2023.3285688]

[60]   Cancela J, Charlafti I, Colloud S, Wu C. Digital health in the era of personalized healthcare: opportunities and challenges for bringing research and patient care to a new level. In: Yogesan K, Brett P, Brett T, Eds. Digital health. Amsterdam: Elsevier; 2021. p. 7-31.

[61]   Sripathi M, Leelavati TS. The fourth industrial revolution: a paradigm shift in healthcare delivery and management. In: Malviya R, Sundram S, Kumar Dhanaraj R, Kadry S, Eds. Digital Transformation in Healthcare 50: Volume 1: IoT, AI and Digital Twin 2024; 67-100.
[http://dx.doi.org/10.1515/9783111327853-003]

[62]   Coffey JD, Christopherson LA, Williams RD, *et al.* Development and implementation of a nurse-based remote patient monitoring program for ambulatory disease management. Front Digit Health 2022 Dec 14; 4: 1052408.
[http://dx.doi.org/10.3389/fdgth.2022.1052408]

[63]   Haddad TC, Maita KC, Inselman JW, *et al.* Patient satisfaction with a multisite, multiregional remote patient monitoring program for acute and chronic condition management: survey-based analysis. J Med Internet Res 2023; 25: e44528.
[http://dx.doi.org/10.2196/44528] [PMID: 37343182]

[64]   Franzoi MA, Ferreira AR, Lemaire A, *et al.* Implementation of a remote symptom monitoring pathway in oncology care: analysis of real-world experience across 33 cancer centres in France and Belgium. Lancet Reg Health Eur 2024; 44: 101005.
[http://dx.doi.org/10.1016/j.lanepe.2024.101005] [PMID: 39444707]

CHAPTER 15

Healthcare Chatbots and Virtual Assistants

Akanksha Sharma[1], Ashish Verma[2], Akhil Sharma[1], Shekhar Singh[3] and Shaweta Sharma[4,*]

[1] *R. J. College of Pharmacy, Raipur, Uttar Pradesh-202165, India*

[2] *Department of Pharmacy, Mangalmay Pharmacy College, Greater Noida, Uttar Pradesh-201306, India*

[3] *Faculty of Pharmacy, Babu Banarasi Das Northern India Institute of Technology, Lucknow, Uttar Pradesh-226028, India*

[4] *Department of Pharmacy, School of Medical and Allied Sciences, Galgotias University, Greater Noida, Uttar Pradesh-201310, India*

Abstract: Healthcare chatbots and virtual assistants are transforming patient care by integrating artificial intelligence (AI) and automation into healthcare systems. Chatbots act as interactive text conversational agents, whereas virtual assistants are more sophisticated, enabling voice interaction and personalized healthcare assistance. These technologies help to improve patient engagement, access to information, and administrative efficiency. AI, machine learning, natural language processing (NLP), and voice recognition play a critical role in helping chatbots and virtual assistants understand and respond to patient needs. Due to their integration with Electronic Health Records (EHRs), these tools are also used in a variety of specializations that allow for seamless communication, personalized symptom checkers, medication management, mental health support, chronic disease management, and even diagnostic assistance. They also enable telemedicine visits and clinical decision support, streamlining the healthcare experience. Despite their potential, challenges remain, including the accuracy of medical information and the need for continuous learning. This chapter discusses the different types of healthcare chatbots and virtual assistants and their applications and technologies; it also highlights the limitations involved in their use.

Keywords: Artificial intelligence, Clinical decision support, Healthcare automation, Healthcare chatbots, Machine learning, Natural language processing, Patient engagement, Virtual assistants.

---
* **Corresponding author Shaweta Sharma:** Department of Pharmacy, School of Medical and Allied Sciences, Galgotias University, Greater Noida, Uttar Pradesh-201310, India; E-mail: shawetasharma@galgotiasuniversity.edu.in

Shaweta Sharma, Akhil Sharma, Shivkanya Fuloria & Anurag Singh (Eds.)
All rights reserved-© 2025 Bentham Science Publishers

INTRODUCTION

Healthcare chatbots and virtual assistants are AI-driven solutions used by healthcare professionals and patients to communicate, making healthcare services more accessible and efficient. Chatbots are essentially text-based systems that answer questions and provide medical advice using natural language processing (NLP), in addition to scheduling appointments and processing user input. Virtual assistants are more advanced types of systems that engage with patients *via* voice and text for personalized support and can integrate with EHRs or medical devices. Such technologies enhance accessibility, create new efficiencies in workflows, and help patients take control of their health. Using artificial intelligence, they function as intermediaries in providing precise, timely, and contextual information, revolutionizing conventional healthcare systems into more economical and patient-centric models [1, 2].

Although chatbots and virtual assistants use AI, they are different in functionality and complexity. Most chatbots will be designed for use cases (symptom checking, appointment setting) and will provide rule-based or AI-based responses. In contrast, virtual assistants offer broader, more dynamic support. They interact with healthcare systems, employ voice recognition, and adjust to user preferences for personalized care. For example, a chatbot can respond to a patient asking about medication dosing. Still, a virtual assistant can remind a patient to take their medication proactively, keep a log of whether they took it, and use the health data to give them insights. Chatbots facilitate simple interactions, whereas virtual assistants have deeper contextual conversations and are often regarded as care companions [3].

Growing Role of AI and Automation in Healthcare

Artificial intelligence (AI) and automation are transforming healthcare by improving efficiency, accuracy, and accessibility. Advancements in AI algorithms can process extensive medical records, aiding in diagnostics, treatment planning, and predictive analytics. Automation helps simplify administrative tasks like appointment scheduling, billing, *etc.*, thus alleviating the burden on the healthcare provider. Machine learning and other technologies make personalized medicine possible, customizing therapy based on individual patient genetic and lifestyle data. In laboratories, robotic process automation (RPA) is used to perform faster and more error-free testing. AI-powered tools within telemedicine enable remote consultations for continuous care. These advances help to respond to issues like dwindling workforce numbers, growing patient loads, and soaring healthcare costs. The integration of AI and automation will lead to quicker, more accurate care and better outcomes, in turn enhancing patient satisfaction in the process [4].

Chatbots and virtual assistants play an important role in the healthcare domain by delivering timely assistance and accurate information to patients. They enable 24/7 access to information, allowing patients to inquire about symptoms, medications, or healthcare services without waiting for a healthcare professional. Virtual assistants take it a step further and provide personal guidance, track chronic conditions, and send reminders for medications or appointments. Such tools promote adherence to treatment plans and enable patients to become active participants in their health management. For healthcare providers, the solution streamlines workflows by automating repetitive tasks, allowing clinicians to devote more time to care needs that require more complex solutions. The use of AI-driven applications enhances healthcare delivery as it becomes increasingly more efficient, accessible, and oriented towards the patient [5].

Significance of Machine-Human Interaction in Healthcare

In healthcare, machine-human interaction is critical for connecting technology with patient care. Integrating machines with human emotions ensures the accuracy of diagnosis, helps in treatment, and satisfies patients. AI-powered chatbots like ChatGPT and virtual assistants make seamless communication possible, assisting people in navigating the healthcare system with ease. Machines can evaluate symptoms and deduce treatments, but humans still enable the contextualization necessary to make ethical decisions. Such collaboration engenders trust, resulting in better health outcomes. The digital transformation of healthcare is inevitable, but striking a balance between the efficiency of machines and the empathy of humans is critical to ensure that high-quality, patient-centered care is provided in the future [6].

TECHNOLOGIES BEHIND HEALTHCARE CHATBOTS AND VIRTUAL ASSISTANTS

Healthcare chatbots and virtual assistants employ Natural Language Processing (NLP) to understand user intent, as shown in Fig. (**1**). Machine Learning (ML) and AI enable chatbots to learn and adapt to healthcare-specific contexts. Voice recognition technology supports seamless speech-to-text and voice synthesis. Integration with EHR/EMR systems ensures personalized patient treatment, and cloud computing gives scalability, interoperability, and secure handling of data [7].

Natural Language Processing (NLP)

NLP empowers chatbots to understand, interpret, and generate human language by analyzing words, phrases, and context. It forms the basis for conversation, allowing virtual assistants to extract meaning from queries, respond in contextually appropriate ways, and support dynamic interactions in healthcare environments [8].

Technologies Behind Healthcare Chatbots and Virtual Assistants

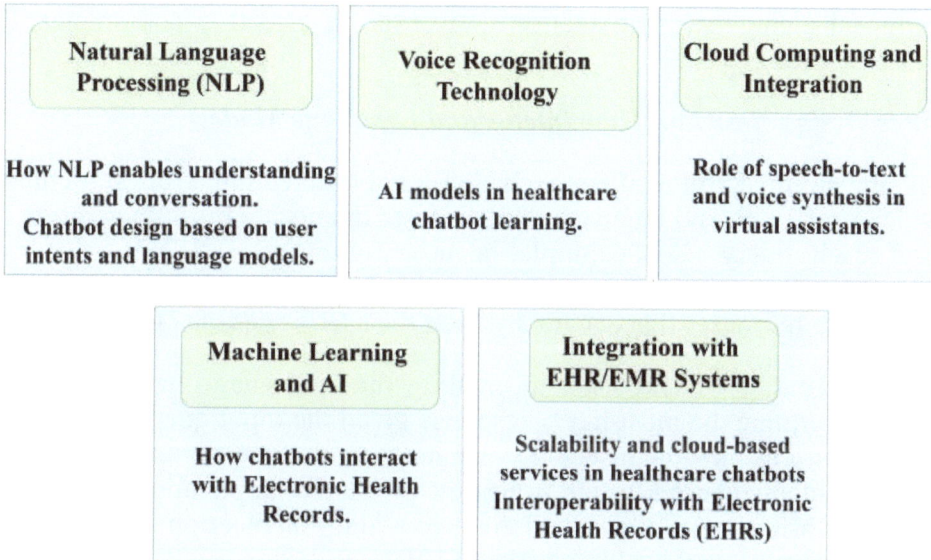

Natural Language Processing (NLP)	Voice Recognition Technology	Cloud Computing and Integration
How NLP enables understanding and conversation. Chatbot design based on user intents and language models.	AI models in healthcare chatbot learning.	Role of speech-to-text and voice synthesis in virtual assistants.

Machine Learning and AI	Integration with EHR/EMR Systems
How chatbots interact with Electronic Health Records.	Scalability and cloud-based services in healthcare chatbots Interoperability with Electronic Health Records (EHRs)

Fig. (1). Technologies involved in healthcare chatbots and virtual assistants.

How NLP Enables Understanding and Conversation?

NLP is vital for the development of chatbots and virtual assistants to interpret and communicate in human languages. It uses a variety of techniques, including tokenization, part-of-speech tagging, named entity recognition, and syntactic parsing, to decompose sentences into machine-processable elements. NLP models convert user input into a structured format so that the chatbot can understand what the words mean. For instance, if a user asks about medication dosage, NLP spots important entities such as "medication" and "dosage" and retrieves relevant information from its knowledge base [9].

NLP enables chatbots to process these nuances, empowering them to disambiguate and understand the context to interpret user intent. When a user presents an ambiguous query, NLP models rely on past interactions, user history, or predetermined patterns to identify the cause. This ability plays a role in allowing virtual assistants to manage conversational subtleties, such as slang, dialects, and different languages, allowing for greater adaptation in diverse healthcare environments [9].

NLP allows dialogue management systems to converse in a coherent context. As users converse with healthcare chatbots, NLP is used to track conversational logic so that the assistant remains consistent over multiple exchanges. NLP also allows these systems to employ sentiment analysis, determining the user's emotional tone to guide appropriate responses, which is vital in healthcare scenarios. Ultimately, NLP enables chatbots to offer precise, personalized, and empathetic responses, thereby enhancing user satisfaction and ensuring effective communication in healthcare settings [10].

Chatbot Design Based on User Intents and Language Models

Designing an impactful healthcare chatbot involves creating a robust architecture based on user intent and language models. User intents are the authorization goals behind each query. For example, a user might ask, "When is my next appointment?" to retrieve appointment details. Knowing these intents is essential for providing responses that accurately meet the user's needs [11].

The large datasets of text used in creating these language models help these chatbots determine the most likely response given the input query. These models look for patterns in how users use language and draw contextually relevant responses. Intent-focused design in healthcare chatbot applications enables them to perform various roles like scheduling, providing medication information, and answering more general health questions [12].

User intent is recognized by means of ML algorithms, assigning the user input into one or more defined groups or intents according to semantic similarity. For instance, when a user poses the question, "How do I manage my diabetes? The chatbot needs to grasp what the user wants. It employs NLP to understand the intent by analyzing the phrasing and context. When the intent is recognized, then the chatbot can either return the most relevant reply or give actionable advice. The chatbot's design often includes fallback mechanisms, such as escalating queries to human healthcare providers when the chatbot cannot interpret complex or urgent situations. It is also important to ensure that the chatbot continues to learn from the interactions and improve its functionality over time to increase its effectiveness. Typically, this process necessitates reinforcement learning and persistent feedback loops that help the model adapt to user behavior and requirements more effectively [13].

Machine Learning and AI

Healthcare chatbots powered by machine learning and AI can improve their responses over time by learning from user interactions as well as expanding datasets. In the field of health care, these technologies facilitate improved forecasting, customized suggestions, and advanced strategic approaches.

AI Models in Healthcare Chatbot Learning

AI models help healthcare chatbots learn from new data, making it possible to refine the chatbot over time. They use deep learning, reinforcement learning, and natural language processing to create data-driven decisions and evolve through interaction with the user. Healthcare chatbots can improve over time in sensing user intent, offering personalized advice, and generating more context-relevant responses [14].

For example, AI models in chatbots can analyze user interaction patterns and detect even subtle trends to build predictions of future needs. In chronic disease management, a chatbot might learn about a patient's medical history, prescriptions, and symptom patterns, offering customized advice based on the patient's particular disease. This personalization enhances the quality of the healthcare delivery process and patient satisfaction [15].

AI can also help chatbots do complex things like diagnosing common health conditions based on the symptoms described or offering personalized wellness tips. The models are trained on huge datasets of medical literature, patient records, and healthcare professionals so that they can provide evidence-based guidance. These are continually updated to ensure that, as new medical research and guidelines are published, they remain part of the chatbot's knowledge to stay up to date on healthcare trends and practices [16].

Chatbots can use reinforcement learning techniques to improve their ability to make decisions by receiving feedback on the results of their interactions. When a chatbot delivers the wrong answer, it can be corrected, and learn from the experience so that future engagements will be better. This cycle of learning enhances the accuracy and competence of AI healthcare chatbots in addressing patients' needs [17].

Voice Recognition Technology

Virtual assistants can read voice commands, which means, as far as hands-free interactions in healthcare go, this is a highly effective technology. This technology facilitates communication between users and systems without requiring typing, enhancing user convenience and accessibility [18].

Role of Speech-to-Text and Voice Synthesis in Virtual Assistants

Speech-to-text and voice synthesis are pivotal components of voice recognition technology that allow healthcare virtual assistants to provide hands-free, accessible services. Speech-to-text conversion enables a virtual assistant to convert verbal commands into text that can be read and processed, including voice commands and questions from patients. This function is especially useful for healthcare facilities where patients may need to enter information or inquire without the ability to type [19].

For instance, a bedridden patient may use voice to inquire about their medication schedule or the status of their health records. Speech-to-text is vital to make sure that the virtual assistant correctly transcribes these voice-based entries into actionable information. This technology is also important for accommodating patients with disabilities, such as those with mobility issues or visual impairments, by offering an alternative to traditional text-based interfaces [20].

Conversely, voice synthesis or text-to-speech (TTS) allows virtual assistants to communicate with users using natural-sounding speech. It improves usability by allowing more human-like interactions. In healthcare applications, it can be used to remind patients about their health issues, explain the medication instructions, provide emotional support, and others. The use of natural-sounding voice synthesis ensures that virtual assistants can communicate with patients in a way that feels familiar and engaging.

Together, speech-to-text and voice synthesis allow healthcare virtual assistants to conduct dynamic, interactive conversations with users. Furthermore, these technologies enable greater healthcare accessibility, particularly through voice-only interactions, allowing patients with physical disabilities or those in challenging environments to easily interface with the system [21].

Integration with EHR/EMR Systems

Chatbots can connect effortlessly with Electronic Health Records (EHR) and Electronic Medical Records (EMR) systems to offer real-time access to patient data, schedule appointments, and health information. This integration enhances patient care by giving healthcare providers and patients timely access to relevant information [22].

How Chatbots Interact with Electronic Health Records?

Chatbots in healthcare are also paired with EHR systems to augment patient welfare, administrative functions, and communication. EHRs are digital versions of patients' medical histories that include diagnoses, treatments, medications, and test results. Chatbots have access to this information to answer patient questions, remind them to take medications, and update appointment schedules [23].

For example, a patient might ask a chatbot about their next doctor's appointment. Being connected to the EHR allows the bot to offer real-time data, such as when, where, and why the visit occurred. Likewise, when patients ask about the medications they are on, the chatbot can pull the information from the EHR, showing dosage, frequency, and possible side effects [24].

Chatbot-EHR integration also supports health practitioners by automating routine tasks and enhancing patient experience. Chatbots can track patient follow-ups; therefore, staff will not miss their patients, thus increasing the workload on medical staff. In addition, chatbots can assist in collecting patient feedback, which can be used as valuable insight in developing healthcare services [25].

Cloud Computing

The cloud computing facility helps healthcare chatbots establish a scalable and flexible infrastructure for handling large datasets and request processing, along with providing the ability for seamless updates and maintenance. Cloud-based tools enable data to be accessed and stored in real time for seamless operations.

Scalability and Cloud-based Services in Healthcare Chatbots

Cloud computing provides healthcare chatbots with the scalability required to meet the demands of growing patient interactions, substantial datasets, and system updates. By leveraging cloud-based infrastructure, chatbots can dynamically scale up or down based on usage, ensuring that the system can handle varying levels of traffic without compromising performance. For instance, healthcare chatbots could potentially receive a higher volume of user requests at critical moments, like flu season or during a health crisis. Cloud services offer the essential resources needed to handle this surge in demand by distributing workloads across various servers, thereby guaranteeing low latency and quick response times [26].

Cloud-based services not only offer a centralized repository for the data to be stored, but they also ensure that patient information is always available to authorized users from multiple devices and locations. Through various devices, *e.g.*, smartphones, tablets, or even desktop computers, healthcare professionals and patients can engage with the chatbot without concern for data access [27].

Moreover, software updates and maintenance are made easy with cloud computing so that the healthcare chatbots stay up to date with all the features, security protocols, and compliance regulations. Cloud services reduce the burden of infrastructure maintenance, allowing healthcare organizations to dedicate their time and resources to providing quality treatment while increasing flexibility and decreasing costs through elements found in cloud computing [28].

Interoperability with Electronic Health Records (EHRs)

Interoperability between healthcare chatbots and EHRs is crucial for enabling seamless communication and data exchange between healthcare providers, patients, and chatbot systems. Interoperability enables healthcare chatbots to retrieve and update patient information in real-time, improving both streamlining care and elevating quality.

EHR-integrated chatbots can communicate with different healthcare applications and maintain the consistency of patient information across these systems. For instance, a chatbot can query a patient's medication history within the EHR to provide dosage information or remind the patient to request refills. Chatbots can ensure patients receive timely information regarding their care, providing communication with systems such as appointment scheduling or laboratory results [29].

Interoperability works only when the chatbot supports standards and protocols used in the industry, like HL7, FHIR, or IHE, which enable disparate systems to communicate the data in a defined, secure, and interoperable way. By ensuring that patient data is interconnected across various platforms, interoperability minimizes errors while boosting care coordination [30].

Chatbots integrated with EHR have the advantage of updating the patient record in real-time. For example, after a patient has had a consultation with a healthcare provider, the chatbot can automatically update the EHR with necessary details, including new medications or treatment plans. It allows all healthcare providers to access up-to-date information about the patient, leading to improved decision-making and fewer medical mistakes [31].

TYPES OF HEALTHCARE CHATBOTS AND VIRTUAL ASSISTANTS

Chatbots and virtual assistants in healthcare have transformed patient care and administration, providing personalized assistance, as depicted in Fig. (**2**). They vary in their functions, such as symptom checkers, medication management, mental health support, health coaching, chronic disease management, patient engagement, administrative support, AI-driven diagnostics, virtual assistants for professionals, and elderly care. They leverage AI to deliver efficient and accessible care and better healthcare experiences.

Healthcare Chatbots and Virtual Assistants

1. Symptom Checkers (WebMD Symptom Checker, Ada Health)	**2.** Medication Management Assistants (Pill Reminder - Meds Alarm, MediSafe)
3. Mental Health Support Bots (Woebot, Wysa)	**4.** Health and Wellness Coaches (MyFitnessPal Assistant, Lark Health)
5. Chronic Disease Management Bots (BlueStar Diabetes Assistant, Livongo)	**6.** Patient Engagement Bots (HealthTap, Florence)
7. Administrative Support Assistants (Amwell Virtual Assistant, QliqSOFT Quincy)	**8.** AI-Driven Diagnostic Assistants (IBM Watson Health Assistant, Babylon Health)
9. Virtual Assistants for Healthcare Professionals (Nuance Dragon Medical Assistant, Suki AI)	**10.** Elderly Care Bots (Examples: Elliq, CareAngel)

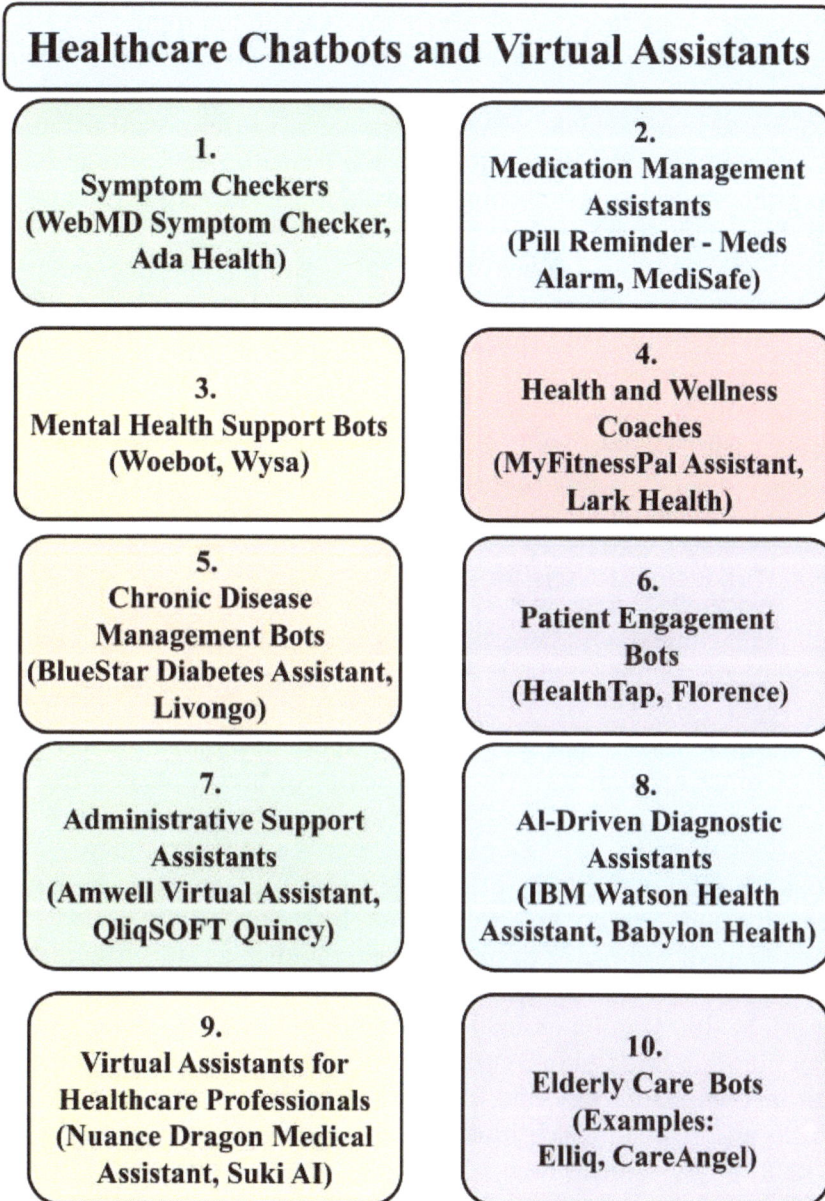

Fig. (2). Various chatbots and virtual assistants in healthcare.

Symptom Checkers

Symptom checkers are AI-based tools that help people evaluate a health condition based on the symptoms that they exhibit. By entering symptoms, users receive potential diagnoses and advice about the next steps, including whether to seek medical care. For example, platforms such as WebMD Symptom Checker and

Ada Health employ advanced algorithms that analyze the input data from users, taking multiple factors into account, such as age, sex, and medical history, to deliver accurate information on potential medical conditions. These tools analyze extensive databases and evidence-based guidelines to offer potential causes based on the given symptoms, thereby improving the triage process and assisting users in assessing the urgency of their symptoms. These tools aren't a substitute for medical professionals, but they provide an initial evaluation that can help guide users to the appropriate type of health care to pursue, saving time and preventing unnecessary visits. For example, WebMD Symptom Checker offers trustworthy health information, while Ada Health provides tailored evaluations powered by machine learning to improve diagnostic accuracy. The accessibility and immediate responses of symptom checkers make them valuable in improving healthcare accessibility, particularly in regions with limited healthcare resources. However, users must be aware that these tools are not a replacement for medical advice, and the final diagnosis should come from a healthcare provider [32, 33].

Medication Management Assistants

Medication management assistants help people stick to their prescribed treatment plans. These chatbots help patients track their medications and make sure they take the correct dose at the right time. A great example includes Pill Reminder - Meds Alarm, MediSafe, which serves as an important tool for those with chronic conditions or other individuals with multiple active prescriptions. They serve as reminders that can help users take their medications on time, which is critical in improving outcomes in the management of conditions such as diabetes, hypertension, or mental health disorders. These features can include reminders for refilling prescriptions and tracking medication history to ensure patients never run out of essential medications. With built-in features such as side effect trackers and medication interaction alerts, these virtual assistants empower users to monitor their general health simultaneously with multiple medications. For example, MediSafe includes a strong community aspect on its platform, allowing users to share their accomplishments and receive encouragement from others as an accountability mechanism. Additionally, these bots give healthcare professionals valuable data to assess adherence to medications. The role of medication management assistants is critical in minimizing medication errors, improving patient outcomes, and encouraging medication adherence practices [34, 35].

Mental Health Support Bots

Mental health support bots offer a safe, judgment-free zone for users to speak about feelings, mental health issues, and stressors. These virtual assistants provide users with coping strategies, guided exercises, and emotional support, which help decrease anxiety, depression, and other mental health challenges. Woebot and Wysa are prime examples of AI-powered mental health assistants that use cognitive behavioral therapy (CBT) principles to engage users. Woebot, for example, uses an empathetic conversational style to encourage users to reflect on their thoughts and behaviors, delivering personalized suggestions to help them cope with the information they provide. It leads users through assessments of how their feelings and thought patterns are contributing to their distress. Wysa, for instance, also employs AI to deliver therapeutic resources such as mindfulness practices, journaling suggestions, and mood monitoring. These bots also involve machine learning to accommodate each individual's needs as they evolve, resulting in a more personalized experience. The advantages of mental health support bots are their availability, which offers 24/7 support, and the anonymity they provide, which encourages individuals who may feel stigmatized to seek help. Although not a replacement for professional therapy, these bots are a way of giving support and early intervention that is readily available to continue in an environment experiencing a growing mental health crisis worldwide [36, 37].

Health and Wellness Coaches

Health and wellness coach bots guide users about exercise, nutrition, and overall health. These virtual assistants assist users in setting and monitoring fitness goals while offering personalized recommendations tailored to individual preferences and progress. These include AI-driven specialists like MyFitnessPal Assistant and Lark Health, combining cutting-edge formulas for personalized exercise regimes and nutrition guidance. MyFitnessPal Assistant, for instance, tracks users' meals, exercises, and calories and provides nutritional advice based on a user's diet and fitness level. Lark Health, by contrast, takes a more holistic approach to wellness, providing coaching in areas such as sleep, stress, and loss. Both platforms use artificial intelligence to log and recommend steps based on users' health, making wellness more attainable. These bots offer motivational and account data using behavioral science and AI so that users ensure they don't deviate from their tasks. They provide reminders, insights, and tips for healthy habits, leading the way for users to a healthier lifestyle. These tools, simply through smartphones, provide continuous support, making health and wellness coaching more cost-effective and scalable, especially for people who would not typically have access to a coach [38].

Chronic Disease Management Bots

The chronic disease management bots are built to assist people with chronic illness in self-monitoring their disease. Examples include BlueStar Diabetes Assistant and Livongo as virtual assistants to facilitate personalized management tools to manage diabetes and hypertension, respectively. These bots monitor essential parameters such as blood glucose levels, medication compliance, and physical activity, providing instant feedback and advice. BlueStar Diabetes Assistant, for example, creates a personalized diabetes care plan for each user and issues insights and alerts when they fall outside certain thresholds, like glucose levels. Livongo, a chronic condition management solution, combines tracking of users' vitals, coaching, and connecting patients to health professionals into an integrated system. They assist patients in self-managing health by delivering practical advice and ongoing assistance, minimizing unnecessary hospital visits. By tracking and analyzing data, they also empower patients to make informed decisions about their health, improving adherence to treatment plans and preventing complications. The integration of these bots with medical devices, like glucometers or blood pressure cuffs, allows for seamless monitoring and enhanced patient care [39].

Patient Engagement Bots

Patient engagement bots enable better communication flow between the healthcare provider and the patient, making them more interactive and involved in their healthcare experience. Such virtual assistants include HealthTap and Florence, which give users personalized health information, help them make appointments, and remind them of follow-ups. HealthTap is a digital platform used by patients to consult with doctors, pose medical inquiries, and receive answers from licensed health professionals. It enables individuals to make educated assessments concerning their well-being by offering access to a system of healthcare specialists for online consultations. In contrast, Florence gives users reminders and tools to track their health, including information on medication adherence, appointment scheduling, and blood pressure monitoring. Utilizing AI, bots can tailor interactions and send messages at the right time to keep patients engaged in health management. Keeping patients informed and reminding them of tasks to complete increases adherence to treatment regimens, improves overall satisfaction, and reduces healthcare costs. Patient engagement bots are widely used in areas such as chronic disease management, preventive care, and general wellness, improving the patient experience while alleviating the administrative burden on care providers [40].

Administrative Support Assistants

Healthcare operations can be automated through administrative support assistants. Some tools, such as Amwell Virtual Assistant and QliqSOFT Quincy, employ AI technology to manage appointment scheduling, billing inquiries, and patient registration. Most of these bots can help the healthcare provider save time and lower the administrative workload by taking care of tasks. For example, the Amwell Virtual Assistant helps to schedule telehealth visits and provides patients with real-time notifications and reminders of their appointments. QliqSOFT Quincy is another tool that helps with patient communication by sending notifications, reminders, and secure messages so patients and healthcare professionals can stay connected. Moreover, administrative support assistants enhance data accuracy by automating information entry and decreasing human error. These bots are game changers for increasing operational efficiency, enhancing patient experience, and lowering healthcare spending, especially in high-volume environments. Optimizing administrative workflows enables healthcare providers to focus on delivering high-quality care while enhancing overall organizational productivity [41, 42].

AI-Driven Diagnostic Assistants

Machine learning and extensive databases of health data are used by AI-enabled diagnosis assistants to help their human counterparts diagnose medical conditions more accurately and efficiently. For instance, IBM Watson Health Assistant and Babylon Health are virtual assistants that apply AI to process patient data and provide diagnostic assistance. IBM Watson Health Assistant can analyze extensive medical literature, research, and patient data, offering healthcare professionals evidence-based recommendations for diagnosis and treatment. Its analytical capability gives it the ability to recognize patterns and make clinical decisions, often guided by complex data sets. Babylon Health operates similarly by using AI to assess symptoms and medical history, offering diagnostic assistance to both patients and doctors. These virtual assistants are trained to recognize the early signs of a variety of diseases so that they can recommend further tests, treatments, or referrals. AI-based diagnostic assistants improve the speed and precision of diagnostic processes, minimizing human errors and assisting healthcare professionals in providing timely interventions. They are revolutionizing diagnosis by delivering speedy access to the oceans of medical knowledge and improving the efficiency and accessibility of health care, particularly in underserved areas [43, 44].

Virtual Assistants for Healthcare Professionals

Virtual assistants for healthcare professionals facilitate the clinical workflow, helping doctors, nurses, and other medical personnel spend more time with patients. AI-enabled tools such as Nuance Dragon Medical Assistant and Suki AI facilitate documentation, management of patient data & decision support. For instance, Nuance Dragon Medical Assistant is a voice-driven AI assistant that enables healthcare providers to create patient notes through voice dictation, thus decreasing time spent on manual documentation. This AI-powered solution interfaces with EHRs to maintain proper and timely documentation of records, thereby fostering efficiency. Also, Suki AI provides voice recognition technology to facilitate clinical documentation and data input. Healthcare professionals save time on administrative work and spend more time attending to patients because they understand medical terminology and integrate with EHRs. Both tools leverage AI to increase productivity, minimize burnout, and improve the accuracy of patient records. The ability to automate repetitive tasks offered by these virtual assistants frees up healthcare professionals' time to provide quality treatment, which, in turn, leads to a better patient experience and healthcare outcomes [45, 46].

Elderly Care Bots

Elderly care bots are made to help older people with daily activities and to help them feel better through reminders, health tracking, and companionship. Virtual assistants like Elliq and CareAngel are specifically tailored to support seniors in managing chronic conditions, staying active, and maintaining social connections. For instance, Elliq is an AI robot that assists older adults with everything from medication reminders to scheduling appointments and exercise regimens. It also serves as a source of entertainment and companionship, combating loneliness and isolation. CareAngel is all about health monitoring; it checks vital signs and gives health advice and reminders for important tasks. These bots often use sensor-based data collection techniques to monitor users' health and activity, enabling real-time sharing with caregivers or healthcare providers. For senior citizens, elderly care bots offer a secure lifestyle by taking care of their everyday needs, which ultimately enhances their quality of life. They also assist caregivers, enabling them to monitor their family members' health from a distance and act appropriately if necessary. Harnessing tech with empathy, these bots are transforming elderly care, enabling seniors to live more independently and with a better quality of life [47, 48].

APPLICATIONS OF CHATBOTS AND VIRTUAL ASSISTANTS IN HEALTHCARE

Chatbots and virtual assistants in healthcare enhance patient interaction, streamline administrative processes, and provide critical clinical support. These technologies improve accessibility to care, reduce the workload on healthcare providers, and empower patients with accurate health information and personalized assistance, as elaborated in Fig. (**3**) [49].

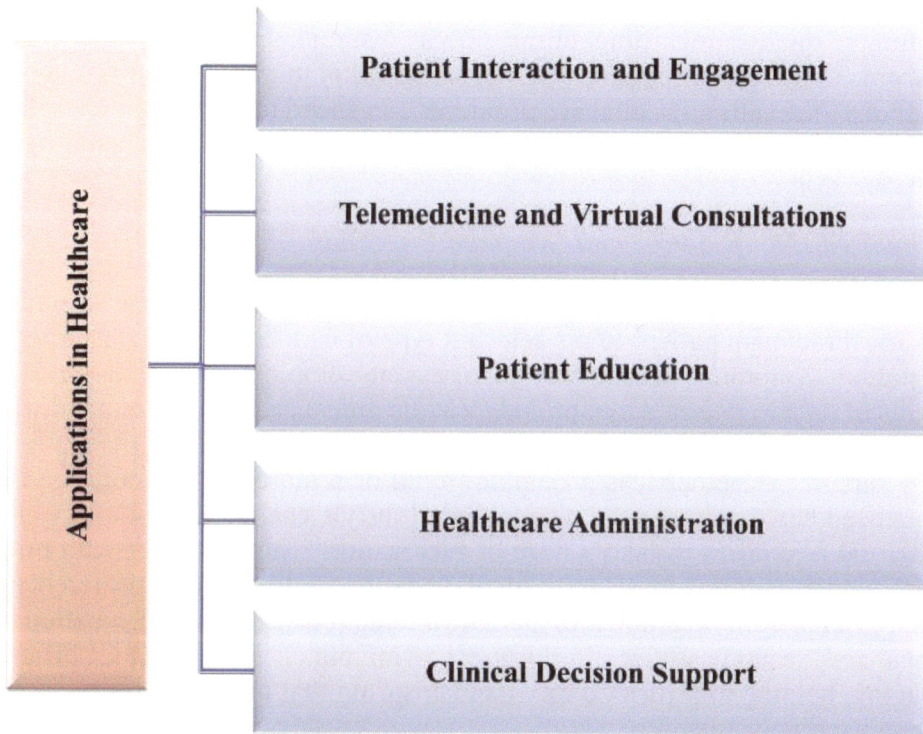

Fig. (3). Application of chatbots and virtual assistants in healthcare.

Patient Interaction and Engagement

Chatbots and virtual assistants greatly enhance patient interaction and engagement, enabling seamless communication between patients and healthcare professionals. Providers can also use these tools to help patients schedule an appointment, issue reminders, and answer frequently asked patient questions, which improves overall patient experience and adherence to care plans. They help patients get easy access to relevant healthcare services directly, without having to interact with human resources, so that healthcare becomes more available and efficient [50].

Appointment Scheduling, Reminders, and Queries

Appointment scheduling is critical for administration functionality, which chatbots facilitate in addition to minimizing wait time and human error. By using chatbots, patients can easily schedule, reschedule, or cancel appointments directly through simple interfaces on websites or apps. These bots can communicate *via* text, email, or even app notifications to remind us, effectively minimizing the number of missed appointments. Automated reminders, customized to patient preferences, can also ensure timely care. Additionally, chatbots provide answers to common queries regarding clinic hours, insurance coverage, and required documents, saving both patient and staff time. This minimizes the frequency of repetitive phone calls so healthcare providers can spend their time on complicated tasks. It also provides convenience and flexibility to patients in scheduling their health care [51].

Personalized Health Advice and Symptom Checking

Chatbots can offer advice tailored to individual needs; they can pose as symptom checkers, directing a patient to the relevant type of care based on the enumeration of reported symptoms. These virtual assistants employ algorithms and large amounts of data to interpret symptoms, provide guidance, and recommend when a patient should seek medical attention. They can help users assess the severity of their symptoms, whether it is a common cold or a more serious condition. The personalized health advice may also include lifestyle change techniques, wellness advice, and reminders to take a dose of medication. These chatbots can provide custom advice tailored to an individual's health conditions and preferences by obtaining data from wearables or patient interactions, making sure patients get personalized, accurate advice. Furthermore, symptom checkers enhance efficiency in triaging, helping to prioritize cases and ensuring that patients who need urgent care receive timely attention [52].

Telemedicine and Virtual Consultations

Chatbots and virtual assistants enhance telemedicine by enabling remote consultations and improving accessibility to healthcare services in rural or underprivileged regions. These tools help connect patients and healthcare providers, allowing virtual consultations that enable patients to receive care without coming to a clinic in person.

Role in Remote Consultations and Triaging

Chatbots and virtual assistants are essential in telemedicine as they act as intermediaries in remote consultations. When patients contact them for advice or consultations, these assistants help assess the case by gathering information about the patient's symptoms, medical history, and concerns. Then, this data is sent to doctors for a faster consultation. Some chatbots come with AI-powered symptom checkers that help the patient decide whether they require medical attention or if their ailment can be treated remotely. The tools are well-suited to triaging patients, allowing healthcare professionals to focus on cases that require direct interaction, while less urgent matters can be solved in digital interactions. This enables telemedicine platforms to work more efficiently and provide faster access to care to patients, alleviating the demand within healthcare facilities [53].

Patient Education

Chatbots and virtual assistants play an integral role in patient education by providing customers with accurate and reliable information about their health. They allow patients to make informed decisions regarding their health by providing evidence-based recommendations on the treatment for various conditions.

Providing Reliable Medical Information

Delivering reliable, up-to-date medical information is one of the major roles of healthcare chatbots. Chatbots have large databases of medical knowledge and can respond to patient questions about specific health conditions, medications, and treatments instantly. These assistants utilize AI and natural language processing to provide patients with straightforward summaries of their medical concerns and possible treatment options. Instead of going to potentially unreliable sources on the Internet for medical advice, patients can get trusted and scientifically backed information delivered directly through a chatbot. These virtual assistants also constantly update their knowledge base to stay abreast of the latest in medical guidelines and research. This helps build trust with patients and allows people to make informed healthcare choices [54].

Education on Medications, Lifestyle Changes, and Disease Management

In addition to general medical information, chatbots can also serve as valuable tools for educating patients about medications, lifestyle changes, and chronic disease management. These virtual assistants can also provide advice on how to take prescribed medications, the possible side effects, and interactions with other drugs. Reminding patients of their medication schedules helps reduce errors and improve adherence to treatment plans. Chatbots can also give personalized lifestyle advice based on the health condition of the patient by recommending dietary changes, exercise routines, or mental health practices. For individuals with chronic diseases such as diabetes or hypertension, chatbots provide the needed support at all times by informing them on self-management methods, tracking symptoms, and even helping with performing physical exercises. By tailoring these recommendations, chatbots help patients proactively manage their health, enhancing their quality of life [55].

Healthcare Administration

Chatbots and virtual assistants contribute to healthcare administration by automating time-consuming administrative tasks. These tools also make healthcare systems more efficient, eliminating errors and leading patients to faster service.

Administrative Tasks

Chatbots increase significant automation in healthcare administration, especially as it relates to patient intake and form filling. These processes have traditionally been manual and subject to human error. Chatbots automate the initial intake of patient data by guiding patients through questions that will lead to accurate data entry. Patients fill out their forms digitally in advance of their appointment at a clinic or hospital, reducing wait time and administrative work. These assistants can verify patient information, check insurance coverage, and confirm appointments, all in a smooth, automated manner. Moreover, chatbots help to perform periodic follow-ups and reminders to complete and submit forms promptly. By automating these repetitive administrative tasks, healthcare staff can focus more on patient care and improve overall operational efficiency [56, 57].

Clinical Decision Support

Healthcare professionals make clinical decisions using chatbots and virtual assistants that analyze patient data to deliver evidence-based recommendations. This can be essential in diagnosing diseases and recommending potential treatments.

Assisting Healthcare Professionals in Diagnosing and Recommending Treatments

In a clinical context, virtual assistants are beneficial providers of decision support. These AI-powered systems assist healthcare professionals by providing real-time analysis of patient data, including symptoms, lab results, and medical histories. Chatbots have access to large medical databases and diagnostic tools, which allow them to determine possible diagnoses given the information provided by the user. They can also recommend treatment options based on the latest medical guidelines and research. Such virtual assistants help ensure that decisions are based on the most accurate and holistic information by supplying relevant insights and evidence to clinicians and vice versa, while also helping to reduce diagnostic errors by ensuring information about patients is cross-examined with medical literature and guidelines. While they cannot substitute for the medical expertise of healthcare providers, chatbots are a fundamental tool for assisting in clinical decision-making, optimizing patient outcomes, and decreasing healthcare expenditure [58].

CHALLENGES ASSOCIATED WITH HEALTHCARE CHATBOTS AND VIRTUAL ASSISTANTS (TABLE 1)

Table 1. Challenges and limitations of healthcare chatbots and virtual assistants.

S. No.	Challenges	Description	References
1	Accuracy and Reliability	Providing accurate medical advice is challenging, as incorrect responses could result in misdiagnosis or even injury.	[59]
2	Limited Understanding of Complex Queries	Virtual assistants often struggle to comprehend nuanced medical questions, leading to suboptimal or generic responses.	[60]
3	User Trust and Acceptance	Patients may be reluctant to share personal health information with chatbots or to consider them more than qualified professionals.	[61]
4	Integration with Existing Healthcare Systems	Chatbots must work seamlessly with Electronic Health Records (EHRs) and other medical databases, which is often challenging due to technical limitations.	[62]
5	Language and Cultural Barriers	Chatbots may not be fully effective across different languages and cultures, limiting their accessibility and accuracy.	[63]
6	Technical Limitations	Restricted by AI capabilities, chatbots may be unable to handle complex medical issues or provide real-time support, especially during emergencies.	[64]
7	Continuous Learning and Updates	Chatbots must be regularly updated with recent medical information, which requires constant monitoring and adaptation to evolving healthcare needs.	[65]

CONCLUSION

Patient care has undergone a paradigm shift with the advent of healthcare chatbots and virtual assistants, as they leverage various sophisticated technologies such as Natural Language Processing (NLP), machine learning, voice recognition, and EHR integration to improve patient care and operational efficiency. These digital solutions can greatly enhance patient engagement, reduce the administrative load, and provide healthcare professionals with support through diagnosis support tools. From symptom checkers to drug reminders, mental health, and chronic disease management, the use of chatbots and virtual assistants is versatile. It provides personalized and instantaneous assistance to patients as well as healthcare providers. Despite their promise, there are challenges to overcome. Issues related to data privacy, accuracy, and the limitations of current AI models in understanding complex medical contexts must be addressed to ensure trust and reliability. The integration of these technologies into existing healthcare systems also raises interoperability concerns. Nevertheless, the growing role of AI and automation in healthcare is apparent, with chatbots and virtual assistants poised to play an integral part in shaping the future of patient care. These tools will not only augment the delivery of healthcare by improving machine-human interaction and support but also facilitate access to better care, save costs, and allow better outcomes. With ongoing innovation and mindful implementation, healthcare chatbots and virtual assistants will evolve further and contribute to the wider goals of accessible, patient-centered care.

REFERENCES

[1]　Ingale V, Wankar B, Jadhav K, Adedoja T, Borate VK, Mali YK. Healthcare is being revolutionized by AI-powered solutions and technological integration for easily accessible and efficient medical care. In: 2024 15th International Conference on Computing, Communication and Networking Technologies (ICCCNT) 2024; 1-6.
[http://dx.doi.org/10.1109/ICCCNT61001.2024.10725646]

[2]　Bhirud N, Tataale S, Randive S, Nahar S. A literature review on chatbots in the healthcare domain. Int J Sci Technol Res 2019; 8(7): 225-31.

[3]　Zhang H, Zheng J. The application analysis of medical chatbots and virtual assistants. Front Soc Sci Technol 2021; 3: 116-4.

[4]　Mohammed MA, Mohammed MA, Mohammed VA. Impact of Artificial Intelligence on the Automation of Digital Health Systems. Int J Softw Eng Appl 2022; 13(6): 23-9.

[5]　Hindelang M, Sitaru S, Zink A. Transforming health care through chatbots for medical history-taking and future directions: comprehensive systematic review. JMIR Med Inform 2024; 12(1): e56628.
[http://dx.doi.org/10.2196/56628] [PMID: 39207827]

[6]　Kela-Madar N, Kela I. The machine-human collaboration in healthcare innovation. In: Brito SM, Ed. Toward Super-Creativity-Improving Creativity in Humans. Machines, and Human-Machine Collaborations. IntechOpen 2019.

[7]　Mendapara H, Digole S, Thakur M, Dange A. An AI-based healthcare chatbot system uses natural language processing. Int J Sci Res Eng Dev 2021; 4(2)

[8]　Chen L, Gu Y, Ji X, *et al.* Extracting medications and associated adverse drug events using a natural language processing system combining knowledge base and deep learning. J Am Med Inform Assoc 2020; 27(1): 56-64.
[http://dx.doi.org/10.1093/jamia/ocz141] [PMID: 31591641]

[9]　Ajmal S, Ahmed AA, Jalota C. Natural language processing in improving information retrieval and knowledge discovery in healthcare conversational agents. J Artif Intell Mach Learn Manag 2023; 7(1): 34-47.

[10]　Ojha R. From algorithms to conversations: The influence of natural language processing on chatbot innovation. Int J Contem Res Multidis 2024; 3(6): 21-27.

[11]　Cahn J. CHATBOT: Architecture, design, & development. University of pennsylvania school of engineering and applied science. Department of Computer and Information Science 2017.

[12]　Babu A, Boddu SB. BERT-Based Medical Chatbot: Enhancing healthcare communication through

natural language understanding. Explor Res Clin Soc Pharm 2024; 13: 100419.
[http://dx.doi.org/10.1016/j.rcsop.2024.100419] [PMID: 38495953]

[13]   Palanichamy H. Contouring a user-centered chatbot for diabetes mellitus. International Journal of High School Research 2022; 4(4): 83-91.
[http://dx.doi.org/10.36838/v4i4.16]

[14]   Alowais SA, Alghamdi SS, Alsuhebany N, *et al.* Revolutionizing healthcare: the role of artificial intelligence in clinical practice. BMC Med Educ 2023; 23(1): 689.
[http://dx.doi.org/10.1186/s12909-023-04698-z] [PMID: 37740191]

[15]   Joshi H. AI and chronic diseases: from data integration to clinical implementation. In: Shah IA, Sial Q, Fateh S, Eds. Generative AI Techniques for Sustainability in Healthcare Security. IGI Global Scientific Publishing 2025; pp. 17-40.

[16]   Kurniawan MH, Handiyani H, Nuraini T, Hariyati RTS, Sutrisno S. A systematic review of artificial intelligence-powered (AI-powered) chatbot intervention for managing chronic illness. Ann Med 2024; 56(1): 2302980.
[http://dx.doi.org/10.1080/07853890.2024.2302980] [PMID: 38466897]

[17]   Coronato A, Naeem M, De Pietro G, Paragliola G. Reinforcement learning for intelligent healthcare applications: A survey. Artif Intell Med 2020; 109: 101964.
[http://dx.doi.org/10.1016/j.artmed.2020.101964] [PMID: 34756216]

[18]   Sezgin E, Huang Y, Ramtekkar U, Lin S. Readiness for voice assistants to support healthcare delivery during a health crisis and pandemic. NPJ Digit Med 2020; 3(1): 122.
[http://dx.doi.org/10.1038/s41746-020-00332-0] [PMID: 33015374]

[19]   Reddy VM, Vaishnavi T, Kumar KP. Speech-to-text and text-to-speech recognition using deep learning. In: 2023 2nd International Conference on Edge Computing and Applications (ICECAA) 2023; 657-66.
[http://dx.doi.org/10.1109/ICECAA58104.2023.10212222]

[20]   Simon C, Rajeswari M. Voice-based virtual assistant with security. In: 2023 Second International Conference on Electronics and Renewable Systems (ICEARS) 2023; 822-7.
[http://dx.doi.org/10.1109/ICEARS56392.2023.10085043]

[21]   Nguyen TS, Nguyen TT, Tran NC, Ta TH, Huynh DK, Nguyen HP. A chatbot application with voice communication for the healthcare system. Tra Vinh Univ J Sci 2024.

[22]   Božić V. Roles of artificial intelligence in various eHealth applications

[23]   Yin R, Neyens DM. Examining how information presentation methods and a chatbot impact the use and effectiveness of electronic health record patient portals: An exploratory study. Patient Educ Couns 2024; 119: 108055.
[http://dx.doi.org/10.1016/j.pec.2023.108055] [PMID: 37976665]

[24]   Sahithya B, Prasad G, Sahithi B, Devarlla AC, Yashavanth TR. Empowering healthcare with AI: Advancements in medical image analysis, electronic health records analysis, and AI-driven chatbots. In: Proc 3rd Int Conf Innovation Technol (INOCON) 2024; 1-7.
[http://dx.doi.org/10.1109/INOCON60754.2024.10511753]

[25]   Blessing J, Christopher G. Artificial intelligence-based chatbot for virtual health consultation. Sci 2024; 2(1): 241-50.

[26]   Chung K, Park RC. Chatbot-based heathcare service with a knowledge base for cloud computing. Cluster Comput 2019; 22(S1): 1925-37.
[http://dx.doi.org/10.1007/s10586-018-2334-5]

[27]   Boppana VR. Future trends in cloud-based CRM solutions for healthcare. EPH-International Journal of Business & Management Science 2023; 9(2): 37-46.
[http://dx.doi.org/10.53555/eijbms.v9i2.177]

[28]   Kar R, Haldar R. Applying chatbots to the internet of things: Opportunities and architectural elements. arXiv preprint arXiv:161103799 2016.

[29]   Olusegun J, Oluwaseyi J, Brightwood S, Temitope OM. Integration of AI with electronic health records: Enhancing clinical workflows, 2024.

[30]   Benson T, Grieve G. Why interoperability is hard. In: Principles of health interoperability. Health information technology standards. Cham: Springer; 2021.
[http://dx.doi.org/10.1007/978-3-030-56883-2_2]

[31]   Yin R. Examining the impact of design features of electronic health records patient portals on the usability and information communication for shared decision making. PhD dissertation. Clemson (SC): Clemson University 2022.

[32]   Abisha D, Mahalakshmi M, Pritiga T, Thanusiya M. Revolutionizing rural healthcare in India: AI-powered chatbots for affordable symptom analysis and medical guidance. In: Proc Int Conf Invent Comput Technol (ICICT) 2024; 181-7.

[33]   Shen C, Nguyen M, Gregor A, Isaza G, Beattie A. Accuracy of a popular online symptom checker for ophthalmic diagnoses. JAMA Ophthalmol 2019; 137(6): 690-2.
[http://dx.doi.org/10.1001/jamaophthalmol.2019.0571] [PMID: 30973602]

[34]   Still CH, Harwell C, Killion C, Sattar A, Viswanath SE. Optimizing Technology to Improve Medication Adherence and BP Control (OPTIMA-BP) Intervention Versus Waitlisted Group in African American Adults with Hypertension: A Randomized Control Trial Protocol. Nurs: Res Rev 2025; 31: 29-41.
[http://dx.doi.org/10.2147/NRR.S491609]

[35]   Kundu S, Chattopadhyay M. Med-Alert: An Android application to increase medication adherence. In: Balas VE, Hassanien AE, Chakrabarti S, Mandal L, Eds. Proc Int Conf Comput Intell Data Sci Cloud Comput (IEM-ICDC) 2021; 455-69.
[http://dx.doi.org/10.1007/978-981-33-4968-1_36]

[36]   Sweeney C, Potts C, Ennis E, *et al.* Can chatbots help support a person's mental health? Perceptions and views from mental healthcare professionals and experts. ACM Trans Comput Healthc 2021; 2(3): 1-15.
[http://dx.doi.org/10.1145/3453175]

[37]   Olawade DB, Wada OZ, Odetayo A, David-Olawade AC, Asaolu F, Eberhardt J. Enhancing mental health with artificial intelligence: current trends and prospects. J Med Surg Public Health 2024; 3: 100099.

[38]   Rios G, O'Hagan E. Consumer- and patient-friendly technology: today and tomorrow. In: Spatz M, Ed. Med Libr Assoc Guide Providing Consumer Patient Health Info 2014 May 1; 57-76.

[39]   Doupis J, Festas G, Tsilivigos C, Efthymiou V, Kokkinos A. Smartphone-Based Technology in Diabetes Management. Diabetes Ther. 2020; 11(3): 607-619.

[40]   Rutledge GW, Wood JC. Virtual health and artificial intelligence: Using technology to improve healthcare delivery. In: Lawless WF, Mittu R, Sofge DA, Eds. Human-Machine Shared Contexts. Academic Press 2020; pp. 169-75.
[http://dx.doi.org/10.1016/B978-0-12-820543-3.00008-0]

[41]   Jayapradha J, Boovaneswari S, Sabarivadivelan S, Uvarajan D, Sarathi S. A Telehealth System Driven by Artificial Intelligence for Effective Patient Consultation and Diagnosis in Hospitals. In: Proc 2023 Int Conf Syst Comput Autom Netw (ICSCAN) 2023; 1-6.
[http://dx.doi.org/10.1109/ICSCAN58655.2023.10395119]

[42]   Drerup B, Espenschied J, Wiedemer J, Hamilton L. Reduced no-show rates and sustained patient satisfaction of telehealth during the COVID-19 pandemic. Telemed e-Health 2021 Dec 1; 27(12): 1409-15.

[43] Aggarwal M, Madhukar M. IBM's Watson analytics for health care: A miracle made true. In: Bhatt CM, Peddoju SK, Eds. Cloud computing systems and applications in healthcare. Hershey (PA): IGI Global; 2017. p. 117-34.
[http://dx.doi.org/10.4018/978-1-5225-1002-4.ch007]

[44] Akila K, Gopinathan R, Arunkumar J, Malar BS. The Role of Artificial Intelligence in Modern Healthcare: Advances, Challenges, and Future Prospects. European Journal of Cardiovascular Medicine. 2025; 15(4): 615-24.

[45] Dowling RA. Ambient clinical documentation shows promise for physicians: Technology may save health care professionals' time and help reduce burnout. Urol Times 2023; 51(11): 34-6.

[46] Thakur A. Market determinants impacting distributed ledger technology and AI-based architectures in the healthcare industry. Int J Bus Anal Intell 2022; 10(2): 36-45.

[47] Coughlin JF, D'Ambrosio LA, Lee C, Kim E. Assistive personal robots for older adults: bridging the divide between robotic technology development and end-users in practical applications. Master's thesis. Cambridge (MA): Massachusetts Institute of Technology 2023.

[48] Dojchinovski D, Ilievski A, Gusev M. Interactive home healthcare system with integrated voice assistant. In: 42nd Intl Conv Info Comm Techn, Elect Microelect (MIPRO); 2019 May 20-24; Opatija, Croatia. IEEE; 2019. p. 284-8.

[49] Bates M. Health care chatbots are here to help. IEEE Pulse 2019; 10(3): 12-4.
[http://dx.doi.org/10.1109/MPULS.2019.2911816] [PMID: 31135345]

[50] Chavali D, Dhiman VK, Katari SC. AI-powered virtual health assistants: transforming patient engagement through virtual nursing. Int J Pharma Sci 2024; 2: 613-24.

[51] Noonia A, Beg R, Patidar A, Bawaskar B, Sharma S, Rawat H. Chatbot vs intelligent virtual assistance. In: Rawat R, Chakrawarti RK, Sarangi SK, Rajavat A, Alamanda MS, Srividya K, Sankaran KS, Eds. Conversational artificial intelligence. Hoboken (NJ): John Wiley & Sons; 2024. p. 655-73.

[52] Polignano M, Narducci F, Iovine A, Musto C, De Gemmis M, Semeraro G. HealthAssistantBot: a personal health assistant for the Italian language. 2020; 8: 107479-97.
[http://dx.doi.org/10.1109/ACCESS.2020.3000815]

[53] Adeghe EP, Okolo CA, Ojeyinka OT. A review of emerging trends in telemedicine: Healthcare delivery transformations. International Journal of Life Science Research Archive 2024; 6(1): 137-47.
[http://dx.doi.org/10.53771/ijlsra.2024.6.1.0040]

[54] Dolianiti F, Tsoupouroglou I, Antoniou P, Konstantinidis S, Anastasiades S, Bamidis P. In: Frasson C, Bamidis P, Vlamos P, Eds. Chatbots in healthcare curricula: the case of a conversational virtual patient. Brain function assessment in learning. BFAL 2020. Lecture notes in computer science, vol. 12462. Cham: Springer; 2020. p. 154-63.
[http://dx.doi.org/10.1007/978-3-030-60735-7_15]

[55] Laymouna M, Ma Y, Lessard D, Schuster T, Engler K, Lebouché B. Roles, users, benefits, and limitations of chatbots in health care: rapid review. J Med Internet Res 2024; 26: e56930.
[http://dx.doi.org/10.2196/56930] [PMID: 39042446]

[56] Malamas N, Papangelou K, Symeonidis AL. Upon improving the performance of localized healthcare virtual assistants. Healthcare (Basel) 2022; 10(1): 99.
[http://dx.doi.org/10.3390/healthcare10010099] [PMID: 35052263]

[57] Singh A, Joshi S, Domb M. Embedded Conversational AI, Chatbots, and NLP to Improve Healthcare Administration and Practices. In: Proc 2nd Int Conf Autom Comput Renew Syst (ICACRS) 2023; 38-45.
[http://dx.doi.org/10.1109/ICACRS58579.2023.10404985]

[58] Khalifa M, Albadawy M, Iqbal U. Advancing clinical decision support: the role of artificial

intelligence across six domains. Comput Methods Programs Biomed Update 2024; 5: 100142.
[http://dx.doi.org/10.1016/j.cmpbup.2024.100142]

[59]   Hayat J, Lari M, AlHerz M, Lari A. The Utility and Limitations of Artificial Intelligence-Powered Chatbots in Healthcare. Cureus 2024; 16(11): e73127.
[http://dx.doi.org/10.7759/cureus.73127] [PMID: 39650926]

[60]   Ouédraogo I. Mobile technology and artificial intelligence for improving health literacy among underserved communities. Université de Bordeaux; Université Nazi Boni (Bobo-Dioulasso, Burkina Faso) 2024.

[61]   Nadarzynski T, Miles O, Cowie A, Ridge D. Acceptability of artificial intelligence (AI)-led chatbot services in healthcare: A mixed-methods study. Digit Health 2019; 5: 2055207619871808.
[http://dx.doi.org/10.1177/2055207619871808] [PMID: 31467682]

[62]   Ittarat M, Cheungpasitporn W, Chansangpetch S. Personalized care in eye health: Exploring opportunities, challenges, and the road ahead for chatbots. J Pers Med 2023; 13(12): 1679.
[http://dx.doi.org/10.3390/jpm13121679] [PMID: 38138906]

[63]   Tseng YC, Jarupreechachan W, Lee TH. Understanding the benefits and design of chatbots to meet the healthcare needs of migrant workers. Proc ACM Hum-Comput Interact 2023 Oct 4; 7(CSCW2): 1-34.
[http://dx.doi.org/10.1145/3610106]

[64]   Chenais G, Lagarde E, Gil-Jardiné C. Artificial intelligence in emergency medicine: viewpoint of current applications and foreseeable opportunities and challenges. J Med Internet Res 2023; 25: e40031.
[http://dx.doi.org/10.2196/40031] [PMID: 36972306]

[65]   Izadi S, Forouzanfar M. Error correction and adaptation in conversational AI: A review of techniques and applications in chatbots. AI 2024; 5(2): 803-41.
[http://dx.doi.org/10.3390/ai5020041]

SUBJECT INDEX

Shaweta Sharma, Akhil Sharma, Shivkanya Fuloria & Anurag Singh (Eds.)
All rights reserved-© 2025 Bentham Science Publishers

www.ingramcontent.com/pod-product-compliance
Lightning Source LLC
Chambersburg PA
CBHW080018240326
41598CB00075B/59